Clinical Approach to Infections in Pregnancy

Clinical Approach to Infections in Pregnancy

Edited by Charlotte Mitchell

STATES
ACADEMIC PRESS

States Academic Press,
109 South 5th Street,
Brooklyn, NY 11249, USA

Visit us on the World Wide Web at:
www.statesacademicpress.com

ISBN: 978-1-63989-778-0

Cataloging-in-Publication Data

Clinical approach to infections in pregnancy / edited by Charlotte Mitchell.
p. cm.
Includes bibliographical references and index.
ISBN 978-1-63989-778-0
1. Communicable diseases in pregnancy. 2. Pregnancy--Complications.
3. Pregnancy--Complications--Treatment. I. Mitchell, Charlotte.
RG578 .C55 2023
618.3--dc23

Table of Contents

Preface

Pregnancy refers to a series and process of changes that occur in a woman's tissues and organs due to the development of a fetus. It causes numerous changes in the body which makes women more vulnerable to various infections. Pregnant women get more severe infections with certain organisms such as hepatitis E virus (HEV), malaria parasites, influenza virus and herpes simplex virus (HSV), than non-pregnant women. Being infected during pregnancy increases the risk of birth defects like blindness or visual impairment, epilepsy, hearing loss and learning difficulties for unborn babies. Antibacterial medications including cephalosporins, penicillins and medicines related to erythromycin are generally regarded as safe to use during pregnancy. This book aims to present a clinical approach to infections in pregnancy. It presents researches and studies performed by experts across the globe. Those in search of information to further their knowledge will be greatly assisted by this book.

The researches compiled throughout the book are authentic and of high quality, combining several disciplines and from very diverse regions from around the world. Drawing on the contributions of many researchers from diverse countries, the book's objective is to provide the readers with the latest achievements in the area of research. This book will surely be a source of knowledge to all interested and researching the field.

In the end, I would like to express my deep sense of gratitude to all the authors for meeting the set deadlines in completing and submitting their research chapters. I would also like to thank the publisher for the support offered to us throughout the course of the book. Finally, I extend my sincere thanks to my family for being a constant source of inspiration and encouragement.

Editor

1

Contribution of Murine Models to the Study of Malaria during Pregnancy

*André Barateiro[1], Marcelo L. M. Pereira[1,2], Sabrina Epiphanio[3] and Claudio R. F. Marinho[1]**

[1] Department of Parasitology, Institute of Biomedical Sciences, University of São Paulo, São Paulo, Brazil, [2] Institute of Biosystems and Integrative Sciences, Faculty of Sciences, University of Lisbon, Lisbon, Portugal, [3] Department of Clinical Analysis and Toxicology, Faculty of Pharmaceutical Sciences, University of São Paulo, São Paulo, Brazil

***Correspondence:**
Claudio R. F. Marinho
marinho@usp.br

Annually, many pregnancies occur in areas of *Plasmodium* spp. transmission, particularly in underdeveloped countries with widespread poverty. Estimations have suggested that several million women are at risk of developing malaria during pregnancy. In particular cases, systemic infection caused by *Plasmodium* spp. may extend to the placenta, dysregulating local homeostasis and promoting the onset of placental malaria; these processes are often associated with increased maternal and fetal mortality, intrauterine growth restriction, preterm delivery, and reduced birth weight. The endeavor to understand and characterize the mechanisms underlying disease onset and placental pathology face several ethical and logistical obstacles due to explicit difficulties in assessing human gestation and biological material. Consequently, the advent of murine experimental models for the study of malaria during pregnancy has substantially contributed to our understanding of this complex pathology. Herein, we summarize research conducted during recent decades using murine models of malaria during pregnancy and highlight the most relevant findings, as well as discuss similarities to humans and the translational capacity of achieved results.

Keywords: murine models, *Plasmodium* spp., malaria, pregnancy, placental malaria

MALARIA IN HUMAN PREGNANCY

Malaria still represents a serious public health issue for several communities distributed worldwide. Estimations from 2017 have shown that at least 219 million cases occurred in areas of *Plasmodium* spp. transmission, in which approximately half a million victims died from the disease (World Health Organization, 2018). These estimations encompass pregnant women, who are particularly more susceptible to developing severe clinical manifestations resulting from malaria in pregnancy (MiP) induced by *Plasmodium* spp. Although outdated, estimations performed by Dellicour et al. (2010) noted 125.2 million pregnancies occurring in malaria-endemic areas. This study came as a follow-up of previous estimations suggesting that 25 million pregnancies occur in areas of *P. falciparum* transmission alone, distributed across sub-Saharan Africa (Desai et al., 2007). Nevertheless, current epidemiologic knowledge is inaccurate and imprecise and might support outdated and underestimated predictions, hiding a much more alarming reality.

This concerning epidemiological scenario highlights the importance of conducting preventive measures to control MiP, which might drastically evolve to placental malaria (PM), a pathology frequently associated with the occurrence of poor outcomes during pregnancy, such as maternal and fetal mortality, intrauterine growth restriction (IUGR), preterm birth and reduced birth weight

(Desai et al., 2007; Umbers et al., 2011; Rogerson et al., 2018). These deleterious consequences affecting both the mother and the growing fetus are reflections of histological and physiological changes occurring within the placenta [recently summarized elsewhere (Sharma and Shukla, 2017)]. One of the key features of *P. falciparum* PM is the accumulation of *P. falciparum*-infected erythrocytes (IE) in the placenta (Beeson et al., 2002; Muthusamy et al., 2004). Upregulation of the VAR2CSA protein, a variant of the highly polymorphic adhesion peptide *P. falciparum* erythrocyte membrane protein 1 (PfEMP1) (Salanti et al., 2003), is responsible for parasite sequestration upon preferential binding to chondroitin sulfate A (CSA), which is abundantly expressed in the placenta (Fried et al., 2006; Muthusamy et al., 2007). Consequently, a severe local inflammatory process is triggered, characterized by the infiltration of monocytes and leukocytes in the placenta and eventual inflammation in response to parasite accumulation (Ismail et al., 2000; Parekh et al., 2010; Lucchi et al., 2011; Souza et al., 2013). This process has been frequently associated with placental histological alterations during MiP, such as dysregulation of placental architecture, formation of syncytial knots, fibrin deposition, necrosis, and placental barrier thickening (Walter et al., 1982; Ismail et al., 2000; Souza et al., 2013), and has been reported to occur during IUGR and preterm delivery, as well as in cases of reduced birth weight (Moormann et al., 1999; Menendez et al., 2000; Rogerson et al., 2003; Umbers et al., 2011).

Although we have obtained substantial knowledge in the field, studies on the epidemiology and pathology of MiP are frequently challenging due to related ethical and logistic difficulties. Long gestational periods, uncontrollable experimental planning, difficult access to biological and placental samples, and critical constraints associated with human experiments represent significant barriers that slow research progress and the understanding of this severe and complex disease. Therefore, alternatives have emerged with the advent of murine models to study MiP that have brought fundamental knowledge to the field. Herein, we have compiled research conducted for the past four decades using experimental rodent models, highlighting the most relevant findings, similarities to humans and, consequently, the translational capacity of achieved results.

HUMAN AND MURINE GESTATION: COMPARISON AND TRANSLATIONAL CHALLENGES FOR THE STUDY OF MiP

Comparative Gestation Development

In parallel with some other features, gestation length and development are somewhat different between human and murine mammals. Human gestation lasts for approximately 38 weeks (three trimesters) in contrast to rodents, in which gestation takes place over a 3-week period (Murray et al., 2010). In addition, there are also slight differences between species regarding the implantation period. Murine implantation takes place between the fourth and fifth days of gestation, somewhat sooner than in humans, in which this phenomenon occurs between the fifth and sixth days (Rossant and Tam, 2017). After implantation, gestation will progress toward a shift in fetal nutritional means. During early gestation in both humans and rodents, the growing fetus will survive through means of histiotrophic nutrition, in which nutrients are acquired by the uptake of substances secreted from the uterine glands present in the endometrium (Burton et al., 2002; Georgiades et al., 2002). However, the nutritional strategy changes around mid-gestation when the maternal blood supply to the placenta is completely established. Accordingly, the nutrient and gas exchanges between the mother and the fetus become functional, marking the onset of placental hemotrophic nutrition (Burton et al., 2001; Georgiades et al., 2002). In humans, this phenomenon occurs between the end of the first and the beginning of the second trimester, while in mice and rats, the same scenario occurs specifically at mid-gestation (between the twelfth and thirteenth days) (Georgiades et al., 2002). This shift in nutritional strategy occurs with the onset of organogenesis and fetal development, after which growth will continue until gestational term is reached.

Comparative Placental Function, Structure, and Histology

Human and murine placentas have a considerable degree of similarity and are nearly identical from physiological and functional perspectives (Rossant and Cross, 2001; Georgiades et al., 2002). In both mammalian species, this transient organ ensures nutrient and gas exchange between the mother and the growing fetus (Lager and Powell, 2012), maintains tolerance to the maternal immune system (Kanellopoulos-Langevin et al., 2003), and works as a physical and immunological barrier against endogenous pathogens (Robbins and Bakardjiev, 2012).

The placentas in both species are discoid organs in which maternal blood coming from the endometrium circulates and is in direct contact with trophoblasts, the fetal-derived cells responsible for regulating most placental physiological functions. In both species, the placenta can be structurally divided into three main areas: (1) an outer layer, consisting of uterine decidual cells and maternal blood vessels; (2) a middle layer, considered the implantation site where the placenta attaches to the uterus; and (3) an inner layer, in which the maternal blood interacts with trophoblasts to promote vital metabolic exchanges [reviewed elsewhere (Georgiades et al., 2002)]. Accordingly, the outer area can be mainly described as being composed by the myometrium and decidua basalis, which are extensively infiltrated by maternal arteries. This area is partially invaded by fetal-derived trophoblasts during the implantation process, which is considerably similar between both mammalian species. Moving toward the inner area of the human placenta, it is possible to distinguish a structural layer with no counterpart in the murine placenta known as the basal plate. This implantation site contains several distinct trophoblast subpopulations, such as extravillous (EVT) and cytotrophoblast (CT) cells. Nevertheless, an analogous area defined as the junctional zone occurs in murine animals, which is populated by specific types of cells such as trophoblast giant cells (TGC) and spongiotrophoblasts (SPG). Inside the placenta, more pronounced differences are observed regarding morphology and structure. The central area, which is commonly referred to as the human fetal placenta, is constituted by villi in an extremely ramified tree-like structure, which increases the contact surface with the maternal blood freely circulating within the intervillous space (IVS) (**Figure 1A**). On the other hand, a similar structure known as the labyrinth develops in mice and rats (**Figures 2A,C**). This impacts maternal blood circulation inside the placenta, where blood stays confined to the tortuous and sinusoidal channels (Rossant and Cross, 2001). Additionally, the surface area contacting the maternal blood is somewhat distinguished between humans and rodents from both cytological and structural perspectives. In the human placenta, maternal blood is separated from fetal capillaries by a single layer of syncytiotrophoblasts (ST), beyond which CT cells are present together with the basal lamina and fetal endothelium (schematically represented in **Figure 3**). According to these characteristics, the human placenta is classified as hemomonochorial (Takata et al., 1997; Georgiades et al., 2002). In opposition, three layers compose the murine labyrinthine wall: one composed of mononuclear trophoblasts dispersed throughout the surface contacting maternal blood and two ST layers definitively separating the maternal and fetal compartments (illustrated in **Figure 3**). Accordingly, murine placentas are classified as hemotrichorial (Takata et al., 1997).

Nevertheless, the structural divergences of human and murine placentas have occurred in parallel with an extensive variety of resident cell populations that are independent of their analogs but not similar in development and characteristics and are equally responsible for the same physiological and functional processes in human, mouse and rat placentas (**Figure 3**).

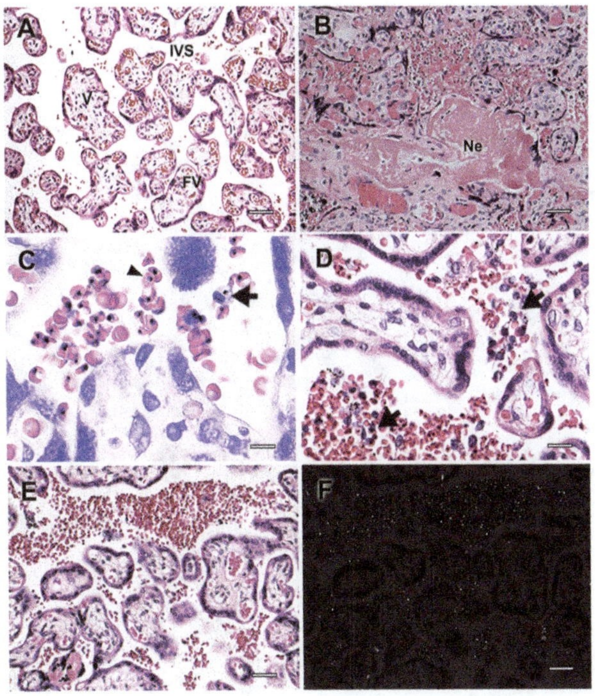

FIGURE 1 | Histologic events associated with placental pathology during human malaria in pregnancy. Placental histologic sections of non-infected **(A)** and *P. falciparum*-infected **(B–F)** women stained with Hematoxylin-Eosin. **(A)** Healthy human placenta without tissue damage and normal architecture in which intervillous spaces (IVS), usually bathed in maternal blood are in contact with placental villi (V), feeding the growing fetus through the fetal vessels (FV). **(B)** *P. falciparum*-infected placentas often characterized by extensive necrotic areas (Ne) and tissue disorganization. **(C,D)** Mononuclear cells infiltrate (arrow) is frequently patent due to the accumulation of parasitized erythrocytes (arrowhead). **(E)** Massive sequestration of *P. falciparum*-infected erythrocytes in the placenta is accompanied by **(F)** the accumulation of hemozoin in the IVS, which can be detected by polarized light microscopy. Scale bars represent **(A,B,E,F)** 100 μm, **(C)** 5 μm, and **(D)** 15 μm. Microscopy pictures were taken by Rodrigo Medeiros de Souza.

Using Murine Models to Study Malaria in Human Pregnancy

It is required that a suitable experimental model includes a group of features that lead to valid and translatable findings. As such, it is pivotal that rodent physiology and genetics, as well as pathologic manifestations during disease, resemble those in humans to a certain extent, ultimately validating them as models for human research (Justice and Dhillon, 2016). Accordingly, after several models were reviewed, mice and rats were validated by Desowitz as suitable to study MiP (Duffy and Fried, 2001) under the assumption that physiological and pathological similarities observed between rodents and humans were sufficient to consider them appropriate to study this disease. Shared placental characteristics, such as hemochorial and discoid structure (Georgiades et al., 2002; Wildman et al., 2006), hemotrophic nutrition (Burton et al., 2001; Georgiades et al., 2002) and analogous placental cell populations (Rossant and Cross, 2001; Georgiades et al., 2002), encourage their usage as models of MiP. These similarities are supported by molecular phylogenetic analysis, which clusters both rodents and humans into the same evolutionary clade (Wildman et al., 2006). The molecular similarities can be extended to immunity, an important aspect to consider when studying a disease in which poor outcomes are predominantly dependent on the host's immune response to malaria (Moormann et al., 1999; Rogerson et al., 2003). Hence, despite controversial discussion, it was shown that patterns of gene expression and biological pathways altered in mouse models of inflammatory diseases were significantly correlated with those from corresponding human conditions (e.g., sepsis) (Takao and Miyakawa, 2015), further supporting the usage of these animals for studying inflammatory diseases such as MiP. Together with the features mentioned above, the short gestational period, capacity for frequent and successive pregnancies, as well as large litter sizes, allow the rapid gathering of a considerable number of biological samples, which makes the rodents a powerful model for studying any pregnancy-related disease.

In addition to host characteristics, parasite intrinsic features are essential to validate experimental models of MiP. Above all, the most relevant features to consider should be the similarities between human and murine parasites cytoadhesion mechanisms. It is well known that the pathogenesis mechanisms involved in severe malaria induced by *P. falciparum* are associated with

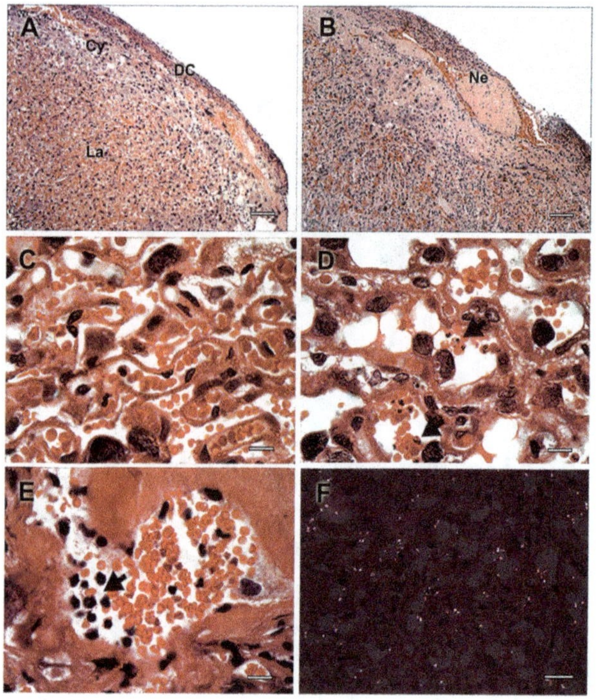

FIGURE 2 | Histologic events associated with placental pathology during murine malaria in pregnancy. Placental histology of non-infected **(A,C)** and *P. berghei*-infected **(B,C,E,F)** mice stained with Hematoxylin-Eosin. **(A)** Healthy placenta with normal histologic structure characterized by normal distribution of layer-specific cell such decidual cells (DC), trophoblastic cells (Cy), and labyrinthic cells (La), having **(C)** a normal labyrinth organization. **(B)** Fibrinoid necrosis (Ne) is depicted in section of *P. berghei*-infected placentas with **(D)** massive tissue disorganization and trophoblast membrane thickening. **(E)** Mononuclear cell infiltrate is visible (arrow), which occurs in response to **(D)** parasite accumulation (arrow) and **(F)** hemozoin deposition observed using polarized light microscopy. Scale bars represent **(A,B)** 100 μm, **(C–E)** 15 μm, and **(F)** 30 μm. Figure was modified from Neres et al. (2008) and Marinho et al. (2009) upon permission granted on behalf of journal's editorial board.

tissue- and organ-specific sequestration of IE (Schofield and Grau, 2005). More specifically, *P. falciparum* MiP may lead to severe PM as a result of IE sequestration in the placenta, which is mediated by the PfEMP1 variant VAR2CSA (which binds to placental CSA). The wide range of PfEMP1 variants known to be encoded by 50–60 *var* genes (Kraemer and Smith, 2006) have no known homologs in murine parasites (Hall et al., 2005). In fact, only some genetic signatures are similar between the murine and human *Plasmodium* species that encode alternate variable surface antigens (VSA), which were grouped in the multigenic *pir* superfamily (*Plasmodium* interspersed repeats) (Janssen et al., 2004; Hall et al., 2005). Nevertheless, murine parasite strains such as *P. berghei* have been shown to accumulate in specific tissues such as brain, fat, lung and spleen in a CD36-dependent and independent manner, which is also a well conserved pathogenesis mechanisms of severe malaria induced by *P. falciparum* (Franke-Fayard et al., 2010). In the same extent, the expression of alternate VSA and the binding capacity to placental CSA observed in murine parasites support the conclusions regarding the similarities between the pathogenesis mechanisms involved in murine and human disease (Hall et al., 2005; Neres et al., 2008; Marinho et al., 2009; Hviid et al., 2010). Distinct mechanisms of pathogenesis might also be directly linked with the biology of the parasites. As such, it is advisable to consider that the usage of murine parasites needs to be adjusted with caution since specific strains might better mimic the distinct diseases associated with the unrelated biology of human parasites (e. g. *P. falciparum* or *P. vivax*). Accordingly, disease severity in mice tends to be higher in *P. berghei* ANKA causing lethal anemia and cerebral malaria in C57BL/6 for instance (resembling *P. falciparum* in humans); however, it has a tropism for reticulocytes (similar to *P. vivax*). Differently, *P. chabaudi* invades mature erythrocytes and is responsible for a less severe pathology shown by the resistance to infection observed in BALB/c and C57BL/6 mice. In the same extent, different parasites might also have different tendencies to accumulation in specific tissues, being better used to study specific diseases and host-pathogen interactions (reviewed in Lamb et al., 2006).

Despite the aforementioned host and parasite characteristics, one must carefully translate findings obtained in murine models to humans, especially regarding preclinical observations, due to the observed differences between both mammals. Nevertheless, the following sections will depict some of the current knowledge acquired using murine models of MiP (research details for each model are presented in **Table 1**) during the past decades while describing the parallel characteristics existing between humans and rodents in regard to poor pregnancy outcomes and MiP placental pathology (summarized list in **Table 2**).

CONTRIBUTION OF MURINE MODELS TO THE STUDY OF MiP

Understanding Recrudescence Using Murine Models of MiP

Currently, we have been facing the emerging problem of drug resistance acquisition observed in *P. falciparum* infections, the outcome of which might be the occurrence of recrudescence (without a new infection episode) as a consequence of subcurative therapy (Cattamanchi et al., 2003; Berrevoets et al., 2013). In addition to treatment incapacity to clear circulating parasites, the immune depression observed in specific situations, such as during pregnancy, might elicit the emergence of recrudescent parasites that are either dormant or at submicroscopic levels (Giobbia et al., 2005; Mayor et al., 2009; Laochan et al., 2015; Al Hammadi et al., 2017; Malvy et al., 2018). In this context, some of the first available studies using murine models of MiP appeared during the early 1980s, when van Zon and Eling first described recrudescence in pregnant mice infected with *P. berghei* (van Zon and Eling, 1980; van Zon et al., 1982). Females of different mouse strains (Swiss, C3H/StZ, BALB/c, and B10LP) challenged with *P. berghei* K173 were treated with chloroquine and sulfadiazine to decrease parasitemia and

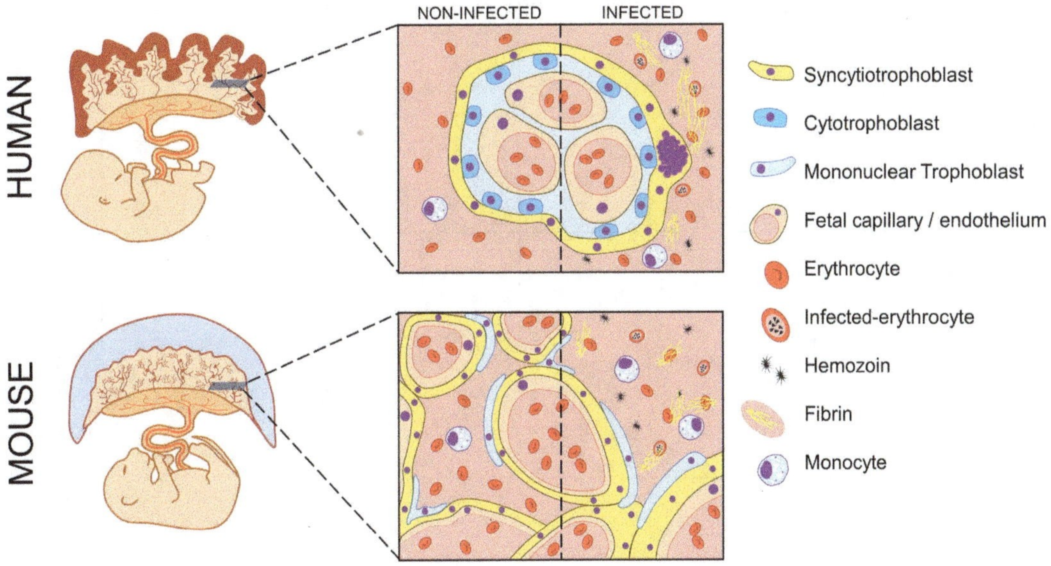

FIGURE 3 | Schematic representation of possible histologic events in human and murine placentas during malaria in pregnancy. Human and murine fetuses are represented with corresponding placentas. Magnification of transversal slices of each placental core illustrate histologic architecture, which widely differs between human placental villi and murine labyrinthine structure. During malaria in pregnancy, both human and murine placentas experience histopathologic manifestations that impair local homeostasis and lead to poor pregnancy outcomes. A comparison between both infected placentas and their non-infected counterparts is depicted. The presence of monocyte infiltrate is visible, which occurs in response to parasite and hemozoin accumulation. Histologic modifications such as fibrin deposition and syncytial knots occur due to the onset of severe local inflammation. Legend of picture components is vertically displayed beside the scheme.

promote the acquisition of immunity before mating. Afterward, pregnancy was shown to induce recrudescence, which was clearly shown to be strain- and gravidity-dependent (van Zon and Eling, 1980) and linked to preterm delivery and maternal mortality (van Zon et al., 1982). Consequently, the pioneering results enabled the authors to draw brief conclusions on similarities observed between human and murine recrudescence by determining that the phenomenon could be associated with (1) the drugs' incapacity to completely clear the parasite in a previous malaria episode and (2) the particular immune status associated with pregnancy, recapitulating the features of recrudescence in human MiP (Giobbia et al., 2005; Al Hammadi et al., 2017; Malvy et al., 2018). Pregnancy-associated immune modulation was then shown to be linked to increased production of corticoids during murine gestation, thereby facilitating the onset of recrudescence (van Zon et al., 1982, 1985). Notwithstanding the relevance of van Zon and coworkers' findings, parasite reappearance in maternal circulation was often ensured by experimental reinfection, raising questions about the translational reliability of murine recrudescence results obtained in these models (van Zon and Eling, 1980; van Zon et al., 1982).

Despite the promising advances made during that period, recrudescence in murine models was poorly addressed until the last decade. Only in 2009, two studies have addressed questions about the topic (Marinho et al., 2009; Megnekou et al., 2009). By reevaluating the pioneering experimental model implemented by van Zon and coworkers, the team of Megnekou addressed the production of specific anti-VSA antibodies in pregnant BALB/c mice immunized against *P. berghei* K173. Although previously immunized, protection was lost during pregnancy due to the recrudescence of parasites expressing specific VSA. Consequently, protection was shown to be gravidity-dependent since the less susceptible multiparous mice have raised antibodies against parasite-specific VSA during their previous pregnancies (Megnekou et al., 2009). However, some parasite reappearances were once again ensured by experimental infections, raising the same translational limitations discussed above. During that same year, a study from Marinho et al. (2009) established a model to study recrudescence in BALB/c mice, however, without recurring to mid-gestation reinfection. Accordingly, non-pregnant mice were infected with *P. berghei* ANKA and administered a subcurative treatment to clear apparent parasitemia. Mice were then mated approximately 1 month later and analyzed for recrudescence, which occurred in up to 58% of pregnant mice from gestational day (G)12 onward (Marinho et al., 2009). Maternal mortality and parasitemia were shown to be increased in primigravidae, which diminished with increased gravidity, supporting the observations of Megnekou et al. (2009) regarding acquired immunity in subsequent pregnancies.

Nevertheless, both recrudescent and newly inoculated parasites constitute a risk for highly susceptible pregnant women (Laochan et al., 2015). Accordingly, a recent study has shown that *P. chabaudi* CB sporozoites are capable of inducing recrudescence in pregnant C57BL/6 mice, being more closely related to the human parasite life cycle. However, poor pregnancy outcomes, such as maternal mortality and reduced birth weight, were likely to occur upon heterologous reinfection with *P. chabaudi* AS rather than in the cases of recrudescence. Preacquired immunity against the recrudescent

TABLE 1 | Summary of the principal findings and observations done using murine models of malaria in pregnancy.

Author(s)	*Plasmodium* strain	Murine strain	Recrudescence	Anemia	Maternal mortality	Abortion Resorption Stillbirth Preterm delivery	Litter size Newborn/fetal weight/health	Placental abnormalities/alterations
van Zon and Eling, 1980	*P. berghei* K173	Swiss Albino C3H/StZ BALB/c B10LP	↑ Primigravidae ↓ multigravidae ↑ due to ↓ immunity	X	↑ In recrudescence ↑ primigravidae	X	X	X
van Zon et al., 1982	*P. berghei* K173	Swiss Albino	→ To pregnancy	X	↑ In recrudescence	Preterm delivery ↑ in recrudescence	X	X
Oduola et al., 1982	*P. berghei* NK65	A/J ICR	→ To pregnancy	↑ In pregnancy	↑ In early infection ↓ in late infection ↑ parturition in late infection	Stillbirth → to early infection	Normal litter size ↓ Weight → to late infection ↑ spleen weight No congenital malaria	Impaired labyrinth structure Trophoblast barrier thickening IEs/Hz MΦ
van Zon et al., 1985	*P. berghei* K173	Swiss Albino B10LP	→ To pregnancy	X	X	X	X	X
Vinayak et al., 1986	*P. berghei* NICD	Swiss Albino	X	X	↑ In early infection Death before parturition	Stillbirth → to mid gestation infection ↑ resorption	↓ Litter size due to resorption ↓ weight ↑ Spleen weight No congenital malaria	Hyperplasia ↓ placental sinusoids IEs/Hz
Oduola et al., 1986	*P. berghei* NK65	Sprague-Dawley ICR	X	X	X	X	X	Hyperplasia Necrosis/fibrin Impaired labyrinth structure Trophoblast barrier thickening IEs/Hz MΦ/Leu
Desowitz et al., 1989	*P. berghei* NYU-2	Wistar	No recrudescence	↑ In pregnancy	↑ In early infection ↓ in mid gestation infection with ↑ parasitemia at term	No preterm delivery	Normal litter size	↑ Placental parasitemia
Hioki et al., 1990	*P. berghei* NK65	BALB/c	X	↑ In pregnancy ↑ in mid gestation infection	↑ In early infection (death before term) ↓ in late infection (live until term)	X	X	X
Pathak et al., 1990	*P. berghei* NICD	Swiss Albino VRC	No recrudescence	X	↑ Maternal mortality ↓ in treated pregnant mice	Stillbirth → to mid gestation infection	↓ Weight ↓ Litter size	Hyperplasia IEs
Pavia and Niederbuhl, 1991	*P. yoelii* YM *P. yoelii* 17X	ICR	No recrudescence	X	↑ Maternal mortality in non-immunized pregnancies ↓ with ↓ parasite virulence	X	Delivery of dead pups in non-immunized pregnancies No congenital malaria	X

(Continued)

TABLE 1 | Continued

Author(s)	*Plasmodium* strain	Murine strain	Recrudescence	Anemia	Maternal mortality	Abortion Resorption Stillbirth Preterm delivery	Litter size Newborn/fetal weight/health	Placental abnormalities/alterations
Tegoshi et al., 1992	*P. berghei* NYU-2	Wistar	X	X	X	X	X	Hyperplasia Necrosis/fibrin Impaired labyrinth structure Trophoblast barrier thickening ↑ IEs after late infection MΦ/Leu
Adachi et al., 2000	*P. berghei* ANKA	BALB/c	X	X	X	X	Congenital malaria	X
Poovassery and Moore, 2006	*P. chabaudi* AS	C57BL/6	X	↑ In pregnancy → to ↑ parasitemia	↑ Mortality → pregnancy	↑ Abortion/resorption at mid gestation → to early infection	↓ Fetal viability	↑ IEs at mid gestation ↓ monocyte accumulation
Neres et al., 2008	*P. berghei* ANKA	BALB/c	X	X	↑ Mortality → pregnancy	↑ Abortion/resorption during infection ↑ preterm delivery during infection	↓ Fetal/birth weight ↓ fetal blood flow/content ↓ viability	Hyperplasia Necrosis/fibrin Impaired labyrinth structure Trophoblast barrier thickening IEs/Hz MΦ ↓ Placental vasculature
Poovassery and Moore, 2009	*P. chabaudi* AS	C57BL/6	X	X	X	↑ Abortion at mid gestation → to early infection	↓ Fetal viability	IEs/Hz
Poovassery et al., 2009	*P. chabaudi* AS	C57BL/6	X	↑ In pregnancy → to ↑ parasitemia	↑ Mortality → pregnancy	↑ Abortion/resorption at mid gestation → to early infection	↓ Fetal viability → to IFN-γ/TNF-α	Fibrin thrombi Placental hemorrhage Impaired labyrinth structure Monocytes/macrophages
Megnekou et al., 2009	*P. berghei* K173	BALB/c	→ To pregnancy ↑ primigravidae	→ To recrudescence	→ To recrudescence ↑ due to ↓ immunity	X	→ To recrudescence ↓ Litter size ↓ Weight	iRBCs/Hz
Marinho et al., 2009	*P. berghei* ANKA	BALB/c	→ To pregnancy	X	→ To recrudescence ↑ primigravidae ↓ multigravidae	X	→ To recrudescence ↓ Litter size ↓ Weight ↓ Primigravidae ↑ Multigravidae	Trophoblast barrier thickening IEs MΦ/Tc/NKc ↓ Placental vascular spaces
Silver et al., 2010	*P. berghei* ANKA	BALB/c	X	X	X	↑ Abortion/resorption at late-gestation → to mid gestation infection	↓ Fetal weight at late gestation ↓ fetal viability	X
Sarr et al., 2012	*P. chabaudi* AS	A/J C57BL/6	X	↑ In pregnant A/J mice when compared to C57BL/6	↑ In pregnant A/J mice when compared to C57BL/6	↑ Abortion/resorption in A/J and C57BL/6	X	↑ Placental IEs in A/J when comparing to C57BL/6

(Continued)

TABLE 1 | Continued

Author(s)	*Plasmodium* strain	Murine strain	Recrudescence	Anemia	Maternal mortality	Abortion Resorption Stillbirth Preterm delivery	Litter size Newborn/fetal weight/health	Placental abnormalities/alterations
Rodrigues-Duarte et al., 2012	*P. berghei* K173 NK65 ANKAΔpm4	C57BL/6	X	X	↑ In pregnant mice infected with *P. berghei* NK65	↑ Stillbirth → mid gestation infection	↓ Fetal weight at late gestation ↓ newborn viability	Necrosis/fibrin Impaired labyrinth structure Trophoblast barrier thickening IEs ↓ Placental vascular spaces
Avery et al., 2012	*P. chabaudi* AS	C57BL/6	X	↑ In pregnancy → to ↑ parasitemia	X	↑ Abortion at mid gestation → to early infection → to coagulation and impaired fibrinolysis	↓ Fetal viability	Necrosis/fibrin Impaired labyrinth structure
Conroy et al., 2013	*P. berghei* ANKA	BALB/c Wildtype $C5aR^{-/-}$	X	X	X	X	↑ Fetal weight and ↑ viability in infected $C5aR^{-/-}$ mice	↑ Placental vascular remodeling in infected $C5aR^{-/-}$ mice
de Moraes et al., 2013	*P. berghei* ANKA	BALB/c ♀ C57BL/6 ♂	X	X	X	X	X	Impaired labyrinth structure Trophoblast barrier thickening Placental vasculature remodeling IEs in ↓ blood flow areas
Barboza et al., 2014	*P. berghei* NK65	C57BL/6 Wildtype $MyD88^{-/-}$	X	X	X	X	↑ Fetal weight in infected $MyD88^{-/-}$ mice ↑ survival in newborn from infected $MyD88^{-/-}$ mice	↑ Placental vascular spaces in infected $MyD88^{-/-}$ mice
Sharma and Shukla, 2014	*P. berghei* NK65	BALB/c	X	X	↓ In pregnant-infected mice treated with CQ/SP	X	↑ Weight and ↑ viability in newborn from mice treated with CQ/SP	↓ IEs, ↓ Hz, and normal placental histology in mice treated with CQ/SP
Lima et al., 2014	*P. berghei* *P. chabaudi*	C57BL/6	X	X	X	X	X	Accumulation of iRBCs mature forms in the placenta IEs uptake by trophoblast
Sarr et al., 2015	*P. chabaudi* AS	A/J C57BL/6	X	X	X	↑ Abortion/resorption in A/J and C57BL/6	X	↑ Tc, Bc, NKc in conceptus from infected A/J and C57BL/6 mice ↑ MΦ in the placental junctional zone of A/J mice Apoptosis present in immune cells and spongiotrophoblast
Sharma et al., 2016	*P. chabaudi* CB *P. chabaudi* AS	C57BL/6	→ To pregnancy → to CB sporozoites	→ To recrudescence → to reinfection	↑ In reinfections but not in recrudescence	↑ Stillbirth in reinfections and → to high parasitemia	Normal litter size ↓ weight and ↓ malaria susceptibility in reinfection	IEs in recrudescence No histologic alterations

(Continued)

TABLE 1 | Continued

Author(s)	*Plasmodium* strain	Murine strain	Recrudescence	Anemia	Maternal mortality	Abortion Resorption Stillbirth Preterm delivery	Litter size Newborn/fetal weight/health	Placental abnormalities/alterations
Barboza et al., 2017	*P. berghei* NK65	C57BL/6 Wildtype TLR2$^{-/-}$ TLR4$^{-/-}$ TLR9$^{-/-}$	×	×	×	×	↑ Fetal weight in infected TLR4$^{-/-}$ mice	IEs MΦ/NΦ/Dc ↑ placental vascular spaces in infected TLR4$^{-/-}$ mice
Rodrigues-Duarte et al., 2018	*P. berghei* NK65	C57BL/6 Wildtype TLR4$^{-/-}$ IFNAR1$^{-/-}$	×	×	×	↓ Stillbirth in TLR4$^{-/-}$ and IFNAR1$^{-/-}$ infected pregnant mice carrying TLR4$^{+/-}$ and IFNAR1$^{+/-}$ progeny	Wildtype and TLR4$^{-/-}$ infected mice with similar litter weight ↑ weight of IFNAR1$^{+/-}$ fetuses from infected IFNAR1$^{-/-}$ mice	×
Barboza et al., 2019	*P. berghei* NK65	C57BL/6 Wildtype MyD88$^{-/-}$	×	×	×	×	↓ Fetal weight in MyD88$^{+/-}$ progeny born from MyD88$^{-/-}$	↓ Placental vascular spaces in MyD88$^{+/-}$ placentas from MyD88$^{-/-}$

The current table content aims to summarize research conducted during the past four decades that was used to inform this review. In summary, Plasmodium and murine strains are described for each reference, as well as observations made regarding pregnancy outcomes and placental histology. Information regarding symbology is depicted as follows: Increased (↑), decreased (↓), associated (→), males (♂), females (♀), infected erythrocytes (IEs), hemozoin (Hz), leukocytes (Leu), monocytes/macrophages (MΦ), T cells (Tc), B cells (Bc), NK cells (NKc), dendritic cells (Dc), neutrophils (NΦ), chloroquine (CQ), sulphadoxine-pyrimethamine (SP).

parasite might justify why only reinfection with heterologous parasite lead to poor pregnancy outcomes. Nonetheless, exposure to heterologous *P. chabaudi* AS ensures newborn protection against postnatal infection, reliably resembling the outcomes of human MiP (Sharma et al., 2016).

Although observed in murine MiP, some studies have reported no recrudescence in protocols of treatment and immunization used in mice to control infection before pregnancy (Pathak et al., 1990; Pavia and Niederbuhl, 1991). Explanations might rely on the (1) drug efficiency to clear circulating parasite, (2) usage of less virulent strains (e.g., *P. berghei* NICD and *P. yoelii* 17X), or (3) less susceptible mice strains (e.g., Swiss Albino VRC). Nonetheless, despite some controversial experimental settings, findings associated with the aforementioned murine models have revealed some hidden biological features associated with malaria recrudescence during pregnancy that otherwise would be impossible to address.

Understanding Poor Pregnancy Outcomes Using Murine Models of MiP

A multitude of outcomes can occur as a result of developing MiP. When considering the areas of *P. falciparum* frequent and stable transmission, pregnancy-associated consequences might depend on several aspects such as infection trimester, gravidity and maternal health status that ultimately dictate the onset of maternal anemia, fetal and maternal mortality, abortion, and reduced birth weight as consequences of IUGR and/or preterm delivery (Desai et al., 2007; Umbers et al., 2011; Rogerson et al., 2018). Outcomes in human pregnancy are accessible for study; however, in addition to ethical constraints, illogical and incorrect correlations might be drawn from imprecise information given by patients enrolling in these prospective studies, such as imprecise time of infection or clinical status. Fittingly, murine models provided the opportunity to investigate MiP outcomes in a controlled experimental setting.

Maternal Anemia

Maternal anemia that develops during MiP is considered a significant risk factor for poor pregnancy outcomes and is closely associated with increased parasite burden and reduced birth weight (Rogerson et al., 2003). Accordingly, several distinct experimental murine models accurately recapitulate anemia observed during human MiP. Similarly, *P. chabaudi* AS infection potentiates the onset of anemia (reduced hematocrit percentage) in pregnant C57BL/6 mice. Anemia was therefore linked to a rapid increase in parasitemia, which peaks abruptly in pregnant mice (Poovassery and Moore, 2006; Poovassery et al., 2009; Avery et al., 2012; Sarr et al., 2012). This phenomenon was also shown to occur in different murine strains, such as BALB/c mice (Hioki et al., 1990) and Wistar rats (Desowitz et al., 1989), infected with *P. berghei* NK65 and NYU-2, respectively, in which hemoglobin and hematocrit decreased as a result of increased parasitemia. Reproducibility of anemia is expected among different experimental models since hemolysis constitutes an intrinsic step in the *Plasmodium* spp. life cycle in both rodents and humans. Nevertheless, this critical parameter has been poorly investigated in murine malaria, in which its

TABLE 2 | Compilation of references mentioning the main pathologic manifestations of malaria in pregnancy observed in humans and murine models.

	Human MiP	Murine MiP
Pregnancy outcome		
Recrudescence	Giobbia et al., 2005; Mayor et al., 2009; Laochan et al., 2015; Al Hammadi et al., 2017; Malvy et al., 2018	van Zon and Eling, 1980; Oduola et al., 1982; van Zon et al., 1982, 1985; Marinho et al., 2009; Megnekou et al., 2009; Sharma et al., 2016
Anemia	Brabin et al., 2001; Rogerson et al., 2003	Oduola et al., 1982; Desowitz et al., 1989; Hioki et al., 1990; Megnekou et al., 2009; Poovassery et al., 2009; Avery et al., 2012; Sarr et al., 2012; Sharma et al., 2016
Maternal mortality	Luxemburger et al., 1997; Brabin et al., 2001; Shulman et al., 2002; Nosten et al., 2004; Menéndez et al., 2008; Rogerson et al., 2018	van Zon and Eling, 1980; Oduola et al., 1982; van Zon et al., 1982; Vinayak et al., 1986; Desowitz et al., 1989; Hioki et al., 1990; Pathak et al., 1990; Pavia and Niederbuhl, 1991; Poovassery and Moore, 2006; Neres et al., 2008; Marinho et al., 2009; Megnekou et al., 2009; Poovassery et al., 2009; Rodrigues-Duarte et al., 2012; Sarr et al., 2012; Sharma and Shukla, 2014; Sharma et al., 2016
Stillbirth	Menendez, 1995; Desai et al., 2007	Oduola et al., 1982; Vinayak et al., 1986; Pathak et al., 1990; Rodrigues-Duarte et al., 2012, 2018; Sharma et al., 2016
Abortion	Desai et al., 2007	Poovassery and Moore, 2006, 2009; Neres et al., 2008; Poovassery et al., 2009; Silver et al., 2010; Avery et al., 2012; Sarr et al., 2012, 2015
Preterm delivery	Menendez et al., 2000; Desai et al., 2007; Moore et al., 2017	van Zon et al., 1982; Neres et al., 2008
Reduced newborn/fetal weight	Menendez et al., 2000; Rogerson et al., 2003; Nosten et al., 2004; Desai et al., 2007; Umbers et al., 2011	Oduola et al., 1982; Vinayak et al., 1986; Pathak et al., 1990; Neres et al., 2008; Marinho et al., 2009; Megnekou et al., 2009; Silver et al., 2010; Rodrigues-Duarte et al., 2012, 2018; Conroy et al., 2013; Barboza et al., 2014, 2017, 2019; Sharma and Shukla, 2014; Sharma et al., 2016
Congenital malaria	Rai et al., 2015; Bhatia et al., 2016	Adachi et al., 2000
Placental histology		
Parasite accumulation	Walter et al., 1982; Beeson et al., 2002; Beeson and Brown, 2004; Muthusamy et al., 2004, 2007	Oduola et al., 1982, 1986; Vinayak et al., 1986; Desowitz et al., 1989; Pathak et al., 1990; Tegoshi et al., 1992; Poovassery and Moore, 2006, 2009; Neres et al., 2008; Marinho et al., 2009; Megnekou et al., 2009; Rodrigues-Duarte et al., 2012; Sarr et al., 2012; de Moraes et al., 2013; Lima et al., 2014; Sharma and Shukla, 2014; Sharma et al., 2016; Barboza et al., 2017
Hemozoin deposition	Bulmer et al., 1993; Ismail et al., 2000	Oduola et al., 1982, 1986; Vinayak et al., 1986; Neres et al., 2008; Megnekou et al., 2009; Poovassery and Moore, 2009
Immune cells infiltrate	Walter et al., 1982; Ordi et al., 1998; Ismail et al., 2000; Rogerson et al., 2007; Othoro et al., 2008; Souza et al., 2013	Oduola et al., 1982, 1986; Tegoshi et al., 1992; Poovassery and Moore, 2006; Neres et al., 2008; Marinho et al., 2009; Poovassery et al., 2009; Barboza et al., 2017
Fibrin Necrosis	Walter et al., 1982; Ismail et al., 2000; Souza et al., 2013	Oduola et al., 1986; Tegoshi et al., 1992; Neres et al., 2008; Poovassery et al., 2009; Avery et al., 2012; Rodrigues-Duarte et al., 2012
Syncytial knots Trophoblast rupture	Ismail et al., 2000; Crocker et al., 2004; Souza et al., 2013	
Trophoblast membrane thickening	Ismail et al., 2000; Souza et al., 2013	Oduola et al., 1982, 1986; Tegoshi et al., 1992; Neres et al., 2008; Marinho et al., 2009; Rodrigues-Duarte et al., 2012; de Moraes et al., 2013; Barboza et al., 2014, 2017, 2019

Distinct pregnancy outcomes and placental histopathologic alterations are depicted. References used to inform this review are cited in the table according to their contribution in unraveling specific clinical and histologic manifestations of both human and murine malaria in pregnancy.

relationship with infection timing, gravidity, and pregnancy outcomes were never addressed as in humans (Brabin et al., 2001; Rogerson et al., 2003).

Maternal Mortality

Maternal mortality seems to be a less frequent outcome in pregnancies complicated by malaria (Menéndez et al., 2008; Rogerson et al., 2018). Maternal death associated with *Plasmodium* spp. infection tends to occur more frequently in areas of low malaria transmission due to the reduced level of premunition (Nosten et al., 2004). Nevertheless, pregnant women with malaria who live in endemic areas are also prone to die due to severe anemia (Brabin et al., 2001; Shulman et al., 2002). Likewise, both pregnant mice and rats infected with murine *Plasmodium* spp. strains were shown to die during gestation, which was dependent on the parasite strain, infection timing, and host intrinsic characteristics. Regarding parasite strains, it was demonstrated that *P. berghei* (van Zon and Eling, 1980; Oduola et al., 1982; van Zon et al., 1982; Vinayak et al., 1986; Desowitz et al., 1989; Hioki et al., 1990; Pathak et al., 1990; Neres et al., 2008; Marinho et al., 2009; Megnekou et al., 2009; Rodrigues-Duarte et al., 2012; Sharma and Shukla, 2014), *P. yoelii* (Pavia and Niederbuhl, 1991), and *P. chabaudi* (Poovassery and Moore, 2006, 2009; Poovassery et al., 2009; Sarr et al., 2012; Sharma et al., 2016) induce maternal death in a considerable variety of experimental settings. However, only one study has directly compared this outcome induced by different parasites, clearly showing increased mortality rates in pregnant C57BL/6 mice infected with *P. berghei* NK65 compared to K173 and ANKAΔpm4 strains (Rodrigues-Duarte et al., 2012). One must consider that mortality rates also depend on host susceptibility to infection since, for instance, pregnant A/J mice experience a higher risk of mortality than C57BL/6 mice when infected with *P. chabaudi* AS (Sarr et al., 2012). These findings support the notion that maternal survival is dependent on both parasite and host intrinsic features. Similarly, mortality was shown to increase in pregnant C57BL/6 and BALB/c mice infected with *P. chabaudi* (Poovassery and Moore, 2006; Poovassery et al., 2009) or *P. berghei* (Neres et al., 2008; Rodrigues-Duarte et al., 2012), respectively, when compared to their non-pregnant counterparts. This is a well-known phenomenon that also occurs in humans who are primarily in areas of unstable malaria transmission (Luxemburger et al., 1997; Nosten et al., 2004). Infection timing was also shown to be linked to maternal mortality, which primarily increases in cases of early gestation infection. This was demonstrated to occur in Wistar rats (Desowitz et al., 1989), as well as in Swiss Albino, A/J, ICR, and BALB/c mice (Oduola et al., 1982; Vinayak et al., 1986; Hioki et al., 1990) infected with *P. berghei*. However, mid-gestation infection was shown to lead to increased survival with a higher number of animals achieving parturition. Interestingly, it is unclear whether this occurs in humans and if first trimester infections lead to increased maternal mortality rates (Desai et al., 2007; Rogerson et al., 2018). Nevertheless, regardless of the infection trimester, mortality is highly dependent on gravidity and is more prevalent in primigravidae than in multiparous women (Menéndez et al., 2008). Equally, mice tend to experience the same effect, which is likely to be dependent on immunity acquired during previous gestations (van Zon and Eling, 1980; Marinho et al., 2009). Accordingly, immunity seems to be pivotal in reduced murine mortality, as ICR mice immunized with attenuated *P. yoelii* before pregnancy had improved survival rates when challenged with the lethal *P. yoelii* 17X strain (Pavia and Niederbuhl, 1991). Although a direct causality has never been proved, increased mortality observed in murine models of MiP seem to be associated with the development of systemic infection measured by increased peripheral parasitemia that correlates with decreased body weight and patent patterns of anemia (Poovassery et al., 2009; Sarr et al., 2012).

Considering the discussion above, it is clear that mortality during pregnancy depends on a wide range of factors that ultimately will affect host survival. Most of them are commonly recapitulated in rodent experimental models in which experiments have contributed with important findings in this regard. However, one must carefully consider the often-fatal outcomes of murine infections induced by highly lethal parasites that are dissimilar to the infrequent lethality observed in human MiP.

In uterus Death and Abortion

In uterus death and abortion are rather infrequent outcomes of pregnancies complicated by malaria. However, there is a clear association between MiP development and stillbirth incidence, which is noted as being higher in women with perceivable placental parasitemia (Desai et al., 2007). In contrast, the association between abortion and MiP seems to be rarely discussed, with only scarce reports of this event occurring in low transmission areas, probably resulting from early trimester infections (Menendez, 1995; Desai et al., 2007). It is important to highlight that logistical constraints imposed by cultural and socioeconomic boundaries are the reason by which it is difficult to assess this particular pregnancy outcome. Interestingly, the incidence of abortion seems to be much more frequent in murine models than in humans. Accordingly, *P. chabaudi* AS infection of pregnant C57BL/6 mice revealed a rather frequent pattern of abortion and reduced fetal viability at mid-gestation (G10-12) when the parasite was inoculated immediately after conception. This event overlaps with the peripheral parasitemia peak and massive accumulation of parasites inside the placenta (Poovassery and Moore, 2006). As expected, the parasitemia peak and abortion were frequently observed in mice having increased production of cytokines in both peripheral blood (e.g., IL-1β and IL-10) and placenta (e.g., IFN-γ) (Poovassery and Moore, 2009). In a follow-up study, it was shown that fetal loss and reduced viability in pregnant C57BL/6 mice infected with *P. chabaudi* AS were markedly influenced by IFN-γ and TNF-α production (Poovassery et al., 2009) and increased coagulopathy and impaired fibrinolysis (Avery et al., 2012). In the same extent, abortion was shown to occur concomitantly with apoptosis of inflammatory cells and spongiotrophoblast in the junctional zone (between the uterus and the labyrinth), which has been discussed to occur in a way that is dependent on TNF-α signaling (Sarr et al., 2015). Altogether, these findings established a clear link between the immune response triggered against malaria and poor pregnancy outcomes. Moreover, models of abortion are also characterized by early infection with *P. chabaudi*, but stillbirth has also been observed in Swiss Albino (Vinayak et al., 1986; Pathak et al., 1990), BALB/c (Neres et al., 2008), and C57BL/6 (Rodrigues-Duarte et al., 2012) mice infected with *P. berghei* at mid-gestation. In these experimental models, reduced fetal viability without clear abortion observed at late gestation somewhat reflects stillbirth occurring in humans during the third gestational trimester (Desai et al., 2007).

Notably, it is important to highlight that translating these findings to human research may raise some serious controversies. Human stillbirth is often described as a dead conceptus that was expelled or removed from the womb 22 weeks after conception, being no longer considered an abortion (less than 22 weeks) (Lawn et al., 2016). In contrast, in the aforementioned murine models, there is no parallel measure at which fetal viability was assessed that considers gestational age. Vaginal secretions containing blood are normally taken as an indicative of early abortion, followed by the observation of necrotic structures (resorptions) that lack fetal or placental morphology (Poovassery and Moore, 2006; Neres et al., 2008). On the other hand, fetal viability is normally evaluated closer to term, after touching *in uterus* or delivered conceptus with pliers. Fetuses that fail to react are considered stillbirths (Neres et al., 2008). Therefore, definitions in these situations are often misleading, and conclusions should be made with extreme caution since abortion and stillbirth etiology may vary between rodent and human MiP.

Preterm Birth

Preterm birth, which encompasses every live birth that occurs before the 37th week of gestation (Goldenberg et al., 2009), is a more frequent consequence and is one of the leading causes of reduced birth weight associated with MiP (Menendez et al., 2000; Desai et al., 2007; Moore et al., 2017). Interestingly, the occurrence of spontaneous delivery in mice or rats in the context of MiP is either poorly addressed or considerably infrequent. One study reported the occurrence of preterm delivery of dead pups from pregnant BALB/c mice infected with *P. berghei* ANKA (Neres et al., 2008). However, this definition does not seem to fit the circumstance since preterm birth assumes that the progeny is born alive before term, which is unlikely to occur before G19 (reviewed elsewhere McCarthy et al., 2018). To the same extent, murine models have been questioned regarding their capacity to reproduce human preterm birth due to inaccurate measurements and non-standardized markers.

In this regard, evaluation of preterm birth in murine models of MiP is probably far from replicating human pathology. However, a better evaluation of this outcome may lead to improved disease models with more reliable translation capacities (McCarthy et al., 2018).

Progeny Outcomes and Development

Progeny outcomes and development will ultimately be severely affected as a result of the aforementioned clinical and obstetric manifestations during MiP. Often resulting from IUGR and/or preterm delivery, reduced birth weight contributes significantly to postnatal mortality and impaired child development across the malaria endemicity spectrum and is clearly more frequent in women during their first pregnancies (Nosten et al., 2004; Desai et al., 2007). It is unclear how MiP truly leads to growth restriction, yet evidences point to a multitude of factors such as angiogenic imbalance, endocrine dysregulation, deficiencies in transplacental nutrient transportation, severe inflammation and placental insufficiency (Umbers et al., 2011). During the 1980s, some studies reported the first observations of altered birth weight in mice suffering from MiP, which was found to be significantly diminished in pups from A/J, ICR (Oduola et al., 1982) and Swiss albino (Vinayak et al., 1986) litters born from mice infected with *P. berghei* NK65 and NICD, respectively. It seems that impaired progeny development is a rather well-conserved outcome of murine MiP since it was reported in BALB/c (Neres et al., 2008; Marinho et al., 2009; Megnekou et al., 2009; Silver et al., 2010) and C57BL/6 (Rodrigues-Duarte et al., 2012; Sharma et al., 2016) mice infected with a wide variety of parasite strains, suggesting the existence of conserved pathogenesis mechanisms (Rodrigues-Duarte et al., 2012). This pathologic outcome seems to be avoided with on-time administration of antimalarial drugs such as chloroquine and sulphadoxine-pyrimethamine, which were shown to abrogate systemic parasitemia, therefore improving offspring weight at delivery (Sharma and Shukla, 2014). Additionally, as it occurs in humans, progeny birth weight improved in mouse multigravidae. This trait was clearly shown to be gravidity-dependent, as pups belonging to the first litter were much smaller on average than those born from subsequent pregnancies when the corresponding dams were induced with MiP by recrudescent *P. berghei* ANKA (Marinho et al., 2009).

Further research conducted in the last decade revealed some hidden aspects of reduced birth weight etiology that would not be revealed without the wide range of genetically manipulated mice strains. Strikingly, it seems that proper fetal development is impaired upon the activation of specific components linked to innate immunity, such as complement system receptor (C5aR), Toll-like receptor 4 (TLR4), type I interferon receptor 1 (IFNAR1), and adaptor protein myeloid differentiation factor 88 (MyD88). BALB/c C5aR$^{-/-}$ (Conroy et al., 2013), C57BL/6 TLR4$^{-/-}$ (Barboza et al., 2017; Rodrigues-Duarte et al., 2018), C57BL/6 IFNAR$^{-/-}$ (Rodrigues-Duarte et al., 2018), and C57BL/6 MyD88$^{-/-}$ (Barboza et al., 2014, 2019) mice were shown to have litters with normal fetal weight, development and survival, even though being infected with *P. berghei* ANKA (in BALB/c) or *P. berghei* NK65 (in C57BL/6). These findings substantially advanced the field by strikingly implying the innate immune system on MiP-associated reduced birth weight pathogenesis, enabling future preclinical trials of anti-inflammatory drugs (e.g., the TLR4 antagonist IAXO) (Barboza et al., 2017) to be used concomitantly with antimalarial therapies to prevent MiP-associated poor pregnancy outcomes. However, progress in this field should also be done with extreme caution due to possible undesired side effects resulting from adjunctive therapies to treat severe malaria such as those observed in trials conducted with anti-TNF-α therapy to treat cerebral malaria and others (van Hensbroek et al., 1996; Varo et al., 2018).

Moreover, the postnatal scenario of human MiP might rarely include the appearance of congenital malaria, whose onset is tightly controlled by transplacental transmission of maternal antibodies to the fetus, resulting in isolated and scarce events often diagnosed as neonatal sepsis (Rai et al., 2015; Bhatia et al., 2016). Conceptus infection might occur due to blood exchanges at delivery or during pregnancy due to loss of villi integrity and syncytium rupture (Crocker et al., 2004; Robbins and Bakardjiev, 2012; Souza et al., 2013). By contrast, the phenomenon is thought to be even rarer in rodents. In related studies, the authors have clearly stated that no congenital malaria was observed, despite an increased fetal spleen weight, which might an indicative of fetal infection (Oduola et al., 1982; Vinayak et al., 1986). However, work by Adachi et al. (2000) addressed this question under the assumption that both mice and rats rarely transmit the parasite to their offspring. Accordingly, the authors detected parasites by nested PCR in a few pups born from pregnant BALB/c mice infected with *P. berghei*. These findings support the rareness of the event due to the lack of a uniform presence of parasites, even in pups within the same litter. The hemotrichorial layer in the murine placenta presents a much thicker barrier against transplacental passage of parasites than the human hemomonochorial placenta (Crocker et al., 2004), which might explain the reduced incidence of murine congenital malaria. Nevertheless, discrepancies in existing reports contraindicate the usage of murine models in this regard, identifying them as unsuitable for studying this rare disease outcome.

In conclusion, one may face challenges when translating pregnancy outcome findings obtained in murine models to human pathology. Nevertheless, significant achievements have been made in recent years, despite the considerable diversity of experimental settings and non-standardized methodologies. Improving them will certainly lead to enriched results and more accurate and meaningful conclusions taken from murine models of MiP.

Understanding Placental Pathology Using Murine Models of MiP

Most of the aforementioned outcomes occurring in pregnancies complicated by malaria are strongly associated with the dysregulation of placental homeostasis due to a significant accumulation of parasite-infected erythrocytes inside this organ, which overlaps with the onset of PM (Sharma and Shukla, 2017). Accordingly, several cytological and histological abnormalities are easily observed in infected placentas in addition to parasite accumulation, such as the malarial pigment hemozoin, immune cells, syncytial knots, fibrin deposition, necrosis and placental barrier thickening (Walter et al., 1982; Ismail et al., 2000; Souza et al., 2013). Although despite being PM hallmarks, not all of these histopathologic features are accurately shown by murine models of MiP (schematically represented in **Figure 3**).

Parasitized Erythrocytes

Parasitized erythrocytes tend to selectively accumulate in the placenta (**Figures 1C,D**), achieving greater parasitemia levels than those observed in the peripheral blood of pregnant infected women (Beeson et al., 2002; Muthusamy et al., 2004). It is unquestionable that murine parasites also accumulate inside the placenta (**Figure 2D**) since a large number of studies of placental histopathology noted this finding for a wide range of strains (**Table 1**). Notably, Poovassery and Moore (2006) have demonstrated that *P. chabaudi* AS parasites also accumulate preferentially inside the placenta of C57BL/6 mice, leading to greater placental parasitemia than that observed in peripheral blood. Interestingly, these murine parasite populations were shown to be mainly constituted by mature forms with an almost null percentage of early ring-stage parasites (Megnekou et al., 2009), which is in line with observations made during *P. falciparum* infections (Beeson et al., 2002). Similarly, intravital microscopy studies performed in placentas from pregnant mice infected either with *P. berghei* or *P. chabaudi* also suggested that those that accumulate are indeed the mature forms of the parasite (Lima et al., 2014), which preferably adhere to the trophoblast in areas of low blood flow inside the maternal blood sinusoids (de Moraes et al., 2013). As observed for *P. falciparum* regarding its preferential adhesion to CSA and controversial binding to hyaluronic acid (HA) (Beeson and Brown, 2004; Muthusamy et al., 2007), the adhesion of *P. berghei* was also shown to be dependent on placental CSA and HA as demonstrated by adhesion assays of mice IEs to placental sections treated with chondroitinase or hyaluronidase (Neres et al., 2008; Marinho et al., 2009). These findings once again support similar pathogenesis mechanisms between human and murine PM despite the lack of known PfEMP1 homologs (Hviid et al., 2010).

The Malarial Pigment Hemozoin

The malarial pigment hemozoin, a byproduct of hemoglobin catabolism performed by *Plasmodium* spp. to detoxify free heme (Olivier et al., 2014), is frequently observed in placentas from infected pregnant women (**Figures 1E,F**) and is often used as an indicator of PM, even in the absence of detectable parasites (Bulmer et al., 1993; Ismail et al., 2000). Similarly, placental infection by murine parasites also leads to hemozoin deposition (**Figure 2F**). Oduola and coworkers first observed this phenomenon in histologic sections of placentas from different murine backgrounds infected with *P. berghei* NK65. Shortly thereafter, the pigment was exclusively observed in maternal blood sinusoids, whose concentrations increased with augmented parasite loads. Accordingly, hemozoin-containing monocytes were also frequently observed (Oduola et al., 1982, 1986). In addition, hemozoin was also detected in trophoblast giant cells, suggesting an active phagocytic process (Poovassery and Moore, 2009). The pigment is frequently detected under polarized light microscopy (Neres et al., 2008; Megnekou et al., 2009) and is used to indicate past-chronic PM in humans according to the diagnostic criteria of Bulmer et al. (1993). To our knowledge, this event was rarely observed in murine models (Oduola et al., 1986). The fact that hemozoin was rarely observed alone in infected placentas suggests that the experimental settings from current models fail to reproduce past-chronic infections and are only able to reproduce acute PM.

Immune Cell Infiltrate

Immune cell infiltrate, which occurs as a response to parasite/hemozoin accumulation inside the placenta (**Figure 1D**), is one of the key hallmarks of the disease and is often associated with poor pregnancy outcomes (Menendez et al., 2000; Rogerson et al., 2003; Umbers et al., 2011). Monocytes/macrophages are the most abundant constituents of these inflammatory infiltrates, and recruitment is widely correlated with placental production of MIP-1α, MCP-1, I-309, and IL-8 chemokines (Abrams et al., 2003). Not surprisingly, the same event was observed in placentas from mice (**Figure 2E**) and rats infected with *P. berghei*, especially in those containing detectable placental parasites (Oduola et al., 1982, 1986; Tegoshi et al., 1992). Notably, the infiltrate, which was mainly composed of monocytes ($CD11b^{+ve}$ cells detected by cytochemistry) and macrophages ($CD11b^{+ve}$ cells detected by cytochemistry and *Cd68-* and *Mgl2*-expressing cells identified by qPCR), was linked to the production of some attractant chemokines, such as MIP-1α and MCP-1 (Neres et al., 2008; Marinho et al., 2009; Sarr et al., 2015; Barboza et al., 2017). However, the event is far from reflecting chronic intervillositis observed in humans (Ordi et al., 1998), probably due to the shorter gestational period in rodents. Additionally, some authors have commented on the scarcity of this event, especially in placentas from C57BL/6 mice infected with *P. chabaudi*, which tend to have fewer accumulated monocytes/macrophages due to reduced placental parasite burden (Poovassery and Moore, 2006; Poovassery et al., 2009). Early reports on different leukocyte populations in infected murine placentas noted the existence of mononuclear (Tegoshi et al., 1992) and polymorphonuclear (Oduola et al., 1986) cells. Molecular biology methods were later used to dissect these cell types, dividing them into dendritic cells (*Mgl2*), neutrophils (*Ncf2*), NK cells (*Klrd1*), T (*Cd3e*), and B (*Cd22*) lymphocytes (gene expression quantification by qPCR) (Marinho et al., 2009; Sarr et al., 2015; Barboza et al., 2017). Remarkably, this is in line with observations performed in human PM regarding the placental accumulation of NK cells, T lymphocytes and other non-specified polymorphonuclear cells (Ordi et al., 2001; Rogerson et al., 2007; Othoro et al., 2008). Nevertheless, despite the clear accumulation of immune cells in murine placentas, its association with poor pregnancy outcomes remains to be elucidated in experimental models that oppose current knowledge of human pathology (Rogerson et al., 2003; Umbers et al., 2011).

Placental Fibrinoid Necrosis

Placental fibrinoid necrosis normally occurs as a consequence of extensive placental tissue damage caused during *Plasmodium* spp. infection (**Figure 1B**). In fact, fibrin deposition is initiated to promote placental tissue repair but soon becomes cytotoxic, leading to necrosis (Walter et al., 1982; Ismail et al., 2000) and poor pregnancy outcomes such as premature delivery and reduced birth weight (Menendez et al., 2000; Avery et al., 2012). Likewise, pioneering studies from the 1980s revealed the presence of fibrinoid necrosis in placental sections from mice and rats infected with *P. berghei*, although without clear conclusions on its consequences (Oduola et al., 1986; Tegoshi et al., 1992). Later, fibrinoid necrosis was reported in placentas from *P. berghei*-infected BALB/c mice (**Figure 2B**), which delivered litters with a patently reduced birth weight phenotype (Neres et al., 2008), and fibrin thrombi in placentas from C57BL/6 mice infected with *P. chabaudi* that experienced spontaneous abortion (Poovassery et al., 2009). Discussion was taken to the point in which fibrin deposition in maternal blood sinusoids would significantly impair placental capability to perform physiological tasks such as respiration and nutrient exchanges, probably due to clotting, blood arrest, necrosis and trophoblast death. In a subsequent study, Avery et al. (2012) showed by western blot that fibrin deposits were increased in placentas from C57BL/6 mice infected with *P. chabaudi*, which occurred in parallel with an upregulation of coagulation-associated genes. These findings established an important association between impaired fibrinolysis and coagulation and the poor pregnancy outcomes of MiP.

Labyrinth Disarrangement

Labyrinth disarrangement will ultimately reflect murine placental dysfunction, which is characterized by particular histological alterations that have considerable differences from human PM, mostly due to the existence of a widely different villi structure (**Figures 1A,B** vs. **Figures 2A–D**). Of note, two features of human PM that have no counterparts in infected murine

BOX 1 | Suggestions to improve future murine models of MiP. Evolution has grouped murine animals and humans in similar phylogenetic clades according to some striking similarities. However, it has also separated them especially from an anatomically perspective. Some differences cannot be surpassed; yet, our understanding of some diseases and complex biological processes can be improved with the refinement of experimental design and standardization of analysis methods when using animal models such as experimental murine models of MiP. As such, our understanding of MiP could be improved by addressing some of the following points:

- Understanding the adhesion mechanism of murine parasite strains.
- Identification of VAR2CSA functional homologs in murine parasites.
- Standardization of protocols using specific species of murine parasites to differently address specific aspects of uncomplicated or severe MiP (e.g., usage of less or more virulent parasite strains, tropism for reticulocytes or mature erythrocytes, preferential tissue for accumulation).
- Standardized definitions and accurate measures for abortion, preterm delivery, stillbirth and placental malaria in the context of murine MiP.
- Investigating the possibility of congenital malaria in murine models of MiP.

placentas are syncytiotrophoblast rupture (previously discussed in the context of congenital malaria) and syncytial knots(Ismail et al., 2000; Souza et al., 2013). These protrusions of syncytial nuclear aggregates, which have been associated with hypoxia and oxidative stress in human placentas (Heazell et al., 2007), were discussed as having no similar structure in murine placentas that could be detected under light or electron microscopy (Tegoshi et al., 1992). Syncytial knots, which are considered an accumulation of degrading nuclei, was once erroneously described as a phenomenon of trophoblast hyperplasia [discussed elsewhere (Heazell et al., 2007)]. To our knowledge, the latter was never clearly discussed in the context of human PM. Accordingly, there are unclear reports of trophoblast hyperplasia occurring in the placentas of mice (Oduola et al., 1986; Vinayak et al., 1986; Pathak et al., 1990; Neres et al., 2008) and rats (Oduola et al., 1986; Tegoshi et al., 1992) infected with *P. berghei*. Nevertheless, evidence of this event includes unclear microscopy images that fail to address the apparent enlargement/swelling of tissue that occurs due to cell proliferation. However, there is a striking thickening of the trophoblast basal membrane that partially overlaps with the concept of tissue swelling. In human PM, this frequent phenomenon can be qualitatively analyzed (Ismail et al., 2000) or more accurately quantified as the distance that separates fetal capillaries from villi outer membrane (Souza et al., 2013). Regardless of the methodology used, this parameter was found to be significantly thicker during human PM and, being discussed as strongly influencing transplacental transport of vital compounds. Similarly, this was qualitatively analyzed and reported in mouse and rat placentas infected with *P. berghei*, which was hypothesized to be a consequence of the fibrotic process resulting from massive tissue repair (Oduola et al., 1986; Tegoshi et al., 1992). Later, some other works have developed methods to indirectly quantify trophoblast thickening, taking advantage of the sinusoidal nature of mouse placentas. Accordingly, maternal blood areas were quantified, and the reduction of vascular spaces in placentas from BALB/c mice infected with *P. berghei* ANKA was considered a proxy for basal membrane thickening (Neres et al., 2008). This supports the conclusion that reduced maternal blood spaces due to trophoblast membrane thickening and maternal sinusoidal remodeling (de Moraes et al., 2013) would ultimately lead to placental insufficiency and impaired transplacental transport of nutrients [discussed elsewhere (Neres et al., 2008; de Moraes et al., 2013)]. The same methodology was further used to determine that distinct parasites inflict different magnitudes of circulatory impairment and membrane thickening in placentas from C57BL/6 mice (Rodrigues-Duarte et al., 2012). The etiology of the event was further addressed in *P. berghei* NK65-infected C57BL/6 TLR4$^{-/-}$ and MyD88$^{-/-}$ KO mice, which had blood sinusoidal areas similar to those observed in non-infected pregnant mice (Barboza et al., 2014, 2017). These findings established a logical link between host innate immunity and placental pathology, once again supporting the notion that outcomes of MiP mostly result from damage and homeostatic dysregulation inflicted mostly by factors of an immunologic nature.

CONCLUSION

Clearly, the development of murine models that recapitulate traits from human MiP has definitively contributed to the current understanding of this disease. However, there are still few reports that truly reveal some of the pathogenesis mechanisms of MiP. Only in the last decade have some studies clearly unraveled some hidden molecular mechanisms of MiP, such as innate immunity activation and its contributions to poor pregnancy outcomes (Poovassery et al., 2009; Conroy et al., 2013; Barboza et al., 2014, 2017, 2019; Rodrigues-Duarte et al., 2018). Indeed, the advent of genetic engineering and the capacity to generate a wide range of knockout mice were definite turning points from which we are still benefiting. Until this point, most studies have tried to establish proper experimental settings that would ultimately validate murine models as suitable for studying MiP. First, striking similarities are observed regarding evolutionary and developmental traits between murine and human placentas, from which one might conclude that physiologically, both would behave in a particularly similar way (Georgiades et al., 2002; Wildman et al., 2006). Additionally, murine parasites exhibit a group of characteristics that support the conclusion that murine pathology would somewhat resemble human MiP, despite the well-known differences between rodent *Plasmodium* species and *P. falciparum* biology (Lamb et al., 2006; Hviid et al., 2010). Nevertheless, one might consider the patent limitations of conclusions regarding disease outcomes, which can later limit the translational capacities of observed results. As such, refinement of experimental design and standardization of methodology is necessary for the improvement of such models (**BOX 1**). Resolving these gaps will certainly enrich research in the field, possibly reaffirming the usage of murine models to address more specific and complex questions implicit in drug preclinical trials and vaccine development (Doritchamou et al., 2017). Research in the field has indeed overcome several milestones due to the usage of rodent models with much progress that is still to come.

AUTHOR CONTRIBUTIONS

AB drafted the manuscript, compiled information from the literature, and designed the figures and tables. MP drafted the manuscript and gathered information from the literature. SE supervised and reviewed the manuscript. CM supervised and reviewed the manuscript and designed the figures and tables.

REFERENCES

Abrams, E. T., Brown, H., Chensue, S. W., Turner, G. D. H., Molyneux, M. E.,

Meshnick, S. R., et al. (2003). Host response to malaria during pregnancy: placental monocyte recruitment is associated with elevated β chemokine expression. *J. Immunol.* 170, 2759–2764. doi: 10.4049/jimmunol.170.5.2759

Adachi, M., Yuda, M., Ando, K., Sakurai, M., and Chinzei, Y. (2000). Scant parasitemia in BALB/c mice with congenital malaria infection. *J. Parasitol.* 86, 1030–1034. doi: 10.1645/0022-3395(2000)086%5B1030%3Aspibcm%5D2.0.co%3B2

Al Hammadi, A., Mitchell, M., Abraham, G. M., and Wang, J. P. (2017). Recrudescence of *Plasmodium falciparum* in a primigravida after nearly 3 years of latency. *Am. J. Trop. Med. Hyg.* 96, 642–644. doi: 10.4269/ajtmh.16-0803

Avery, J. W., Smith, G. M., Owino, S. O., Sarr, D., Nagy, T., Mwalimu, S., et al. (2012). Maternal malaria induces a procoagulant and antifibrinolytic state that is embryotoxic but responsive to anticoagulant therapy. *PLoS One* 7:e31090. doi: 10.1371/journal.pone.0031090

Barboza, R., Hasenkamp, L., Barateiro, A., Murillo, O., Peixoto, E. P. M., Lima, F. A., et al. (2019). Fetal-derived MyD88 signaling contributes to poor pregnancy outcomes during gestational malaria. *Front. Microbiol.* 10:68. doi: 10.3389/fmicb.2019.00068

Barboza, R., Lima, F. A., Reis, A. S., Murillo, O. J., Peixoto, E. P. M., Bandeira, C. L., et al. (2017). TLR4-mediated placental pathology and pregnancy outcome in experimental malaria. *Sci. Rep.* 7, 1–12. doi: 10.1038/s41598-017-08299-x

Barboza, R., Reis, A. S., Silva, L. G., Da Hasenkamp, L., Pereira, K. R. B., Câmara, N. O. S., et al. (2014). MyD88 signaling is directly involved in the development of murine placental malaria. *Infect. Immun.* 82, 830–838. doi: 10.1128/IAI.01288-1213

Beeson, J. G., Amin, N., Kanjala, M., and Rogerson, S. J. (2002). Selective accumulation of mature asexual stages of plasmodium falciparum -infected erythrocytes in the placenta. *Infect. Immun.* 70, 5412–5415. doi: 10.1128/IAI.70.10.5412

Beeson, J. G., and Brown, G. V. (2004). Plasmodium falciparum–infected erythrocytes demonstrate dual specificity for adhesion to hyaluronic acid and chondroitin sulfate a and have distinct adhesive properties. *J. Infect. Dis.* 189, 169–179. doi: 10.1086/380975

Berrevoets, M. A. H., Sprong, T., Meis, J. F., and Dofferhoff, A. S. M. (2013). Plasmodium falciparum malaria recrudescence occurring 2.5 years after leaving an endemic country. *Neth. J. Med.* 71, 426–428.

Bhatia, R., Rajwaniya, D., and Agrawal, P. (2016). Congenital malaria due to plasmodium vivax infection in a neonate. *Case Rep. Pediatr.* 2016, 1–2. doi: 10.1155/2016/1929046

Brabin, B. J., Hakimi, M., and Pelletier, D. (2001). An analysis of anemia and pregnancy-related maternal mortality. *J. Nutr.* 131, 604S–615S. doi: 10.1093/jn/131.2.697S

Bulmer, J. N., Rasheed, F. N., Francis, N., Morrison, L., and Greenwood, B. M. (1993). Placental malaria.1. Pathological Classification. Histopathology 22, 211–218.

Burton, G. J., Hempstock, J., and Jauniaux, E. (2001). Nutrition of the human fetus during the first trimester - a review. *Placenta* 22, 70–76. doi: 10.1053/plac.2001.0639

Burton, G. J., Watson, A. L., Hempstock, J., Skepper, J. N., and Jauniaux, E. (2002). Uterine glands provide histiotrophic nutrition for the human fetus during the first trimester of pregnancy. *J. Clin. Endocrinol. Metab.* 87, 2954–2959. doi: 10.1210/jcem.87.6.8563

Cattamanchi, A., Kyabayinze, D., Hubbard, A., Rosenthal, P. J., and Dorsey, G. (2003). Distinguishing recrudescence from reinfection in a longitudinal antimalarial drug efficacy study: comparison of results based on genotyping of MSP-1. MSP-2, and GLURP. *Am. J. Trop. Med. Hyg.* 68, 133–139. doi: 10.1186/1475-2875-5-127

Conroy, A. L., Silver, K. L., Zhong, K., Rennie, M., Ward, P., Sarma, J. V., et al. (2013). Complement activation and the resulting placental vascular insufficiency drives fetal growth restriction associated with placental malaria. *Cell Host Microbe* 13, 215–226. doi: 10.1016/j.chom.2013.01.010

Crocker, I. P., Walraven, G., Tanner, O. M., Baker, P. N., Myers, J. E., and Bulmer, J. N. (2004). Syncytiotrophoblast degradation and the pathophysiology of the malaria-infected placenta. *Placenta* 25, 273–282. doi: 10.1016/j.placenta.2003.09.010

de Moraes, L. V., Tadokoro, C. E., Gómez-Conde, I., Olivieri, D. N., and Penha-Gonçalves, C. (2013). Intravital placenta imaging reveals microcirculatory dynamics impact on sequestration and phagocytosis of plasmodium-infected erythrocytes. *PLoS Pathog.* 9:e1003154. doi: 10.1371/journal.ppat.1003154

Dellicour, S., Tatem, A. J., Guerra, C. A., Snow, R. W., and Ter Kuile, F. O. (2010). Quantifying the number of pregnancies at risk of malaria in 2007: a demographic study. *PLoS Med.* 7:e1000221. doi: 10.1371/journal.pmed.1000221

Desai, M., ter Kuile, F. O., Nosten, F., McGready, R., Asamoa, K., Brabin, B., et al. (2007). Epidemiology and burden of malaria in pregnancy. *Lancet Infect. Dis.* 7, 93–104. doi: 10.1016/S1473-3099(07)70021-X

Desowitz, R. S., Shida, K. K., Pang, L., and Buchbinder, G. (1989). Characterization of a model of malaria in the pregnant host: plasmodium berghei in the white rat. *Am. J. Trop. Med. Hyg.* 41, 630–634. doi: 10.4269/ajtmh.1989.41.630

Doritchamou, J., Teo, A., Fried, M., and Duffy, P. E. (2017). Malaria in pregnancy: the relevance of animal models for vaccine development. *Lab Anim.* 46, 388–398. doi: 10.1038/laban.1349

Duffy, P. E., and Fried, M. (2001). "Malaria in pregnancy," in *Deadly Parasite, Susceptible Host*, 1st Edn, eds P. E. Duffy and M. Fried (London: Taylor & Francis).

Franke-Fayard, B., Fonager, J., Braks, A., Khan, S. M., and Janse, C. J. (2010). Sequestration and tissue accumulation of human malaria parasites: can we learn anything from rodent models of malaria? *PLoS Pathog.* 6:e1001032. doi: 10.1371/journal.ppat.1001032

Fried, M., Domingo, G. J., Gowda, C. D., Mutabingwa, T. K., and Duffy, P. E. (2006). Plasmodium falciparum: chondroitin sulfate A is the major receptor for adhesion of parasitized erythrocytes in the placenta. *Exp. Parasitol.* 113, 36–42. doi: 10.1016/j.exppara.2005.12.003

Georgiades, P., Fergyson-Smith, A. C., and Burton, G. J. (2002). Comparative developmental anatomy of the murine and human definitive placentae. *Placenta* 23, 3–19. doi: 10.1053/plac.2001.0738

Giobbia, M., Tonon, E., Zanatta, A., Cesaris, L., Vaglia, A., and Bisoffi, Z. (2005). Late recrudescence of Plasmodium falciparum malaria in a pregnant woman: a case report. *Int. J. Infect. Dis.* 9, 234–235. doi: 10.1016/j.ijid.2004.08.002

Goldenberg, R., Culhane, J., and Iams, J. (2009). Preterm birth 1: epidemiology and causes of preterm birth. *Obstet. Anesth.* 371, 75–84. doi: 10.1111/j.1440-1754.2012.02536.x

Hall, N., Marianna, K., Raine, J. D., Carlton, J. M., Kooij, T. W. A., Berriman, M., et al. (2005). A comprehensive survey of the plasmodium life cycle by genomic. transcriptomic, and proteomic analyses. *Science* 307, 82–86. doi: 10.1126/science.1103717

Heazell, A. E. P., Moll, S. J., Jones, C. J. P., Baker, P. N., and Crocker, I. P. (2007). Formation of syncytial knots is increased by hyperoxia. hypoxia and reactive oxygen species. *Placenta* 28, S33–S40. doi: 10.1016/j.placenta.2006.10.007

Hioki, A., Hioki, Y., and Ohtomo, H. (1990). Influence of pregnancy on the course of malaria in mice infected with plasmodium berghei. *J. Protozool.* 37, 163–167. doi: 10.1111/j.1550-7408.1990.tb01121.x

Hviid, L., Marinho, C. R. F., Staalsoe, T., and Penha-Gonçalves, C. (2010). Of mice and women: rodent models of placental malaria. *Trends Parasitol.* 26, 412–419. doi: 10.1016/j.pt.2010.04.010

Ismail, M. R., Ordi, J., Menendez, C., Ventura, P. J., Aponte, J. J., Kahigwa, E., et al. (2000). Placental pathology in malaria: a histological, immunohistochemical, and quantitative study. *Hum. Pathol.* 31, 85–93. doi: 10.1016/S0046-8177(00)80203-80208

Janssen, C. S., Phillips, R. S., Turner, M. R., and Barret, M. P. (2004). Plasmodium interspersed repeats: the major multigene superfamily of malaria parasites. *Nucleic Acids Res.* 32, 5712–5720. doi: 10.1093/nar/gkh907

Justice, M. J., and Dhillon, P. (2016). Using the mouse to model human disease: increasing validity and reproducibility. *Dis. Model. Mech.* 9, 101–103. doi: 10.1242/dmm.024547

Kanellopoulos-Langevin, C., Caucheteux, S. M., Verbeke, P., and Ojcius, D. M. (2003). Tolerance of the fetus by the maternal immune system: role of inflammatory mediators at the feto-maternal interface. *Reprod. Biol. Endocrinol.* 1, 1–6. doi: 10.1186/1477-7827-1-121

Kraemer, S. M., and Smith, J. D. (2006). A family affair: var genes, PfEMP1 binding, and malaria disease. *Curr. Opin. Microbiol.* 9, 374–380. doi: 10.1016/j.mib.2006.06.006

Lager, S., and Powell, T. L. (2012). Regulation of nutrient transport across the placenta. *J. Pregnancy* 2012, 1–14. doi: 10.1155/2012/179827

Lamb, T. J., Brown, D. E., Potocnik, A. J., and Langhorne, J. (2006). Insights into the immunopathogenesis of malaria using mouse models. *Expert Rev. Mol. Med.* 8, 1–22. doi: 10.1017/S1462399406010581

Laochan, N., Zaloumis, S., Imwong, M., Lek-Uthai, U., Brockman, A., Sriprawat, K., et al. (2015). Intervals to *Plasmodium falciparum* recurrence after anti-malarial treatment in pregnancy: a longitudinal prospective cohort. *Malar. J.* 14:221. doi: 10.1186/s12936-015-0745-749

Lawn, J. E., Blencowe, H., Waiswa, P., Amouzou, A., Mathers, C., Hogan, D., et al. (2016). Stillbirths: rates, risk factors, and acceleration towards 2030. *Lancet* 387, 587–603. doi: 10.1016/S0140-6736(15)00837-835

Lima, F. A., Gómez-Conde, I., Videira, P. A., Marinho, C. R. F., Olivieri, D. N., and Tadokoro, C. E. (2014). Intravital microscopy technique to study parasite dynamics in the labyrinth layer of the mouse placenta. *Parasitol. Int.* 63, 254–259. doi: 10.1016/j.parint.2013.06.012

Lucchi, N. W., Sarr, D., Owino, S. O., Mwalimu, S. M., Peterson, D. S., and Moore, J. M. (2011). Natural hemozoin stimulates syncytiotrophoblast to secrete chemokines and recruit peripheral blood mononuclear cells. *Placenta* 32, 579–585. doi: 10.1016/j.placenta.2011.05.003

Luxemburger, C., Ricci, F., Nosten, F., Raimond, D., Bathet, S., and White, N. J. (1997). The epidemiology of severe malaria in an area of low transmission in Thailand. *Trans. R. Soc. Trop. Med. Hyg.* 91, 256–262. doi: 10.1016/S0035-9203(97)90066-3

Malvy, D., Torrentino-Madamet, M., L'Ollivier, C., Receveur, M. C., Jeddi, F., Delhaes, L., et al. (2018). Plasmodium falciparum recrudescence two years after treatment of an uncomplicated infection without return to an area where malaria is endemic. *Antimicrob. Agents Chemother.* 62, 1–5. doi: 10.1128/AAC.01892-1817

Marinho, C. R. F., Neres, R., Epiphanio, S., Gonçalves, L. A., Catarino, M. B., and Penha-Gonçalves, C. (2009). Recrudescent *Plasmodium berghei* from pregnant mice displays enhanced binding to the placenta and induces protection in multigravida. *PLoS One* 4:e5630. doi: 10.1371/journal.pone.0005630

Mayor, A., Serra-Casas, E., Bardají, A., Sanz, S., Puyol, L., Cisteró, P., et al. (2009). Sub-microscopic infections and long-term recrudescence of Plasmodium falciparum in Mozambican pregnant women. *Malar. J.* 8, 1–10. doi: 10.1186/1475-2875-8-9

McCarthy, R., Martin-Fairey, C., Sojka, D. K., Herzog, E. D., Jungheim, E. S., Stout, M. J., et al. (2018). Mouse models of preterm birth: suggested assessment and reporting guidelines†. *Biol. Reprod.* 99, 922–937. doi: 10.1093/biolre/ioy109

Megnekou, R., Hviid, L., and Staalsoe, T. (2009). Variant-specific immunity to Plasmodium berghei in pregnant mice. *Infect. Immun.* 77, 1827–1834. doi: 10.1128/IAI.01321-1328

Menendez, C. (1995). Malaria during pregnancy: a priority area of malaria research and control. *Parasitol* 11, 178–183. doi: 10.1016/0169-4758(95)80151-0

Menendez, C., Ordi, J., Ismail, M. R., Ventura, P. J., Aponte, J. J., Kahigwa, E., et al. (2000). The impact of placental malaria on gestational age and birth weight. *J. Infect. Dis.* 181, 1740–1745. doi: 10.1086/315449

Menéndez, C., Romagosa, C., Ismail, M. R., Carrilho, C., Saute, F., Osman, N., et al. (2008). An autopsy study of maternal mortality in Mozambique: the contribution of infectious diseases. *PLoS Med.* 5:e44. doi: 10.1371/journal.pmed.0050044

Moore, K. A., Simpson, J. A., Wiladphaingern, J., Min, A. M., Pimanpanarak, M., Paw, M. K., et al. (2017). Influence of the number and timing of malaria episodes during pregnancy on prematurity and small-for-gestational-age in an area of low transmission. *BMC Med.* 15:117. doi: 10.1186/s12916-017-0877-6

Moormann, A. M., Sullivan, A. D., Rochford, R. A., Chensue, S. W., Bock, P. J., Nyirenda, T., et al. (1999). Malaria and pregnancy: placental cytokine expression and its relationship to intrauterine growth retardation. *J. Infect. Dis.* 180, 1987–1993. doi: 10.1086/315135

Murray, S. A., Morgan, J. L., Kane, C., Sharma, Y., Heffner, C. S., Lake, J., et al. (2010). Mouse gestation length is genetically determined. *PLoS One* 5:e12418. doi: 10.1371/journal.pone.0012418

Muthusamy, A., Achur, R. N., Bhavanandan, V. P., Fouda, G. G., Taylor, D. W., and Gowda, D. C. (2004). Plasmodium falciparum-infected erythrocytes adhere both in the intervillous space and on the villous surface of human placenta by binding to the low-sulfated chondroitin sulfate proteoglycan receptor. *Am. J. Pathol.* 164, 2013–2025. doi: 10.1016/S0002-9440(10)63761-63763

Muthusamy, A., Achur, R. N., Valiyaveettil, M., Botti, J. J., Taylor, D. W., Leke, R. F., et al. (2007). Chondroitin sulfate proteoglycan but not hyaluronic acid is the receptor for the adherence of Plasmodium falciparum-infected erythrocytes in human placenta, and infected red blood cell adherence up-regulates the receptor expression. *Am. J. Pathol.* 170, 1989–2000. doi: 10.2353/ajpath.2007.061238

Neres, R., Marinho, C. R. F., Gonçalves, L. A., Catarino, M. B., and Penha-Gonçalves, C. (2008). Pregnancy outcome and placenta pathology in Plasmodium berghei ANKA infected mice reproduce the pathogenesis of severe malaria in pregnant women. *PLoS One* 3:e1608. doi: 10.1371/journal.pone.0001608

Nosten, F., Rogerson, S. J., Beeson, J. G., McGready, R., Mutabingwa, T. K., and Brabin, B. (2004). Malaria in pregnancy and the endemicity spectrum: what can we learn? *Trends Parasitol.* 20, 425–432. doi: 10.1016/j.pt.2004.06.007

Oduola, A. M. J., Holbrook, T. W., Galbraith, R. M., Bank, H., and Spicer, S. S. (1982). Effects of malaria (*Plasmodium berghei*) on the maternal-fetal relationship in mice. *J. Protozool.* 29, 77–81. doi: 10.1111/j.1550-7408.1982.tb02883.x

Oduola, A. M. J., Phillips, J. H., Spicer, S. S., and Galbraith, R. M. (1986). *Plasmodium berghei* - histology. immunocytochemistry, and ultrastructure of the placenta in rodent malaria. *Exp. Parasitol.* 62, 181–193. doi: 10.1016/0014-4894(86)90022-6

Olivier, M., Van Den Ham, K., Shio, M. T., Kassa, F. A., and Fougeray, S. (2014). Malarial pigment hemozoin and the innate inflammatory response. *Front. Immunol.* 5:25. doi: 10.3389/fimmu.2014.00025

Ordi, J., Ismail, M. R., Ventura, P. J., Kahigwa, E., Hirt, R., Cardesa, A., et al. (1998). Massive chronic intervillositis of the placenta associated with malaria infection. *Am. J. Surg. Pathol.* 22, 1006–1011. doi: 10.1097/00000478-199808000-00011

Ordi, J., Menendez, C., Ismail, M. R., Ventura, P. J., Palacín, A., Kahigwa, E., et al. (2001). Placental malaria is associated with cell-mediated inflammatory responses with selective absence of natural killer cells. *J. Infect. Dis.* 183, 1100–1107. doi: 10.1086/319295

Othoro, C., Moore, J. M., Wannemuehler, K. A., Moses, S., Lal, A., Otieno, J., et al. (2008). Elevated gamma interferon-producing NK cells, CD45RO memory-like T cells, and CD4 T cells are associated with protection against malaria infection in pregnancy. *Infect. Immun.* 76, 1678–1685. doi: 10.1128/IAI.01420-1427

Parekh, F. K., Davison, B. B., Gamboa, D., Hernandez, J., and Branch, O. L. H. (2010). Placental histopathologic changes associated with subclinical malaria infection and its impact on the fetal environment. *Am. J. Trop. Med. Hyg.* 83, 973–980. doi: 10.4269/ajtmh.2010.09-0445

Pathak, G., Asnani, P. J., and Vinayak, V. K. (1990). Effect of prior eradication of Plasmodium berghei infection on the foetal development and parasitaemic levels under the stress of pregnancy. *J. Hyg. Epidemiol. Microbiol. Immunol.* 34, 139–146.

Pavia, C. S., and Niederbuhl, C. J. (1991). Immunization and protection against malaria during murine pregnancy. *Am. J. Trop. Med. Hyg.* 44, 176–182. doi: 10.4269/ajtmh.1991.44.176

Poovassery, J., and Moore, J. M. (2006). Murine malaria infection induces fetal loss associated with accumulation of *Plasmodium chabaudi* AS-infected erythrocytes in the placenta. *Infect. Immun.* 74, 2839–2848. doi: 10.1128/IAI.74.5.2839-2848.2006

Poovassery, J., and Moore, J. M. (2009). Association of malaria-induced murine pregnancy failure with robust peripheral and placental cytokine responses. *Infect. Immun.* 77, 4998–5006. doi: 10.1128/IAI.00617-619

Poovassery, J. S., Sarr, D., Smith, G., Nagy, T., and Moore, J. M. (2009). Malaria-induced murine pregnancy failure: distinct roles for IFN-γ and TNF. *J. Immunol.* 183, 5342–5349. doi: 10.4049/jimmunol.0901669

Rai, P., Majumdar, K., Sharma, S., Chauhan, R., and Chandra, J. (2015). Congenital malaria in a neonate: case report with a comprehensive review on differential diagnosis, treatment and prevention in Indian perspective. *J. Parasit. Dis.* 39, 345–348. doi: 10.1007/s12639-013-0342-341

Robbins, J. R., and Bakardjiev, A. I. (2012). Pathogens and the placental fortress. *Curr. Opin. Microbiol.* 15, 36–43. doi: 10.1016/j.mib.2011.11.006

Rodrigues-Duarte, L., De Moraes, L. V., Barboza, R., Marinho, C. R., Franke-Fayard, B., Janse, C. J., et al. (2012). Distinct placental malaria pathology caused by different *Plasmodium berghei* lines that fail to induce cerebral malaria in the C57BL/6 mouse. *Malar. J.* 11, 1–9. doi: 10.1186/1475-2875-11-231

Rodrigues-Duarte, L., Pandya, Y., Neres, R., and Penha-Gonçalves, C. (2018). Fetal and maternal innate immunity receptors have opposing effects in severity of experimental malaria in pregnancy: beneficial roles for fetal-derived TLR4 and IFNAR1. *Infect. Immun.* 86, IAI.708–IAI.717. doi: 10.1128/IAI.00708-717

Rogerson, S. J., Desai, M., Mayor, A., Sicuri, E., Taylor, S. M., and van Eijk, A. M. (2018). Burden, pathology, and costs of malaria in pregnancy: new developments for an old problem. *Lancet Infect. Dis.* 18, e107–e118. doi: 10.1016/S1473-3099(18)30066-30065

Rogerson, S. J., Hviid, L., Duffy, P. E., Leke, R. F., and Taylor, D. W. (2007). Malaria in pregnancy: pathogenesis and immunity. *Lancet Infect. Dis.* 7, 105–117. doi: 10.1016/S1473-3099(07)70022-70021

Rogerson, S. J., Pollina, E., Getachew, A., Tadesse, E., Lema, V. M., and Molyneux, M. E. (2003). Placental monocyte infiltrates in response to Plasmodium falciparum malaria infection and their association with adverse pregnancy outcomes. *Am. J. Trop. Med. Hyg.* 68, 115–119. doi: 10.4269/ajtmh.2003.68.1.0680115

Rossant, J., and Cross, J. C. (2001). Placental development: lessons from mouse mutants. *Nat. Rev. Genet.* 2, 538–548. doi: 10.1038/35080570

Rossant, J., and Tam, P. P. L. (2017). New insights into early human development: lessons for stem cell derivation and differentiation. *Cell Stem Cell* 20, 18–28. doi: 10.1016/j.stem.2016.12.004

Salanti, A., Staalsoe, T., Lavstsen, T., Jensen, A. T. R., Sowa, M. P. K., Arnot, D. E., et al. (2003). Selective upregulation of a single distinctly structured var gene in chondroitin sulphate A-adhering *Plasmodium falciparum* involved in pregnancy-associated malaria. *Mol. Microbiol.* 49, 179–191. doi: 10.1046/j.1365-2958.2003.03570.x

Sarr, D., Bracken, T. C., Owino, S. O., Cooper, C. A., Smith, G. M., Nagy, T., et al. (2015). Differential roles of inflammation and apoptosis in initiation of mid-gestational abortion in malaria-infected C57BL/6 and A/J mice. *Placenta* 36, 738–749. doi: 10.1016/j.placenta.2015.04.007

Sarr, D., Smith, G. M., Poovassery, J. S., Nagy, T., and Moore, J. M. (2012). Plasmodium chabaudi AS induces pregnancy loss in association with systemic pro-inflammatory immune responses in A/J and C57BL/6 mice. *Parasite Immunol.* 34, 224–235. doi: 10.1111/j.1365-3024.2012.01355.x

Schofield, L., and Grau, G. E. (2005). Immunological processes in malaria pathogenesis. *Nat. Rev. Immunol.* 5, 722–735. doi: 10.1038/nri1686

Sharma, A., Conteh, S., Langhorne, J., and Duffy, P. E. (2016). Heterologous infection of pregnant mice induces low birth weight and modifies offspring susceptibility to malaria. *PLoS One* 11:e0160120. doi: 10.1371/journal.pone.0160120

Sharma, L., and Shukla, G. (2014). Treatment of pregnant BALB/c mice with sulphadoxine pyrimethamine or chloroquine abrogates Plasmodium berghei induced placental pathology. *Parasitol. Int.* 63, 49–56. doi: 10.1016/j.parint.2013.08.016

Sharma, L., and Shukla, G. (2017). Placental malaria: a new insight into the pathophysiology. *Front. Med.* 4:117. doi: 10.3389/fmed.2017.00117

Shulman, C. E., Dorman, E. K., and Bulmer, J. N. (2002). Malaria as a cause of severe anaemia in pregnancy. *Lancet* 360:494. doi: 10.1016/s0140-6736(02)09662-9

Silver, K. L., Zhong, K., Leke, R. G. F., Taylor, D. W., and Kain, K. C. (2010). Dysregulation of angiopoietins is associated with placental malaria and low birth weight. *PLoS One* 5:e9481. doi: 10.1371/journal.pone.0009481

Souza, R. M., Ataíde, R., Dombrowski, J. G., Ippólito, V., Aitken, E. H., Valle, S. N., et al. (2013). Placental histopathological changes associated with plasmodium vivax infection during pregnancy. *PLoS Negl. Trop. Dis.* 7:e2071. doi: 10.1371/journal.pntd.0002071

Takao, K., and Miyakawa, T. (2015). Genomic responses in mouse models greatly mimic human inflammatory diseases. *Proc Natl Acad Sci.* 112, 1167–1172. doi: 10.1073/pnas.1401965111

Takata, K., Fujikura, K., and Shin, B.-C. (1997). Ultrastructure of the rodent placental labyrinth: a site of barrier and transport. *J. Reprod. Dev.* 43, 13–24. doi: 10.1262/jrd.43.13

Tegoshi, T., Desowitz, R. S., Pirl, K. G., Maeno, Y., and Aikawa, M. (1992). Placental pathology in plasmodium berghei-infected Rats. *Am. J. Trop. Med. Hyg.* 47, 643–651. doi: 10.4269/ajtmh.1992.47.643

Umbers, A. J., Aitken, E. H., and Rogerson, S. J. (2011). Malaria in pregnancy: small babies, big problem. *Trends Parasitol.* 27, 168–175. doi: 10.1016/j.pt.2011.01.007

van Hensbroek, M. B., Palmer, A., Onyiorah, E., Schneider, G., Jaffar, S., Dolan, G., et al. (1996). The effect of a monoclonal antibody to tumor necrosis factor on survival from childhood cerebral malaria. *J. Infect. Dis.* 174, 1091–1097. doi: 10.1093/infdis/174.5.1091

van Zon, A. A. J. C., and Eling, W. M. C. (1980). Pregnancy associated recrudescence in murine malaria (*Plasmodium berghei*). *Tropenmed. Parasitol.* 31, 402–408.

van Zon, A. A. J. C., Eling, W. M. C., and Hermsen, C. C. (1985). Pregnancy-induced recrudescences strengthen malarial immunity in mice infected with *Plasmodium berghei*. *Parasitology* 91, 9–17. doi: 10.1017/s003118200005647x

van Zon, A. A. J. C., Eling, W. M. C., Hermsen, C. C. R., and Koekkoek, A. A. G. M. (1982). Corticosterone regulation of the effector function of malarial immunity during pregnancy. *Infect. Immun.* 36, 484–491. doi: 10.1016/j.scitotenv.2015.10.076

Varo, R., Crowley, V. M., Sitoe, A., Madrid, L., Serghides, L., Kain, K. C., et al. (2018). Adjunctive therapy for severe malaria: a review and critical appraisal. *Malar. J.* 17, 1–18. doi: 10.1186/s12936-018-2195-2197

Vinayak, V. K., Pathak, G., Asnani, P. J., Jain, S., and Malik, A. K. (1986). Influence of malarial infection on the maternal-foetal relationship in pregnant mice. *Aust. J. Exp. Biol. Med. Sci.* 64, 223–227. doi: 10.1038/icb.1986.24

Walter, P. R., Garin, Y., and Blot, P. (1982). Placental pathologic changes in malaria: a histologic and ultrastructural study. *Am. J. Pathol.* 109, 330–342.

Wildman, D. E., Chen, C., Erez, O., Grossman, L. I., Goodman, M., and Romero, R. (2006). Evolution of the mammalian placenta revealed by phylogenetic analysis. *Proc. Natl. Acad. Sci. U.S.A.* 103, 3203–3208. doi: 10.1073/pnas.0511344103

World Health Organization (2018). *World Malaria Report 2018*. Geneva: WHO.

2

The Identification and Genetic Characterization of Parechovirus Infection among Pediatric Patients with Wide Clinical Spectrum in Chongqing, China

Xiao-Ai Zhang[1†], Rui-Qiu Zhao[2†], Jin-Jin Chen[1†], Yang Yuan[1], Xiang Tang[2], Zi-Wei Zhou[1], Luo Ren[2], Qin-Bin Lu[3], Yu-Na Wang[1], Hai-Yang Zhang[1], Pan-He Zhang[1], Li-Qun Fang[1], Hai-Sheng Zhou[4,5], En-Mei Liu[2], Hong-Mei Xu[2] and Wei Liu[1,6*]*

[1] State Key Laboratory of Pathogen and Biosecurity, Beijing Institute of Microbiology and Epidemiology, Beijing, China, [2] Children's Hospital of Chongqing Medical University, Chongqing, China, [3] Department of Laboratorial Science and Technology, School of Public Health, Peking University, Beijing, China, [4] Key Laboratory of Dermatology, Anhui Medical University, Hefei, China, [5] Department of Biochemistry and Molecular Biology, Anhui Medical University, Hefei, China, [6] Beijing Key Laboratory of Vector Borne and Natural Focus Infectious Diseases, Beijing, China

***Correspondence:**
Hong-Mei Xu
xuhongm0095@sina.com
Wei Liu
lwbime@163.com;
liuwei@bmi.ac.cn

† These authors have contributed equally to this work

Human parechoviruses (HPeVs) are important causes of infection in children. However, without a comprehensive and persistent surveillance, the epidemiology and clinical features of HPeV infection remain ambiguous. We performed a hospital-based surveillance study among three groups of pediatric patients with acute respiratory infection (Group 1), acute diarrhea (Group 2), and hand, foot and mouth disease (Group 3) in Chongqing, China, from 2009 to 2015. Among 10,212 tested patients, 707 (6.92%) were positive for HPeV, with the positive rates differing significantly among three groups (Group 1, 3.43%; Group 2, 14.94%; Group 3, 3.55%; $P < 0.001$). The co-infection with other pathogens was detected in 75.2% (531/707) of HPeV-positive patients. Significant negative interaction between HPeV and Parainfluenza virus (PIV) ($P = 0.046$, OR = 0.59, 95% CI = 0.34–0.98) and positive interactions between HPeV and Enterovirus (EV) ($P = 0.015$, OR = 2.28, 95% CI = 1.23–4.73) were identified. Among 707 HPeV-positive patients, 592 (83.73%) were successfully sequenced, and 10 genotypes were identified, with HPeV1 ($n = 396$), HPeV4 ($n = 86$), and HPeV3 ($n = 46$) as the most frequently seen. The proportion of genotypes differed among three groups ($P < 0.001$), with HPeV1 and HPeV4 overrepresented in Group 2 and HPeV6 overrepresented in Group 3. The spatial patterns of HPeV genotypes disclosed more close clustering of the currently sequenced strains than those from other countries/regions, although they were indeed mixed. Three main genotypes (HPeV1, HPeV3, and HPeV4) had shown distinct seasonal peaks, highlighting a bi-annual cycle of all HpeV and two genotypes (HPeV 1 and HPeV 4) with peaks in odd-numbered years and with peaks in even-numbered years HPeV3. Significantly higher HPeV1 viral loads were associated with severe diarrhea in Group 2 ($P = 0.044$), while associated with HPeV single infection than HPeV-EV coinfection among HFMD patients ($P = 0.001$). It's concluded that HPeV infection was correlated with wide clinical spectrum in pediatric patients with a high variety of genotypes determined. Still no clinical significance can be confirmed, which warranted more molecular surveillance in the future.

Keywords: parechovirus, epidemiology, respiratory infection, acute diarrhea, hand foot and mouth disease

INTRODUCTION

Human parechoviruses (HPeVs) are small, non-enveloped RNA viruses closely related to enteroviruses (EVs) in the *Picornaviridae* family. The *Parechovirus* genus currently contains 6 species, Parechovirus A to F.[1] Among them Parechovirus A is the only species of *Parechovirus* genus which infects humans (de Crom et al., 2016b). Similar to Enterovirus, Parechovirus A causes frequent infection in children, presenting with a wide clinical spectrum that spanned from asymptomatic infection, mild illness, to severe diseases (Cordey et al., 2015). To date, a total of 19 HPeV genotypes (HPeV1–HPeV19) had been identified, with their causative illness also differing among the determined types (Shakeel et al., 2017). HPeV genotypes 1, 3, and 6 are most commonly associated with human disease (de Crom et al., 2016b; Olijve et al., 2018). Of particular interest is HPeV3, which has been suggested as a leading cause of sepsis-like illness and central nervous system infection in neonates and young infants (Boivin et al., 2005; Olijve et al., 2018). The circulation of HPeV in China has been previously studied with small sample size and short duration, and mostly limited to diarrhea (Lin et al., 2008; Shan et al., 2009; Li et al., 2010; Cai et al., 2014). Without a comprehensive and persistent surveillance, the epidemiological and genetic characteristics of HPeV infection remain ambiguous. The present study was designed to systematically investigate the prevalence, epidemiological feature, and genetic diversity of HPeV in pediatric patients in China through a long-lasting surveillance period in three groups of patients.

MATERIALS AND METHODS

Patient Recruitment

During 2009–2015, a hospital-based surveillance study was performed at the Children's hospital, Chongqing Medical University (CHCMU), the largest children's hospital in southwestern China, serving patients with a wide geographic range across central and western China. Since 2009, a laboratory surveillance has been performed to detect the viral infections in three groups of patients, i.e., with acute respiratory tract infection (ARTI), acute diarrhea, or hand, foot and mouth disease (HFMD). The ARTI was defined on the basis of acute disease onset with symptoms of cough, rhinorrhea and/or dyspnea, and/or fever of $> 37.5°C$. Fever caused by known chronic medical conditions was excluded. The pneumonia was defined by the presence of patchy alveolar opacities on chest radiographs, in addition to symptoms of cough, dyspnea (lower chest wall indrawing), or tachypnea. Hospitalized patients with moderate, severe, and critical severe pneumonia were diagnosed as severe ARTI. Diarrhea was defined as > 3 loose stools in the previous 24 h. Patients who had confirmed inflammatory bowel disease, celiac disease, cystic fibrosis, food intolerance, or patients who had any apparent clinical respiratory signs or symptoms were excluded. Severe diarrhea was defined as ≥ 5 loose stools in the previous 24 h. HFMD were diagnosed according to the guidelines released by the Ministry of Health of the People's Republic of China.[2] Severe HFMD was defined if one of the following complications were additionally presented: encephalitis, meningitis, AFP, or cardiorespiratory failure. Before the surveillance was started, the staff that participated in the study had undergone training to be qualified for recruiting patients, sample collection, and test following the standard operating procedures (SOP) developed by Beijing Institute of Microbiology and Epidemiology. The tested specimen included nasopharyngeal swab (NPAs) for patients with ARTI and stool for patients with diarrhea or HFMD. All the samples were required to be collected on patients' admission into the hospital. A standardized questionnaire was used to obtain the patients' information from medical records, including demographic data, underlying medical conditions, symptoms and signs, routine blood test results, radiographic findings, and disease outcome. This study was performed with the approval of the Ethics Review Committee of CHCMU, and in accordance with the approved SOP throughout the years. At recruitment, written informed consent was obtained from all guardians of participants.

Laboratory Detection

Viral RNA/DNA was isolated from stool or swab samples using QIAamp Viral RNA Mini Kit (Qiagen, Germantown, MD, United States) according to the manufacturer's instructions. All samples were screened for HPeV using real-time RT-PCR assay targeting the 5′untranslated region (UTR) as previously described (Benschop et al., 2008). All HPeV positive samples were amplified for the viral protein (VP) 1 or VP3/VP1 genes using nested RT-PCR or touch-down RT-PCR approach for genotyping as previously described (Benschop et al., 2006; Harvala et al., 2008; Cristanziano et al., 2015; Brouwer et al., 2019; Pietsch and Liebert, 2019; **Supplementary Table 1**). All the amplicons were subject to sequencing and BLAST analysis.

[1]https://talk.ictvonline.org/

[2]http://www.moh.gov.cn/publicfiles/business/htmlfiles/mohyzs/s3586/201004/46884.htm

For all the NPA samples collected from patients with ARTI, influenza virus (IFV), metapneumovirus (MPV), respiratory syncytial virus (RSV), parainfluenza virus (PIV), human rhinovirus (HRV), and coronavirus (CoV) were tested by reverse transcriptase polymerase chain reaction (RT-PCR), and human bocavirus (HBoV) and human adenovirus (HadV) were tested by performing polymerase chain reaction (PCR) as described previously (Xu et al., 2000; Gunson et al., 2005; Tiveljung-Lindell et al., 2009). Five viral enteric pathogens were tested for the stool specimens collected from patients with acute diarrhea. Rotavirus A antigen was tested by enzyme-linked immunosorbent assay. Testing of norovirus (NoV), HadV, astrovirus (AstV), and sapovirus (SaV) was performed by PCR or RT-PCR (Rohayem et al., 2004; Qu et al., 2007; Stals et al., 2009). The stool samples from HFMD patients had been simultaneously tested for enterovirus (EV) by using real-time RT-PCR (Verstrepen et al., 2002). All steps of the nucleic acid extraction and RT-PCR/PCR test were conducted in parallel with positive and negative controls.

The HpeV viral load was determined by using the same primers and probes as for detection. Plasmids containing known copy number of amplification targets were applied in real-time RT-PCR test to generate a standard curve for quantification of test samples. Positive and negative controls were included. The copy number of virus expressed as copies/mL was determined by comparison with a serially diluted plasmid standard of known concentration. All samples were quantified in at least duplicate wells.

Phylogenetic Analysis

The sequences obtained from the study were submitted to NCBI with the GenBank Accession Numbers MT700562-MT700938 and MT702393-MT702579. Genomic sequences were assembled using Lasergene's DNA SeqMan software (version 7.1.0, DNA Star Inc., Madison, WI, United States). The phylogenetic trees were constructed with maximum likelihood method with 1,000 replicates using MEGA 7.0.

Statistical Analysis

Descriptive statistics were performed for categorical variables as frequencies and proportions or rates, and continuous variables were expressed as medians and interquartile ranges. The non-parametric test with Mann-Whitney *U*-test method was used to compare the differences of continuous variables between different groups. Pearson chi-square test or Fisher exact test was performed to compare the differences of categorical variables. Logistic regression models were used to determine the association between clinical characteristics and HPeV infection. Odds ratio (OR) and its 95% CI were estimated using maximum likelihood method. The viral loads were estimated for their association with age, sex, disease severity, and single/co-infection by multiple linear regression analysis. Statistical analysis was performed using R software (version 3.5.3). The interactions between HPeV and each of the other detected viruses was explored at the scale of individual hosts as previously described (Nickbakhsh et al., 2019).

RESULTS

Detection of HPeV in Three Groups of Patients

Altogether 10,212 pediatric patients, including 3,438 hospitalized patients with ARTI (Group 1), 3,059 with acute diarrhea (Group 2), and 3,715 with HFMD (Group 3), met the inclusion criteria and were recruited into the study (**Supplementary Table 2**). The age of Group 3 was significantly higher than that of Group 1 and Group 2 ($P < 0.001$), while sex was comparable among three groups. In total, 6.92% (707/10212) of patients were positive for HPeV (**Table 1** and **Figure 1A**), with the positive rates differing significantly among three groups (3.43%, 118/3,438 for Group 1, 14.94%, 457/3,059 for Group 2, and 3.55%, 132/3,715 for Group 3, $P < 0.001$). The co-infections were counted by positive test for HPeV and any one of the other tested viruses. Both rates of single infection (1.72%, 176/10,212) and co-infection involving HPeV (5.20%, 531/10,212) differed among three groups, with the highest co-infection rate/single infection rate ratio observed for Group 3 (3.28% vs. 0.27%, $P < 0.001$; **Table 1**).

For Group 1, the 118 HPeV-positive patients were younger than the 3,320 negative patients ($P = 0.002$, **Table 2**). Compared with those with HPEV single infection, although the coinfection with other respiratory viruses was related to an increased frequency of cough (95.51%), moist rales (92.13%), and dyspnea (17.98%), none of the difference attained significant level. Co-infection of HPeV with other viruses occurred mostly for RSV (31, 34.83%), HRV (29, 32.58%), and PIV (26, 29.21%) (**Supplementary Table 3** and **Supplementary Figure 1A**). Co-infection of HPeV with other two viruses occurred mostly for HpeV-RV-NoV ($n = 61$) (**Supplementary Figure 1B**). Co-infection of HPeV with other three viruses (RV-NoV-AstV, RV-SaV-NoV, IFV-HBoV-HRV, HAdV-RV-NoV, RSV-IFV-HRV, RSV-PIV-HBoV) were also observed in 10 patients (**Supplementary Figure 1C**). The interaction analysis between HPeV and other respiratory viruses disclosed significant negative interaction between HPeV and PIV, when HPeV was used as response virus (dependent variable), and PIV was used as the responsive explanatory virus (independent variable) ($P = 0.046$, OR = 0.59, 95% CI = 0.34–0.98) (**Supplementary Table 4**).

For Group 2, the 457 HPeV-positive patients were younger compared with 2,602 HPeV-negative patients ($P < 0.001$, **Table 1**). The 137 patients with HPeV-single infection were younger than the 320 patients with HPeV co-infection ($P < 0.001$). Although less vomiting was observed from HPeV-positive patients than those negative (36.98% vs. 47.58%, $P < 0.001$), HPeV coinfection indeed had higher frequency of vomiting than HPeV single infection (21.90% vs. 43.44%, $P < 0.001$). The co-infection occurred mostly between HPeV and NoV (233, 72.81%), RV (138, 43.13%), and SaV (16, 5.00%) (**Supplementary Figure 1** and **Supplementary Table 3**).

For Group 3, the 132 HPeV-positive patients were younger than the 3,583 HPeV-negative patients ($P < 0.001$, **Table 2**).

TABLE 1 | The detection and genotyping of HPeVs in three cohorts of pediatric patients.

Characteristics	Total (n = 10212)	Group 1$ (n = 3438)	Group 2$ (n = 3059)	Group 3$ (n = 3715)	*P*-value
All HpeV infected patients	707(6.92)	118 (3.43)	457 (14.94)	132 (3.55)	<0.001$
Single infection	176 (1.72)	29 (0.84)	137 (4.48)	10 (0.27)	<0.001$
Coinfection	531 (5.20)	89 (2.59)	320 (10.46)	122 (3.28)	
Age groups (months)					<0.001#
0–6	166 (7.97)	59 (4.27)	101 (15.93)	6 (8.96)	
7–12	224 (9.47)	38 (4.77)	172 (14.74)	34 (8.46)	
13–24	152 (5.56)	11 (2.15)	92 (10.03)	49 (3.76)	
25–36	42 (2.59)	5 (1.96)	13 (7.56)	24 (2.01)	
37–48	16 (2.34)	4 (2.30)	7 (9.59)	5 (1.14)	
48–60	3 (0.96)	0 (0)	1 (2.78)	2 (1.06)	
>60	5 (1.21)	1 (0.44)	1 (1.67)	3 (2.44)	
Sex, boy	440 (6.71)	77 (3.40)	277 (14.87)	86 (3.53)	0.695$
Year of disease					<0.001$
2009	49 (6.56)	4 (2.76)	42 (15.56)	3 (0.90)	
2010	132 (5.21)	16 (3.59)	66 (11.66)	50 (3.28)	
2011	124 (7.95)	21 (3.01)	99 (16.98)	4 (14.34)	
2012	116 (8.40)	21 (3.97)	81 (13.64)	14 (5.43)	
2013	125 (10.02)	14 (2.77)	95 (23.51)	16 (4.73)	
2014	111 (6.85)	19 (3.54)	55 (12.97)	37 (5.60)	
2015	50 (4.46)	23 (3.97)	19 (8.72)	8 (2.47)	
HpeV genotype					P_{total} < 0.001$ $P_{singleinfection}$ = 0.187$ $P_{coinfection}$ < 0.001$
HPeV1	396 (3.88)	87 (2.53)	252 (8.24)	57 (1.53)	<0.001$
Single infection	120 (1.18)	21 (0.61)	93 (3.04)	6 (0.16)	
Coinfection	276 (2.70)	66 (1.92)	159 (5.2)	51 (1.37)	
HPeV2	1 (0.01)	0 (0)	1 (0.03)	0 (0)	NA
Single infection	0 (0)	0 (0)	0 (0)	0 (0)	
Coinfection	1 (0.01)	0 (0)	1 (0.03)	0 (0)	
HPeV3	46 (0.45)	3 (0.09)	31 (1.01)	12 (0.32)	0.541#
Single infection	8 (0.08)	0 (0)	7 (0.23)	1 (0.03)	
Coinfection	38 (0.37)	3 (0.09)	24 (0.78)	11 (0.3)	
HPeV4	86 (0.84)	7 (0.2)	65 (2.12)	14 (0.38)	0.015#
Single infection	23 (0.23)	3 (0.09)	20 (0.65)	0 (0)	
Coinfection	63 (0.62)	4 (0.124)	45 (1.47)	14 (0.38)	
HPeV5	18 (0.18)	0 (0)	11 (0.36)	7 (0.19)	1.000 #
Single infection	4 (0.04)	0 (0)	3 (0.1)	1 (0.03)	
Coinfection	14 (0.14)	0 (0)	8 (0.26)	6 (0.16)	
HPeV6	40 (0.39)	8 (0.23)	13 (0.42)	19 (0.51)	0.038#
Single infection	3 (0.03)	2 (0.06)	1 (0.03)	0 (0)	
Coinfection	37 (0.36)	6 (0.17)	12 (0.39)	19 (0.51)	
HPeV7	2 (0.02)	0 (0)	1 (0.03)	1 (0.03)	NA
Single infection	0 (0)	0 (0)	0 (0)	0 (0)	
Coinfection	2 (0.02)	0 (0)	1 (0.03)	1 (0.03)	
HPeV8	3 (0.03)	0 (0)	2 (0.07)	1 (0.03)	NA
Single infection	2 (0.02)	0 (0)	2 (0.07)	0 (0)	
Coinfection	1 (0.01)	0 (0)	0 (0)	1 (0.03)	
HPeV10	3 (0.03)	0 (0)	2 (0.07)	1 (0.03)	NA
Single infection	1 (0.01)	0 (0)	1 (0.03)	0 (0/0)	
Coinfection	2 (0.02)	0 (0)	1 (0.03)	1 (0.03)	

(Continued)

TABLE 1 | Continued

Characteristics	Total (*n* = 10212)	Group 1$ (*n* = 3438)	Group 2$ (*n* = 3059)	Group 3$ (*n* = 3715)	*P*-value
HPeV14	7 (0.07)	0 (0)	6 (0.20)	1 (0.03)	NA
Single infection	0 (0)	0 (0)	0 (0)	0 (0)	
Coinfection	7 (0.07)	0 (0)	6 (0.20)	1 (0.03)	
Untyped*	115 (1.13)	13 (0.38)	81 (2.65)	21 (0.56)	0.601#
Single infection	18 (0.18)	3 (0.09)	13 (0.42)	2 (0.05)	
Coinfection	97 (0.95)	10 (0.29)	68 (2.22)	19 (0.51)	

Data are n (detection rate%) unless otherwise indicated.
$Group 1: pediatric patients with respiratory illness; Group 2: pediatric patients with acute diarrhea; Group 3: pediatric patients with Hand foot and mouth disease. The P-value was calculated by comparing Group 1, Group 2, and Group 3 as a general. Proportions may not total 100 because of rounding. There were 10 patients coinfected with two genotypes of HPeVs, including HPeV1-HPeV4 coinfection in 7 patients in Group 2, HPeV1-HPeV4 coinfection in 1 patient in Group 3, HPeV3-HPeV6 coinfection in 1 patient in Group 2, and HPeV1-HPeV5 coinfection in 1 patient in Group 3.
#Fisher-test, two-sided.
$Chi-square test, two-sided.
**Due to genotyping failure.*

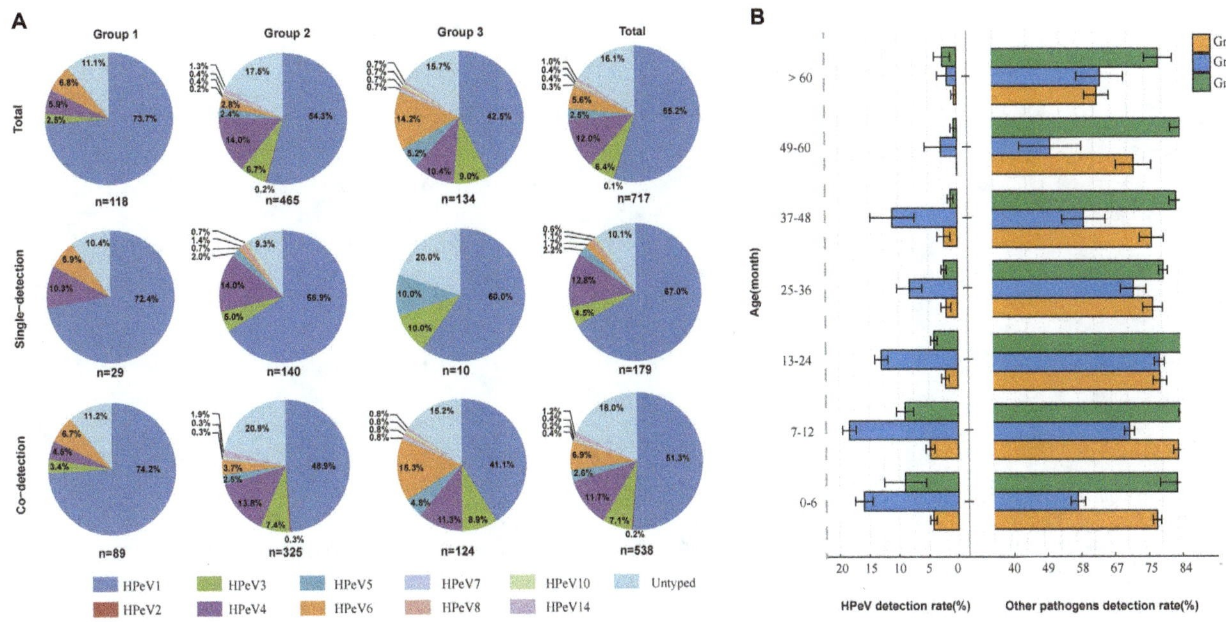

FIGURE 1 | The single infection and co-infection pattern, phylogenetic analysis of all the HPeV, and the age specific pattern of HPeV among three groups of pediatric patients. **(A)** HPeV single infection and co-infection rate and co-infection pattern between each HPeV genotype and the predominant viruses among three groups of pediatric patients. There were 10 patients coinfected with two genotypes of HPeVs, including HPeV1-HPeV4 coinfection in 7 patients in Group 2, HPeV1-HPeV4 coinfection in 1 patient in Group 3, HPeV3-HPeV6 coinfection in 1 patient in Group 2, and HPeV1-HPeV5 coinfection in 1 patient in Group 3. **(B)** The age specific pattern of HPeV and other viruses infection among three groups of pediatric patients. Group 1: patients with acute respiratory tract infection (ARTI), Group 2: patients with acute diarrhea, Group 3: patients with hand foot and mouth disease (HFMD).

The 10 patients with HPeV-single infection were younger than those with co-infection (*P* = 0.010). Compared with the HPeV-negative patients, only digestive system complication was significantly overrepresented in the HPeV-positive patients. More presence of neurological complication was observed from patients with HPeV-coinfection than from those with single infection (47.54% vs. 10.00%, *P* = 0.049). It's noteworthy in one child with nervous system syndromes, untyped HPeV was detected with all other pathogens tested to be negative. The interaction analysis revealed significant positive interactions between HPeV and EV, when HPeV was used as the responsive virus (dependent variable) and EV was used as the explanatory virus (independent variable) (*P* = 0.015, OR = 2.28, 95% CI = 1.23–4.73) (**Supplementary Table 4**).

The Genotype and Genetic Characteristics of HPeV-Positive Patients

From the 707 HPeV-positive patients, 592 (83.73%) were successfully sequenced for VP1 or VP3/VP1 nucleotide sequences, and 10 genotypes of HPeV were identified. There

TABLE 2 | The demographic and clinical characteristics of the HPeV infected patients compared with non-infected.

Variable	HPeV-positive			HPeV-negative	*P*-value	
	Subtotal	Single-detection	Co-detection		HPeV-positive vs. HPeV-negative	Single-infection vs. co-infection
Group 1	**(*n* = 118)**	**(*n* = 29)**	**(*n* = 89)**	**(*n* = 3,320)**		
Age, months (median, IQR)*	6.5 (4.0 – 10.0)	6.0 (4.0 – 10.0)	7.0 (4.0 – 10.0)	9.0 (4.0 – 21.0)	0.002	0.958
Sex, boy (%)#	77 (65.25)	17 (58.62)	60 (67.42)	2, 186 (65.84)	0.859	0.388
Clinical manifestation						
Cough#	111 (94.07)	26 (89.66)	85 (95.51)	3, 131 (94.31)	0.912	0.480
Moist rales#	107 (90.68)	25 (86.21)	82 (92.13)	2, 985 (89.91)	0.86	0.950
Pneumonia#	107 (90.68)	25 (86.21)	82 (92.13)	2, 985 (89.91)	0.785	0.558
Asthma#	89 (75.42)	22 (75.86)	67 (75.28)	2, 480 (74.72)	0.083	1.000
Rhinorrhoea#	58 (49.15)	14 (48.28)	44 (49.44)	1, 549 (46.66)	0.809	0.813
Bronchitis#	22 (18.64)	5 (17.24)	17 (19.10)	668 (20.12)	1.000	1.000
Dyspnea#	20 (16.95)	4 (13.79)	16 (17.98)	535 (16.11)	0.694	0.823
Rhonchi#	8 (6.78)	2 (6.90)	6 (6.74)	399 (12.02)	0.593	0.913
Sore throat#	5 (4.24)	1 (3.45)	4 (4.49)	131 (3.95)	0.721	1.000
Group 2	**(*n* = 457)**	**(*n* = 137)**	**(*n* = 320)**	**(*n* = 2,602)**		
Age, months (median, IQR)*	8.7 (6.3 – 13.1)	7.8 (5.4 – 11.0)	9.4 (6.8 – 13.2)	10.8 (6.7 – 16.2)	<0.001	<0.001
Sex, boy (%)#	277 (60.61)	88 (64.23)	189 (59.06)	1, 586 (60.95)	0.891	0.300
Clinical manifestation						
Diarrhea times ≥ 5#	294 (64.33)	80 (58.39)	214 (66.88)	1, 636 (62.87)	0.551	0.083
Vomiting#	169 (36.98)	30 (21.90)	139 (43.44)	1, 238 (47.58)	<0.001	<0.001
Respiratory symptoms#	141 (30.85)	40 (29.20)	101 (31.56)	887 (34.09)	0.177	0.616
Group 3	**(*n* = 132)**	**(*n* = 10)**	**(*n* = 122)**	**(*n* = 3583)**		
Age, months (median, IQR)*	15.6 (12.0 – 24.8)	11.0 (7.7 – 12.9)	16.1 (12.0 – 25.8)	25.6 (17.0 – 36.0)	<0.001	0.010
Sex, boy (%)#	86 (65.15)	7 (70.00)	79 (64.75)	2, 350 (65.59)	0.918	1.000
Clinical manifestation						
Neurological complications#	59 (44.70)	1 (10.00)	58 (47.54)	1, 477 (41.22)	0.426	0.049
Respiratory complications#	7 (5.30)	0 (0)	7 (5.74)	208 (5.81)	0.808	1.000
Digestive complications#	6 (4.55)	1 (10.00)	5 (4.10)	56 (1.56)	0.023	0.383
Circulatory complications#	5 (3.79)	0 (0)	5 (4.10)	176 (4.91)	0.556	1.000

Data are n (%) unless otherwise indicated.
**Mann-Whitney U-test.*
#Chi-square test, two-sided. Single infection refers to the single positive detection of HPeV among all the tested viruses in the group of patients; coinfection refers to the positive detection of HPeV and other tested viruses in the group of patients.

were 10 patients coinfected with two genotypes of HPeVs, including HPeV1-HPeV4 coinfection in 7 patients in Group 2, HPeV1-HPeV4 coinfection in 1 patient in Group 3, HPeV3-HPeV6 coinfection in 1 patient in Group 2, and HPeV1-HPeV5 coinfection in 1 patient in Group 3. Thus, 602 HPeV genotypes from 592 patients were used for the final analysis. HPeV-1 was the most common genotype (n = 396), followed by HPeV4 (n = 86), HPeV3 (n = 46), and HPeV6 (n = 40) (**Table 1** and **Figure 2**). Other uncommon genotypes included HPeV5 (n = 18), HPeV14 (n = 7), HPeV8 (n = 3), HPeV10 (n = 3), HPeV7 (n = 2), and HPeV2 (n = 1). The proportion of genotypes differed among three groups ($P < 0.001$), with HPeV1 and HPeV4 overrepresented among diarrhea patients and HPeV6 overrepresented among HFMD (**Figure 1**).

Phylogenetic trees were constructed based on the HPeV VP1 nucleotide sequences obtained from current study and extracted from GenBank. The spatial patterns of the genetic clustering were identified for each genotype. For HPeV1, two branches, HPeV1A and HPeV1B, were formed, and the strains from our three patient groups were located in both HPeV1A and HPeV1B (**Figure 3A**). For HPeV2, three branches were formed and one strain in 2013 (FX/130905/2013) from Group 2 of our study was located in Cluster 2, together with the strains from Malawi, India, and Australia (**Figure 3B**). As recently described, 2 HPeV-3 lineages have been identified (Elling et al., 2019) and all the current strains were distributed in Cluster 2.2 together with strains from United States and Japan (**Figure 3C**). For HPeV4, most current strains were in Cluster 1 (**Figure 4A**). For HPeV5, our strains were located in Cluster 1 (**Figure 4B**). For HPeV6, our strains were located in Cluster 1 and Cluster 3 (**Figure 4C**). The HPeV7 strains from our study were close to Pakistan strain, which collectively formed Cluster 2 (**Figure 4D**). For both HPeV10 and HPeV14, our strains were close to Hong Kong strain (**Figure 4D**). The HPeV8 strains from the current study were exclusively located in Cluster 3 (**Figure 3D**).

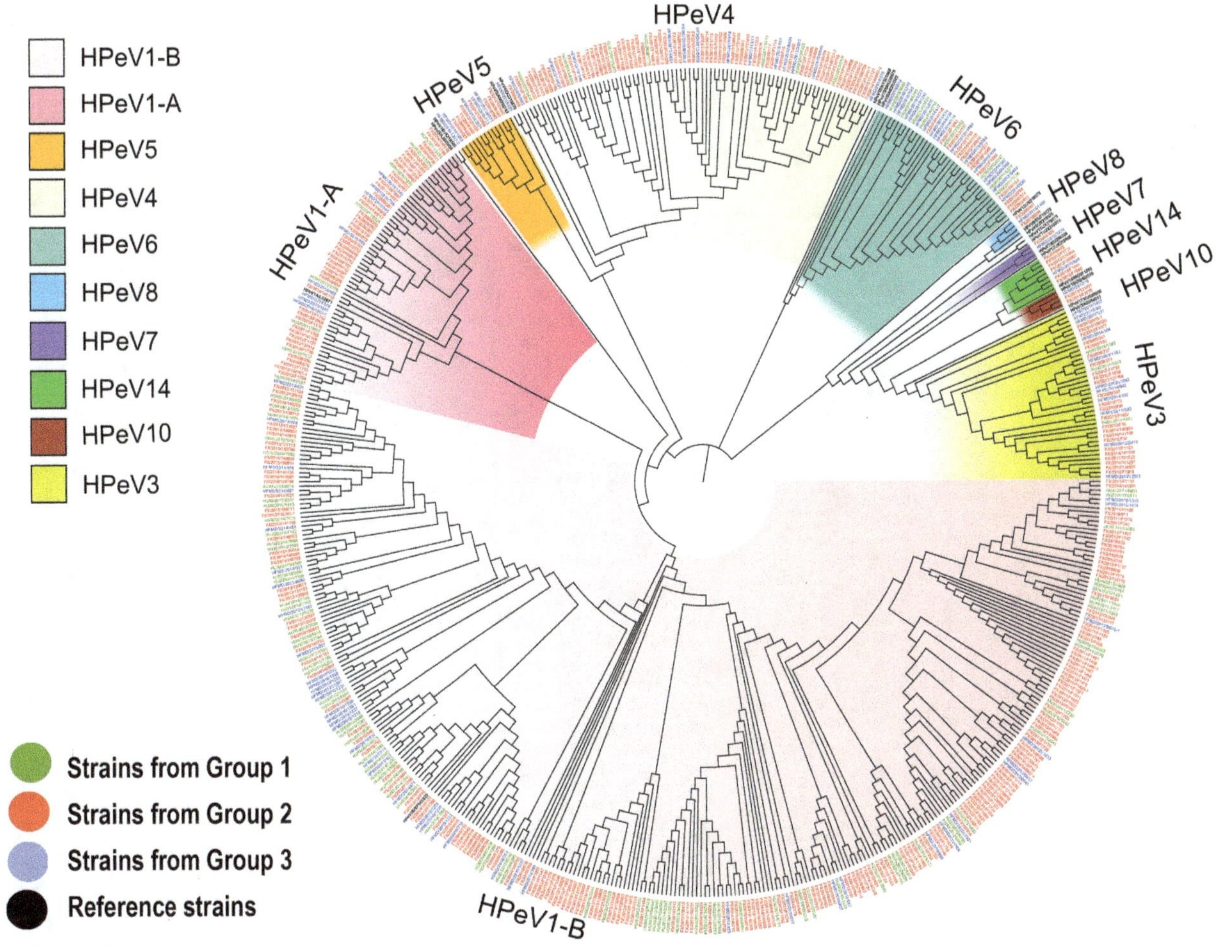

FIGURE 2 | Phylogenetic analysis of all the HPeV strains from our study based on the compete VP1 sequence. The phylogenetic trees were constructed with maximum likelihood method with 1,000 replicates using MEGA 7.0. The strains of black names in the figure were the reference strains (HPeV1A/L02971, HPeV1B/EF051629, HPeV2/AJ005695, HPeV3/AB084913, HPeV4/DQ315670, HPeV5/AM235749, HPeV6/AB252582, HPeV7/EU556224, HPeV8/EU716175, HPeV9/JX219575, HPeV10/GQ402516, HPeV11/JX219574, HPeV12/JX219566, HPeV13/JX219579, HPeV14/MG571809, HPeV15/JX219573, HPeV16/JX219580, HPeV17/KU885089, HPeV18/KY931660, and HPeV19/MH339678). The strains of green names with the beginning of "HUXI" were isolated from patients with Group 1 (patients with acute respiratory tract infection). The strains of red names with the beginning of "FX" were isolated from Group2 (patients with diarrhea). The strains of blue names with the beginning of "HFMD" were isolated from Group3 (patients with hand-foot-mouth disease).

The determined clusters were also analyzed for their proportion that differed according to the year of sampling and disease severity. We observed significant difference in the composition of clusters only within HpeV1A along the study years, that altered from 100% of Cluster1.1 in 2009 to 100% of Cluster1.3 in 2015 ($P < 0.001$, **Supplementary Table 5** and **Supplementary Figure 2**). No significant difference was observed for the proportion of clusters regarding the disease severity (**Supplementary Tables 5,6** and **Supplementary Figures 2, 3**).

The Age Specific Pattern of HPeV Infection

The positive rate of HPeV started to increase after birth to the highest level at the 7–12 months group, then gradually decreased until at a plain level at 25–36 months, with the low level maintained, except with a slight rebound at 37–48 months group for Group 2 (**Figure 1B**). This was highly similar with the age-specific trend of other detected viral pathogen in Group 1, but not the viral pathogens in Group 2 or 3, where their highest positive rate was observed in the 13–24-month age (**Figure 1B**). The three most common genotypes, HPeV1, HPeV3, and HPeV4, revealed the same trend that increased after birth to the highest positive level at 7–12 months (**Supplementary Table 7**).

The Temporal Pattern of HPeV Infection

During the study period from 2009 to 2015, a biannual cycle of circulation was observed for HPeV infections, i.e., peaks of infections occurred in even-numbered years in Group 1 and Group 3, while in odd-numbered years in Group 2 (**Supplementary Figures 4A,B**). Similar results were observed for HPeV1 (**Supplementary Figure 5A**), which showed similar peaks of infection every 2 years. HPeV3 is unusual in exhibiting

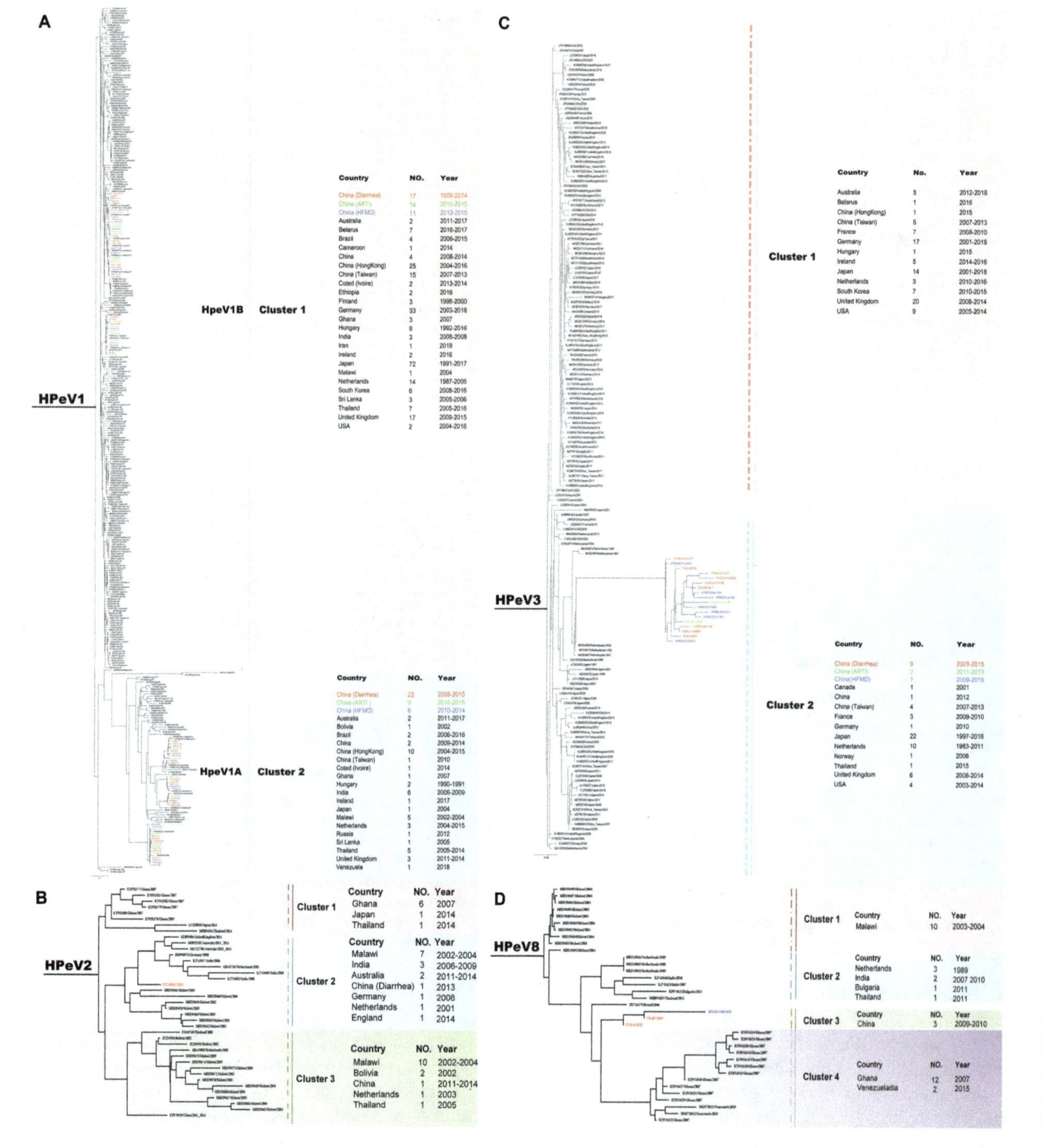

FIGURE 3 | Phylogenetic analysis of all the HPeV1-3 and 8 strains based on the compete VP1 sequence. **(A)** Phylogenetic analysis of representative HPeV1 strains based on the compete VP1 sequence. **(B)** Phylogenetic analysis of all the HPeV2 strains based on the compete VP1 sequence. **(C)** Phylogenetic analysis of representative HPeV3 strains based on the compete VP1 sequence. **(D)** Phylogenetic analysis of all the HPeV8 strains based on the compete VP1 sequence. The phylogenetic trees were constructed with maximum likelihood method with 1,000 replicates using MEGA 7.0. The strains of black names were downloaded from GenBank and others were from our study. The strains of green names with the beginning of "HUXI" were isolated from Group 2 (patients with acute respiratory tract infection). The strains of red names with the beginning of "FX" were isolated from Group 2 (patients with diarrhea). The strains of blue names with the beginning of "HFMD" were isolated from Group 3 (patients with hand-foot-mouth disease).

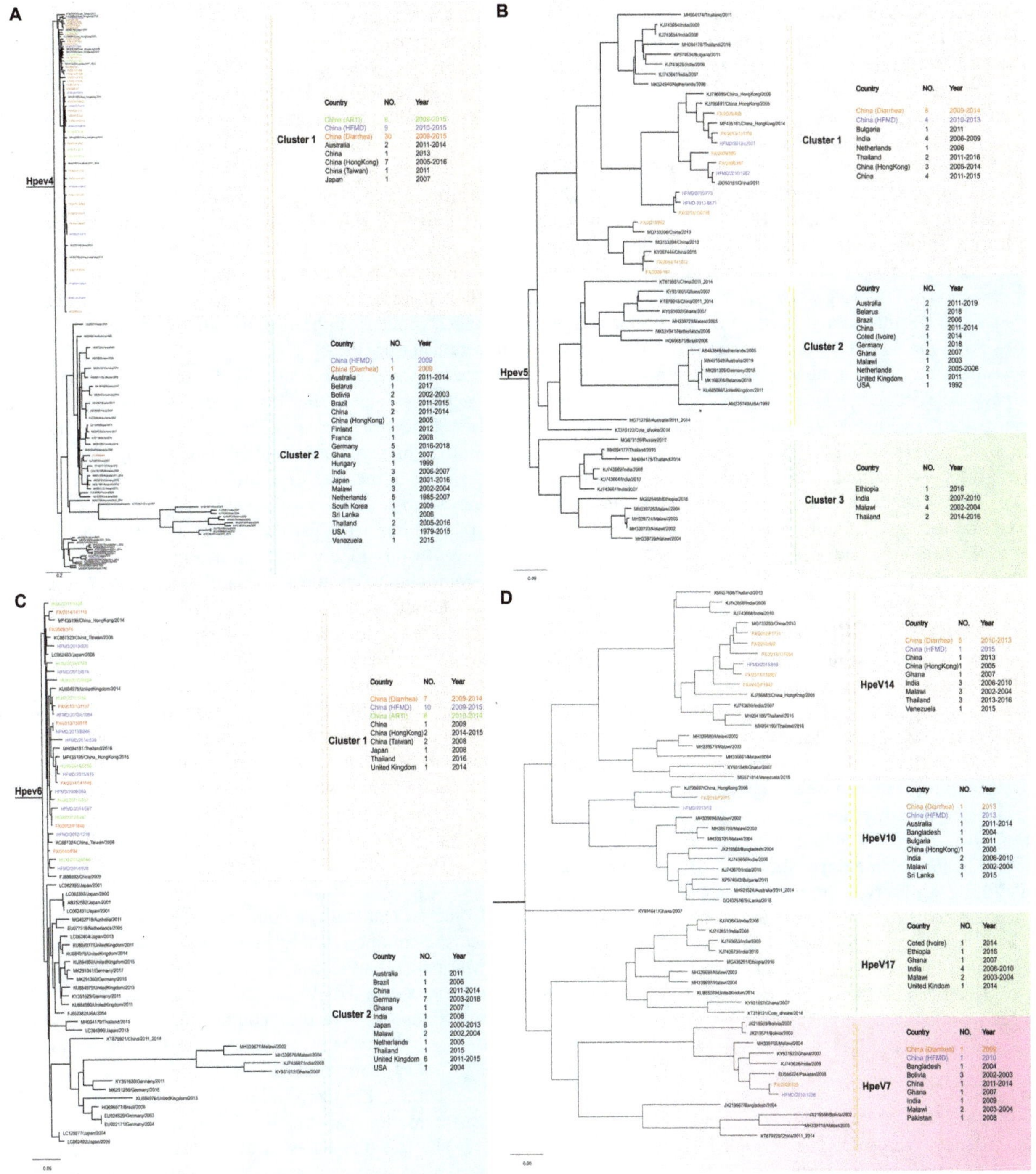

FIGURE 4 | Phylogenetic analysis of all the HPeV4–7, HPeV10, and HPeV14 strains based on the compete VP1 sequence. **(A)** Phylogenetic analysis of representative HPeV4 strains based on the compete VP1 sequence. **(B)** Phylogenetic analysis of representative the HPeV5 strains based on the compete VP1 sequence. **(C)** Phylogenetic analysis of representative HPeV6 strains based on the compete VP1 sequence. **(D)** Phylogenetic analysis of representative HPeV7, HPeV10, and HPeV14 strains based on the compete VP1 sequence. The phylogenetic trees were constructed with maximum likelihood method with 1,000 replicates using MEGA 7.0. The strains of black names were downloaded from GenBank and others were from our study. The strains of green names with the beginning of "HUXI" were isolated from Group 1 (patients with acute respiratory tract infection). The strains of red names with the beginning of "FX" were isolated from Group 2 (patients with diarrhea). The strains of blue names with the beginning of "HFMD" were isolated from Group 3 (patients with hand-foot-mouth disease).

a biannual cycle of infections, for which the circulation peaked in even-numbered years in Group 2 and Group 3, while the opposite was observed in Group 1 (**Supplementary Figures 5C,D**). For HPeV4, all three groups were characterized by bi-annual cycles of infections with the circulation peaked in even-numbered years (**Supplementary Figure 5E**).

For Group 2, an obvious seasonal pattern was observed in that higher positive rates were observed in summer (6.00%, 37.24%) or autumn (5.22%, 23.43%) than those in spring (0.98%, 6.20%) and winter (1.27%, 5.45%) ($P < 0.001$) (**Supplementary Table 8** and **Supplementary Figure 4C**). A major peak was observed during June–October, demonstrated by remarkably higher infection rates, suggesting the possibility of outbreak occurrence during this period. Less obvious seasonal pattern was observed for Group 1 and Group 3, partially owing to the small positive number. The three most common genotypes, HPeV1, HPeV3, and HPeV4 revealed distinct seasonal patterns, with HPeV1 and HPeV4 largely mimicking the seasonal pattern of all HPeV genotypes (**Supplementary Figures 5B,F**). By contrast, HPeV3 had displayed a biannual cycle of infections, with spring and autumn–winter peaks observed in Group 2, and a single peak observed for Group 1 (in summer) and Group 3 (in winter), respectively (**Supplementary Figure 5D**).

Viral Loads and Clinical Phenotypes

Viral loads of three common genotypes, HpeV1, HPeV3, and HPeV4, were measured and related to age, sex, disease severity, and single/co-infection for three types of diseases separately (**Supplementary Tables 9–11**). It's disclosed that higher viral loads of HPeV1 were significantly associated with severe diarrhea than the mild diarrhea ($P = 0.044$), and also significantly more associated with HPeV single infection than HPeV-EV coinfection among HFMD patients ($P = 0.001$) (**Supplementary Table 9**). Higher viral loads of HPeV3 were observed in male than the female patients with acute diarrhea ($P = 0.035$) (**Supplementary Table 10**). The viral load was also evaluated in corresponding to the days since disease onset, which revealed no significant trend of decreasing as the disease progressed (**Supplementary Table 12**).

DISCUSSION

In the current 6-year study, we identified HPeV infection in 6.92% of the pediatric patients with ARTI, acute diarrhea, and HFMD, with comparable levels across the studied years, indicating its persistent circulation in the surveillance region. The current positive rate of 3.55% for HPeV in HFMD patients was comparable with those of previous studies [4.5% in EV negative HFMD patients in China (Li et al., 2019), 2.55% in Japan (Ito et al., 2010)]. While positive detection of HPeV in 14.94% of the pediatric diarrhea was lower than previous studies in Shanghai, China (55%) (Zhong et al., 2011) and in Europe (29.4%) (Zhang et al., 2011), but higher than that studies in Korea (11.1%) (Seo et al., 2015) and Hong Kong (2.3%) (Chiang et al., 2017). However, the comparison among various studies should be explained with caution because the prevalence differed remarkably regarding the patients' demography, and it also varied depending on the sampling season and residential areas and the detection methods. As has been shown in the current results, the highest infection rate occurred in the age group of 7–12 months and decreased thereafter to a significantly lower level at 24 months, which is consistent with the serological data from Europe and Japan showing that 90% of infants have been infected with at least one HPeV subtype by the age of 2 years (Olijve et al., 2018). However, compared with the commonly seen viruses that were causative of the currently studied diseases, the age with peaking HPeV detection was younger, probably indicating its different manner of acquiring infection at early life.

Studies investigating more than one type of diseases would be helpful in elucidating disease caution of HPeV infections; however, they are scarcely performed. In one study performed on more than one type of patients in Hong Kong (Cabrerizo et al., 2017), 2.3% of the 3911 examined children had HPeV infection. The infected children mostly manifested with upper respiratory tract infection, acute gastroenteritis, and maculopapular rash, however, with no comparison made between patients with different clinical features (Chiang et al., 2017). A Spanish study simultaneously detected HPeV RNA in patients with encephalitis/meningoencephalitis and clinical sepsis, however, with no further genotyping efforts (Cabrerizo et al., 2017). Here by a comparison among case groups of varying clinical spectrum, we found that HPeV1 and HPeV4 were more likely to be identified from acute diarrhea compared with respiratory illness, while HPeV3 was more likely to be identified from acute diarrhea and severe HFMD compared with respiratory illness. This is partially consistent with previous research showing the association between the HPeV1 or HPeV3 infection and acute gastroenteritis (Pham et al., 2011; Zhang et al., 2011).

In the present study, 8 common respiratory viruses in ARTI patients, 5 common viruses in diarrhea patients, and all EVs in HFMD patients were concurrently detected. Only 176 (24.8%) cases had single HPeV infection and the other 75.2% had co-infections. This rate of coinfection was comparable with 60.0% in patients with acute bronchiolitis or pneumonia in Hong Kong (Chiang et al., 2017), 67% in respiratory specimens in the United Kingdom (Harvala et al., 2008), and 71.4% in gastroenteritis patients in North of China (Zhang et al., 2011). The fact that HPeV is often concurrently detected with other viruses has made it difficult to draw conclusions about its pathogenicity merely from PCR-based prevalence studies. Studies comparing HPeV RNA in cases and controls (Zhang et al., 2011) or the detection of the HPeV genome in CSF or other aseptic samples (Boivin et al., 2005; Olijve et al., 2018) can help to settle that issue. Very few clinical studies have evaluated the clinical significance of HPeV viral loads and the findings on this issue so far were inconsistent. In a group of neonates and young infants, higher viral load of HPeV3 in serum was observed in younger age and higher disease severity; however, no such correlation was observed in stool (Aizawa et al., 2016). Other studies reported no correlation between viral load and infection (Zhang et al., 2011) or severity of symptoms (Wildenbeest et al., 2014), both with small sample size and lacking multivariate analysis. Here by performing multivariate analysis to fully consider the effect from demographic factors, we found significant association between higher viral loads of HPeV1 and more severe diarrhea, which indicated a possible pathogenesis role of HPeV1 in the severe diarrhea. To support this finding, we also observed significantly higher positive rate of HPeV in diarrhea than the HFMD patients, when the latter group can act as an internal control without presenting diarrhea, since the same specimen type of stool were tested in both groups. Therefore, according to the "internal symptomatic controls" theory for human bocavirus posed by Allander (2008), a link between HPeV1 and severe diarrhea might be supported by the current findings. For HFMD disease, although HPeV is often co-detected with EV, we indeed determined higher viral loads in HPeV single infection than HPeV-EV coinfection, highlighting the possible role as a cause of HFMD in children. Still studies comparing HPeV in cases and asymptomatic controls may offer further evidence. On the other hand, no decline of viral load was shown as the days from disease onset, indicating a long-term persistence of viral shedding after disease onset. All these findings, taken together, could argue for a causal relationship between HPeV and the clinical disease, which, however, need to be confirmed by further case-control study or serological study, as well as molecular diagnostics of the virus in blood.

Variable results have been reported regarding the seasonality of HPeV infection, revealing a large disparity across studies. In Thailand, the biannual peaks of HPeV infection in the rainy (Jun–Aug) and winter (Nov–Jan) months had been reported (Malasao et al., 2019), while in Spain had been reported in spring and autumn (Cabrerizo et al., 2017). In Italy and Denmark, both EV and HPeV had been suggested to follow a similar seasonal pattern with a single peak during the summer and autumn (Nielsen et al., 2013; Bubba et al., 2017); in Hong Kong, inconsistent seasonal pattern was also observed between HPeV and EV, which occurred in the autumn–winter seasons and in summer and autumn, respectively (Chiang et al., 2017). Meteorological factors are likely to modulate the infection of EV, from direct influence on viral survival to indirect effects on human susceptibility. Despite various reports regarding the seasonality of HPeV infection, few studies have explored the seasonality for HPeV genotypes, and only with the commonly seen genotypes investigated. HPeV1 infections followed a clear seasonal pattern (September–April) in Finland during each individual year from 1995 to 2000 (Tauriainen et al., 2007). With respect to HPeV-3, previous studies had reported the biannual intervals for the infections (Harvala et al., 2011; van der Sanden et al., 2013; Jeziorski et al., 2015). In the current surveillance city, Chongqing, a seasonal peaking of all HPeV was observed in summer and autumn, with the seasonal pattern more obvious in patients with ARTI and acute diarrhea than in those with HFMD. However, three main genotypes (HPeV1, HPeV3, and HPeV4) had shown distinct seasonal peaks, highlighting a bi-annual cycles of all HpeV and two genotypes (HPeV 1 and HPeV 4) with peaks in odd-numbered years, whereas with peaks in even-numbered years HPeV3, as has been reported widely elsewhere (Tapia et al., 2008; Piralla et al., 2012; Schuffenecker et al., 2012; Ghanem-Zoubi et al., 2013; Harvala et al., 2014; Jeziorski et al., 2015; Vergnano et al., 2015). The reasons for this phenomenon underlying the bi-annual cycle of HPeV infections and its much greater frequency in the odd or even years thus remain to be determined. In addition, further investigation is warranted to decipher how the meteorological factors, such as temperature, humidity, and precipitation, might determine the seasonality and periodicity of HPeV infections with wider geographic range.

Importantly, the current study added to the limited sequence analysis on HPeVs, based on a broad collection of HPeVs strains circulating in China. Our study showed that 10 HPeV genotypes and different sublineages belonging to HPeV1, HPeV4, and HPeV6 were co-circulating in China, with two rare genotypes, HPeV7 and HPeV10, reported in China for the first time. Each of the currently determined genotpes, HPeV1, HPeV4, and HPeV6, were grouped into at least two clusters, with no specific temporal or geographic patterns. Strains that belonged to a single genetic lineage of HPeV were also found in both the respiratory and enteric tracts. Considering the wide distribution available from previous publication that reported HPeV1 in Japan and India (Patil et al., 2018; Pham et al., 2019), HPeV4 in Thailand and Netherlands (de Crom et al., 2016a; Malasao et al., 2019), HPeV6 in United Kingdom and Japan (Harvala et al., 2008; Pham et al., 2019), it's hypothesized that these three HPeVs might be prevalent in children world-wide. Seven other HPeV genotypes (HPeV2, HPeV3, HPeV5, HPeV7, HPeV8, HPeV10, and HPeV14) that were determined in this study were less closely related to the strains found in other regions, possibly indicating spatial differences in the genetic or pathogenic nature of this agent. It is also possible that the observed genetic diversity and the origin of variant strains are limited by the lack of these uncommon HPeV sequences that are available from different regions, which need a larger collection of sequences to be accumulated for analysis. Moreover, the large amounts of untyped HPeVs warrant further sequencing efforts, in order to identify emerging or recombinants HPeV variants with epidemic potential (Pham et al., 2019).

Our study was subject to several limitations. First, we failed to identify a detectable etiology in more than 21% of cases although with multiple tests of viruses. This limitation seemed to be common to surveillance studies with similar study design. Thus, the single infection of HPeV might be a mixed infection with other undetermined pathogens. Second, causal relationships cannot be determined merely from positive detection of HPeVs. This is especially true for HPeV due to its high coinfection rate with other commonly seen pathogens. The clinical spectrum of HPeV and the role that it plays in disease remain to be clarified. Third, although with wide clinical spectrum, the important disease category, sepsis, and meningoencephalitis in neonates and young infants were not included in the study, due to the difficulties in collecting samples from those children undergoing emergency situations.

CONCLUSION

In conclusion, the current study based on a comparative analysis of multiple case types and through a long-term surveillance had determined the epidemiological, genetic, and clinical characteristics of HPeV infection in China. The findings have important implications in projecting the expected disease burden and designing interventions aiming to decrease transmission in the vulnerable population. Still, extended surveillance beyond 2015 in wider areas and among various clinical phenotypes might help to acquire an in-depth understanding of its dynamic epidemic features and full spectrum of clinical syndromes. Further investigations are required to determine whether the differentially clustered strains were relevant to their replication, persistence, or pathogenesis.

AUTHOR CONTRIBUTIONS

WL and X-AZ contributed to organizing and supervising the whole study and were also responsible for the funding acquisition. X-AZ, R-QZ, J-JC, YY, XT, and Z-WZ conducted the experiments. Q-BL, Y-NW, H-YZ, P-HZ, and L-QF analyzed the data. X-AZ, R-QZ, and J-JC drafted the manuscript. WL, H-MX, E-ML, and H-SZ mainly contributed to designing the experiments and data analysis. All authors contributed to the article and approved the final manuscript.

ACKNOWLEDGMENTS

We are grateful to all the subjects, their families, and collaborating clinicians for their participation.

SUPPLEMENTARY MATERIAL

Supplementary Figure 1 | The co-infection between HPeV and other pathogens. **(A)** The co-infection between HPeV and one other pathogen among three groups of pediatric patients. **(B)** The number co-infection between HPeV and two other pathogens. **(C)** The number co-infection between HPeV and three other pathogens.

Supplementary Figure 2 | Phylogenetic analysis of all the HPeV1 strains based on the compete VP1 sequence. **(A)** The whole phylogenetic tree of HPeV1. **(B)** The detailed phylogenetic tree for Cluster 2. **(C)** The detailed phylogenetic tree for Cluster 1. The strains of green names with the beginning of "HUXI" were isolated from patients with Group 1 (patients with acute respiratory tract infection). The strains of red names with the beginning of "FX" were isolated from Group 2 (patients with diarrhea). The strains of blue names with the beginning of "HFMD" were isolated from Group 3 (patients with hand-foot-mouth disease).

Supplementary Figure 3 | Phylogenetic analysis of all the HPeV3 strains based on the compete VP1 sequence. **(A)** The whole phylogenetic tree of HPeV3. **(B)** The detailed phylogenetic tree for Cluster 1. **(C)** The detailed phylogenetic tree for Cluster 2. The strains of green names with the beginning of "HUXI" were isolated from patients with Group 1 (patients with acute respiratory tract infection). The strains of red names with the beginning of "FX" were isolated from Group 2 (patients with diarrhea). The strains of blue names with the beginning of "HFMD" were isolated from Group 3 (patients with hand-foot-mouth disease).

Supplementary Figure 4 | The temporal pattern of HPeV infection. **(A)** The relation between year and HPeV genotypes among all pediatric patients. **(B)** Annual patterns of detected HPeV. **(C)** The relation between season and HPeV detection rate among three groups of pediatric patients. Group 1: patients with acute respiratory tract infection (ARTI), Group 2: patients with acute diarrhea, Group 3: patients with hand, foot and mouth disease (HFMD).

Supplementary Figure 5 | The temporal pattern of HPeV1, HPeV3, and HPeV4 infection. **(A)** Annual patterns of HPeV1. **(B)** The relation between year and HPeV1 genotypes among all pediatric patients. **(C)** Annual patterns of detected HPeV3. **(D)** The relation between year and HPeV3 genotypes among all pediatric patients. **(E)** Annual patterns of detected HPeV4. **(F)** The relation between year and HPeV4 genotypes among all pediatric patients. Group 1: patients with acute respiratory tract infection (ARTI), Group 2: patients with acute diarrhea, Group 3: patients with hand, foot and mouth disease (HFMD).

REFERENCES

Aizawa, Y., Suzuki, Y., Watanabe, K., Oishi, T., and Saitoh, A. (2016). Clinical utility of serum samples for human parechovirus type 3 infection in neonates and young infants: the 2014 epidemic in Japan. *J. Infect.* 72, 223–232. doi: 10.1016/j.jinf.2015.10.010

Allander, T. (2008). Human bocavirus. *J. Clin. Virol.* 41, 29–33. doi: 10.1016/j.jcv.2007.10.026

Benschop, K. S., Schinkel, J., Minnaar, R. P., Pajkrt, D., Spanjerberg, L., Kraakman, H. C., et al. (2006). Human parechovirus infections in Dutch children and the association between serotype and disease severity. *Clin. Infect. Dis.* 42, 204–210. doi: 10.1086/498905

Benschop, K., Molenkamp, R., van der Ham, A., Wolthers, K., and Beld, M. (2008). Rapid detection of human parechoviruses in clinical samples by real-time PCR. *J. Clin. Virol.* 41, 69–74. doi: 10.1016/j.jcv.2007.10.004

Boivin, G., Abed, Y., and Boucher, F. D. (2005). Human parechovirus 3 and neonatal infections. *Emerg. Infect. Dis.* 11, 103–105. doi: 10.3201/eid1101.040606

Brouwer, L., Karelehto, E., Han, A. X., Thomas, X. V., Bruning, A. H. L., Calis, J. C. J., et al. (2019). High frequency and diversity of parechovirus A in a cohort of Malawian children. *Arch. Virol.* 164, 799–806. doi: 10.1007/s00705-018-04131-7

Bubba, L., Martinelli, M., Pellegrinelli, L., Primache, V., Tanzi, E., Pariani, E., et al. (2017). A 4-year study on epidemiologic and molecular characteristics of human parechoviruses and enteroviruses circulating in children younger than 5 years in northern Italy. *Pediatr. Infect. Dis. J.* 36, 13–19. doi: 10.1097/inf.0000000000001344

Cabrerizo, M., íaz-Cerio, M. D., Muñoz-Almagro, C., Rabella, N., Tarragó, D., Romero, M. P., et al. (2017). Molecular epidemiology of enterovirus and parechovirus infections according to patient age over a 4-year period in Spain. *J. Med. Virol.* 89, 435–442. doi: 10.1002/jmv.24658

Cai, X. Y., Wang, Q., Lin, G. Y., Cai, Z. W., Lin, C. X., Chen, P. Z., et al. (2014). Respiratory virus infections among children in South China. *J. Med. Virol.* 86, 1249–1255. doi: 10.1002/jmv.23931

Chiang, G. P. K., Chen, Z., Chan, M. C. W., Lee, S. H. M., Kwok, A. K., Yeung, A. C. M., et al. (2017). Clinical features and seasonality of parechovirus infection in an Asian subtropical city, Hong Kong. *PLoS One* 12:e0184533. doi: 10.1371/journal.pone.0184533

Cordey, S., L'Huillier, A. G., Turin, L., Gervaix, A., Posfay Barbe, K., and Kaiser, L. (2015). Enterovirus and *Parechovirus viraemia* in young children presenting to the emergency room: Unrecognised and frequent. *J. Clin. Virol.* 68, 69–72. doi: 10.1016/j.jcv.2015.05.003

Cristanziano, V. D., Böttcher, S., Diedrich, S., Timmen-Wego, M., Knops, E., Lübke, N., et al. (2015). Detection and characterization of enteroviruses and parechoviruses in healthy people living in the South of Côte d'Ivoire. *J. Clin. Virol.* 71, 40–53. doi: 10.1016/j.jcv.2015.08.004

de Crom, S. C., Rossen, J. W., de Moor, R. A., Veldkamp, E. J., van Furth, A. M., and Obihara, C. C. (2016a). Prospective assessment of clinical symptoms associated with enterovirus and parechovirus genotypes in a multicenter study in Dutch children. *J. Clin. Virol.* 77, 15–20. doi: 10.1016/j.jcv.2016.01.014

de Crom, S. C., Rossen, J. W., van Furth, A. M., and Obihara, C. C. (2016b).

Enterovirus and parechovirus infection in children: a brief overview. *Eur. J. Pediatr.* 175, 1023–1029. doi: 10.1007/s00431-016-2725-7

Elling, R., Böttcher, S., du Bois, F., Müller, A., Prifert, C., Weissbrich, B., et al. (2019). Epidemiology of human parechovirus type 3 upsurge in 2 hospitals, Freiburg, Germany, 2018. *Emerg. Infect. Dis.* 25, 1384–1388. doi: 10.3201/eid2507.190257

Ghanem-Zoubi, N., Shiner, M., Shulman, L. M., Sofer, D., Wolf, D., Marva, E., et al. (2013). Human parechovirus type 3 central nervous system infections in Israeli infants. *J. Clin. Virol.* 58, 205–210. doi: 10.1016/j.jcv.2013.06.001

Gunson, R. N., Collins, T. C., and Carman, W. F. (2005). Real-time RT-PCR detection of 12 respiratory viral infections in four triplex reactions. *J. Clin. Virol.* 33, 341–344. doi: 10.1016/j.jcv.2004.11.025

Harvala, H., Calvert, J., Van Nguyen, D., Clasper, L., Gadsby, N., Molyneaux, P., et al. (2014). Comparison of diagnostic clinical samples and environmental sampling for enterovirus and parechovirus surveillance in Scotland, 2010 to 2012. *Euro. Surveill.* 19:20772. doi: 10.2807/1560-7917.es2014.19.15.20772

Harvala, H., McLeish, N., Kondracka, J., McIntyre, C. L., McWilliam Leitch, E. C., Templeton, K., et al. (2011). Comparison of human parechovirus and enterovirus detection frequencies in cerebrospinal fluid samples collected over a 5-year period in edinburgh: HPeV type 3 identified as the most common picornavirus type. *J. Med. Virol.* 83, 889–896. doi: 10.1002/jmv.22023

Harvala, H., Robertson, I., McWilliam Leitch, E. C., Benschop, K., Wolthers, K. C., Templeton, K., et al. (2008). Epidemiology and clinical associations of human parechovirus respiratory infections. *J. Clin. Microbiol.* 46, 3446–3453. doi: 10.1128/jcm.01207-08

Ito, M., Yamashita, T., Tsuzuki, H., Kabashima, Y., Hasegawa, A., Nagaya, S., et al. (2010). Detection of human parechoviruses from clinical stool samples in Aichi, Japan. *J. Clin. Microbiol.* 48, 2683–2688. doi: 10.1128/jcm.00086-10

Jeziorski, E., Schuffenecker, I., Bohrer, S., Pain, J. B., Segondy, M., and Foulongne, V. (2015). Relevance of human parechovirus detection in cerebrospinal fluid samples from young infants with sepsis-like illness. *J. Clin. Lab. Anal.* 29, 112–115. doi: 10.1002/jcla.21737

Li, K., Lin, X. D., Chen, Y. P., Liu, Q., Wang, W., Plyusnin, A., et al. (2019). Identification of norovirus and human parechovirus in patients with hand, foot and mouth disease syndrome. *Pediatr. Infect. Dis. J.* 38, 1079–1084. doi: 10.1097/inf.0000000000002459

Li, X., Chen, J., Kong, M., Su, X., Zou, M., Zhang, H., et al. (2010). WUPyV in children with acute respiratory tract infections, China. *Emerg. Infect. Dis.* 16, 735–736. doi: 10.3201/eid1604.100011

Lin, F., Zheng, M., Li, H., Zheng, C., Li, X., Rao, G., et al. (2008). WU polyomavirus in children with acute lower respiratory tract infections, China. *J. Clin. Virol.* 42, 94–102. doi: 10.1016/j.jcv.2007.12.009

Malasao, R., Khamrin, P., Kumthip, K., Ushijima, H., and Maneekarn, N. (2019). Molecular epidemiology and genetic diversity of human parechoviruses in children hospitalized with acute diarrhea in Thailand during 2011-2016. *Arch. Virol.* 164, 1743–1752. doi: 10.1007/s00705-019-04249-2

Nickbakhsh, S., Mair, C., Matthews, L., Reeve, R., Johnson, P. C. D., Thorburn, F., et al. (2019). Virus-virus interactions impact the population dynamics of influenza and the common cold. *Proc. Natl. Acad. Sci. U.S.A.* 116, 27142–27150. doi: 10.1073/pnas.1911083116

Nielsen, A. C., Böttiger, B., Midgley, S. E., and Nielsen, L. P. (2013). A novel enterovirus and parechovirus multiplex one-step real-time PCR-validation and clinical experience. *J. Virol. Methods* 193, 359–363. doi: 10.1016/j.jviromet.2013.06.038

Olijve, L., Jennings, L., and Walls, T. (2018). Human parechovirus: an increasingly recognized cause of sepsis-like illness in young infants. *Clin. Microbiol. Rev.* 31:e00047-17. doi: 10.1128/cmr.00047-17

Patil, P. R., Ganorkar, N. N., and Gopalkrishna, V. (2018). Epidemiology and genetic diversity of human parechoviruses circulating among children hospitalised with acute gastroenteritis in Pune, Western India: a 5-years study. *Epidemiol. Infect.* 146, 11–18. doi: 10.1017/s095026881700262x

Pham, N. T. K., Thongprachum, A., Shimizu, Y., Trinh, Q. D., Okitsu, S., Komine-Aizawa, S., et al. (2019). Diversity of human parechovirus in infants and children with acute gastroenteritis in Japan during 2014-2016. *Infect. Genet. Evol.* 75:104001. doi: 10.1016/j.meegid.2019.104001

Pham, N. T., Takanashi, S., Tran, D. N., Trinh, Q. D., Abeysekera, C., Abeygunawardene, A., et al. (2011). Human parechovirus infection in children hospitalized with acute gastroenteritis in Sri Lanka. *J. Clin. Microbiol.* 49, 364–366. doi: 10.1128/jcm.02151-10

Pietsch, C., and Liebert, U. G. (2019). Genetic diversity of human parechoviruses in stool samples, Germany. *Infect. Genet. Evol.* 68, 280–285. doi: 10.1016/j.meegid.2019.01.007

Piralla, A., Furione, M., Rovida, F., Marchi, A., Stronati, M., Gerna, G., et al. (2012). Human parechovirus infections in patients admitted to hospital in Northern Italy, 2008-2010. *J. Med. Virol.* 84, 686–690. doi: 10.1002/jmv.23197

Qu, X. W., Duan, Z. J., Qi, Z. Y., Xie, Z. P., Gao, H. C., Liu, W. P., et al. (2007). Human bocavirus infection, People's Republic of China. *Emerg. Infect. Dis.* 13, 165–168. doi: 10.3201/eid1301.060842

Rohayem, J., Berger, S., Juretzek, T., Herchenröder, O., Mogel, M., Poppe, M., et al. (2004). A simple and rapid single-step multiplex RT-PCR to detect Norovirus, Astrovirus and Adenovirus in clinical stool samples. *J. Virol. Methods* 118, 49–59. doi: 10.1016/j.jviromet.2004.01.016

Schuffenecker, I., Javouhey, E., Gillet, Y., Kugener, B., Billaud, G., Floret, D., et al. (2012). Human parechovirus infections, Lyon, France, 2008-10: evidence for severe cases. *J. Clin. Virol.* 54, 337–341. doi: 10.1016/j.jcv.2012.04.016

Seo, J. H., Yeom, J. S., Youn, H. S., Han, T. H., and Chung, J. Y. (2015). Prevalence of human parechovirus and enterovirus in cerebrospinal fluid samples in children in Jinju, Korea. *Korean J. Pediatr.* 58, 102–107.doi:10.3345/kjp.2015.58.3.102

Shakeel, S., Dykeman, E. C., White, S. J., Ora, A., Cockburn, J. J. B., Butcher, S. J., et al. (2017). Genomic RNA folding mediates assembly of human parechovirus. *Nat. Commun.* 8:5. doi: 10.1038/s41467-016-0011-z

Shan, T. L., Guo, W., Cui, L., Shang, X. G., Dai, X. Q., Yuan, C. L., et al. (2009). The first detection of human parechovirus infections in China. *J. Clin. Virol.* 45, 371–372. doi: 10.1016/j.jcv.2009.05.033

Stals, A., Baert, L., Botteldoorn, N., Werbrouck, H., Herman, L., Uyttendaele, M., et al. (2009). Multiplex real-time RT-PCR for simultaneous detection of GI/GII noroviruses and murine norovirus 1. *J. Virol. Methods* 161, 247–253. doi: 10.1016/j.jviromet.2009.06.019

Tapia, G., Cinek, O., Witsø, E., Kulich, M., Rasmussen, T., Grinde, B., et al. (2008). Longitudinal observation of parechovirus in stool samples from Norwegian infants. *J. Med. Virol.* 80, 1835–1842. doi: 10.1002/jmv.21283

Tauriainen, S., Martiskainen, M., Oikarinen, S., Lönnrot, M., Viskari, H., Ilonen, J., et al. (2007). Human parechovirus 1 infections in young children–no association with type 1 diabetes. *J. Med. Virol.* 79, 457–462. doi: 10.1002/jmv.20831

Tiveljung-Lindell, A., Rotzén-Ostlund, M., Gupta, S., Ullstrand, R., Grillner, L., Zweygberg-Wirgart, B., et al. (2009). Development and implementation of a molecular diagnostic platform for daily rapid detection of 15 respiratory viruses. *J. Med. Virol.* 81, 167–175. doi: 10.1002/jmv.21368

van der Sanden, S. M., Koopmans, M. P., and van der Avoort, H. G. (2013). Detection of human enteroviruses and parechoviruses as part of the national enterovirus surveillance in the Netherlands, 1996-2011. *Eur. J. Clin. Microbiol. Infect. Dis.* 32, 1525–1531. doi: 10.1007/s10096-013-1906-9

Vergnano, S., Kadambari, S., Whalley, K., Menson, E. N., Martinez-Alier, N., Cooper, M., et al. (2015). Characteristics and outcomes of human parechovirus infection in infants (2008-2012). *Eur. J. Pediatr.* 174, 919–924. doi: 10.1007/s00431-014-2483-3

Verstrepen, W. A., Bruynseels, P., and Mertens, A. H. (2002). Evaluation of a rapid real-time RT-PCR assay for detection of enterovirus RNA in cerebrospinal fluid specimens. *J. Clin. Virol.* 25, S39–S43. doi: 10.1016/s1386-6532(02)00032-x

Wildenbeest, J. G., Benschop, K. S., Minnaar, R. P., Bouma-de Jongh, S., Wolthers, K. C., and Pajkrt, D. (2014). Clinical relevance of positive human parechovirus type 1 and 3 PCR in stool samples. *Clin. Microbiol. Infect.* 20, 640–647. doi: 10.1111/1469-0691.12542

Xu, W., McDonough, M. C., and Erdman, D. D. (2000). Species-specific identification of human adenoviruses by a multiplex PCR assay. *J. Clin. Microbiol.* 38, 4114–4120. doi: 10.1128/jcm.38.11.4114-4120.2000

Zhang, D. L., Jin, Y., Li, D. D., Cheng, W. X., Xu, Z. Q., Yu, J. M., et al. (2011). Prevalence of human parechovirus in Chinese children hospitalized for acute gastroenteritis. *Clin. Microbiol. Infect.* 17, 1563–1569. doi: 10.1111/j.1469-0691.2010.03390.x

Zhong, H., Lin, Y., Sun, J., Su, L., Cao, L., Yang, Y., et al. (2011). Prevalence and genotypes of human parechovirus in stool samples from hospitalized children in Shanghai, China, 2008 and 2009. *J. Med. Virol.* 83, 1428–1434. doi: 10.1002/jmv.22114

3

Sequelae of Fetal Infection in a Non-Human Primate Model of Listeriosis

Bryce Wolfe[1,2]*, *Andrea R. Kerr*[3], *Andres Mejia*[2], *Heather A. Simmons*[2], *Charles J. Czuprynski*[4] and *Thaddeus G. Golos*[2,3,5]

[1] *Department of Pathology and Laboratory Medicine, University of Wisconsin - Madison, Madison, WI, United States,* [2] *Wisconsin National Primate Research Center, University of Wisconsin - Madison, Madison, WI, United States,* [3] *Department of Comparative Biosciences, School of Veterinary Medicine, University of Wisconsin - Madison, Madison, WI, United States,* [4] *Department of Pathobiological Sciences, School of Veterinary Medicine, University of Wisconsin -Madison, Madison, WI, United States,* [5] *Department of Obstetrics and Gynecology, University of Wisconsin - Madison, Madison, WI, United States*

Correspondence:
Bryce Wolfe
bryce.wolfe@wisc.edu

Listeria monocytogenes (Lm) is a common environmental bacterium that thrives on vegetation and soil matter, but can infect humans if contaminated food products are ingested, resulting in severe disease in immunosuppressed populations, including pregnant women and newborns. To better understand how the unique immunological milieu of pregnancy increases susceptibility to infection, we study listeriosis in cynomolgus macaques, a non-human primate that closely resembles humans in placentation and in the physiology, and immunology of pregnancy. Non-human primates are naturally susceptible to Lm infection, and spontaneous abortions due to listeriosis are known to occur in outdoor macaque colonies, making them ideal models to understand the disease pathogenesis and host-pathogen relationship of listeriosis. We have previously shown that Lm infection in the first trimester has a high rate of miscarriage. This study expands on our previous findings by assessing how the quantity of Lm as well as stage of pregnancy at the time of exposure may influence disease susceptibility. In the current study we inoculated a cohort of macaques with a lower dose of Lm than our previous study and although this did not result in fetal demise, there was evidence of *in utero* inflammation and fetal distress. Animals that were reinfected with an equivalent or higher dose of the same strain of Lm resulted in approximately half of cases continuing to term and half ending in fetal demise. These cases had inconsistent bacterial colonization of the fetal compartment, suggesting that Lm does not need to directly infect the placenta to cause adverse pregnancy outcomes. Timed surgical collection of tissues following inoculation demonstrated that transmission from mother to fetus can occur as soon as 5 days post-inoculation. Lastly, third trimester inoculation resulted in pregnancy loss in 3 out of 4 macaques, accompanied by characteristic pathology and Lm colonization. Collectively, our studies demonstrate that common laboratory culture tests may not always recover Lm despite known maternal ingestion. Notably, we also find it is possible for maternal infection to resolve in some cases with no discernible adverse outcome; however, such cases had evidence of a sterile intrauterine inflammatory response, with unknown consequences for fetal development.

Keywords: listeriosis, pregnancy, histopathology, cytokines, non-human primate, fetal infection

INTRODUCTION

Listeriosis remains a public health concern for pregnant individuals, despite efforts in surveillance, reporting, public awareness campaigns, and implementation of safety measures by industry and agriculture (Tappero et al., 1995; Pohl et al., 2019). A foodborne disease caused by the bacterium *Listeria monocytogenes* (Lm), listeriosis can result in miscarriage, stillbirth, preterm birth, or neonatal infection (Craig et al., 2019). Lm is able to survive in a wide range of environments, including at refrigeration temperature. Common sources of infection include unpasteurized dairy products and ready-to-eat foods, although less common items such as caramel-coated apples have been responsible for human outbreaks (Glass et al., 2015). It can lead to a particularly insidious disease because symptoms may be mild, mistaken for the flu, or masked by morning sickness, resulting in delayed diagnosis and treatment. The United States' Centers for Disease Control and Prevention (CDC) reports that 1 in 6 cases of listeriosis in the U.S. is associated with pregnancy (Centers for Disease Control and Prevention, 2019) and that nearly one quarter of pregnancy-associated cases result in fetal loss or death of the newborn (Centers for Disease Control and Prevention, 2016). Most data concerning the course and nature of human infection come from retrospective clinical cases, identified based on symptoms, positive bacterial cultures, or adverse pregnancy outcomes. The first prospective clinical study, the Multicentric Observational NAtional Study on LISteriosis and ListeriA (MONALISA), found that the disease burden of listeriosis is higher than previously estimated: particularly, that more than 80% of infected mothers experienced major fetal or neonatal complications, and that the rate of fetal loss was significantly greater at <29 weeks of gestation (Charlier et al., 2017). Underreporting of pregnancy-associated listeriosis is very likely due to undiagnosed asymptomatic illness, unreported/unrecognized early miscarriage, misdiagnosed stillbirths, and difficulty in positively identifying Lm by standard laboratory culture, and Gram stain (Kylat et al., 2016).

Our current study addresses these limitations using a macaque model of infection, which allows for experimental manipulation, including a predetermined dose and timing of exposure, in a system highly relevant to the unique structure and physiology of human pregnancy (Lamond and Freitag, 2018; Lowe et al., 2018). Previously we found that dams given an inoculum of 10^7 CFUs Lm in the first trimester of pregnancy resulted in rapid infection and fetal demise, accompanied by diffuse bacterial colonization of the maternal-fetal interface (Wolfe et al., 2017). The objectives of the current study were to determine how a milder exposure changes the disease trajectory and outcome, and if increasing gestational age or previous infection influences susceptibility. We gave dams a single dose of 10^6 CFUs Lm in the first trimester. Exposure to $<10^7$ CFUs Lm in a single dose did not result in acute pregnancy loss. In subsequent pregnancies, we gave dams an equivalent or higher dose of Lm than previously administered. We find that re-exposure following a previous infection resulted in a lower rate of bacterial colonization, but could still induce adverse pregnancy outcomes associated with a sterile inflammatory response in the placenta and fetus. Because the maternal-fetal interface is not in a static state as pregnancy progresses, we next assessed third trimester infection to determine if increasing gestational age may enhance or mitigate Lm virulence. Our results demonstrate that infection with 10^7 CFUs Lm in late gestation results in a lower bacterial burden and slightly higher rate of fetal survival compared to the same dose in early gestation (33 vs. 20%, respectively), but does not mitigate against adverse pregnancy outcomes, which remain severe and can occur in as few as 4 days following exposure.

Abbreviations: CFUs, colony forming units; GD, gestational day; Lm, *Listeria monocytogenes;* MFI, maternal-fetal interface; PCA, principle component analysis; WNPRC, Wisconsin National Primate Research Center.

MATERIALS AND METHODS

Ethics Statement

The cynomolgus macaques (*Macaca fascicularis*) in this study were cared for by the staff at the Wisconsin National Primate Research Center (WNPRC) according to the regulations and guidelines of the University of Wisconsin Institutional Animal Care and Use Committee which approved this study, and adheres to principles described in the National Research Council's Guide for the Care and Use of Laboratory Animals.

Animals and Breeding

Adult female cynomolgus monkeys maintained at the WNPRC were cohoused with compatible males and observed daily for menses and copulation. Pregnancy was detected by ultrasound examination of the uterus approximately 18 to 20 days following the predicted day of ovulation. The day of gestation when pregnancy was detected was estimated based on previous experience and published data describing cynomolgus macaque fetal size during gestation (Tarantal and Hendrickx, 1988). Ultrasound examination of the uterus was done weekly or biweekly to monitor placental and fetal growth until the day of Lm inoculation, and every 2–3 days or daily after inoculation to assess fetal vital signs.

Inoculation With *L. monocytogenes*

At varied days of gestation in the first trimester (between days 36 to 50) or third trimester (between days 110 to 135 [full term is day 165]), monkeys were sedated, the uterus was examined by ultrasound to confirm a viable pregnancy, and a single dose between 10^6 and 10^8 colony forming units (CFUs) log-phase cells of strain LM2203 (serotype 4b, derived from an outbreak of listeriosis among pregnant women in Winston-Salem, North Carolina in the year 2000 MacDonald et al., 2005), were administered in 10 ml of whipping cream via a soft intragastric feeding tube as previously described (Smith et al., 2003). For each inoculation, Lm was cultured at 37°C in Tryptic Soy Broth (Becton Dickinson, Sparks, MD). 500 ul of the inoculum was diluted in phosphate-buffered saline (PBS; Catalog #P5368, Sigma-Aldrich, St. Louis, MO), plated on Trypticase soy agar with 5% sheep blood (Becton Dickinson, Sparks, MD), and incubated at 37°C to confirm the dose given to each animal as CFUs of Lm per milliliter. Six monkeys were given a whipping cream inoculum without Lm in an identical manner to be included as uninfected controls.

Fecal Shedding

Before and after inoculation, fecal samples were collected from cage pans to monitor fecal shedding of Lm. Schedules of sample collection are described in the legend to **Figure 1**. Serial dilutions

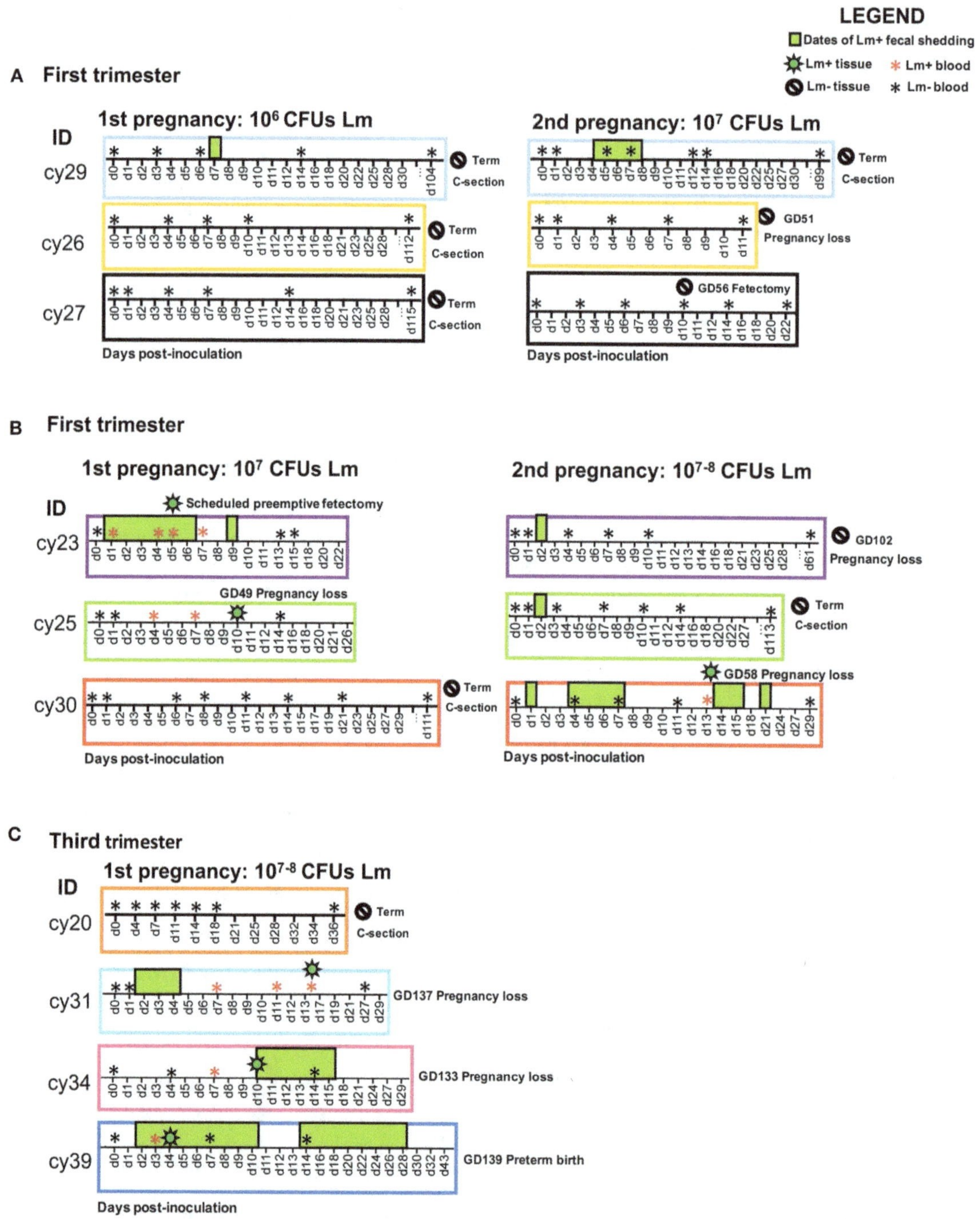

FIGURE 1 | Experimental timelines for each cohort showing animal ID, sample collections, and pregnancy outcome. The x-axis displays post-inoculation days. The following symbols indicate events on the timeline: positive blood culture (red asterisk), negative blood culture (black asterisk), positive tissue culture (green bacteria), negative tissue culture (negative sign), and positive fecal culture (green box). Fecal samples were collected on each date shown on the timeline; dates without a green box denote negative fecal cultures, and absent dates indicate that no samples were collected. Overlapping symbols indicate concurrent events. **(A)** First trimester cohort: 10^6 CFUs Lm initial dose; 10^7 CFUs Lm reexposure. **(B)** First trimester cohort: 10^7 CFUs Lm initial dose; 10^7 CFUs Lm reexposure. **(C)** Third trimester cohort: 10^7–10^8 CFUs Lm dose.

in PBS of fecal samples were plated in duplicate on modified Oxford agar plates (Kang and Fun, 1999) and the number of colonies was determined using ImageJ colony-counting software (https://imagej.nih.gov/ij/plugins/colony-counter.html) after 24 to 48 h of incubation at 37°C.

Bacteremia Monitoring

Peripheral blood samples were collected periodically for aerobic and anaerobic cultures to detect bacteremia as previously described (Lancaster, 2015) and processed on a BD Bactec 9,050 blood culture system (Becton Dickinson Diagnostic Systems, Sparks, MD) in the Clinical Pathology Laboratory at the University of Wisconsin—Madison School of Veterinary Medicine. Bactec Peds Plus/F blood culture bottles aseptically inoculated with 3 ml sample per bottle were incubated at 35°C until a positive signal was observed or for a maximum of 5 days. Bottles that did not signal positive at the end of 5 days were Gram-stained and sub-cultured to two chocolate agar plates (Remel, Lenexa, KS). Subcultures were incubated for 24–48 h aerobically at 35°C in 5% CO2 and anaerobically in an anaerobic chamber (SHEL LAB, Cornelius, OR) at 35°C in 80% N2, 5% H2, and 5% CO2 for verification of true or false negativity. Positive blood cultures were Gram-stained and subcultured to a blood agar plate supplemented with 5% sheep blood, chocolate agar, eosin methylene blue agar, and Columbia nalidixic acid agar (Remel, Lenexa, KS), and incubated at 35°C for 24–28 h in 5% CO2. An anaerobic subculture was also performed and incubated in an anaerobic chamber for 24–48 h as indicated above. Recovered isolates were identified by matrix-assisted laser desorption-ionization time-of-flight (MALDI-TOF) mass spectrometry (Bruker Daltonics, Billerica, MA). Sample extraction and strain identification was performed following the manufacturer's instruction. A score of >2 indicated secure genus and probable species identification.

Surgery and Tissue Processing

Ultrasound examination of the uterus was done 1 to 3 times per week after Lm dosing to monitor fetal well-being and confirm fetal heartbeat and umbilical blood flow. When fetal demise was indicated by absence of heartbeat, fetal and maternal tissues were promptly collected at laparotomy. The entire conceptus (decidua, placenta, fetal membranes, umbilical cord, amniotic fluid, and fetus) was removed by uterotomy. These were survival surgeries for the dams. The fetus was dissected into ~4-mm coronal segments, and alternating segments were fixed and embedded for histology (see below), or homogenized for bacteriological analysis on blood agar plates as previously described (Poulsen et al., 2013).

Histology and Histopathological Scoring

Dissected tissues were fixed in 2 to 4% paraformaldehyde for 24 to 72 h, rinsed in PBS, and stored in 70% ethanol until processed and embedded in paraffin. Paraffin sections were stained with hematoxylin and eosin (H&E) and Gram-stained using standard methods. Lm was confirmed by chromogenic immunohistochemistry with *Listeria* O antiserum (Difco Laboratories' rabbit polyclonal antibody against the somatic O antigen of *Listeria* serogroup 4). Stained sections were then examined and scored by WNPRC veterinary pathologists. Gram-stained slides were digitally scanned by the Wisconsin State Lab of Hygiene and analyzed using Aperio eSlide Manager with ImageScope 12.4 software (Leica Biosystems Inc. Buffalo Grove, IL). Scatterplot graphs of histological scores were prepared using GraphPad Prism version 8.0 (GraphPad Software, La Jolla, CA).

Cytokine/Chemokine Expression

Homogenized tissue samples were analyzed for cytokine expression by Luminex multiplex assay (Luminex Corporation, Austin, TX) with an NHP-validated kit containing CCL5/Regulated on Activation, Normal T cell Expressed and Secreted (RANTES), interleukin-1 beta (IL1b), IL-1 receptor antagonist (IL1ra), IL-2, IL-4, IL-6, IL-8, IL-10, IL-12, IL-13, IL-15, IL-16, IL-17 alpha, IL-18, IL-21, IL-23, IL-33, fibroblast growth factor 2 (FGF-2), granulocyte colony-stimulating factor (G-CSF), granulocyte macrophage-colony stimulating factor (GM-CSF), granzyme A, interferon gamma (IFN-g), monocyte chemoattractant protein (MCP)-1, monocyte inflammatory protein (MIP)-1alpha, MIP-1beta, perforin, soluble CD40 Ligand (sCD40L), soluble FAS ligand (sFASL), tumor necrosis factor alpha (TNFa), and vascular endothelial growth factor (VEGF) (Milliplex Non-Human Primate Cytokine and Chemokine Panel, Millipore, Billerica, MA). Cytokine and chemokine concentrations were quantified using the Bioplex 200 system (Biorad, Hercules, CA). Concentrations were normalized to the protein levels in each homogenate using a Thermo Scientific Pierce Micro BCA Protein Assay Kit (Catolog #23235, Thermo Fisher Scientific, Waltham, MA). Values were log-transformed and hierarchical clustering of principle components was performed using ClustVis (Metsalu and Vilo, 2015).

RESULTS

Pregnancy Outcomes With 10^6 Lm

All three dams continued to term with no evident fetal infection and no evident colonization of the maternal reproductive tract (**Table 1**; **Figure 1A**). There was sporadic maternal fecal shedding, but none of the dams showed signs of illness such as inappetence, fever, or bacteremia. Tissues collected at cesarean section appeared grossly normal in all cases. Microscopically, however, all cases had histologic signs of inflammation, including decidual fibrinoid necrosis, neutrophilic villitis with villous necrosis, neutrophilic chorioamnionitis, fetal hepatitis, and increased numbers of intra-alveolar squamous cells and cellular debris consistent with fetal distress *in utero* (**Figures 2A,B**). The placenta from case cy29.1 also had evidence that basal plate infarction and bleeding into the intervillous space had occurred earlier in gestation, with focal but extensive areas of organized fibrin and hemosiderin deposition. Cases cy29.1 and cy26.1 had moderate numbers of lymphocytes and plasma cells within the basal plate and placental villi, which is indicative of a chronic inflammatory response. After grading for extent and severity of histopathology, all cases from this cohort scored higher than age-matched controls (**Figure 3**: Lower dose vs. Control). Consistent with this trend, placenta samples from this cohort had increased levels of several pro-inflammatory cytokines, including RANTES,

TABLE 1 | Overview of treatment groups and outcomes.

Treatment	Trimester	Cohort	Outcome	ID	Gestation at inoculation	Maternal age	Maternal weight (kg)	Confirmed total dose Lm	Dose by weight (Lm/kg)	Peak maternal temperature (°F)	Gestation at collection	Duration	Fetal sex	Fetal weight (kg)
Lm	1	10^6, first exposure	Fetal survival	cy29.1	44	6	3.74	1.64E+06	4.39E+05	101	148	104	M	0.32
Lm	1	10^6, first exposure	Fetal survival	cy26.1	40	7	4.2	2.80E+06	6.67E+05	100.5	152	112	F	0.34
Lm	1	10^6, first exposure	Fetal survival	cy27.1	39	7	4.5	2.60E+06	5.78E+05	101.4	154	115	F	0.45
Lm	1	10^7, first exposure	Pregnancy loss	cy19.1	40	9	5.74	2.47E+07	4.30E+06	102.1*	48	8	x	0.004
Lm	1	10^7, first exposure	Pregnancy loss	cy21.1	36	6	3.35	1.23E+07	3.67E+06	101.4	50	14	x	0.019
Lm	1	10^7, first exposure	Pregnancy loss	cy23.1	41	7	5.03	1.52E+07	3.02E+06	101	46	5	x	(–)
Lm	1	10^7, first exposure	Pregnancy loss	cy25.1	39	6	3.32	1.60E+07	4.82E+06	102.9*	50	11	x	(–)
Lm	1	10^7, first exposure	Fetal survival	cy30.1	43	13	3.45	1.65E+07	4.78E+06	101.1	154	111	M	0.33
Lm	1	10^7, re-exposure	Fetal survival	cy29.2	47	7	4.66	1.34E+07	2.88E+06	101	145	98	F	0.33
Lm	1	10^7, re-exposure	Pregnancy loss	cy26.2	40	8	4.78	2.00E+07	4.18E+06	98.9	51	11	x	(–)
Lm	1	10^7, re-exposure	Timed fetectomy	cy27.2	46	8	4.44	1.13E+07	2.55E+06	98.6	56	10	x	0.0101
Lm	1	10^7, re-exposure	Pregnancy loss	cy23.2	41	8	5.2	1.20E+07	2.31E+06	101.2	102	61	x	0.098
Lm	1	10^7, re-exposure	Fetal survival	cy25.2	39	7	3.9	2.00E+07	5.13E+06	99.7	153	114	M	0.34
Lm	1	10^8, re-exposure	Pregnancy loss	cy30.2	45	14	4.16	1.40E+08	3.37E+07	99.1	58	13	x	0.0115
Lm	3	10^7, first exposure	Fetal survival	cy20.1	110	5	5.92	1.60E+07	2.70E+06	100.3	146	36	M	0.34
Lm	3	10^7, first exposure	Pregnancy loss	cy31.1	123	6	4	1.60E+07	4.00E+06	101	137	14	M	0.27
Lm	3	10^7, first exposure	Pregnancy loss	cy34.1	123	9	5.34	1.12E+07	2.10E+06	96.6	133	10	M	0.21
Lm	3	10^8, first exposure	Pregnancy loss	cy39.1	135	5	3.86	2.33E+08	6.04E+07	101.2	139	4	M	0.25
None	1	Control	Normal	cy24c	42	8	4.38	n/a	n/a	99.3	57	15	x	0.008
None	1	Control	Normal	cy27c	41	6	4.14	n/a	n/a	99.9	51	10	x	0.006
None	1	Control	Normal	cy35c	46	5	2.68	n/a	n/a	99.5	51	5	x	0.003
None	1	Control	Normal	cy26c	38	6	3.86	n/a	n/a	99.7	55	17	x	0.02
None	3	Control	Normal	cy35c	141	6	3.54	n/a	n/a	98.6	154	13	M	0.31
None	3	Control	Normal	cy33	124	10	8.15	n/a	n/a	97.9	152	28	F	0.34
None	3	Control	Normal	cy38	115	5	4.03	n/a	n/a	99.9	137	22	F	0.31
None	3	Control	Normal	cy31c	133	9	4.36	n/a	n/a	98.1	137	4	M	0.296

Cynomolgus macaque females reach maturity around age 4, are fertile until approximately age 24, and have an average lifespan of 30 years.

*Maternal fever.

x, too early in gestation to determine.

(–), not recorded.

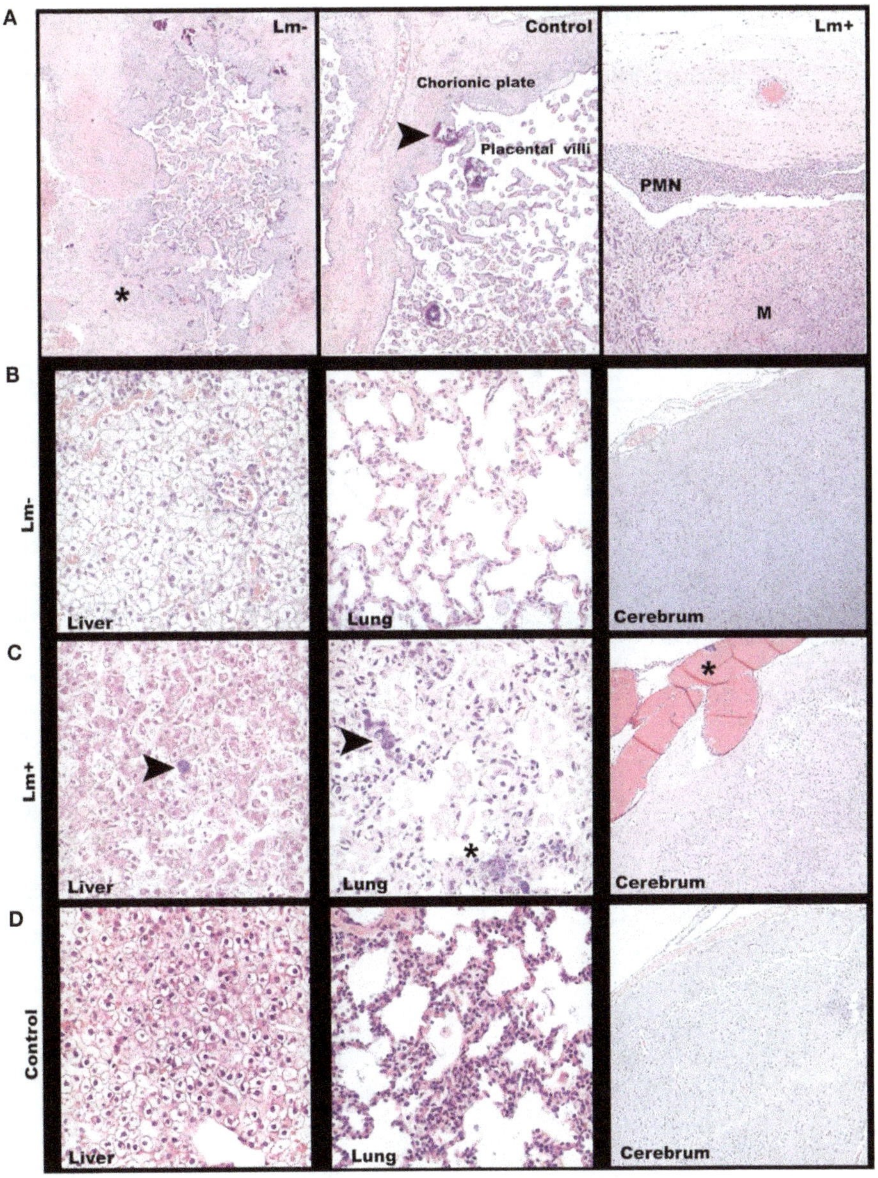

FIGURE 2 | Third trimester histology. **(A)** Maternal-fetal interface. Left: A focus of avascular villi entrapped in fibrin (asterisk) in a placenta from a dam exposed to Lm but without discernible infection. Cy29.1 H&E, 2x. Center: Normal placenta with incidental multifocal mineralization (arrowhead). Cy33. H&E, 40x. Right: Lm-infected placenta with acute subchorionic neutrophilic (PMN) inflammation and intervillous microabscesses (M). Cy31. H&E, 2x. **(B)** Representative tissue findings in Lm-inoculated animals who did not show clinical signs of infection. Left: Fetal liver with mild diffuse subcapsular neutrophil infiltration, intravascular and perivascular neutrophils. Cy27.1. H&E 40x. Center: Fetal lung with rare squamous cells in alveoli. Cy26.1. H&E 40x. Right: Fetal cerebrum with no significant findings Cy26.1. H&E, 10x. **(C)** Representative tissue findings in Lm-infected animals. Left: Lm+ Fetal liver with intralesional bacteria (arrow). Cy31. H&E, 10x. Center: Lm+ fetal lung with intravascular bacteria (arrow) and alveolus with luminal bacteria, neutrophils, squamous cells, and cellular debris. Cy31. H&E, 40x. Right: Lm+ fetal cerebrum with an intravascular bacterial embolus (asterisk). Cy31. H&E, 10x. **(D)** Representative tissue findings in control animals. Left: Control fetal liver. Cy33. H&E, 40x. Center: Control fetal lung. Occasional interalveolar squamous cells are an incidental finding commonly seen in cesarean deliveries. Cy33. H&E, 40x. Right: Control fetal cerebrum. Cy33. H&E, 10x.

perforin, and granzyme A. Anti-inflammatory IL-1RA, which antagonizes IL1b, was highest in controls and lowest with Lm infection. Placentas from pregnancies that received Lm but continued to term C-section had levels of IL-1RA higher than samples from Lm+ cases of pregnancy loss, but lower than age-matched controls (**Figure 4**).

Pregnancy Outcomes Following Re-infection

Inoculation with the same strain of Lm in a subsequent pregnancy resulted in fetal demise in 3 of 5 dams: cy26.2 at gestation day (gd)51 (11 days post-inoculation), cy30.2 at gd58 (13 days post-inoculation), and cy23.2 at gd102 (61 days

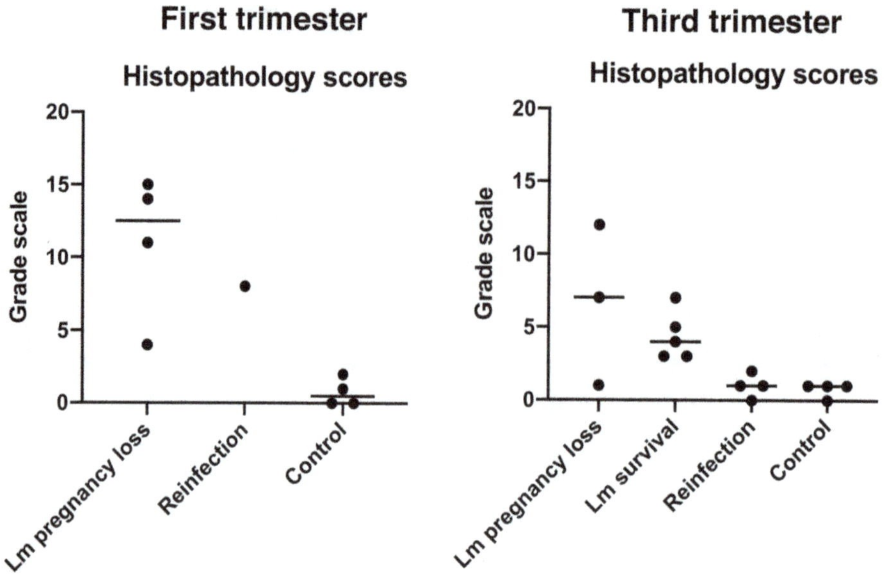

FIGURE 3 | Histopathology scores. Each dot represents the final score from a single case. Final scores were calculated from the sum of abnormal histological findings noted in both fetal and maternal-fetal interface tissues. Central black lines indicate the average score of a group.

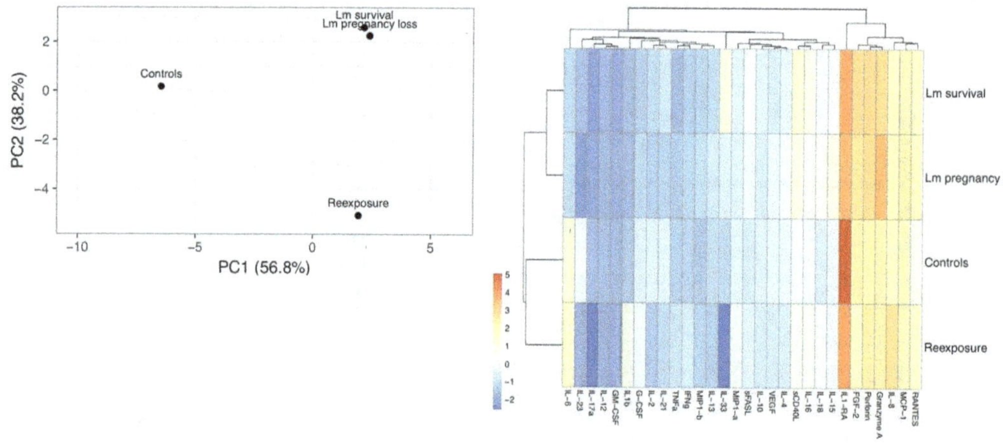

FIGURE 4 | Cytokine cluster analysis of third trimester placenta samples. **(A)** Principle component analysis based on the variation between subgroups. Original values were ln(x + 1)-transformed. Singular value decomposition with imputation was used to calculate principal components. X and Y axes show principal component 1 and principal component 2 that explain 56.4 and 37.2% of the total variance, respectively. **(B)** Heat map showing relative expression of all 30 cytokines assayed. Original values were ln(x + 1)-transformed. Pareto scaling was applied to rows. Both rows and columns were clustered using Manhattan distance and average linkage. Dendrograms indicate tightness of clusters.

post-inoculation) (**Figure 1B**). In this cohort, two received an Lm dose equivalent to their first exposure (cy26.2, cy29.2), and three received a higher dose (cy23.2, cy25.2, cy30.2) (**Table 1**). We were unable to culture bacteria (Lm) from the maternal-fetal interface in two cases (cy26.2 and cy23.2), and one of the dams (cy26.2) had no detectable Lm shedding or signs of infection prior to first trimester miscarriage. In this case (cy26.2), placental and fetal tissues were not available for analysis due to maternal placentophagy following spontaneous abortion. Cy23.2 had Lm-positive maternal fecal shedding and miscarried in the second trimester. Tissues examined from cy23.2 demonstrated mild histopathology, with multifocal neutrophilic villitis in the placenta and diffuse lymphoplasmacytic deciduitis. The fifth dam (cy30.2) received a higher dose in her second pregnancy (10^8 CFUs) and spontaneously aborted at gd58 (13 days post-inoculation), accompanied by fecal shedding, maternal bacteremia, and tissue colonization and histopathology characteristic of listeriosis (**Figures 1B, 5, 6**). The remaining two cases, cy29.2 and cy25.2, continued uneventfully to term. On histological examination, the placenta from cy29.2 showed basal plate infarcts with hemosiderin, indicating prior hemorrhage, and the placenta from cy25.2 had focal villous infarcts with

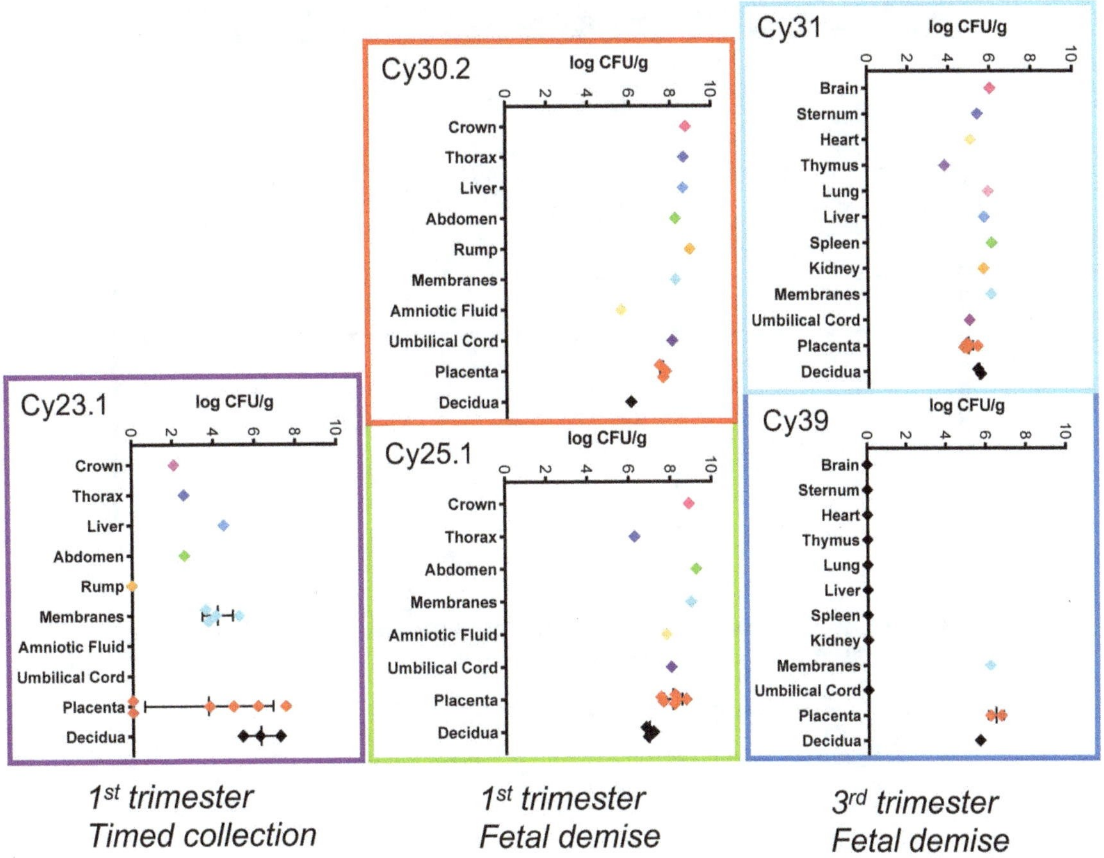

FIGURE 5 | Tissue bacterial burden Bacterial burden of Lm from individual pregnancies. The y-axis shows tissues and the x-axis shows the bacterial burden in colony forming units per gram (CFUs/g) in log scale for each tissue. Central black lines indicate the mean CFUs/g for replicate samples.

lymphoplasmacytic deciduitis. Interestingly, placenta samples from this cohort did not cluster with control samples by PCA plot and showed a shift in cytokine expression distinct from the other cohorts (**Figure 4**).

Timed Surgical Collection Following Inoculation to Assess Timing of Colonization

We performed pre-emptive surgery and sample collection shortly following inoculation to assess early events at the maternal-fetal interface. We assessed first time exposure (cy23.1) and re-exposure (cy27.2). Tissues collected at post-inoculation day 5 (cy23.1) showed that replicate decidua biopsies had a consistently high bacterial burden (5–7 log CFUs/g) whereas replicate placenta biopsies had more variable colonization (0–8 log CFUs/g). Of these, 2 of 6 replicates yielded no culturable Lm. There was moderate colonization of the amniotic membranes (3–6 log CFUs/g), and no culturable bacteria in the amniotic fluid (**Figures 1B, 5**), suggesting that surgery had interrupted colonization of the fetal compartment. Once the placenta has been breached, Lm characteristically colonizes highly vascular tissues of the fetus including developing bone, lung, spleen, and liver (**Figure 7**). The most heavily infected fetal organ in case cy23.1 was liver, with a bacterial burden equivalent to that of the amniotic membranes (**Figure 5**). All fetal tissues in this case had a bacterial burden several logs lower than cases which had fetal death *in utero* and an incubation duration longer than 5 days (1st trimester timed collection vs. 1st trimester fetal demise). Consistent with interrupted infection at this early timepoint, there was no discernable histopathology or inflammation in the fetus (data not shown). Tissues at the maternal-fetal interface demonstrated necrosuppurative arteritis in the decidua and multifocal suppurative necrosis of placental septa and anchoring villi, with a laterally dissecting hemorrhage and focal abscessation of a basal vein. Of note, cy23.1 tested positive for Lm in both fecal and blood cultures the day after inoculation. In contrast, cy27.2 had no maternal fecal shedding or bacteremia, and tissue samples at day 10 post-inoculation yielded no positive cultures and no evident histopathology (**Figure 1A**; **Table 2**).

Third Trimester Infection

We assessed third trimester pregnancy outcomes following infection with the same clinical strain of Lm. Two of three monkeys given 10^7 CFUs Lm in the third trimester of pregnancy had a stillbirth between 10 and 14 days post-inoculation. A fourth monkey received 10^8 CFUs and gave birth prematurely

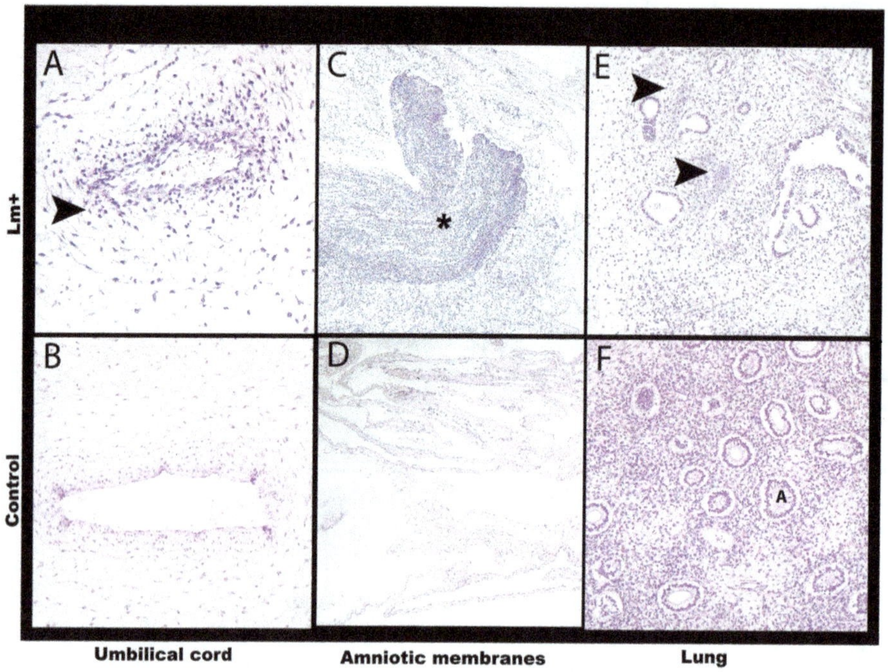

FIGURE 6 | Histology of the first trimester Lm infection. **(A)** Umbilical cord. Neutrophilic umbilical arteritis. Arrow points to clustered neutrophils. Cy30.2. H&E, 20x. **(B)** Control umbilical cord. Cy26c H&E, 20x. **(C)** Amniotic membranes with Gram-positive bacteria and neutrophilic infiltrate (asterisk). Cy30.2. H&E, 4x. **(D)** Control amniotic membranes. Cy26c H&E, 20x. **(E)** Fetal lung with listerial infiltration of pulmonary interstitium between alveoli. Arrows point to bacterial foci. Cy30.2 H&E, 20x. **(F)** Control fetal lung. A indicates alveolus. Cy26c H&E, 20x.

at 4 days post-inoculation. All three of these cases had Lm+ maternal fecal shedding, bacteremia, and tissue colonization (**Figures 1C, 5**). The most severe pathologic changes were seen in the stillbirth cases, characterized by neutrophilic deciduitis, suppurative villitis, and chorioamnionitis at the maternal-fetal interface, and fetal hepatitis and pulmonary congestion with neutrophils (**Figure 2C**). The preterm infant had Lm-positive cultures only within the amniotic membranes, placenta, and decidua, and no discernible inflammatory reaction or pathologic changes in the fetus (**Table 2**). The lack of fetal colonization is likely due to the occurrence of preterm birth before Lm could traffic to the fetal compartment, consistent with our observation that cy23.1 had a comparatively low fetal bacterial burden at post-inoculation day 5 (**Figure 5**). One dam (cy20) showed no evidence of maternal infection and continued to term uneventfully, but examination of tissues after surgical collection demonstrated villous necrosis of the placenta as well as fetal hepatitis, neither of which have been noted in age-matched control tissues. All third trimester placentas had variable mineralization, also seen in healthy controls, and the degree of mineralization most strongly associated with increasing gestational age. Focal placental infarction with few scattered neutrophils and focal areas of decidual necrosis is also an incidental finding in the third trimester (**Figure 2D**). Areas of infarction and mineralization are a normal consequence of cell death and ischemia due to the nature of the placenta as a temporary fetal organ that undergoes senescence as it nears parturition.

DISCUSSION

It is known that listeriosis causes adverse pregnancy outcomes, including miscarriage, stillbirth, and neonatal infection (Hof, 2003; Lamont et al., 2011; World Health Organization, 2018). Our research aims to clarify the course of infection, as well as the histological and cellular sequelae, which cannot be readily studied in human pregnancy. We have previously described the course of infection following a first-time exposure in the first trimester of pregnancy in a non-human primate model, resulting in acute infection and loss of the pregnancy between 1 and 2 weeks post-inoculation (Wolfe et al., 2017). Here we employed the same clinical isolate of Lm to determine how a lower initial dose impacts disease pathogenesis and pregnancy outcomes, if the virulence of our strain of Lm depends on gestational age, and whether or not prior exposure influences the immune response with reinfection in a subsequent pregnancy. Our previous study showed that the first trimester of pregnancy is keenly sensitive to infection, which caused fetal demise in 4 out of 4 monkeys following inoculation with 10^7 CFUs Lm. With the lower dose given in this study, we hypothesized that we would observe a long incubation period followed by acute fetal infection, which is thought to occur in human outbreaks based on retrospective surveys, clinical cases and estimated exposure dates (Goulet et al., 2013). However, we found that inoculation with 10^6 CFUs Lm in the first trimester did not result in latent maternal infection, nor in acute or chronic fetal infection. All 3 monkeys progressed to term C-section without

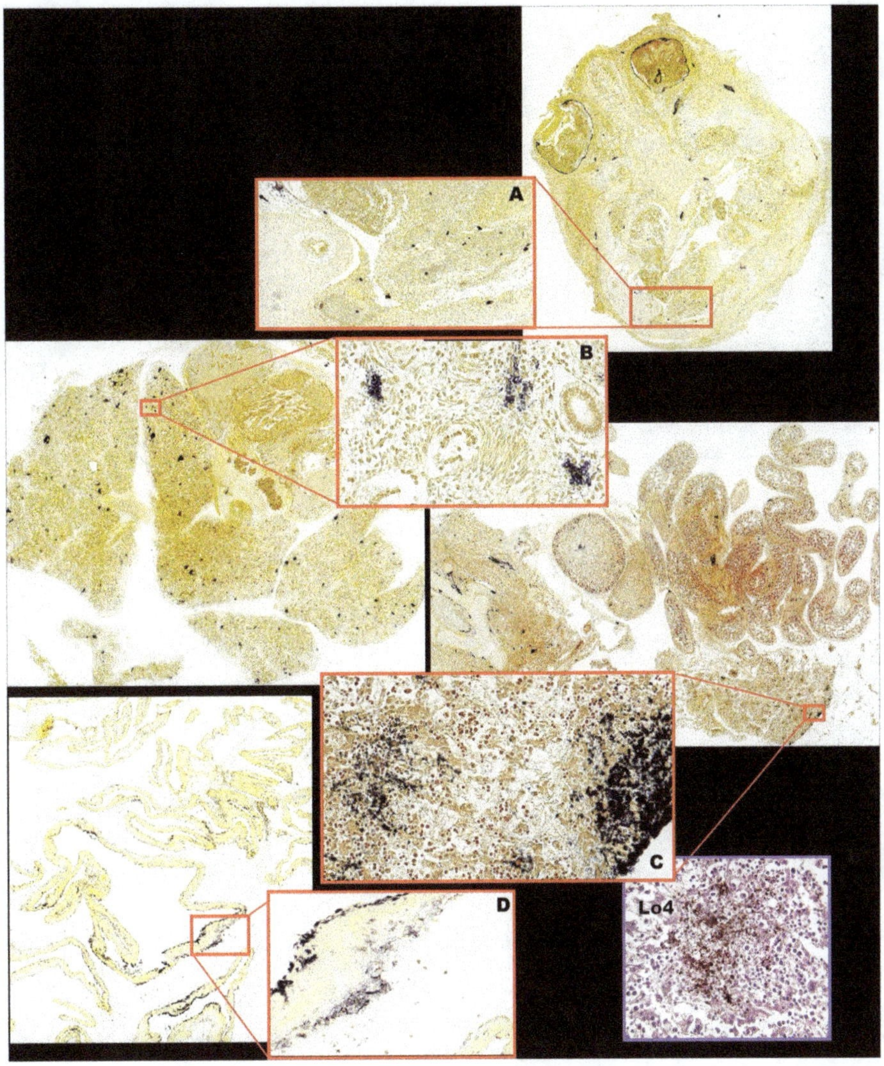

FIGURE 7 | Fetal bacterial distribution with Lm infection in the first trimester (Cy25.1). **(A)** Fetal cranium with large clusters of Gram-positive rods within the ocular musculature, diffusely within the nasal sinus and nasal cartilage, multifocally within the neural tissue, periosteum of the skull, and within the dermis, and subcutaneous tissues. Gram stain, 2x (inset 10x). **(B)** Fetal lung with multiple foci of intravascular bacteria. Gram stain, 2x (inset 40x). **(C)** Fetal liver, vertebrae, intestines, kidney, and adrenal gland, with multiple foci of bacterial colonization of the kidney, adrenal gland, intestinal serosa, hepatic capsule and interstitium, periosteum, and perichondrium. Gram stain, 2x (inset liver 40x). **(D)** Fetal membranes (chorioamniotic membranes) with multiple foci of Gram-positive bacteria. Gram stain 2x (inset 10x). Inset (Lo4): Immunohistochemical staining of fetal liver confirming Lm-positive foci.

adverse events. Infant weights remained comparable to controls, and there were no gross abnormalities. None of the sampled tissues had Gram-positive stained or culturable Lm. Interestingly, however, histological examination of tissues following surgical collection revealed lesions consistent with chronic inflammation and intrauterine bleeding, not found in gestational age-matched control samples, as well as a shift in the placenta toward a pro-inflammatory cytokine profile.

We next examined the impact of gestational age on infection susceptibility and pregnancy outcomes. Following the same experimental paradigm as before, we observed an adverse outcome in 3 out of 4 monkeys given 10^7-10^8 CFUs Lm in the third trimester. Two spontaneously aborted at 10- and 14-days post-inoculation with significant inflammation of the maternal and fetal tissues, a tissue bacterial burden comparable to that seen in the first trimester, and histological evidence of fetal hepatitis and pneumonia. The third (cy39.1) delivered a premature infant 4 days post-inoculation. Although the fourth (cy20.1) continued to term C-section, there was evidence of fetal distress *in utero* and abnormal placental necrosis. At 10^7 CFUs Lm, our combined studies show a survival rate of 1/3 in the third trimester and 1/5 in the first trimester. Our findings of fewer stillbirths yet still severe outcomes in later pregnancy are consistent with reports that fetal survival odds increase with gestational age, potentially due to an improved fetal immune response (Wadhwa and Smith, 2017). It will be intriguing for future studies to assess the development

TABLE 2 | Histopathology score chart.

Treatment (Tissue +/−)	Trimester	ID	Maternal-Fetal Interface						Fetal					TOTAL
			Lymphocytic and neutrophilic deciduitis	Decidual fibrinoid necrosis	Placental villous necrosis	Neutrophilic villitis	Neutrophilic chorio-amnionitis	MFI score	Funisitis	Hepatitis	Splenitis	Pulmonary congestion with neutrophils	Fetal score	
Control	1	cy24c						0					0	0
Control	1	cy27c						0					0	0
Control	1	cy26c	x					1					0	1
Control	1	cy35c	x		x			2					0	2
Lm (+)	1	cy23.1	x		x	xx		4					0	4
Lm (+)	1	cy30.2	xxx			xxx	xx	8					0	8
Lm (+)	1	cy21.1	xx	x	x	xx	x	7		xxx		x	4	11
Lm (+)	1	cy25.1	xx	xx	x	xx	xxx	10	x	xxx			4	14
Lm (+)	1	cy19.1	xx	xx	xxx	xxx	x	11	x	xx		x	4	15
Lm (−)	1	cy27.2						0					0	0
Lm (−)	1	cy26.2	x	x	n/a	n/a	n/a	n/a	n/a	n/a	n/a	n/a	n/a	n/a
Lm (−)	2	cy23.2	x*			x		2					0	2
Lm (−)	3	cy26.1	x*			x	x	3					0	3
Lm (−)	3	cy29.1	xx*		xx			4			x		1	5
Lm (−)	3	cy27.1	xx	xx	xx			6		x			1	7
Lm (−)	3	cy29.2	x					1					0	1
Lm (−)	3	cy25.2	x*					1					0	1
Lm (+)	3	cy39.1				x		1					0	1
Lm (−)	3	cy20.1			x			1		x			1	2
Lm (−)	3	cy30.1			xx	xx		4				x	1	5
Lm (+)	3	cy34.1	xx	xx		xx		6		x			1	7
Lm (+)	3	cy31.1	xxx			xx	xxx	8		x		xxx	4	12
Control	3	cy35c						0					0	0
Control	3	cy33c		x				1					0	1
Control	3	cy38c		x				1					0	1
Control	3	cy31c		x				1					0	1

*Histological scores for samples from the maternal-fetal interface and fetal tissues are presented as the sum of discrete pathologies noted by WNPRC board-certified veterinary pathologists on examination of H&E stained sections. Cases are organized by cohort and trimester at the time of tissue collection. ID ending in "c" indicates control, "1" indicates first pregnancy, and "2" indicates second pregnancy. Case cy26.2 had no identifiable uterine contents following spontaneous abortion, and n/a indicates these samples could not be analyzed for discrete histopathology. *Presence of plasma cells (indicative of a chronic inflammatory response).*

Score criteria are as follows:

X, mild (rare single scattered cells throughout the histologic section or multiple clusters of 4–10 cells; findings impact 0–25% of thesection).

XX, moderate (1–2 clusters of 10–20 cells or diffuse cell infiltration; findings impact 26–50% of thesection).

XXX, severe (1–2 clusters of more than 20 cells; findings impact more than 50% of thesection).

and adult health of infants known to have survived a pregnancy impacted by listeriosis.

Despite moderate to severe inflammation at the maternal-fetal interface, there was frequently minimal to absent fetal immune response detected by histologic examination (**Table 2**: cy23.1, cy30.1, cy34.1, cy26.1, cy26.1, cy27.1). The capacity for a fetal immune response emerges as pregnancy progresses with the development of hematopoietic and lymphoid organs (Chougnet, 2018). Differentiated immune cells, including neutrophils, macrophages, B cells, and T cells, can be observed by the late second to early third trimester, but these cells appear to be geared toward immunosuppression rather than defense against non-self-entities, and evidence suggests that the fetal immune system functions distinctly differently from that of adults as well as newborns, given its *in utero* niche and need to coexist with the maternal immune system (Makori et al., 2003; McGovern et al., 2017). An absence of fetal inflammatory response in the first trimester can be attributed to early gestational age and a lack of infiltration by maternal immune cells. At later stages of pregnancy, this may be due to fetal death or expulsion of uterine contents occurring before tissue-level changes caused by a cellular defense response can be observed. Similar to our early pregnancy study, we observed a fairly short incubation period of 4–14 days, which may be strain-dependent.

To determine if prior exposure to Lm confers protection or causes sensitization to subsequent exposures, we re-inoculated dams with an equivalent or higher dose of the same clinical isolate of Lm at approximately the same gestational day during a second pregnancy. We hypothesized first-time exposure would elicit a maternal immune response that would provide subsequent protection. Re-exposure resulted in a lower rate of pregnancy loss than first-time exposure, which is consistent with observations in livestock (Fensterbank, 1987), however we did not identify a clear association between initial response and secondary response that would have allowed us to predict the pregnancy outcomes of specific individuals. For example, cy25 lost her first pregnancy to Lm infection and then carried her second pregnancy to term despite reinfection, suggesting protection. In contrast, cy23 also had fulminant tissue colonization and maternal bacteremia in her first pregnancy, yet lost her second pregnancy to Lm infection. Cy30 and cy26 each had successful first pregnancies but miscarried their second, while cy29 successfully carried both pregnancies to term despite culture-positive maternal Lm infection each time. In total, re-exposure resulted in fetal demise in 3 out of 5 cases. Two of these cases (cy30.2 and cy23.2) could be diagnostically attributed to listeriosis. We did not recover Lm from the third case (cy26.2). While this case cannot be diagnostically attributed to listeriosis because all bacterial cultures and histologic stains for Lm were negative, it is possible that Lm does not need to directly infect the reproductive tract to induce adverse pregnancy outcomes. Peripheral immune cell activation following maternal infection may induce a signaling cascade of pro-inflammatory cytokines or other cellular responses contributing to the incidence of spontaneous abortion and preterm birth (Rowe et al., 2012).

The rate of miscarriage in this study exceeds the rate of spontaneous abortion at WNPRC's breeding colony of macaques, which were not used in these experimental studies. The breeding colony at WNPRC serves as an excellent control for infection studies because these animals are housed indoors and protected from environmental exposures. According to colony management records, the rate of spontaneous abortion in the colony per year is around 1 in 25 pregnancies. Less than 1% of these could be attributed to spontaneous ascending bacterial infection associated with fecal or vaginal flora. Prior to initiation of this study, there were no positive Lm culture results in the WNPRC database, which spans 35+ years of clinical and pathological results. All WNPRC animals and aborted tissues receive gross and histologic evaluation with appropriate bacteriological and viral testing. Additionally, our studies on listeriosis to-date have included a total of 10 designated control monkeys who underwent the same treatments and procedures as our experimental animals, except that they did not receive Lm in the inoculum. None of the control pregnancies in our current or previous studies have resulted in an adverse outcome, which suggests that maternal exposure to Lm, even without detectable reproductive tract colonization, has a detrimental impact on pregnancy health.

A preliminary assessment of cytokine expression in placenta samples from our cohorts shows that exposure to Lm alters the balance of pro- vs anti-inflammatory mediators at the maternal-fetal interface. Principle component analysis (PCA) can be used to visualize the degree of variability between sample sets and is particularly useful in demonstrating general relationships among subgroups based on multivariate data (Helmy et al., 2012). Because cytokines are not expressed in isolation, rather many are pleiotropic, act upon one another, and have the capacity to be pro-inflammatory or anti-inflammatory depending on the context and presence other cytokines, we therefore wanted to perform an exploratory cluster analysis to evaluate how much variation between our cohorts could be identified based on their overall pattern of cytokine expression. On PCA plot, Lm samples cluster apart from control samples. Given the inflammatory tissue response induced by Lm infection, this confirms expectations. Notably, Lm pregnancy loss samples had reduced IL-1RA expression, which has been linked to an impaired primary immune response and increased susceptibility to Lm infection (Irikura et al., 1999). Placenta samples from dams who received Lm yet went on to have uneventful pregnancies (Lm survival) clustered more closely to Lm pregnancy loss samples than to controls. Intriguingly, Lm survival samples had greater IL-1RA expression than Lm pregnancy loss samples, yet lower than controls. This suggests that the histopathology observed in the Lm survival cohort may be underpinned by responsive cell signaling. On the same plot, placentas from dams re-exposed to Lm in a subsequent pregnancy clustered apart from all other groups, suggesting a distinct secondary response. Hierarchical clustering based on cytokine expression demonstrates that exposure to Lm alters the chemical milieu of the placenta even in cases without adverse pregnancy outcomes. It will be enlightening to confirm these trends pending a larger study with additional samples, and to further evaluate this dataset in relation to cytokine signaling from the maternal decidua and fetal amniotic membranes. We cannot say if the Lm survival cohort's sterile yet inflammatory intrauterine environment would have an impact on infant development, behavior, or health in later life, as this study was not designed to explore that question. Retrospective studies on the long-term morbidity and neurodevelopment of survivors of prenatal listeriosis are mixed (Evans et al., 1984; Bortolussi and Mailman, 2011) and more definitive studies assessing prenatal programming from a pregnancy impacted by maternal Lm infection would be valuable.

Diagnosing Lm infection prior to an adverse event such as stillbirth or preterm birth continues to be difficult and inconsistent based on patient presentation and laboratory results (Charlier et al., 2014). A retrospective study at a hospital in Israel found that listeriosis is simultaneously underdiagnosed and overtreated (Fouks et al., 2018): over the course of five years, more than one hundred pregnant women who received a diagnosis of suspected listeriosis did not subsequently have a Lm+ culture, while 7 patients who had culture-confirmed Lm had not initially received a diagnosis of suspected listeriosis. One of the advantages of our model is that we can assess infection outcomes given a known bacterial quantity and timing of exposure. Although we directly administered a known amount of Lm to the maternal gastrointestinal tract, we note inconsistent fecal shedding of bacteria, clinical signs, and disease course. In some cases, we were unable to grow colonies on blood agar plates even though microscopy showed Gram-positive rods in tissues, and in other cases we did not observe Gram-positive rods despite Lm-positive cultures. In several cases, we had Lm-positive maternal samples, yet did not recover Lm from fetal or maternal-fetal interface samples through assay, culture, or cold enrichment. It has been reported that Lm is capable of entering a viable but non-culturable (VBNC) state (Highmore et al., 2018) which could complicate diagnostics, and Gram-staining can yield false results if artifacts are introduced or errors are made in specimen collection and processing (Samuel et al., 2016). Another cause for discrepancy with Lm detection across samples may be the characteristically multifocal pattern of listerial colonization: within the same tissue, we observe infiltration of some regions but not others. As we collect biopsies, it is possible that one contains a focus of Lm while another does not. In cases with maternal bacteremia and extensive tissue colonization, we had no difficulty identifying Lm; rather it was the cases in which there was light maternal fecal shedding and minimal colonization of maternal organs that proved more ambiguous. In these cases, we hypothesize that Lm was restricted from the intrauterine compartment, and that histologically-evident placental and fetal pathologies resulted from an immune response to infection, as opposed to direct infection. Maternal bacteremia was our strongest predictor of an adverse outcome and associated fetal histopathology. The pregnancies of dams who became bacteremic consistently ended in acute fetal demise shortly after initial detection of bacteremia, and all of these cases had bacterial colonization of the maternal-fetal interface, in contrast to dams with positive fecal cultures but no bacteremia, indicating that hematologic trafficking is critical for Lm to reach the reproductive tract. Identifying accurate and reliable markers of early infection that can be tested *in utero* remains an important goal to prevent the unnecessary use of antibiotics while at the same time ensuring that patients genuinely at risk of pre- and perinatal listeriosis can be promptly recognized and treated.

Based on our findings, prior maternal exposure does not appear to be predictive of disease susceptibility or pregnancy outcome, nor does the timing or duration of maternal shedding of Lm. Interindividual variation in response to transmissible disease is notable in humans, and no doubt factors into the range of outcomes observed in nonhuman primates as well (Casadevall and Pirofski, 2018). Confounding factors such as environment, diet, exercise, comorbidities and prior medical treatment plausibly may be ruled out given the controlled conditions of indoor housing and colony management at WNPRC facilities. We documented fetal sex and maternal age, weight, and body temperature, and these do not appear to correlate with pregnancy outcome. Maternal temperatures were, on average, mildly elevated following Lm inoculation, and two dams had clinical fever, but this was neither pathognomonic nor predictive of infection. We took into account the range of maternal body size by calculating the Lm dose per kilogram, and individual dams proved susceptible to different doses. Some, like cy34.1, had pregnancy loss with 2^6 Lm/kg, whereas cy30.1 tolerated 4^6 Lm/kg without pregnancy loss. Like humans, monkeys are genetically diverse and it is possible that disease resilience is driven by genomic differences or microbiome composition (Namasivayam et al., 2019), or that social dynamics play a role in immune programming (Snyder-Mackler et al., 2016). Individual determinants of disease remain an important area of study.

Although we observed fewer adverse pregnancy outcomes in our cohort of monkeys that received a lower dose of Lm, we cannot conclude and do not suggest that we have found any safe level of exposure to Lm. It is evident that different bacterial strains, environmental conditions, and individual susceptibility can alter Lm virulence and infection kinetics (Vázquez-Boland et al., 2001; Smith et al., 2008). Our study instead offers evidence that maternal Lm infection which spares the fetus still impacts the placenta, creating a more pro-inflammatory intrauterine environment, and reiterates that Lm is a pathogen of serious consequence. Ongoing studies from these same cohorts examining the maternal and fetal cellular response to listeriosis, including transcriptomic changes, post-transcriptional modifications, and host microbiome shifts, aim to shed light on the determinants of disease susceptibility vs. resilience.

AUTHOR CONTRIBUTIONS

BW, CC, and TG contributed to the conception and design of the study. BW organized experiments, quantified bacterial burden, produced figures, and wrote the first draft of the manuscript. HS and AM collected, read, and scored histological specimens. HS photographed H&E sections. AK curated, scanned, and analyzed Gram-stained specimens. BW, HS, and TG wrote sections of the manuscript. All authors contributed to manuscript revision, read, and approved the submitted version.

ACKNOWLEDGMENTS

We thank the WNPRC Veterinary, Scientific Protocol Implementation, Colony Services, and Pathology Services staff for assistance with animal procedures, including breeding, ultrasound monitoring, and sample collection. We thank Sophia Kathariou of North Carolina State University for generous donation of clinical strain LM2203, Nan Faith of UW-Madison School of Veterinary Medicine for assistance with microbiology, Faye Hartmann of UW-Madison Veterinary Care's Diagnostic Microbiology for assistance with blood cultures, Greg Wiepz at WNPRC for assistance with specimen processing and cytokine measurements, Mike Meyer, Troy Thoong, and Anna Marie Rowell at WNPRC for assistance with specimen processing and colony counting, Beth Gray of UW-Madison Research Animal Resources Center for assistance and training with Gram staining, and Ruth Sullivan of UW-Madison School of Veterinary Medicine for assistance with slide interpretation.

REFERENCES

Bortolussi, R., and Mailman, T. L. (2011). *Infectious Diseases of the Fetus and Newborn*. 7th ed. Philadelphia, PA: Elsevier Saunders.

Casadevall, A., and Pirofski, L. (2018). What is a host? attributes of individual susceptibility. *Infect. Immun.* 86, e00636-17. doi: 10.1128/IAI.00636-17

Centers for Disease Control and Prevention (2016). *Listeriosis Information for Health Professionals and Laboratories*. Available online at: https://www.cdc.gov/listeria/technical.html (accessed December 12, 2016).

Centers for Disease Control and Prevention (2019). *Prevent Infections During Pregnancy*. Available online at: https://www.cdc.gov/features/prenatalinfections/index.html (accessed June 19. 2019).

Charlier, C., Goffinet, F., Azria, E., Leclercq, A., and Lecuit, M. (2014). Inadequate management of pregnancy-associated listeriosis: lessons from four case reports. *Clin. Microbiol. Infect.* 20, 246–249. doi: 10.1111/1469-0691.12281

Charlier, C., Perrodeau, É., Leclercq, A., Cazenave, B., Pilmis, B., Henry, B., et al. (2017). Clinical features and prognostic factors of listeriosis: the MONALISA national prospective cohort study. *Lancet Infect. Dis.* 17, 510–519. doi: 10.1016/S1473-3099(16)30521-7

Chougnet, C. (2018). Human fetal immune cells fight back. *Sci. Trans. Med.* 10:aat3910. doi: 10.1126/scitranslmed.aat3910

Craig, A. M., Dotters-Katz, S., Kuller, J. A., and Thompson, J. L. (2019). Listeriosis in pregnancy: a review. *Obstet. Gynecol. Survey* 74, 362–368. doi: 10.1097/OGX.0000000000000683

Evans, J. R., Allen, A. C., Bortolussi, R., Issekutz, T. B., and Stintson, D. A. (1984). Follow-up study of survivors of fetal and early onset neonatal listeriosis. *Clin Invest Med.* 7, 329–334.

Fensterbank, R. (1987). Vaccination with a Listeria strain of reduced virulence against experimental Listeria abortion in goats. *Annal. Vet. Res.* 18, 415–419.

Fouks, Y., Amit, S., Many, A., Haham, A., Mandel, D., and Shinar, S. (2018). Listeriosis in pregnancy: under-diagnosis despite over-treatment. *J. Perinatol.* 38, 26–30. doi: 10.1038/jp.2017.145

Glass, K. A., Golden, M. C., Wanless, B. J., Bedale, W., and Czuprynski, C. (2015). Growth of *Listeria monocytogenes* within a caramel-coated apple microenvironment. *mBio.* 6:e01232-15. doi: 10.1128/mBio.01232-15

Goulet, V., King, L. A., Vaillant, V., and de Valk, H. (2013). What is the incubation period for listeriosis? *BMC Infect. Dis.* 13:11. doi: 10.1186/1471-2334-13-11

Helmy, A., Antoniades, C. A., Guilfoyle, M. R., Carpenter, K. L. H., and Hutchinson, P. J. (2012). Principal component analysis of the cytokine and chemokine response to human traumatic brain injury. *PLoS ONE* 7:e39677. doi: 10.1371/journal.pone.0039677

Highmore, C. J., Warner, J. C., Rothwell, S. D., Wilks, S. A., and Keevil, C. W. (2018). Viable-but-Nonculturable *Listeria monocytogenes* and *Salmonella enterica* Serovar Thompson Induced by Chlorine Stress Remain Infectious. *mBio.* 9. doi: 10.1128/mBio.00540-18

Hof, H. (2003). History and epidemiology of listeriosis. *FEMS Immunol. Med. Microbiol.* 35, 199–202. doi: 10.1016/S0928-8244(02)00471-6

Irikura, V. M., Hirsch, E., and Hirsh, D. (1999). Effects of interleukin-1 receptor antagonist overexpression on infection by *Listeria monocytogenes*. *Infect. Immun.* 67, 1901–1909.

Kang, D. H., and Fun, D. Y. (1999). Thin agar layer method for recovery of heat-injured *Listeria monocytogenes*. *J. Food Pro.* 62, 1346–1349. doi: 10.4315/0362-028X-62.11.1346

Kylat, R. I., Bartholomew, A., Cramer, N., and Bader, M. Y. (2016). Neonatal listeriosis: uncommon or misdiagnosed? *J. Neonatal. Perinatal. Med.* 9, 313–316. doi: 10.3233/NPM-16915121

Lamond, N. M., and Freitag, N. E. (2018). Vertical transmission of *Listeria monocytogenes*: probing the balance between protection from pathogens and fetal tolerance. *Pathogens.* 7:E52. doi: 10.3390/pathogens7020052

Lamont, R. F., Sobel, J., Mazaki-Tovi, S., Kusanovic, J. P., Vaisbuch, E., Kim, S. K., et al. (2011). Listeriosis in human pregnancy: a systematic review. *J Perinat Med.* 39, 227–236. doi: 10.1515/jpm.2011.035

Lancaster, D. P. (2015). Blood volume required for detection of low levels and ultralow levels of organisms responsible for neonatal bacteremia by use of Bactec Peds Plus/F, Plus Aerobic/F medium, and the BD Bactec FX system: an *in vitro* study. *J. Clin. Microbiol.* 53, 3609–3613. doi: 10.1128/JCM.01706-15

Lowe, D. E., Robbins, J. R., and Bakardjiev, A. I. (2018). Animal and human tissue models of vertical *Listeria monocytogenes* transmission and implications for other pregnancy-associated infections. *Infect. Immun.* 89:IAI.00801-17. doi: 10.1128/IAI.00801-17

MacDonald, P. D., Whitwam, R. E., Boggs, J. D., MacCormack, J. N., Anderson, K. L., Reardon, J. W., et al. (2005). Outbreak of listeriosis among Mexican immigrants as a result of consumption of illicitly produced Mexican-style cheese. *Clin. Infect. Dis.* 40, 677–82. doi: 10.1086/427803

Makori, N., Tarantal, A. F., Lu, F. X., Rourke, T., Martas, M. L., McChesney, M. B., et al. (2003). Functional and morphological development of lymphoid tissues and immune regulatory and effector function in rhesus monkeys: cytokine-secreting cells, immunoglobulin-secreting cells, and CD5. B-1 cells appear early in fetal development. *Clin. Diagnos. Lab. Immunol.* 10, 140–153. doi: 10.1128/CDLI.10.1.140-153.2003

McGovern, N., Shin, A., Low, G., Low, D., Duan, K., Yao, L. J., et al. (2017). Human fetal dendritic cells promote prenatal T-cell immune suppression through arginase-2. *Nature* 546, 662–666. doi: 10.1038/nature22795

Metsalu, T., and Vilo, J. (2015). Clustvis: a web tool for visualizing clustering of multivariate data using principal component analysis and heatmap. *Nucleic Acids Res.* 43, W566–W570. doi: 10.1093/nar/gkv468

Namasivayam, S., Kauffman, K. D., McCulloch, J. A., Yuan, W., Thovarai, V., Mittereder, L. R., et al. (2019). Correlation between disease severity and the intestinal microbiome in mycobacterium tuberculosis-infected rhesus macaques. *mBio.* doi: 10.1128/mBio.01018-19

Pohl, A. M., Pouillot, R., Bazaco, M. C., Wolpert, B. J., Healy, J. M., Bruce, B. B., et al. (2019). Differences among incidence rates of invasive listeriosis in the U.S. foodnet population by age, sex, race/ethnicity, and pregnancy status, 2008–2016. *Foodborne Pathog. Dis.* 16, 290–297. doi: 10.1089/fpd.2018.2548

Poulsen, K. P., Faith, N. G., Steinberg, H., and Czuprynski, C. J. (2013). Bacterial load and inflammation in fetal tissues is not dependent on IL-17a or IL-22 in 10-14 day pregnant mice infected with *Listeria monocytogenes*. *Microb. Pathog.* 56, 47–45. doi: 10.1016/j.micpath.2012.11.003

Rowe, J. H., Ertelt, J. M., Xin, L., and Way, S. S. (2012). *Listeria monocytogenes* cytoplasmic entry induces fetal wastage by disrupting maternal Foxp3+ regulatory T cell-sustained fetal tolerance. *PLoS Pathog.* 8:e1002873. doi: 10.1371/journal.ppat.1002873

Samuel, L. P., Balada-Llasat, J. M., Harrington, A., and Cavagnolo, R. (2016). Multicenter assessment of gram stain error rates. *J. Clin. Microbiol.* 54, 1442–1447. doi: 10.1128/JCM.03066-15

Smith, M. A., Takeuchi, K., Anderson, G., Ware, G. O., McClure, H. M., Raybourne, R. B., et al. (2008). Dose-response model for *Listeria monocytogenes*-induced stillbirths in nonhuman primates. *Infect. Immun.* 76, 726–731. doi: 10.1128/IAI.01366-06

Smith, M. A., Takeuchi, K., Brackett, R. E., McClure, H. M., Raybourne, R. B., Williams, K. M., et al. (2003). Nonhuman primate model for *Listeria monocytogenes*-induced stillbirths. *Infect. Immun.* 71, 1574–1579. doi: 10.1128/IAI.71.3.1574-1579.2003

Snyder-Mackler, N., Sanz, J., Kohn, J. N., Brinkworth, J. F., Morrow, S., Shaver, A. O., et al. (2016). Social status alters immune regulation and response to infection in macaques. *Science* 354, 1041–1045. doi: 10.1126/science.aah3580

Tappero, J. W., Schuchat, A., Deaver, K. A., Mascola, L., and Wenger, J. D. (1995). Reduction in the incidence of human listeriosis in the United States. Effectiveness of prevention efforts? the listeriosis study group. *JAMA.* 273, 1118–1122. doi: 10.1001/jama.1995.03520380054035

Tarantal, A. F., and Hendrickx, A. G. (1988). Characterization of prenatal growth and development the crab-eating macaque (Macaca fascicularis) by ultrasound. *Anat. Rec.* 222, 177–184. doi: 10.1002/ar.1092220210

Vázquez-Boland, J. A., Kuhn, M., Berche, P., Chakraborty, T., Dominguez-Bernal, G., Goebel, W., et al. (2001). Listeria pathogenesis and molecular virulence determinants. *Clin. Microbiol. Rev.* 14, 584–640. doi: 10.1128/CMR.14.3.584-640.2001

Wadhwa, D. R., and Smith, M. A. (2017). Pregnancy-related listeriosis. *Birth Defects Res.* 109, 324–335. doi: 10.1002/bdr2.1012

Wolfe, B., Wiepz, G. J., Schotzko, M., Bondarenko, G. I., Durning, M., Simmons, H. A., et al. (2017). Acute fetal demise with first trimester maternal infection resulting from *Listeria monocytogenes* in a nonhuman primate model. *mBio.* 8. doi: 10.1128/mBio.01938-16

World Health Organization (2018). *Fact Sheets: Listeriosis.* Available online at: https://www.who.int/news-room/fact-sheets/detail/listeriosis (accessed February 20, 2018).

4

Maternal-Fetal Conflict during Infection: Lessons from a Mouse Model of Placental Malaria

*Yash Pandya and Carlos Penha-Gonçalves**

Instituto Gulbenkian de Ciência, Oeiras, Portugal

***Correspondence:**
Carlos Penha-Gonçalves
cpenha@igc.gulbenkian.pt

Infections that reach the placenta via maternal blood can target the fetal-placental barrier and are associated with reduced birth weight, increased stillbirth, miscarriage and perinatal mortality. Malaria during pregnancy can lead to infection of the placental tissue and to adverse effects on the unborn child even if the parasite is successfully cleared, indicating that placental sufficiency is significantly compromised. Human samples and animal models of placental malaria have been used to unravel mechanisms contributing to this insufficiency and have implicated molecular pathways related to inflammation, innate immunity and nutrient transport. Remarkably, fetal TLR4 was found to take part in placental responses that protect the fetus, in contrast to maternal TLR4 responses that presumably preserve the mother's health but result in reduced fetal viability. We propose that this conflict of fetal and maternal responses is a determinant of the clinical outcomes of placental malaria and that fetally derived trophoblasts are on the front lines of this conflict.

Keywords: placenta, malaria, maternal-fetal conflict, toll-like receptors, pregnancy

1. INTRODUCTION

Pregnant women are at a higher risk of malaria infection (Espinosa et al., 2000; Lindsay et al., 2000). Infection by *Plasmodium falciparum* contributes to adverse outcomes including premature delivery, intra-uterine growth restriction, stillbirth and perinatal death alongside worsened maternal anemia and increased maternal parasite loads (Menendez et al., 2000; Crocker et al., 2004). These outcomes have been found to occur in pregnancies several months after clearance of the parasite, illustrating that treatment of the infection alone may be of little benefit (Schmiegelow et al., 2017).

Placental infection is a key determinant of these outcomes and the molecular basis of placental malaria pathology has been intensively studied (recently reviewed by Fried and Duffy, 2017). Parasite sequestration in the placenta is the primary pathological event, and, in the case of *Plasmodium falciparum*, is primarily mediated by infected erythrocytes binding to chondroitin sulfate A on the surface of syncytiotrophoblasts (Fried and Duffy, 1996; Abrams et al., 2003; Miller et al., 2013; Moya-Alvarez et al., 2014). Interactions between infected erythrocytes and placental tissue trigger significant infiltration of maternal inflammatory cells (Fried and Duffy, 2017) and alterations in the profile of cytokines secreted in the placenta, namely increases in TNFα and IFN-γ which are linked to adverse pregnancy outcomes (Moormann et al., 1999; Muehlenbachs et al., 2007).

Placentas from infected women show functional alterations including reduction in the activity of system A, a group of sodium dependent amino acid transporters which actively uptake small amino acids into the trophoblast layer (Boeuf et al., 2013). Placental glucose transporter activity is reduced when infection is accompanied by intervillositis (Chandrasiri et al., 2013). Malaria also reduces placental megalin, a transporter for a vast array of proteins (Lybbert et al., 2016). These nutrient transport pathways depend on an adequate placental blood supply to function effectively and placentas from women infected with malaria exhibit reduced placental perfusion (Dorman et al., 2002; Brabin and Johnson, 2005), impaired trophoblast invasion (Umbers et al., 2013), and alterations in various angiogenic factors within the placenta (Ataíde et al., 2015) which corroborates suboptimal placental perfusion.

More recently, a prospective study revealed that blood levels of L-arginine, a precursor to the potent vasodilator nitric oxide, were reduced in women with placental malaria while levels of dimethylarginine, an inhibitor of nitric oxide biosynthesis, were increased. These changes were strongly correlated with worse birth outcomes (McDonald et al., 2018). Earlier studies have highlighted a potential role for vascular endothelial growth factor (VEGF) and its receptors in the response to placental malaria in primigravid mothers, with soluble receptors for VEGF being more abundantly expressed in the placenta. This further implicates circulatory impairments in the disease pathology and provides the first evidence that placental responses to infection may not be in harmony with maternal responses, as maternal cells in the placenta showed elevated VEGF levels whereas fetal syncytiotrophoblasts produced more sVEGFR1, reducing VEGF bioavailability (Muehlenbachs et al., 2006).

These findings suggest that the intertwining of inflammatory signals, vasoregulatory systems, and nutrient transport pathways in the placenta are critical components of human placental malaria pathophysiology. However, experimental demonstration of the pathogenic mechanisms operating in the placenta relies on available mouse models of disease. In this perspective article we explore evidence generated from a mouse model of acute placental malaria that highlights the role of toll-like receptor 4 (TLR4) in controlling the outcomes of pregnancy ergo providing an interesting example of infection provoking conflict between the mother and the unborn child.

2. PATHOGENESIS OF MURINE ACUTE PLACENTAL MALARIA

Several murine experimental systems have been used to model specific aspects of malaria in pregnancy, but extrapolations to human disease should be considered with caution (Hviid et al., 2010). These experimental systems model different aspects of malaria in pregnancy, including: use of recrudescent *Plasmodium berghei* ANKA to study maternal susceptibility to infection (Marinho et al., 2009); a system using *P. berghei* K173 strains to infect mice both prior to and during gestation as would occur in high transmission settings (Van Zon and Eling, 1980); and a system making use of *Plasmodium chabaudi* which allows for the study of infections in early stages of pregnancy (Poovassery et al., 2009). Here, we will focus on a model which makes use of *Plasmodium berghei* infection during gestation and which models acute malaria during pregnancy in women. Briefly, infecting naïve, primigravid BALB/c females with 10^6 *P. berghei ANKA* infected erythrocytes intra-venously on the 13th day of gestation results in severe disease outcomes, such as intra-uterine growth restriction, decreased fetal viability, post-natal growth impairment and increased maternal parasitemia and anemia (Neres et al., 2008). Similar results are obtained with the use of the NK65, K173 and ANKApm4 lines of *P. berghei* in primigravid C57BL/6 mice, following the same mating and dosage protocols (Rodrigues-Duarte et al., 2012). Examination of the placentas with acute infection revealed an accumulation of infected erythrocytes and hemozoin in the blood sinusoids (Sharma et al., 2012b), thickening of the labyrinthine zone, deposits of hemozoin, fibrinoid necrosis, hyperplasia of the syncytiotrophoblasts, reduced blood sinusoid area, and a significant infiltration of maternal macrophages and monocytes (Neres et al., 2008).

This model has allowed investigation of the underpinnings of placental dysfunction, particularly by linking inflammatory responses to alterations in angiogenic and vasoregulatory pathways. This is illustrated by descriptions of increases in the amounts of angiopoietin 1 and in the ratio of angiopoietin 1 to angiopoietin 2 in infected placentas belonging to viable, low birth weight offspring (Silver et al., 2010) as well as by the reduced expression of bradykinin receptor B2 and NOS3 genes, both known to be involved in vasodilatory responses (de Moraes et al., 2018). Human studies have also revealed that infection with *P. falciparum* during pregnancy increases levels of these angiopoietins and complement C5a while reducing nitric oxide bioavailability (Conroy et al., 2013; McDonald et al., 2018). Genetically ablating C5a receptor in mice infected with *P. berghei* during pregnancy increased placental vascular branching and ameliorated the increase in resistance to flow caused by infection (Conroy et al., 2013). Similar results were obtained by dietary supplementation with L-arginine, a nitric oxide precursor (McDonald et al., 2018). Furthermore, intra-vital imaging (Lima et al., 2014) has revealed how infected erythrocytes accumulate in areas of slower flow in the placental labyrinth, possibly adhering to, or being phagocytosed by, the syncytiotrophoblasts and suggesting that infection impairs local circulatory regulation (de Moraes et al., 2013). Additionally, oxidative stress has been implicated in malaria during pregnancy, with a combination of increased lipid perodixation (Sharma et al., 2012a), decreased catalase activity and increases in apoptosis markers being observed in the placentas of infected mice while the absence of alterations in Fas expression and Caspase 8 indicate that the damage caused is primarily via the mitochondrial pathway of apoptosis (Sharma et al., 2012b). Treating the infected mice with chloroquine or with sulfadoxine pyrimethamine abrogated oxidative stress, apoptosis, and placental damage, consequently improving birth weight. Interestingly, anti-malarial treatment of mice with placental malaria did not improve fetal survival, indicating that placental insufficiency is not recoverable by parasite clearance alone (Sharma and Shukla, 2014). This raises the possibility that innate immune stimulation during pregnancy results in enduring placental dysfunction. Here, we argue that responses mediated by Toll-like receptors (TLRs), particularly

TLR4, have a decisive impact on the development of placental pathologies during infection.

3. TLR4, MALARIA, AND PREGNANCY

TLRs are a class of pattern recognition receptors involved in the detection of, and in the response to, pathogen and damage associated molecular patterns (PAMPs and DAMPs) by activation of downstream signaling pathways which induce immunity mediators including pro-inflammatory cytokines and interferons. TLR signaling makes use of either of two adaptor proteins, MyD88 or TRIF, with TLR4 being unique in its ability to use both of these pathways (**Figure 1D**) (Lu et al., 2008; Kawasaki and Kawai, 2014).

TLRs play a significant role in the response to malaria infection, participating in the recognition of glycosylphosphatidylinositol anchors, peroxiredoxin and fibrinogen/hemozoin complexes as well as host derived microvesicles and heme (Eriksson et al., 2014; Gazzinelli et al., 2014) (**Figure 1C**). TLR4 polymorphisms have also been associated with disease severity, particularly the hyporesponsive polymorphisms *Tlr4* Asp299Gly and *Tlr4* Thr399Ile which predispose children to severe malaria (Schmitt et al., 2002; Mockenhaupt et al., 2006a). However, contrasting results suggested that these polymorphisms may be beneficial in adults (Esposito et al., 2012; Basu et al., 2014) and a recent meta-analysis found no association between *Tlr4* Asp299Gly and the outcomes of malaria (Dhangadamajhi et al., 2017). In mice, TLR4 has been implicated in dendritic and mast cell activation during malaria (Furuta et al., 2008; Seixas et al., 2009), potentially contributing to the resistance of DBA/2 mice to infection with *P. yoelii*, although TLR4 has not been linked to the pathology of experimental cerebral malaria (Togbe et al., 2007).

3.1. TLR4 in Pregnancy

Several TLRs are expressed in fetally derived placental tissues and surrounding maternal tissue Koga and Mor (2010) but cumulative evidence suggests a specific role for TLR4 in the outcomes of pregnancy. It has been observed that fetoplacental TLR4 expression is decreased in miscarriages (Kolben et al., 2019) and in preeclampsia patients (Kulikova et al., 2016), while the *Tlr4* Asp299Gly polymorphism in the fetus is associated with severe prematurity (Rey et al., 2008). In contrast, increases in TLR4 expression on maternal monocytes, which may be responding to fibrinogen, are correlated with spontaneous preterm labor (Pawelczyk et al., 2010; Al-ofi et al., 2014), and increased expression in maternal decidua has been linked to recurrent miscarriages (Li et al., 2016). These data suggest that the role of maternal and fetal TLR4 in pregnancy may be in opposition, with reductions in fetal activity and/or increases in maternal activity being detrimental to the outcomes of the pregnancy.

Various mouse models have illustrated the role of TLR4 in pregnancy associated infections and disorders, including malaria (Barboza et al., 2017; Rodrigues-Duarte et al., 2018), bacterial infections (Liu et al., 2007; Arce et al., 2012; Chin et al., 2016), lipopolysaccharide exposure (Breen et al., 2012; Wahid et al., 2015) and uterine ischemia (Thaete et al., 2013). It should be noted that these studies (barring that by Rodrigues-Duarte et al., 2018) have focused on completely eliminating TLR4 signaling and, consequently, do not differentiate between fetal and maternal TLR4 responses. Furthermore, increased fetal TLR4 activity has been found in models of maternal ethanol-induced inflammation (Zheng et al., 2014) as well as in maternal cigarette smoke exposure (Chan et al., 2016). These studies support that maternal factors may be contributing to alterations in fetal innate immune responses as well as having direct impacts on the outcomes of pregnancy. Still, in all of these cases, the downstream actions of TLR4 are yet to be fully understood.

3.2. TLR4 in Placental Malaria

The role of TLR4 in malaria during pregnancy has also been examined in genetic association studies. The *Tlr4* Asp299Gly and *Tlr4* Thr399Ile maternal polymorphisms appeared more frequently in women who had a higher parasitemia and severe anemia, and translated to a significantly increased risk of low birth weight. They had no impact on prematurity, viability or the incidence of placental malaria (Mockenhaupt et al., 2006b), suggesting that maternal TLR4 takes part in responding to infection, but may not be linked to severe placental dysfunction during malaria. In mice, examination of TLR4 was preceded by work on MyD88, which was shown to contribute to reductions in placental vascular space and fetal weight (Barboza et al., 2014). Genetic ablation of several TLRs which use this adaptor protein demonstrated that alterations in vascular space, TNFα production and detrimental outcomes are directly linked to TLR4 (Barboza et al., 2017).

Genetic ablation of TLR4 confers striking protection from fetal death induced in murine placental malaria. The roles played by fetally derived placental cells in protecting fetal viability were discerned by comparing pregnancy outcomes when the fetal placenta either expressed TLR4 or did not. As expected, we observed improvements in fetal viability in TLR4KO females which were carrying TLR4KO offspring, suggesting that the TLR4 response to infection was deleterious to the fetuses, as observed in the other mouse models of disease during pregnancy mentioned above. Unexpectedly, TLR4KO females carrying placentas expressing fetally derived TLR4 showed further improvements in the outcomes of pregnancy with stillbirth rates similar to those of uninfected mothers (Rodrigues-Duarte et al., 2018). This showed that TLR4 in the fetal compartment was protective for the litter, whereas having it in the maternal compartment was harmful, a conflict which is yet to be investigated in other infections. Although the mechanism behind this protection has not been fully elucidated, alterations in glucose (Chandrasiri et al., 2013) and amino acid (Boeuf et al., 2013) transport, observed using human samples from malaria infected individuals, suggest that a conflict may arise over the allocation of metabolic resources. On the other hand, altered nitric oxide bioavailability (McDonald et al., 2018) and VEGF levels further point toward a role for fetal TLR4 responses in regulating placental perfusion.

While other models of infection during pregnancy have not yet been interrogated in a manner which allows for the

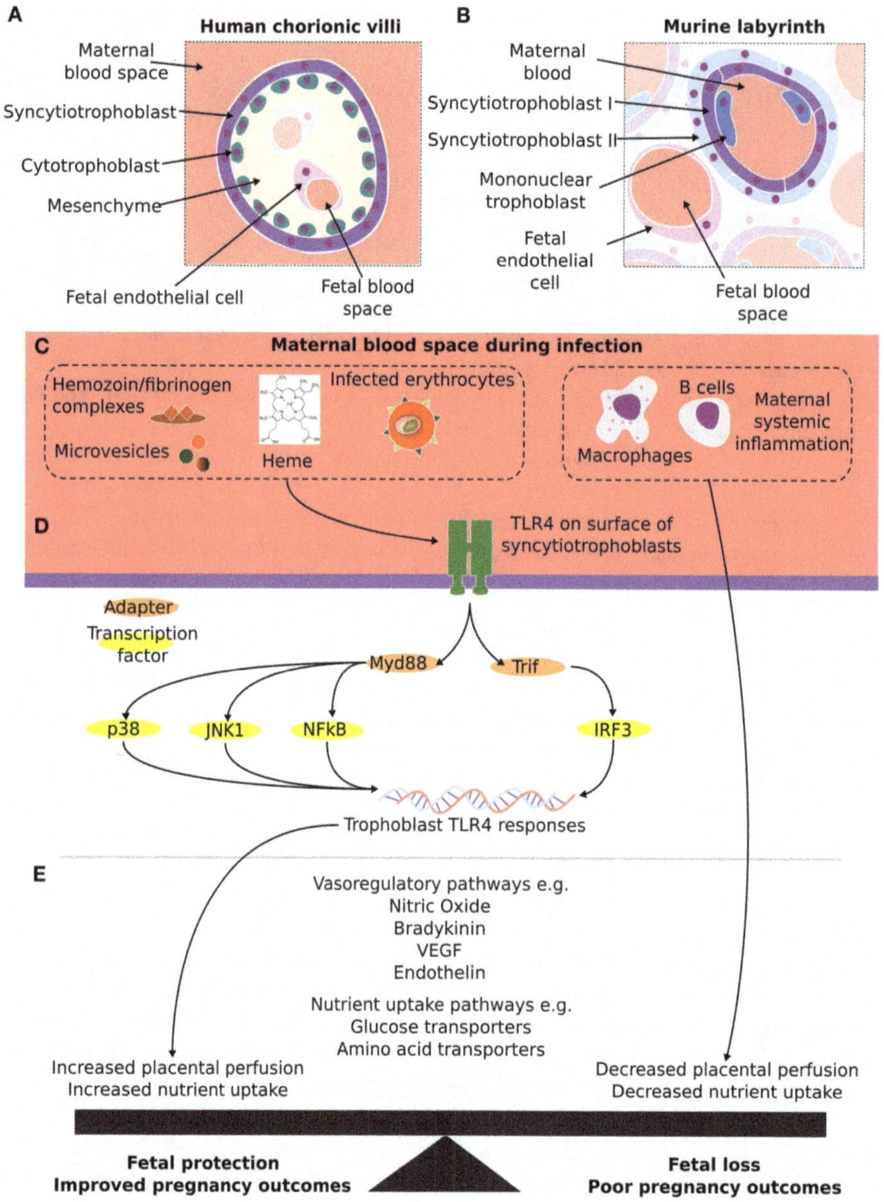

FIGURE 1 | (A) Cross section of a human placental terminal chorionic villus, which is part of highly branched tree of fetally derived tissue anchored in the chorionic plate and surrounded by maternal blood. At the terminal chorionic villi, the placental barrier is composed by the endothelial cells enclosed in mesenchyme followed by a layer of cytotrophoblasts and an outermost layer of syncytiotrophoblasts in contact with maternal blood. **(B)** Cross section of the analogous murine tissue, the placental labyrinth where the maternal fetal barrier is made up of a layer of fetal capillary endothelial cells, two layers of syncytiotrophoblasts and a discontinuous layer of mononuclear trophoblasts that is in direct contact with maternal blood. **(C)** In both the human and murine placentas, fetally derived syncytiotrophoblasts come into direct contact with maternal blood, an important similarity, as during a malaria infection, these are the fetal cells exposed to maternal inflammatory mediators and to components of parasite origin such as infected erythrocytes and microvesicles. **(D)** TLR4 detects and responds to several of these stimuli via either MyD88 or TRIF, activating several transcriptional factors including p38 and IRF3. **(E)** Transcriptional changes in the syncytiotrophoblast contribute to alterations in local production of vasoactivators such as nitric oxide, bradykinin and endothelin as well as altering nutrient transport pathways in a manner which result in fetal protection. In contrast, maternal responses impair these pathways and worsen the outcomes of pregnancy.

disentanglement of fetal and maternal responses, there are strong similarities between the impact of malaria infection on placental TLR4 and the impact of a variety of other pathogens. In wild type mice infected with *P. berghei*, the amount of TLR4 protein detected in the placenta is significantly increased (Barboza et al., 2017), a pattern which is replicated with *Campylobacter rectus*, *Porphyromonas gingivalis* (Arce et al., 2009) and murine cytomegalovirus infections (Liao et al., 2018). It would be particularly important to determine if the maternal component is responsible for the outcomes of these infections and assess the impact of maintaining the fetal response. Bearing in mind that the first point of contact for fetally derived TLR4 with infectious agents in the maternal blood is at the placental barrier, examining fetally derived placental cells may be key to better understand the conflict with maternal responses.

4. PRIMARY TROPHOBLAST RESPONSES TO INFECTION

The fetal cell type directly in contact with maternal blood in both humans and mice are the syncytiotrophoblasts. They are responsible for the exchange of nutrients and waste, as well as forming the barrier between maternal and fetal circulation (Zeldovich et al., 2013; Blackburn, 2015; Maltepe and Fisher, 2015) (**Figures 1A,B**). While TLRs are found in fetally derived cells in the placenta (Koga and Mor, 2010), their expression and activity is greatly altered in placental cell lines, showing a lack of suitability for examining certain aspects of trophoblast behavior (Amirchaghmaghi et al., 2013; Gierman et al., 2015), and highlighting a requirement for the employment of primary cultures.

Although they are rarely used for studies with malaria (Lucchi et al., 2006, 2008), primary human trophoblasts have been successfully isolated and used to examine responses to a variety of infectious agents such as *Brucella spp.*, zika virus and *Toxoplasma gondii* (Salcedo et al., 2013; Aagaard et al., 2017; Ander et al., 2018), the latter being further examined in villous explants (Ander et al., 2018). This experimental system has also been used to study *Trypanosoma cruzi* infection (Díaz-Luján et al., 2016; Medina et al., 2018; Triquell et al., 2018), which is known to provoke changes in several immune related genes during pregnancy (Juiz et al., 2018). Trophoblasts are reported to show changes in amino acid and glucose uptake in response to lipopolysaccharide (a TLR4 ligand) (Liong and Lappas, 2017), pathways which are also altered in human placental malaria samples (Boeuf et al., 2013; Chandrasiri et al., 2013). Therefore, the use of primary human trophoblasts to study responses to malaria infection may provide insights into the pathology of placental malaria.

As an alternative, murine trophoblasts, isolated from term placentas or of stem cell origin, represent a powerful tool for studying infection during pregnancy. TLR4 responses have been examined in cell culture studies using *P. berghei*. These studies have revealed a reduction in the amount of trophoblast-associated parasite in absence of TLR4 as well as marked reduction in the expression of *Ifnar1* in these cells (Rodrigues-Duarte et al., 2018). Along the same lines, *Listeria monocytogenes* has been shown to be taken up by trophoblast giant cells in a MAPK dependent manner, using innate sensing systems heavily influenced by TLR2, subsequently downregulating HO-1 and resulting in cell death (Hashino et al., 2015). In a study not linked to TLRs, trophoblasts exposed to *Toxoplasma gondii* have been demonstrated to undergo apoptosis as well as alter production of various cytokines, with increased oxidative stress and subsequent mitochondrial damage (Liu et al., 2013; Xu et al., 2015). Thus, it is clear that trophoblasts respond to pathogens infecting maternal blood, raising the interesting possibility that they are the initiators of fetal protective responses in placental infections, particularly when the pathogens do not cross the placental barrier.

5. CONCLUDING REMARKS

It is expected that a variety of pathways are impacted upon during placental infection, affecting inflammatory responses, nutrient transport and vasoregulatory responses, and contributing to placental insufficiency that leads to poor pregnancy outcomes. A key finding from the acute murine placental malaria model has been the importance of TLR4 in the determination of the outcomes of pregnancy. Interestingly, this trait is shared with several other models of disease in pregnancy that also show signs of placental dysfunction. The strong pathological similarities between these models supports the proposal that innate immune recognition by the placental tissue may improve fetal survival in other infections.

Taken together, the work highlighted here leads us to propose that maternally driven TLR4 responses to malaria infections, and other illnesses during pregnancy, are deleterious for the fetus, impairing nutrient/waste exchange, hampering placental perfusion and worsening the outcomes of pregnancy. In contrast, feto-placental TLR4 responses are protective, as demonstrated by Rodrigues-Duarte et al. (2018) and may compensate for the maternal actions by activating mechanisms to increase nutrient uptake and placental perfusion (**Figure 1E**). This re-inforces the notion that malaria infection induces maternal-fetal conflict, as proposed by Muehlenbachs et al. (2006), in their examination of soluble VEGF receptor 1 in human placental malaria, but further hints that fetal responses which preserve placental function are initiated by innate immune recognition and downstream signaling to effector mediators in trophoblasts.

The syncytiotrophoblasts are at the front line of this conflict between mother and fetus and their examination, using *in vitro* and *in vivo* experimental systems, as well as in human tissue samples, will be required for the identification of critical components of the fetal protective responses. Making use of the vast range of existing genetic mouse models in conjunction with the gamut of infection systems which have been developed for the study of pathological pregnancies, will provide a clearer understanding of the mechanisms that protect from adverse outcomes of pregnancy.

AUTHOR CONTRIBUTIONS

YP contributed to writing the paper. CP-G contributed to writing the paper.

REFERENCES

Aagaard, K. M., Lahon, A., Suter, M. A., Arya, R. P., Seferovic, M. D., Vogt, M. B., et al. (2017). Primary human placental trophoblasts are permissive for zika virus (ZIKV) replication. *Sci. Rep.* 7, 1–14. doi: 10.1038/srep41389

Abrams, E. T., Brown, H., Chensue, S. W., Turner, G. D., Tadesse, E., Lema, V. M., et al. (2003). Host response to malaria during pregnancy: placental monocyte recruitment is associated with elevated chemokine expression. *J. Immunol.* 170, 2759–2764. doi: 10.4049/jimmunol.170.5.2759

Al-ofi, E., Coffelt, S. B., and Anumba, D. O. (2014). Fibrinogen, an endogenous ligand of Toll-like receptor 4, activates monocytes in pre-eclamptic patients. *J. Reprod. Immunol.* 103, 23–28. doi: 10.1016/j.jri.2014.02.004

Amirchaghmaghi, E., Taghavi, S. A., Shapouri, F., Saeidi, S., Rezaei, A., and Aflatoonian, R. (2013). The role of toll like receptors in pregnancy. *Int. J. Fertil. Steril.* 7, 147–154.

Ander, S. E., Rudzki, E. N., Arora, N., Sadovsky, Y., Coyne, C. B., and Boyle, J. P. (2018). Human placental syncytiotrophoblasts restrict toxoplasma gondii attachment and replication and respond to infection by producing immunomodulatory chemokines. *MBio* 9, 1–14. doi: 10.1128/mBio.01678-17

Arce, R. M., Barros, S. P., Wacker, B., Peters, B., Moss, K., and Offenbacher, S. (2009). Increased TLR4 expression in murine placentas after oral infection with periodontal pathogens. *Placenta* 30, 156–162. doi: 10.1016/j.placenta.2008.11.017

Arce, R. M., Caron, K. M., Barros, S. P., and Offenbacher, S. (2012). Toll-like receptor 4 mediates intrauterine growth restriction after systemic Campylobacter rectus infection in mice. *Mol. Oral Microbiol.* 27, 373–381. doi: 10.1111/j.2041-1014.2012.00651.x

Ataíde, R., Murillo, O., Dombrowski, J. G., Souza, R. M., Lima, F. A., Lima, G. F. et al. (2015). Malaria in pregnancy interacts with and alters the angiogenic profiles of the placenta. *PLoS Negl. Trop. Dis.* 9:e0003824. doi: 10.1371/journal.pntd.0003824

Barboza, R., Lima, F. A., Reis, A. S., Murillo, O. J., Peixoto, E. P. M., Bandeira, C. L., et al. (2017). TLR4-mediated placental pathology and pregnancy outcome in experimental malaria. *Sci. Rep.* 7:8623. doi: 10.1038/s41598-017-08299-x

Barboza, R., Reis, A. S., da Silva, L. G., Hasenkamp, L., Pereira, K. R. B., Câmara, N. O. S., et al. (2014). MyD88 signaling is directly involved in the development of murine placental malaria. *Infect. Immun.* 82, 830–838. doi: 10.1128/IAI.01288-13

Basu, S., Hubbard, B., and Shevach, E. M. (2014). Foxp3-mediated inhibition of Akt inhibits Glut1 (glucose transporter 1) expression in human T regulatory cells. *J. Leukoc. Biol.* 97, 2–6. doi: 10.1189/jlb.2AB0514-273RR

Blackburn, D. G. (2015). Evolution of vertebrate viviparity and specializations for fetal nutrition: a quantitative and qualitative analysis. *J. Morphol.* 276, 961–990. doi: 10.1002/jmor.20272

Boeuf, P., Aitken, E. H., Chandrasiri, U., Chua, C. L., McInerney, B., McQuade, L., et al. (2013). Plasmodium falciparum malaria elicits inflammatory responses that dysregulate placental amino acid transport. *PLoS Pathog.* 9:e1003153. doi: 10.1371/journal.ppat.1003153

Brabin, B. J., and Johnson, P. M. (2005). Placental malaria and pre-eclampsia through the looking glass backwards? *J. Reprod. Immunol.* 65, 1–15. doi: 10.1016/j.jri.2004.09.006

Breen, K., Brown, A., Burd, I., Chai, J., Friedman, A., and Elovitz, M. A. (2012). TLR-4-dependent and -independent mechanisms of fetal brain injury in the setting of preterm birth. *Reprod. Sci.* 19, 839–850. doi: 10.1177/1933719112438439

Chan, Y. L., Saad, S., Pollock, C., Oliver, B., Al-Odat, I., Zaky, A. A., et al. (2016). Impact of maternal cigarette smoke exposure on brain inflammation and oxidative stress in male mice offspring. *Sci. Rep.* 6, 1–12. doi: 10.1038/srep25881

Chandrasiri, U. P., Chua, C. L., Umbers, A. J., Chaluluka, E., Glazier, J. D., Rogerson, S. J., et al. (2013). Insight into the pathogenesis of fetal growth restriction in placental malaria: decreased placental glucose transporter isoform 1 expression. *J. Infect. Dis.* 209, 1663–1667. doi: 10.1093/infdis/jit803

Chin, P. Y., Dorian, C. L., Hutchinson, M. R., Olson, D. M., Rice, K. C., Moldenhauer, L. M., et al. (2016). Novel toll-like receptor-4 antagonist (+)-naloxone protects mice from inflammation-induced preterm birth. *Sci. Rep.* 6, 1–13. doi: 10.1038/srep36112

Conroy, A. L., Silver, K. L., Zhong, K., Rennie, M., Ward, P., Sarma, J. V., et al. (2013). Complement activation and the resulting placental vascular insufficiency drives fetal growth restriction associated with placental malaria. *Cell Host Microbe* 13, 215–226. doi: 10.1016/j.chom.2013.01.010

Crocker, I. P., Tanner, O. M., Myers, J. E., Bulmer, J. N., Walraven, G., and Baker, P. N. (2004). Syncytiotrophoblast degradation and the pathophysiology of the malaria-infected placenta. *Placenta* 25, 273–282. doi: 10.1016/j.placenta.2003.09.010

de Moraes, L. V., Barateiro, A., Sousa, P. M., and Penha-Gonçalves, C. (2018). Bradykinin sequestration by plasmodium berghei infected erythrocytes conditions B2R signaling and parasite uptake by fetal trophoblasts. *Front. Microbiol.* 9:3106. doi: 10.3389/fmicb.2018.03106

de Moraes, L. V., Tadokoro, C. E., Gómez-Conde, I., Olivieri, D. N., and Penha-Gonçalves, C. (2013). Intravital placenta imaging reveals microcirculatory dynamics impact on sequestration and phagocytosis of Plasmodium-infected erythrocytes. *PLoS Pathog.* 9:e1003154. doi: 10.1371/journal.ppat.1003154

Dhangadamajhi, G., Kar, A., Rout, R., and Dhangadamajhi, P. (2017). A meta-analysis of TLR4 and TLR9 SNPs implicated in severe malaria. *Rev. Soc. Bras. Med. Trop.* 50, 153–160. doi: 10.1590/0037-8682-0475-2016

Díaz-Luján, C., Triquell, M. F., Castillo, C., Hardisson, D., Kemmerling, U., and Fretes, R. E. (2016). Role of placental barrier integrity in infection by *Trypanosoma cruzi*. *Acta Trop.* 164, 360–368. doi: 10.1016/j.actatropica.2016.09.021

Dorman, E. K., Shulman, C. E., Kingdom, J., Bulmer, J. N., Mwendwa, J., Peshu, N., and Marsh, K. (2002). Impaired uteroplacental blood flow in pregnancies complicated by falciparum malaria. *Ultrasound Obstet. Gynecol.* 19, 165–170. doi: 10.1046/j.0960-7692.2001.00545.x

Eriksson, E., Sampaio, Natália, G., and Schofield, L. (2014). Toll-like receptors and malaria - sensing and susceptibility. *J. Trop. Dis.* 2, 1–7. doi: 10.4172/2329-891X.1000126

Espinosa, F. M., Alecrim, W. D., and Daniel-Ribeiro, C. T. (2000). Attraction of mosquitoes to pregnant women. *Lancet* 356:685. doi: 10.1016/S0140-6736(05)73838-1

Esposito, S., Molteni, C. G., Zampiero, A., Baggi, E., Lavizzari, A., Semino, M., et al. (2012). Role of polymorphisms of toll-like receptor (TLR) 4, TLR9, toll-interleukin 1 receptor domain containing adaptor protein (TIRAP) and FCGR2A genes in malaria susceptibility and severity in Burundian children. *Malar. J.* 11:196. doi: 10.1186/1475-2875-11-196

Fried, M., and Duffy, P. E. (1996). Adherence of plasmodium falciparum to chondroitin sulfate A in the human placenta. *Science* 272, 1502–1504. doi: 10.1126/science.272.5267.1502

Fried, M., and Duffy, P. E. (2017). Malaria during pregnancy. *Cold Spring Harb. Perspect. Med.* 7:a025551. doi: 10.1101/cshperspect.a025551

Furuta, T., Imajo-Ohmi, S., Fukuda, H., Kano, S., Miyake, K., and Watanabe, N. (2008). Mast cell-mediated immune responses through IgE antibody and Toll-like receptor 4 by malarial peroxiredoxin. *Eur. J. Immunol.* 38, 1341–1350. doi: 10.1002/eji.200738059

Gazzinelli, R. T., Kalantari, P., Fitzgerald, K. A., and Golenbock, D. T. (2014). Innate sensing of malaria parasites. *Nat. Rev. Immunol.* 14, 744–757. doi: 10.1038/nri3742

Gierman, L. M., Stødle, G. S., Tangerås, L. H., Austdal, M., Olsen, G. D., Follestad, T., et al. (2015). Toll-like receptor profiling of seven trophoblast cell lines warrants caution for translation to primary trophoblasts. *Placenta* 36, 1246–1253. doi: 10.1016/j.placenta.2015.09.004

Hashino, M., Tachibana, M., Nishida, T., Hara, H., Tsuchiya, K., Mitsuyama, M., et al. (2015). Inactivation of the MAPK signaling pathway by Listeria monocytogenes infection promotes trophoblast giant cell death. *Front. Microbiol.* 6:1145. doi: 10.3389/fmicb.2015.01145

Hviid, L., Marinho, C. R., Staalsoe, T., and Penha-Gonçalves, C. (2010). Of mice and women: rodent models of placental malaria. *Trends Parasitol.* 26, 412–419. doi: 10.1016/j.pt.2010.04.010

Juiz, N. A., Torrejón, I., Burgos, M., Torres, A. M., Duffy, T., Cayo, N. M., et al. (2018). Alterations in placental gene expression of pregnant women with chronic chagas disease. *Am. J. Pathol.* 188, 1345–1353. doi: 10.1016/j.ajpath.2018.02.011

Kawasaki, T., and Kawai, T. (2014). Toll-like receptor signaling pathways. *Front. Immunol.* 5:461. doi: 10.3389/fimmu.2014.00461

Koga, K., and Mor, G. (2010). Toll-like receptors at the maternal-fetal interface in normal pregnancy and pregnancy disorders. *Am. J. Reprod. Immunol.* 63, 587–600. doi: 10.1111/j.1600-0897.2010.00848.x

Kolben, T. M., Rogatsch, E., Hester, A., Kuhn, C., Schmoeckel, E., Czogalla, B., et al. (2019). Involvement of ILR4α and TLR4 in miscarriages. *J. Reprod. Immunol.* 131, 36–43. doi: 10.1016/j.jri.2018.12.001

Kulikova, G. V., Nizyaeva, N. V., Nagovitsina, M. N., Lyapin, V. M., Loginova, N. S., Kan, N. E., et al. (2016). Specific features of TLR4 expression in structural elements of placenta in patients with preeclampsia. *Bull. Exp. Biol. Med.* 160, 718–721. doi: 10.1007/s10517-016-3259-8

Li, P., Wu, H. L., and Dong, B. H. (2016). Relationship between TLR4 and CCL2 expression and recurrent spontaneous abortion. *Genet. Mol. Res.* 15, 1–8. doi: 10.4238/gmr.15016882

Liao, Y., nan Zhang, Y., lou Liu, X., yuan Lu, Y., lin Zhang, L., Xi, T., et al. (2018). Maternal murine cytomegalovirus infection during pregnancy up-regulates the gene expression of toll-like receptor 2 and 4 in placenta. *Curr. Med. Sci.* 38, 632–639. doi: 10.1007/s11596-018-1924-z

Lima, F. A., Gómez-Conde, I., Videira, P. A., Marinho, C. R., Olivieri, D. N., and Tadokoro, C. E. (2014). Intravital microscopy technique to study parasite dynamics in the labyrinth layer of the mouse placenta. *Parasitol. Int.* 63, 254–259. doi: 10.1016/j.parint.2013.06.012

Lindsay, S., Ansell, J., Selman, C., Cox, V., Hamilton, K., and Walraven, G. (2000). Effect of pregnancy on exposure to malaria mosquitoes. *Lancet* 355:1972. doi: 10.1016/S0140-6736(00)02334-5

Liong, S., and Lappas, M. (2017). Lipopolysaccharide and double stranded viral RNA mediate insulin resistance and increase system a amino acid transport in human trophoblast cells *in vitro*. *Placenta* 51, 18–27. doi: 10.1016/j.placenta.2017.01.124

Liu, H., Redline, R. W., and Han, Y. W. (2007). Fusobacterium nucleatum induces fetal death in mice via stimulation of TLR4-mediated placental inflammatory response. *J. Immunol.* 179, 2501–2508. doi: 10.4049/jimmunol.179.4.2501

Liu, T., Zhang, Q., Liu, L., Xu, X., Chen, H., Wang, H., et al. (2013). Trophoblast apoptosis through polarization of macrophages induced by Chinese Toxoplasma gondii isolates with different virulence in pregnant mice. *Parasitol. Res.* 112, 3019–3027. doi: 10.1007/s00436-013-3475-3

Lu, Y. C., Yeh, W. C., and Ohashi, P. S. (2008). LPS/TLR4 signal transduction pathway. *Cytokine* 42, 145–151. doi: 10.1016/j.cyto.2008.01.006

Lucchi, N. W., Koopman, R., Peterson, D. S., and Moore, J. M. (2006). Plasmodium falciparum-infected red blood cells selected for binding to cultured syncytiotrophoblast bind to chondroitin sulfate A and induce tyrosine phosphorylation in the syncytiotrophoblast. *Placenta* 27, 384–394. doi: 10.1016/j.placenta.2005.04.009

Lucchi, N. W., Peterson, D. S., and Moore, J. M. (2008). Immunologic activation of human syncytiotrophoblast by *Plasmodium falciparum*. *Malar J.* 7:42. doi: 10.1186/1475-2875-7-42

Lybbert, J., Gullingsrud, J., Chesnokov, O., Turyakira, E., Dhorda, M., Guerin, P. J., et al. (2016). Abundance of megalin and Dab2 is reduced in syncytiotrophoblast during placental malaria, which may contribute to low birth weight. *Sci. Rep.* 6:24508. doi: 10.1038/srep24508

Maltepe, E., and Fisher, S. J. (2015). Placenta: the forgotten organ. *Annu. Rev. Cell Dev. Biol.* 31, 523–552. doi: 10.1146/annurev-cellbio-100814-125620

Marinho, C. R., Neres, R., Epiphanio, S., Gonçalves, L. A., Catarino, M. B., and Penha-Gonçalves, C. (2009). Recrudescent Plasmodium berghei from pregnant mice displays enhanced binding to the placenta and induces protection in multigravida. *PLoS ONE* 4:e5630. doi: 10.1371/journal.pone.0005630

McDonald, C. R., Cahill, L. S., Gamble, J. R., Elphinstone, R., Gazdzinski, L. M., Zhong, K. J., et al. (2018). Malaria in pregnancy alters l-arginine bioavailability and placental vascular development. *Sci. Transl. Med.* 10:eaan6007. doi: 10.1126/scitranslmed.aan6007

Medina, L., Castillo, C., Liempi, A., Herbach, M., Cabrera, G., Valenzuela, L., et al. (2018). Differential infectivity of two Trypanosoma cruzi strains in placental cells and tissue. *Acta Trop.* 186, 35–40. doi: 10.1016/j.actatropica.2018.07.001

Menendez, C., Ordi, J., Ismail, M. R., Ventura, P. J., Aponte, J. J., Kahigwa, E., et al. (2000). The impact of placental malaria on gestational age and birth weight. *J. Infect. Dis.* 181, 1740–1745. doi: 10.1086/315449

Miller, L. H., Ackerman, H. C., Su, X. z., and Wellems, T. E. (2013). Malaria biology and disease pathogenesis: insights for new treatments. *Nat. Med.* 19, 156–167. doi: 10.1038/nm.3073

Mockenhaupt, F. P., Cramer, J. P., Hamann, L., Stegemann, M. S., Eckert, J., Oh, N. R., et al. (2006a). Toll-like receptor (TLR) polymorphisms in African children: common TLR-4 variants predispose to severe malaria. *Proc. Natl. Acad. Sci. U.S.A.* 103, 177–182. doi: 10.1073/pnas.0506803102

Mockenhaupt, F. P., Hamann, L., von Gaertner, C., Bedu-Addo, G., von Kleinsorgen, C., Schumann, R. R., et al. (2006b). Common polymorphisms of toll-Like receptors 4 and 9 are associated with the clinical manifestation of malaria during pregnancy. *J. Infect. Dis.* 194, 184–188. doi: 10.1086/505152

Moormann, A. M., Sullivan, A. D., Rochford, R. A., Chensue, S. W., Bock, P. J., Nyirenda, T., et al. (1999). Malaria and pregnancy: placental cytokine expression and its relationship to intrauterine growth retardation. *J. Infect. Dis.* 180, 1987–1993. doi: 10.1086/315135

Moya-Alvarez, V., Abellana, R., and Cot, M. (2014). Pregnancy-associated malaria and malaria in infants: an old problem with present consequences. *Malar. J.* 13:271. doi: 10.1186/1475-2875-13-271

Muehlenbachs, A., Fried, M., Lachowitzer, J., Mutabingwa, K., and Duffy, P. E. (2007). Genome-wide expression analysis of placental malaria reveals features of lymphoid neogenesis during chronic infection. *J. Immunol.* 179, 557–565. doi: 10.4049/jimmunol.179.1.557

Muehlenbachs, A., Mutabingwa, T. K., Edmonds, S., Fried, M., and Duffy, P. E. (2006). Hypertension and maternal-fetal conflict during placental malaria. *PLoS Med.* 3:e446. doi: 10.1371/journal.pmed.0030446

Neres, R., Marinho, C. R., Gonçalves, L. A., Catarino, M. B., and Penha-Gonçalves, C. (2008). Pregnancy outcome and placenta pathology in *Plasmodium berghei* ANKA infected mice reproduce the pathogenesis of severe malaria in pregnant women. *PLoS ONE* 3:e1608. doi: 10.1371/journal.pone.0001608

Pawelczyk, E., Nowicki, B. J., Izban, M. G., Pratap, S., Sashti, N. A., Sanderson, M., et al. (2010). Spontaneous preterm labor is associated with an increase in the proinflammatory signal transducer TLR4 receptor on maternal blood monocytes. *BMC Pregnancy Childbirth* 10:66. doi: 10.1186/1471-2393-10-66

Poovassery, J. S., Sarr, D., Smith, G., Nagy, T., and Moore, J. M. (2009). Malaria-induced murine pregnancy failure: distinct roles for IFN- and TNF. *J. Immunol.* 183, 5342–5349. doi: 10.4049/jimmunol.0901669

Rey, G., Skowronek, F., Alciaturi, J., Alonso, J., Bertoni, B., and Sapiro, R. (2008). Toll receptor 4 Asp299Gly polymorphism and its association with preterm birth and premature rupture of membranes in a South American population. *Mol. Hum. Reprod.* 14, 555–559. doi: 10.1093/molehr/gan049

Rodrigues-Duarte, L., de Moraes, L. V., Barboza, R., Marinho, C. R., Franke-Fayard, B., Janse, C. J., et al. (2012). Distinct placental malaria pathology caused by different Plasmodium berghei lines that fail to induce cerebral malaria in the C57BL/6 mouse. *Malar. J.* 11:231. doi: 10.1186/1475-2875-11-231

Rodrigues-Duarte, L., Pandya, Y., Neres, R., and Penha-Gonçalves, C. (2018). Fetal and maternal innate immunity receptors have opposing effects in severity of experimental malaria in pregnancy: beneficial roles for fetal-derived TLR4 and IFNAR1. *Infect. Immun.* 86:e00708-17. doi: 10.1128/IAI.00708-17

Salcedo, S. P., Chevrier, N., Lacerda, T. L., Ben Amara, A., Gerart, S., Gorvel, V. A., et al. (2013). Pathogenic brucellae replicate in human trophoblasts. *J. Infect. Dis.* 207, 1075–1083. doi: 10.1093/infdis/jit007

Schmiegelow, C., Matondo, S., Minja, D. T. R., Resende, M., Pehrson, C., Nielsen, B. B., et al. (2017) *Plasmodium falciparum* infection early in pregnancy has profound consequences for fetal growth. *J. Infect. Dis.* 216, 1601–1610. doi: 10.1093/infdis/jix530

Schmitt, C., Humeny, A., Becker, C. M., Brune, K., and Pahl, A. (2002). Polymorphisms of TLR4: rapid genotyping and reduced response to lipopolysaccharide of TLR4 mutant alleles. *Clin. Chem.* 48, 1661–1667.

Seixas, E., Moura Nunes, J. F., Matos, I., and Coutinho, A. (2009). The interaction between DC and Plasmodium berghei/chabaudi-infected erythrocytes in mice involves direct cell-to-cell contact, internalization and TLR. *Eur. J. Immunol.* 39, 1850–1863. doi: 10.1002/eji.200838403

Sharma, L., Kaur, J., Rishi, P., and Shukla, G. (2012a). Plasmodium berghei: influence of infection on the oxidant and antioxidants levels in pregnant BALB/c mice. *Exp. Parasitol.* 131, 215–222. doi: 10.1016/j.exppara.2012.04.005

Sharma, L., Kaur, J., and Shukla, G. (2012b). Role of oxidative stress and apoptosis in the placental pathology of plasmodium berghei infected mice. *PLoS ONE* 7:e32694. doi: 10.1371/journal.pone.0032694

Sharma, L., and Shukla, G. (2014). Treatment of pregnant BALB/c mice with sulphadoxine pyrimethamine or chloroquine abrogates Plasmodium berghei induced placental pathology. *Parasitol. Int.* 63, 49–56. doi: 10.1016/j.parint.2013.08.016

Silver, K. L., Zhong, K., Leke, R. G., Taylor, D. W., and Kain, K. C. (2010). Dysregulation of angiopoietins is associated with placental malaria and low birth weight. *PLoS ONE* 5:e9481. doi: 10.1371/journal.pone.0009481

Thaete, L. G., Qu, X. W., Jilling, T., Crawford, S. E., Fitchev, P., Hirsch, E., et al. (2013). Impact of toll-like receptor 4 deficiency on the response to uterine ischemia/reperfusion in mice. *Reproduction* 145, 517–526. doi: 10.1530/REP-12-0433

Togbe, D., Schofield, L., Grau, G. E., Schnyder, B., Boissay, V., Charron, S., et al. (2007). Murine cerebral malaria development is independent of toll-like receptor signaling. *Am. J. Pathol.* 170, 1640–1648. doi: 10.2353/ajpath.2007.060889

Triquell, M. F., Díaz-Luján, C., Romanini, M. C., Ramirez, J. C., Paglini-Oliva, P., Schijman, A. G., et al. (2018). Nitric oxide synthase and oxidative-nitrosative stress play a key role in placental infection by *Trypanosoma cruzi*. *Am. J. Reprod. Immunol.* 80, 1–12. doi: 10.1111/aji.12852

Umbers, A. J., Stanisic, D. I., Ome, M., Wangnapi, R., Hanieh, S., Unger, H. W., et al. (2013). Does malaria affect placental development? Evidence from *in vitro* models. *PLoS ONE* 8:e55269. doi: 10.1371/journal.pone.0055269

Van Zon, A. A., and Eling, W. M. (1980). Depressed malarial immunity in pregnant mice. *Infect. Immun.* 28, 630–632.

Wahid, H. H., Dorian, C. L., Chin, P. Y., Hutchinson, M. R., Rice, K. C., Olson, D. M., et al. (2015). Toll-like receptor 4 is an essential upstream regulator of on-time parturition and perinatal viability in mice. *Endocrinology* 156, 3828–3841. doi: 10.1210/en.2015-1089

Xu, X., He, L., Zhang, A., Li, Q., Hu, W., Chen, H., et al. (2015). *Toxoplasma gondii* isolate with genotype Chinese 1 triggers trophoblast apoptosis through oxidative stress and mitochondrial dysfunction in mice. *Exp. Parasitol.* 154, 51–61. doi: 10.1016/j.exppara.2015.04.008

Zeldovich, V. B., Clausen, C. H., Bradford, E., Fletcher, D. A., Maltepe, E., Robbins, J. R., et al. (2013). Placental syncytium forms a biophysical barrier against pathogen invasion. *PLoS Pathog.* 9:e1003821. doi: 10.1371/journal.ppat.1003821

Zheng, D., Li, Y., He, L., Tang, Y., Li, X., Shen, Q., et al. (2014). The protective effect of astaxanthin on fetal alcohol spectrum disorder in mice. *Neuropharmacology* 84, 13–18. doi: 10.1016/j.neuropharm.2014.04.013

5

Effect of Sublethal Prenatal Endotoxaemia on Murine Placental Transport Systems and Lipid Homeostasis

*Mila W. Reginatto[1], Klaus Novaes Fontes[1], Victoria R. S. Monteiro[1], Natalia L. Silva[1], Cherley Borba Vieira Andrade[1], Hanailly Ribeiro Gomes[1], Guinever E. Imperio[1,2,3], Flavia Fonseca Bloise[1], George Eduardo Gabriel Kluck[4], Georgia Correa Atella[4], Stephen G. Matthews[2,3,5,6], Enrrico Bloise[7] and Tania M. Ortiga-Carvalho[1]**

[1]Laboratory of Translational Endocrinology, Institute of Biophysics Carlos Chagas Filho, Universidade Federal do Rio de Janeiro, Rio de Janeiro, Brazil, [2]Department of Physiology, Faculty of Medicine, University of Toronto, Toronto, ON, Canada, [3]Lunenfeld-Tanenbaum Research Institute of Medical, Sinai Health System, Toronto, ON, Canada, [4]Laboratory of Lipids and Lipoproteins Biochemistry, Institute of Medical Biochemistry Leopoldo de Meis, Universidade Federal do Rio de Janeiro, Rio de Janeiro, Brazil, [5]Department of Obstetrics and Gynecology, Faculty of Medicine, University of Toronto, Toronto, ON, Canada, [6]Department of Medicine, Faculty of Medicine, University of Toronto, Toronto, ON, Canada, [7]Department of Morphology, Universidade Federal de Minas Gerais, Belo Horizonte, Brazil

***Correspondence:**
Tania M. Ortiga-Carvalho
taniaort@biof.ufrj.br

Infection alters the expression of transporters that mediate the placental exchange of xenobiotics, lipids and cytokines. We hypothesized that lipopolysaccharide (LPS) modifies the expression of placental transport systems and lipid homeostasis. LPS (150 μg/kg; i.p.) treatments were administered for 4 h or 24 h, animals were euthanized at gestational days (GD) 15.5 or 18.5, and maternal blood, fetuses and placentae were collected. Increased rates of fetal demise were observed at GD15.5 following LPS treatment, whereas at GD18.5, high rates of early labour occurred and were associated with distinct proinflammatory responses. Lipopolysaccharide did not alter ATP-binding cassette (ABC) transporter mRNA expression but decreased fatty acid binding protein associated with plasma membrane (*Fabppm*) at GD15.5 (LPS-4 h) and increased fatty acid translocase (*Fat/Cd36*) mRNA at GD18.5 (LPS-4 h). At the protein level, breast cancer-related protein (Bcrp) and ABC sub-family G member 1 (Abcg1) levels were decreased in the placental labyrinth zone (Lz) at GD15.5, whereas P-glycoprotein (P-gp) and Bcrp Lz-immunostaining was decreased at GD18.5. In the placental junctional zone (Jz), P-gp, Bcrp and Abcg1 levels were higher at GD18.5. Specific maternal plasma and placental changes in triacylglycerol, free fatty acid, cholesterol, cholesterol ester and monoacylglycerol levels were detected in a gestational age-dependent manner. In conclusion, LPS-increased risk of fetal death and early labour were associated with altered placental ABC and lipid transporter expression and deranged maternal plasma and placental lipid homeostasis. These changes may potentially modify fetal xenobiotic exposure and placental lipid exchange in cases of bacterial infection.

Keywords: lipopolysaccharide, ATP binding cassette transporters, P-glycoprotein, breast cancer resistance protein, cholesterol, ABC sub-family G member 1, fatty acid binding protein associated with plasma membrane, FAtty acid translocase

INTRODUCTION

Global estimates indicate that more than 15 million babies are born preterm every year (Harrison and Goldenberg, 2016). Preterm birth (PTB) occurs at higher rates in low- and middle-income countries and may range from 5 to 18% of all pregnancies worldwide (Goldenberg et al., 2009). Of particular importance, low-income countries have a higher incidence of histological chorioamnionitis (HCA)-related genitourinary (retrograde or ascending bacterial) and malarial (haematogenous) infections. These infections may lead to severe systemic and placental inflammatory response (Bloise et al., 2010; Novembri et al., 2011; Fontes et al., 2019) and become important triggers of inflammatory PTB pathways (Challis et al., 2009; Conti et al., 2015; Harrison and Goldenberg, 2016). Other routes/risk factors for infection-associated PTB include maternal periodontal disease, transplacental transfer of pathogens, iatrogenic infection from complicating amniocentesis or chorionic villous sampling (Conti et al., 2015; Nadeau et al., 2016).

The most common microbes observed in HCA are the gram-negative bacteria *Ureaplasma urealyticum, Mycoplasma hominis,* and *Escherichia coli* (Conti et al., 2015). Lipopolysaccharide (LPS), an endotoxin enriched in the cell wall of gram-negative bacteria, binds Toll-like receptor 4 (Tlr-4) and is widely used to model gram-negative bacterial infections (Beutler et al., 2003). Studies in mice have shown that LPS exposure alters the fetal-placental unit in a gestational age-dependent manner. In early pregnancy, it induces embryonic loss (Ogando et al., 2003) or miscarriage (Leazer et al., 2002), whereas in mid-pregnancy, it causes fetal death, fetal growth restriction (Guo et al., 2013) and fetal brain injury (Elovitz et al., 2011).

Infection and inflammation have the potential to disrupt the syncytiotrophoblast barrier by modulating the expression and function of ATP-binding cassette (ABC) transporters (Lye et al., 2015; Bloise et al., 2016; Do Imperio et al., 2018). These proteins are active transmembrane efflux transport systems that control the biodistribution of clinically relevant endogenous and exogenous substrates across the maternal-fetal interface. Examples of endogenous substrates include nutrients (cholesterol and other lipids), metabolites (bilirubin- and bile salt-conjugated compounds and oxysterols), steroid hormones (glucocorticoids, mineralocorticoids, oestrogens, progestogens, and androgens) and immunological factors (cytokines and chemokines). Examples of exogenous substrates include therapeutic drugs (antibiotics, antiretrovirals, synthetic glucocorticoids and NSAIDs) and environmental toxins (organochlorine and organophosphorus pesticides, ivermectin and bisphenol A). As a result, ABC transporters limit the transfer of potentially harmful substrates to the foetus and control transplacental passage of nutrients (mostly lipids) and other maternally derived substances in a gestational age-dependent manner (Imperio et al., 2018). In addition, the biodistribution of cytokines and chemokines within gestational tissues is modulated by the actions of placental ABC transporters and, as such, may be involved in the pathogenesis of PTB.

Importantly, cultured human primary villous trophoblast cells exposed to LPS and to the viral double-stranded RNA analogue polyinosinic:polycytidylic acid (polyI:C) exhibit markers of insulin resistance and increased amino acid uptake (Liong and Lappas, 2017). Treatment of trophoblast cells with cytokines, such as interleukin (IL)-1β and IL-6, elicited similar responses (Jones et al., 2009; Aye et al., 2013) indicating that infection may alter placental nutrient uptake and fetal transfer. However, the effect of infection on placental lipid uptake and fetal transfer is less well understood.

In the present study, we determined whether LPS challenge at different stages of gestation modulates the levels of selected ABC transporters in the placenta, which in turn might alter fetal exposure to potentially harmful substrates. Furthermore, we investigated the maternal plasma and placental levels of lipid fractions and the mRNA expression of key placental lipid transporters in dams exposed to a sublethal LPS dose to elucidate the possible effects of LPS on altering lipid homeostasis related or unrelated to placental ABC transporter-mediated lipid exchange. We hypothesized that LPS exposure modifies the expression of key placental ABC and lipid transporters, as well as maternal and placental lipid homeostasis in a gestational age-dependent manner.

MATERIALS AND METHODS

Animal Experiments and Study Design

This study was approved by the Animal Care Committee of the Health Sciences Center, Federal University of Rio de Janeiro (CEUA-190/13) and registered within the Brazilian National Council for Animal Experimentation Control. The study complied with the "Principles of Laboratory Animal Care" generated by the National Society for Medical Research and the United States. National Academy of Sciences Guide for the Care and Use of Laboratory Animals.

Virgin female and male C57BL/6 mice (8–10 weeks of age) were housed in a temperature-controlled room (23°C) on a 12/12 h light/dark cycle, with free access to fresh food and water. Female mice in the oestrous phase (identified by vaginal cytology) were time-mated with C57BL/6 males and assigned (gestational day (GD) 0.5) to different groups. Lipopolysaccharide (Sigma, *E. coli* 055:B5; 150 μg/kg; intraperitoneal injection, i.p., in a single dose) or vehicle (i.p. injection of a single dose) was administered to mice in mid- (GD14.5/15.5) or late- (GD17.5/18.5) pregnancy for 24 or 4 h, respectively. Animals were euthanized at GD15.5 or GD18.5 at the end of the 4 or 24 h treatments with a single dose of LPS/vehicle, and maternal blood, fetuses and placentae were collected. **Supplementary Figure 1** summarizes the design of the study. Of importance, LPS was specifically chosen to mimic bacterial infection during pregnancy, because LPS induction of Tlr-4 activation by intrauterine microbes poses the greatest risk for pregnancy complications such as HCA and PTB (Conti et al., 2015; Firmal et al., 2020).

Fetal and placental tissues were weighed, and three placentae per litter were selected for further study. The selection was based on placentae with weights closest to the mean, an approach that we and others have used previously (Festing, 2006; Coan et al., 2008; Bloise et al., 2012; Fontes et al., 2019; Connor et al., 2020). The LPS dose (150 µg/kg) was selected because it has previously been shown to cause an acute maternal inflammatory response with less than 50% fetal death in mid-pregnancy at 4 h after treatment (Bloise et al., 2013).

Quantitative PCR

Total placental RNA was extracted using TRIzol reagent according to the manufacturer's instructions (Life Technologies, CA, United States). The total RNA concentration was assessed using a nanophotometer (Implen, Munchen, Germany), and samples with RNA purity (260/280 absorbance) ratios ranging between 1.8 and 2.0 and with proven RNA integrity (confirmed through gel electrophoresis) were included in the study. Total RNA (1 µg) was reverse transcribed into cDNAs using the High Capacity cDNA Reverse Transcription Kit (Applied Biosystems, São Paulo, Brazil) according to the manufacturer's instructions.

The mRNA levels of selected ABC transporters, lipid metabolism-related genes, proinflammatory cytokines and chemokines (**Supplementary Table 1**) were evaluated using qPCR according to the manufacturer's recommendations (EVAGREEN; Solis Byodine, EUA) and using the Master Cycler Realplex system (Eppendorf, Germany) with the following cycling conditions: combined initial denaturation steps at 50°C (2 min) and 95°C (10 min), followed by 40 cycles of denaturation at 95°C (15 s), annealing at 60°C (30 s) and extension at 72°C (45 s). Relative gene expression was quantified using the $2^{-\Delta\Delta C_q}$ method (Livak and Schmittgen, 2001). Assays with 95–105% efficiency were considered acceptable.

Gene expression was normalized to the geometric mean of selected reference genes in each experimental group, which exhibited stable expression levels following LPS challenge (**Supplementary Table 1**). The geometric mean expression of *B2m* and *β-actin* genes was used to normalize mRNA expression at GD15.5, whereas the geometric mean expression of *Gapdh* and *Ywhaz* reference genes was used to normalize mRNA expression at GD18.5. Intron-spanning primers, reverse transcriptase-negative samples and a melting curve analysis obtained for each qPCR were used to exclude DNA contamination.

Histological and Immunohistochemical Staining

Placental discs were fixed with 4% buffered paraformaldehyde, dehydrated with increasing concentrations of ethanol, diaphanized in xylene, embedded in paraffin and sectioned (5 µm) using a Rotatory Microtome CUT 5062 (Slee Medical GmbH, Germany) for periodic acid-Schiff (PAS) staining and immunohistochemistry as previously described (Fontes et al., 2019).

Briefly, PAS staining was performed by oxidizing placental sections with 0.5% periodic acid (Sigma-Aldrich, Missouri, United States) for 15 min. Sections were washed with distilled water and incubated (10 min at room temperature) with Schiff's reagent (Merck, Germany), followed by hematoxylin (Proquímios, Rio de Janeiro, Brazil) staining. The junctional zone (Jz) interface between the maternal and fetal placental cellular components was visually identified, and the area of each region of interest, the Jz and the labyrinth zone (Lz), was measured using ImageJ software (National Institutes of Health, Maryland, United States).

Immunohistochemistry was performed by incubating sections with Tris-EDTA buffer (pH 9.0) for 15 min, followed by immersion in sodium citrate buffer (pH 6.0) for 8 min (in a microwave). Sections were immersed in a bovine serum albumin (BSA3% - in PBS) solution to block nonspecific antibody binding sites and then incubated with primary antibodies against P-glycoprotein (P-gp-1:500; Santa Cruz Biotechnology, Texas, United States), breast cancer resistance protein (Bcrp-1:100; Merck Millipore, Massachusetts, United States) or ABC sub-family G member 1 (Abcg1, 1:200; Abcam Plc, United Kingdom) overnight at 4°C. BSA (3% - in PBS) solution was incubated with negative control sections instead of primary antibodies. Sections were then washed with PBS (3 × 5 min) and incubated with a biotin-conjugated secondary antibody (SPD-060 - Spring Bioscience, California, United States) for 1 h followed by an incubation for 1 h with streptavidin (SPD-060 - Spring Bioscience, California, United States). The reaction was halted with 3, 3-diaminobenzidine (SPD-060 - Spring Bioscience, California, United States) followed by hematoxylin (Proquímios, Brazil) staining.

Digital images of histological staining were acquired using a high-resolution Olympus DP72 camera (Olympus Corporation, Japan) attached to the Olympus BX53 microscope (Olympus Corporation, Japan). P-gp, Bcrp and Abcg1 staining were quantified using Image-Pro Plus 5.0 software (Media Cybernetics, Maryland, United States), where the percentage of stained tissue area was calculated and negative spaces were excluded. In each experimental group, 30 digital images per placenta (15 digital images for each labyrinthine and spongiotrophoblast area) were evaluated (Fontes et al., 2019).

Lipid Analysis

Lipid extraction and analysis were performed using the method described by Bligh and Dyer (1959) with some modifications. Maternal plasma (30 µl) and placentae (10 mg) were separately mixed with a solution containing chloroform (1 ml), methanol (2 ml) and water (0.8 ml) with intermittent shaking. After 2 h, the solution was centrifuged (1,500 g, 20 min, 4°C; Sorvall RC-5b; Sorvall Centrifuge, Newtown, CT, United States), the supernatant was collected, and a water-chloroform solution (1:1 v/v) was added. The mixture was shaken and centrifuged (1,500 g, 20 min, 4°C), and the organic phase was removed and dried under nitrogen gas. The lipid classes were separated by one-dimensional thin layer chromatography (TLC) for neutral lipids using a solution containing hexane, diethyl ether and acetic acid (60:40:1 v/v). Plates were immersed in a solution composed of 3% CuSO4 and 8% H3PO4 (v/v; 10 s) and then heated (110°C, 10 min; Ruiz and Ochoa, 1997). Thin layer chromatography plates were analyzed by densitometry using ImageMaster Total Lab 4.1 software (Total Lab Ltd., Newcastle, United Kingdom). Standards for each lipid species were used to identify different lipid classes (Sigma-Aldrich, Sao Paulo, Brazil). Their IDs and catalogue numbers are as follows: triacylglycerol, 1, 3-dipalmitoyl-2-oleoylglycerol, #D2157; cholesteryl ester, cholesteryl oleate, #C9253; free fatty acids, palmitic acid, #76119; cholesterol, #C8667; and monoacylglycerol, #M2140.

A TLC plate with a standard curve for each of the lipid species was developed to quantify the lipid classes. Densitometric units from the standard curve were compared with densitometric units from the samples (which were already normalized to the unit of tissue or amount of plasma). Thin layer chromatography plates were developed in the mobile phase for 1 h. **Supplementary Figures 2, 3** show the TLC plates with plasma and placenta samples from different groups.

Measurement of Plasma Cytokine and Chemokine Levels

Maternal plasma was collected by cardiac puncture, transferred into heparinized tubes on ice, centrifuged (1,077 g, 15 min) and frozen (−80°C). The levels of interleukin (Il)-1β, Il-6, monocyte chemoattractant protein-1 (Mcp-1/Ccl2) and chemokine (C-X-C motif) ligand 1 (Cxcl1) were assessed using the MILLIPLEX-MAP kit Cytokine/Chemokine Magnetic Bead Panel (MCYTOMAG-70K, Merck Millipore, Germany) according to the manufacturer's recommendations. Fluorescence intensity was detected using a Luminex 200™ system (Merck Millipore, Massachusetts, United States).

Statistical Analysis

Normality tests were applied followed by Student's *t*-test or the nonparametric Mann–Whitney test to compare two variables. Pregnancy parameters were evaluated using the mean value of placentae/fetuses in each litter and not individuals (Festing, 2006). For qPCR, PAS/immunohistochemistry, lipid fraction analysis and cytokine/chemokine measurements, three placentae with the closest weight to the mean placental weight within each litter were selected, i.e., one placenta w. Thus, "n" represents the number of litters (Festing, 2006; Coan et al., 2008; Bloise et al., 2013; Fontes et al., 2019; Connor et al., 2020). Values for all data are presented as the means ± SEM. GraphPad Prism 6 software (GraphPad Software, Inc., San Diego, CA, United States) was used to conduct statistical analyses, and differences were considered significant when $p < 0.05$.

RESULTS

Acute Sublethal Effects of LPS on Pregnancy Outcomes

The sublethal LPS treatment elicited different pregnancy outcomes that varied according to the time of exposure and gestational age. At GD15.5, LPS at 4 h induced the death of 26% of fetuses, whereas at 24 h, an 84% fetal death rate was observed. Conversely, the same LPS dosage induced only 1 and 2% fetal death rates at GD18.5 after 4 h and 24 h of LPS exposure, respectively. However, a sublethal LPS treatment for 24 h in late pregnancy (GD18.5) induced a 64% increase in early labour compared to controls, i.e., fourteen of twenty-two dams exhibited signs of labour within 24 h (**Table 1**), i.e., exhibited the presence of one or more offspring (live or dead) in the cage, or exhibited abrupt weight loss concomitant with signs of maternal cannibalism in the cage (McCarthy et al., 2018) and, therefore, were not included in the study. Importantly, the average gestation length for C57BL/6 mice is 19.25 days (range GD18-22; Murray et al., 2010; Fontes et al., 2019), whereas PTB in C57BL/6 mice may occur prior to GD18 (Fontes et al., 2019). Since we were unable to determine the precise birth time within the 24 h limit of LPS treatment (i.e., GD17.5 or GD18.5) in our cohort, we opted to designate this mode of labour as early rather than preterm as a precaution. Of importance, the high percentage of fetal death at GD15.5 and the induction of early labour at GD18.5 prevented us from conducting further placental analysis in the 24 h groups. Thus, all following analyses were performed in tissues from fetuses that did not show signs of death and from dams that did not undergo early labour.

Maternal and Placental Proinflammatory/Morphological Responses to Acute Sublethal LPS Exposure

Maternal plasma levels of cytokines/chemokines associated with the pathogenesis of PTB, including Il-1β, Il-6, chemokine (C-X-C motif) ligand 1 (Cxcl1) and Mcp-1/Ccl2 (Khan and Hay, 2015; Hayward et al., 2016), were assessed in dams following sublethal LPS exposure (4 h) at GD15.5 and GD18.5. At GD15.5, maternal plasma levels of Il-1β ($p < 0.01$), Il-6 ($p < 0.01$), Cxcl1 ($p < 0.0001$) and Ccl2 ($p < 0.01$) were increased compared to the control group (**Figures 1A–D**). At GD18.5, we observed increased maternal plasma Il-6 ($p < 0.001$), Cxcl1 ($p < 0.01$) and Ccl2 levels ($p < 0.001$; **Figures 1F–H**), (LPS) challenge whereas Il-1β levels remained unchanged (**Figure 1E**).

In the placenta, the expression of the Il-6 and Cxcl1 ($p < 0.05$) mRNA was significantly increased following LPS challenge at GD 15.5 and GD 18.5 (**Figure 2**). In contrast, Ccl2 mRNA expression was unchanged at GD15.5, but increased at GD18.5 ($p < 0.0001$; **Figure 2B**). Placental weight was decreased 4 h after LPS exposure at GD18.5, compared to controls (**Table 1**). This led us to investigate whether LPS would elicit changes in the placental proportions of Lz and Jz. No differences in gross placental morphology, including changes in Lz and Jz areas, were identified in any of the groups investigated (**Figure 3**).

Gestational Age-Dependent Sublethal LPS Effects on Placental ABC Transporters

To investigate how bacterial infection impacts placental efflux transport potential, we investigated the expression of the of *Abca1*, *Abcb1a*, *Abcb1b*, *Abcb4*, *Abcc2*, *Abcc5*, *Abcf2*, *Abcg1* and *Abcg2* mRNAs in the mouse placenta at GD15.5 or GD18.5

TABLE 1 | Pregnancy outcomes following sublethal LPS challenge in mid and late pregnancy.

LPS injection	Groups	Exposure (h)	N (Dams)	Early labour %	Fetal death %	Fetal weight (mg)	Placental weight (mg)	F:P ratio
E15.5	Control	4	8	0	10(8/81)	410 ± 30	95 ± 2	4.3 ± 0.35
	LPS		8	0	36(19/53)	400 ± 30	90 ± 3	4.3 ± 0.12
E14.5	Control	24	6	0	3(1/30)	–	–	–
	LPS		4	0	87(20/23)	–	–	–
E18.5	Control	4	9	0	0(0/35)	1.149 ± 50	80 ± 0.9	14.16 ± 0.6
	LPS		10	0	1(1/68)	1.145 ± 40	90* ± 2.0	12.80 ± 0.64
E17.5	Control	24	12	0	2.5(2/80)	1.130 ± 50	82 ± 0.9	13.39 ± 0.54
	LPS		22	64(14/22)	2.0(1//51)	950* ± 60	92* ± 3	10.72** ± 0.72

Statistics: Student's t-test. $^{*}p < 0.05$; $^{**}p < 0.01$.

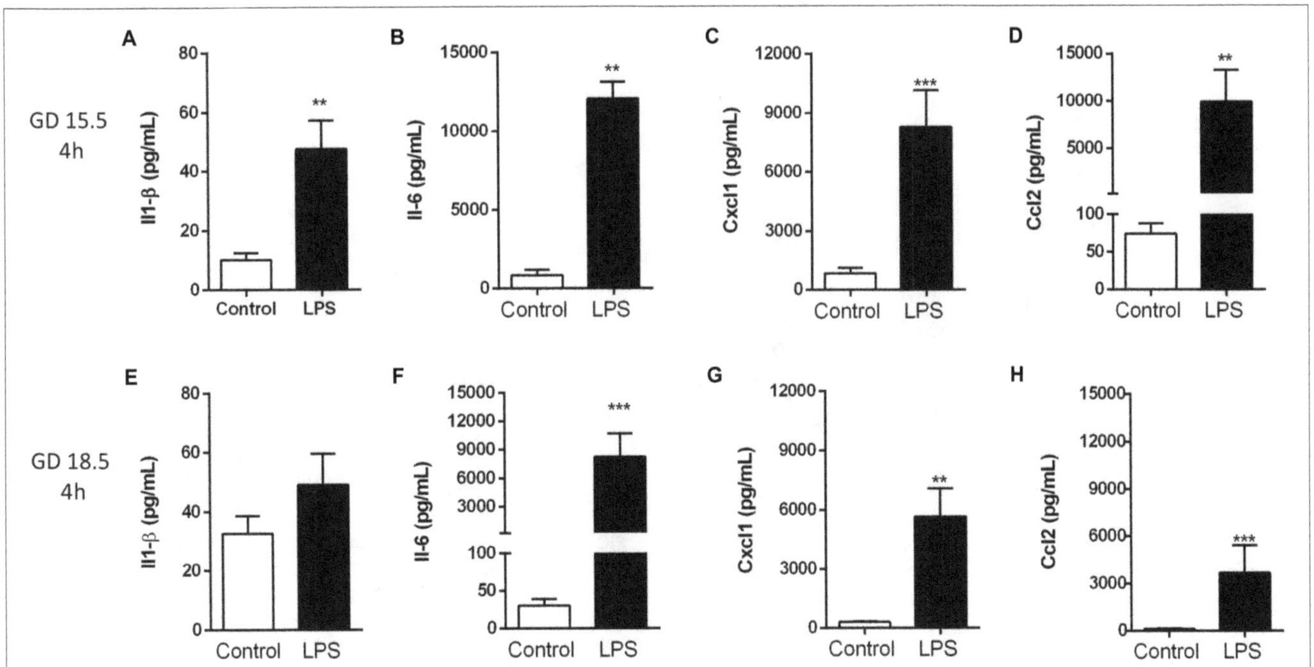

FIGURE 1 | Lipopolysaccharide (4 h) elicited an acute maternal inflammatory response at GD 15.5 and 18.5. Maternal plasma levels of Il-1β **(A,E)**, Il-6 **(B,F)**, Cxcl1 **(C,G)** and Ccl2 **(D,H)** in dams at GD15.5 (control group, $n = 8$, LPS group, $n = 8$) and GD18.5 (control group, $n = 9$, LPS group, $n = 10$), respectively. Statistical analysis: unpaired Student's *t*-test (GD15.5 and 18.5: Il1-β and Ccl2) or Mann-Whitney nonparametric test (GD15.5: Il-6 and Cxcl1; GD 18.5: Il-6). $^{**}p < 0.01$ and $^{***}p < 0.001$.

following LPS challenge (4 h). These specific ABC transporter genes were selected based on evidence showing their sensitivity to infection in other models and/or based on their importance to placental and yolk sac barrier function (Bloise et al., 2016; Do Imperio et al., 2018; Fontes et al., 2019; Martinelli et al., 2020a,b). We did not observe significant differences after LPS treatments (4 h) at GD15.5 and GD18.5 (**Figure 4**).

P-gp and Bcrp are key multidrug resistance transporters that have been shown to play roles in fetal protection, whereas the lipid transporter Abcg1 is important for fetal lipid transfer. Therefore, these three ABC transporters were specifically chosen for further examination. P-gp immunostaining was detected in the cellular membrane of labyrinthine cells, with variable staining in the cellular membrane and cytoplasm of spongiotrophoblast cells (**Figure 5**). Using a semiquantitative analysis, we identified no differences in P-gp staining after LPS administration (4 h) at GD. 15.5 in the Lz and Jz (**Figures 5A–H**). Reduced P-gp staining intensity was observed in the Lz at GD18.5 ($p < 0.01$) after LPS administration (4 h), compared to controls (**Figures 5I–L**). In contrast, P-gp intensity in spongiotrophoblast cells was higher at GD18.5 ($p < 0.05$) 4 h after LPS exposure (**Figures 5M–P**).

Breast cancer-related protein exhibited a similar placental distribution pattern, but with faint and variable nuclear staining in labyrinthine cells. Generally, greater Bcrp cytoplasmic labelling was observed in labyrinthine and spongiotrophoblast cells compared to P-gp-labeled placental cells (**Figure 6**). The Bcrp staining intensity in the Lz was reduced at GD15.5 ($p < 0.05$) and at GD 18.5 ($p < 0.0001$; **Figures 6A–D,I–L**). We identified no differences in Bcrp staining after LPS administration (4 h)

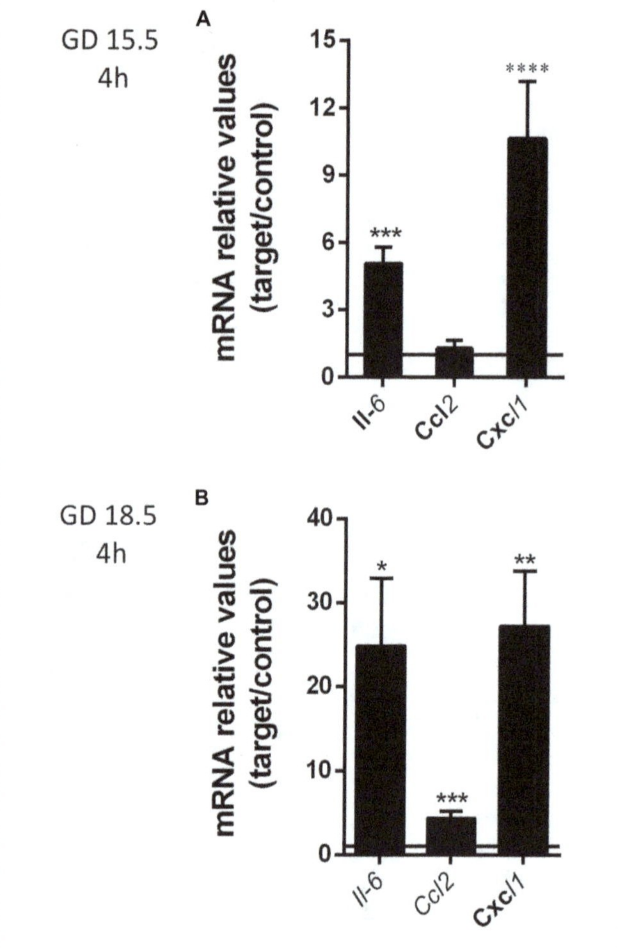

FIGURE 2 | Lipopolysaccharide insult (4 h) elicited an increase in selected placental cytokine/chemokine levels at GD 15.5 and 18.5. mRNA levels of placental *Il6*, *Ccl2* and *Cxcl1* at GD 15.5 **(A)** control group, $n = 8$, LPS group, $n = 8$ and GD 18.5 **(B)** control group, $n = 9$, LPS group, $n = 10$, 4 h after LPS exposure. Gene expression was normalized to the levels of the reference genes *B2m* and *βactin* **(A)**, or *Gapdh* and *Ywhaz* **(B)**. Statistical analysis: GD 15.5: Student's *t*-test and GD 18.5: Student's *t*-test. $^{*}p < 0{,}05$; $^{**}p < 0.01$; $^{***}p < 0.001$; and $^{****}p < 0.0001$. Line shows the expression levels of the control group.

A

GD 15.5/4h

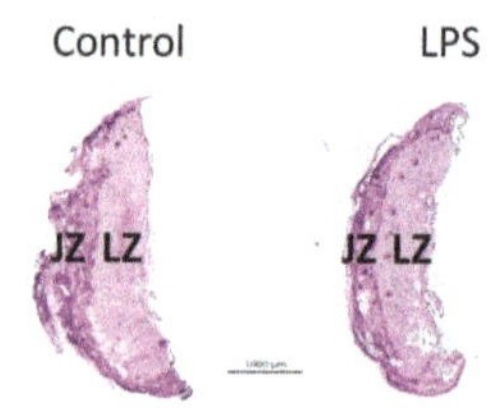

Placental Compartment	Area (Median-IQR)	*P* value
Labyrinth Zone (Lz)	3.4 (2.5-5.5) (control) 3.5 (2.8-4.0) (LPS)	> 0.99
Junctional Zone (Jz)	3.3 (2.4-3.8) (control) 2.0 (1.5-2.4) (LPS)	0.09

B

GD 18.5/4h

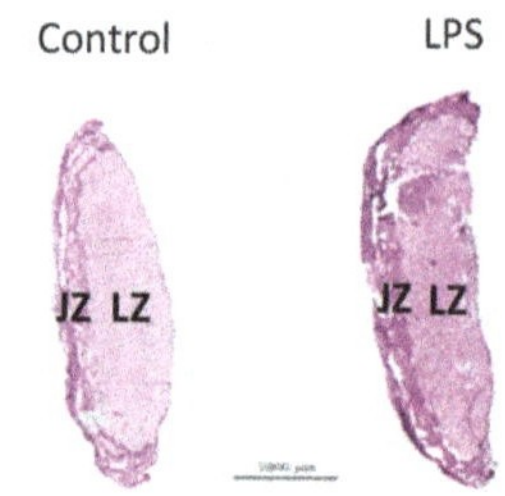

Placental Compartment	Area (Median-IQR)	*P* value
Labyrinth Zone (Lz)	4.7 (2.9-5.6) (control) 2.9 (2.2-3.6) (LPS)	0.15
Junctional Zone (Jz)	1.8 (1.6-1.9) (control) 1.3 (1.0-1.7) (LPS)	0.18

FIGURE 3 | Lipopolysaccharide (4 h) does not alter placental gross morphology. Analysis in the placental proportions of labyrinth (Lz) and junctional zone (Jz) of dams at GD15.5 **(A)** and 18.5 **(B)**, 4 h after LPS exposure. Periodic acid-Schiff staining of control and LPS-treated mice evaluating Lz and Jz areas. $n = 5$/group. Statistical analysis: Mann-Whitney nonparametric test.

at GD. 15.5 in the Lz and Jz (**Figures 6E–H**). In contrast, Bcrp intensity in Jz were higher at GD18.5 ($p < 0.05$) 4 h after LPS exposure (**Figures 6M–P**).

The lipid transporter Abcg1 was predominantly localized to cellular membranes in the Lz and Jz, with some variable cytoplasmic staining throughout these layers (**Figure 7**). A lower Abcg1 staining intensity was observed in labyrinth cells at GD 15.5 ($p < 0.05$), whereas at GD18.5, it remained unchanged (**Figures 7A–D,I–L**). No differences in the levels of Abcg1 in spongiotrophoblast cells of the Jz were identified at GD15.5 after LPS treatment (**Figures 7E–H**). However, when we evaluated at GD 18.5, Abcg1 levels were higher after LPS treatment ($p < 0.01$, **Figures 7M–P**).

Supplementary Figures 4–6 depict higher magnification photomicrographies of placental P-gp, Bcrp and Abcg1 staining, respectively.

LPS Alters Maternal and Placental Lipid Homeostasis Throughout Pregnancy

Since we observed an inhibitory effect of LPS on Abcg1 expression (a lipid transporter) in the Lz, we investigated the impact of sublethal LPS exposure (4 h) on the maternal plasma and placental levels of various lipid classes (triacylglycerol, free fatty acids, cholesterol ester, cholesterol, monoacylglycerol, and phospholipids) at GDs 15.5 and 18.5.

We observed significant alterations in placental lipid levels following sublethal LPS challenge. Triacylglycerol, free fatty acid, cholesterol ester and free cholesterol levels were decreased at GD15.5 compared to the control groups ($p < 0.01$, **Table 2**), whereas triacylglycerol, free fatty acid, free cholesterol, monoacylglycerol and phospholipid levels were increased at GD18.5 compared to the control groups ($p < 0.05$, **Table 3**). The levels of the lipid classes monoacylglycerol and phospholipid remained unchanged at GD15.5 (**Table 2**), whereas cholesterol ester levels did not exhibit alterations at GD18.5 (**Table 3**).

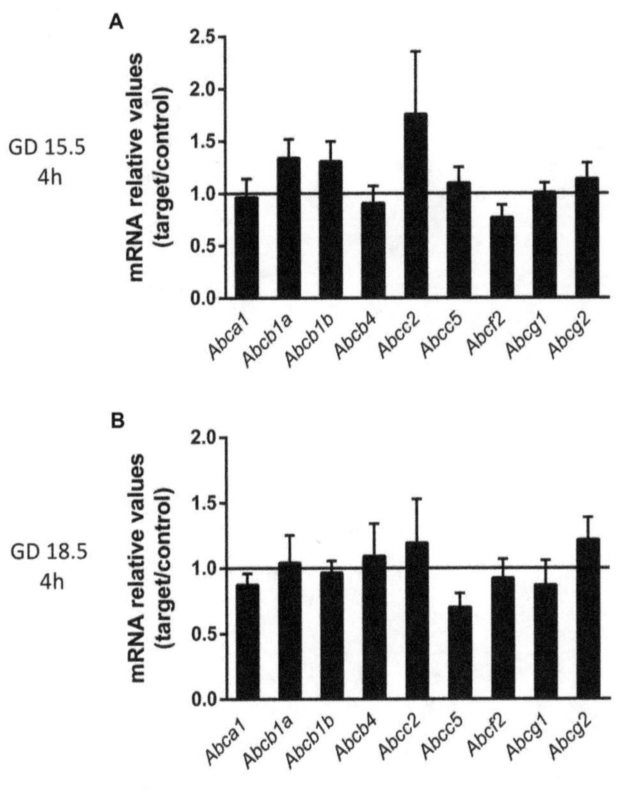

FIGURE 4 | Sublethal LPS challenge (4 h) does not alter the expression of key ABC transporter genes at GDs 15.5 and 18.5. **(A)** Placental levels of the *Abca1*, *Abcb1a*, *Abcb1b*, *Abcb4*, *Abcc2*, *Abcc5*, *Abcf2*, *Abcg1,* and *Abcg2* mRNA at GD15.5 **(A)** and at GD18.5 **(B)**, 4 h after sublethal LPS administration. 15.5/4 h: $n = 8$ (control group); $n = 8$ (LPS group). 18.5/4 h: $n = 9$ (control group); $n = 10$ (LPS group). Gene expression was normalized to the levels of the reference genes **(A)** *B2m* and *βactin* or **(B)** *Gapdh* and *Ywhaz*. Statistical analysis: GD 15.5: Student's *t* test and GD 18.5: Student's *t*-test (*Abcb1b*, *Abcb4*, *Abcc5*, *Abcf2*, and *Abcg1*) and Mann-Whitney nonparametric test (*Abca1*, *Abcb1a*, *Abcc2*, and *Abcg2*). Line shows the expression levels of the control group.

We detected increased triacylglycerol levels and decreased free fatty acid and cholesterol ester levels in the maternal plasma from the LPS-exposed group at GD15.5 compared to the control group ($p < 0.001$, **Table 4**). At GD18.5, the triacylglycerol levels were decreased in the LPS group compared to the control group ($p < 0.05$, **Table 5**). No differences were observed in the levels of free cholesterol, monoacylglycerol and phospholipid classes at either gestational age, whereas the cholesterol ester contents remained unchanged at GD18.5 (**Table 5**).

Placental mRNA expression of key lipid transporters and lipid metabolism-related genes following sublethal LPS treatments was assessed. At GD15.5 (4 h), LPS exposure resulted in lower fatty acid binding protein associated with plasma membrane (*Fabppm*) mRNA levels ($p < 0.05$), whereas at GD18.5 (4 h), increased placental fatty acid translocase (*Fat/Cd36*) levels ($p < 0.01$) were detected (**Figures 8A,B**). The mRNA expression of other lipid transporters and metabolism-related genes, such as *Pparg*, fatty acid transporter family protein (*Fatp1*) and lipase lipoprotein (*Lpl*), remained unchanged throughout pregnancy.

DISCUSSION

We have documented the effects of sub-lethal LPS on placental ABC transporters and lipid homeostasis. Lipopolysaccharide caused substantial fetal death at GD15.5 and triggered early labour in late pregnancy (GD18.5) without inducing fetal demise. These effects were likely mediated by distinct maternal and placental cytokine/chemokine responses to LPS throughout pregnancy and were associated with distinct expression profiles of placental efflux and lipid transporters, as well as changes in maternal and placental lipid levels.

Our present findings showing a greater fetal demise susceptibility to LPS at GD15.5 are consistent with previous studies from our group (Bloise et al., 2013). However, here, we also show that sublethal LPS challenge in late pregnancy increased early labour, probably by intensifying the maternal and placental output of labour-inducing cytokines and chemokines. Our data are consistent with one study conducted in rats showing that LPS treatment (24 h) at GD18.5 induced early labour in 55% of pregnancies (Toyama et al., 2015), a percentage similar to the value reported in our study (64%). Furthermore, LPS administration in late gestation decreased the fetal weight, stimulated placental growth and reduced the F:P weight ratio. These changes might indicate an impairment of placental nutrient transport efficiency that prevents fetuses from attaining optimal growth potential (Bloise et al., 2014; Khan and Hay, 2015; Toyama et al., 2015; Hayward et al., 2016) and predisposing them to poor long-term health outcomes (Bloise et al., 2014).

Acute sublethal LPS exposure during pregnancy elicited an intense maternal and placental proinflammatory response, which varied across pregnancy. We observed a marked increase in a number of key proinflammatory factors (IL-6 and Cxcl1 and Ccl2) related to PTB. In contrast, plasma Il-1β levels and placental levels of the Ccl2 mRNA were not consistently affected by LPS, since they did exhibit a gestational age-dependent expression profile. IL-1β, IL-6 and IL-8 are commonly upregulated by infection and induce prostaglandin (PG)E2 and $PGF_{2\alpha}$ production to stimulate myometrial contractility and PTB (Kim et al., 2004; Vrachnis et al., 2012; Khan and Hay, 2015). Ccl2 is subsequently upregulated in the human myometrium during preterm and term labour and recruits infiltrating leukocytes into the myometrium to amplify local inflammation and trigger the onset of labour (Shynlova et al., 2009). Ccl2 also induces the expression of proinflammatory cytokines, prostaglandins and leukotrienes in the myometrium during late pregnancy (Gibb, 1998; Whittle et al., 2000). Importantly, Tlr4 activation induces the myometrial production of Il-1β, Il-6 and Ccl2 *via* nuclear factor-κB (NF-κB) and p38 mitogen-activated protein kinase activation (Chen et al., 2020).

In the present study, LPS stimulated placental Ccl2 expression in a gestational time-dependent manner, suggesting that this cytokine may participate in the pathogenesis of infective chorioamnionitis and the induction of early labour. Furthermore, our data extracted from pregnancies that did not undergo early labour and at an earlier time point (4 h) indicate that a lack of Il-1β upregulation in these pregnancies may have

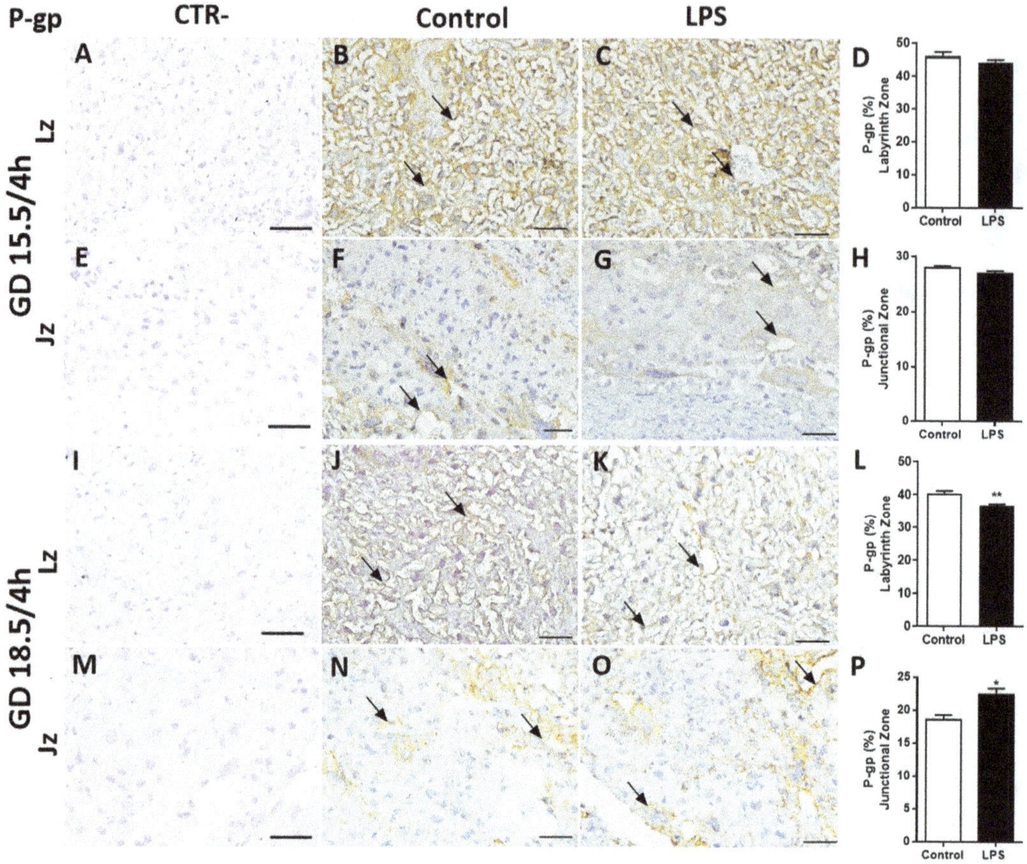

FIGURE 5 | Lipopolysaccharide challenge modulates P-gp protein in the mouse placenta. Representative photomicrographies of immunohistochemistry (arrows) and semiquantitative analysis of P-gp in the labyrinth zone (Lz) and junctional zone (Jz) at GD 15.5/4 h **(A–H)** and GD 18.5/4 h **(I–P)** after LPS administration (4 h). Graphs represent the % of positively stained cells. *n* = 5/group. Scale bar = 50 μm). Statistical analysis: Student's *t*-test. $^*p < 0,05$; $^{**}p < 0.01$.

been important in preventing an earlier onset of labour. Future studies comparing the maternal and placental inflammatory responses of pregnancies that did and did not undergo LPS-induced early labour are required to test this hypothesis.

We evaluated the mRNA and protein expression/localization of selected ABC transporters involved in the biodisposition of clinically relevant substrates across pregnancy to understand how a sublethal bacterial infection alters placental efflux transport potential. As shown in our previous study, a sublethal LPS challenge (150 μg/kg) impairs placental P-gp activity at GD15.5 (4 h) in C57BL/6 mice, with no changes in placental *Abcb1a* and *Abcb1b* mRNA levels (Bloise et al., 2013). In the present study, no changes in P-gp-encoding genes (*Abcb1a* and *Abcb1b*) were observed at GD15.5 and GD18.5 (4 h), however, lower labyrinthine P-gp staining intensity at GD18.5 (4 h) was detected. Placental levels of P-gp and its encoding genes are developmentally regulated in both rodents and humans, i.e., expression decreases towards term (Kalabis et al., 2005; Lye et al., 2013) resulting in reduced fetal protection against P-gp substrates in late pregnancy. Based on our results, a late-term bacterial infection may further decrease this already limited P-gp-mediated barrier function. These changes will likely increase the levels of cytokines and chemokines within gestational tissues, causing fetal demise and morbidity and/or inducing preterm/early labour pathways.

The results from the present and previous studies suggest that bacterial infection has the potential to increase fetal accumulation of P-gp substrates (cytokines, chemokines, endogenous and synthetic glucocorticoids, antibiotics, antiretrovirals, etc.; Bloise et al., 2016) both in earlier stages of pregnancy due to impaired placental P-gp activity (Bloise et al., 2013) and in later stages of pregnancy by decreasing labyrinthine-P-gp expression. These changes will likely increase the levels of cytokines and chemokines within gestational tissues, causing fetal demise and morbidity and/or inducing preterm/early labour pathways.

Consistent with our data, P-gp is downregulated in (1) human first trimester placental explants exposed to LPS (Lye et al., 2015), (2) human PTB placentae with chorioamnionitis (Do Imperio et al., 2018), (3) placentae from pregnant malaria-infected C57BL/6 mice exhibiting high rates of PTB (Fontes et al., 2019), and (4) placentae from pregnant ZIKV-infected mice (Andrade et al., 2021). Furthermore, P-gp activity is impaired in the developing fetal blood brain barrier of pregnant

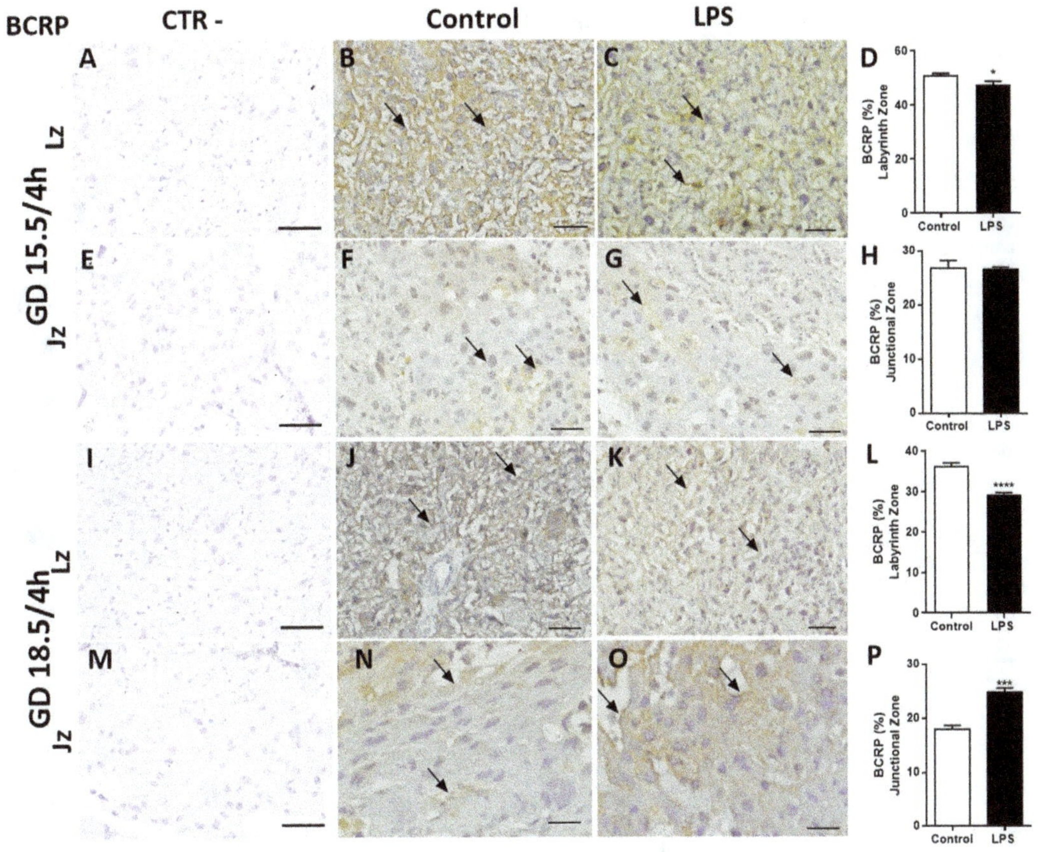

FIGURE 6 | Lipopolysaccharide challenge modulates breast cancer-related protein (Bcrp) protein in the mouse placenta. Representative photomicrographies of immunohistochemistry (arrows) and semiquantitative analysis of Bcrp in the labyrinth zone (Lz) and junctional zone (Jz) at GD 15.5/4 h **(A–H)** and GD 18.5/4 h **(I–P)** after LPS administration (4 h). Graphs represent the % of positively stained cells. n = 5/group. Scale bar = 50 μm). Statistical analysis: Student's t-test. *p < 0,05; ***p < 0.001; ****p < 0.0001.

C57BL/6 mouse exposed to PolyI:C, a TLR3 viral mimic (Bloise et al., 2017). Together, these studies suggest that lower placental *Abcb1b* and P-gp levels are associated with increased risk of infection-driven PTB (Do Imperio et al., 2018; Fontes et al., 2019) and/or earlier labour and delivery. The effects of lower placental P-gp levels on fetal health and postnatal development require further investigation.

A lower level of Bcrp immunostaining was observed in the Lz at GDs 15.5 and 18.5, following LPS exposure. Placental Bcrp levels have been shown to be downregulated in human first trimester placental explants treated with LPS (Lye et al., 2015), in malaria-infected murine placentae (Fontes et al., 2019) and in HTR8/SVneo (human extravillous trophoblast-like) cells exposed to either LPS or to the TLR8 viral mimic single stranded RNA (ssRNA; Lye et al., 2019). Thus, different infective agents/challenges during pregnancy, including bacterial infection, have the potential to increase fetal accumulation of Bcrp substrates during pregnancy. However, Bcrp was upregulated in human PTB placentae with chorioamnionitis (Do Imperio et al., 2018) which is commonly induced by polymicrobial infection (Conti et al., 2015), and after treatment of trophoblastic cells with PGE2 (Mason et al., 2014), indicating that the nature of infective/inflammatory stimuli determines the trophoblastic-Bcrp modulatory response. Furthermore, in the present study, we focused in the effects of LPS rather than infection of different strains of gram-bacteria related to PTB and chorioamnionitis. It is possible that infection by different bacterial strains or by polymicrobial infection would impose distinct responses in placental cytokine and transporter levels.

Interestingly, the P-gp, Bcrp and Abcg1 staining intensity in the spongiotrophoblast was higher at GD18.5 following LPS (4 h) administration but not different at GD15.5. The role of ABC transporters in spongiotrophoblast cells is far less understood. Breast cancer-related protein immunolocalization has been previously reported in spongiotrophoblasts, which remained unaltered in pregnancies in which the mother underwent nutritional manipulations (Connor et al., 2020). Spongiotrophoblasts comprise the mouse placental Jz and provide structural support for the growth of the labyrinthine villi and limit fetal endothelium overgrowth (Silva and Serakides, 2016). However, very little is known about the possible functions of ABC transporters in the mouse Jz and how infection and inflammation impact Jz function.

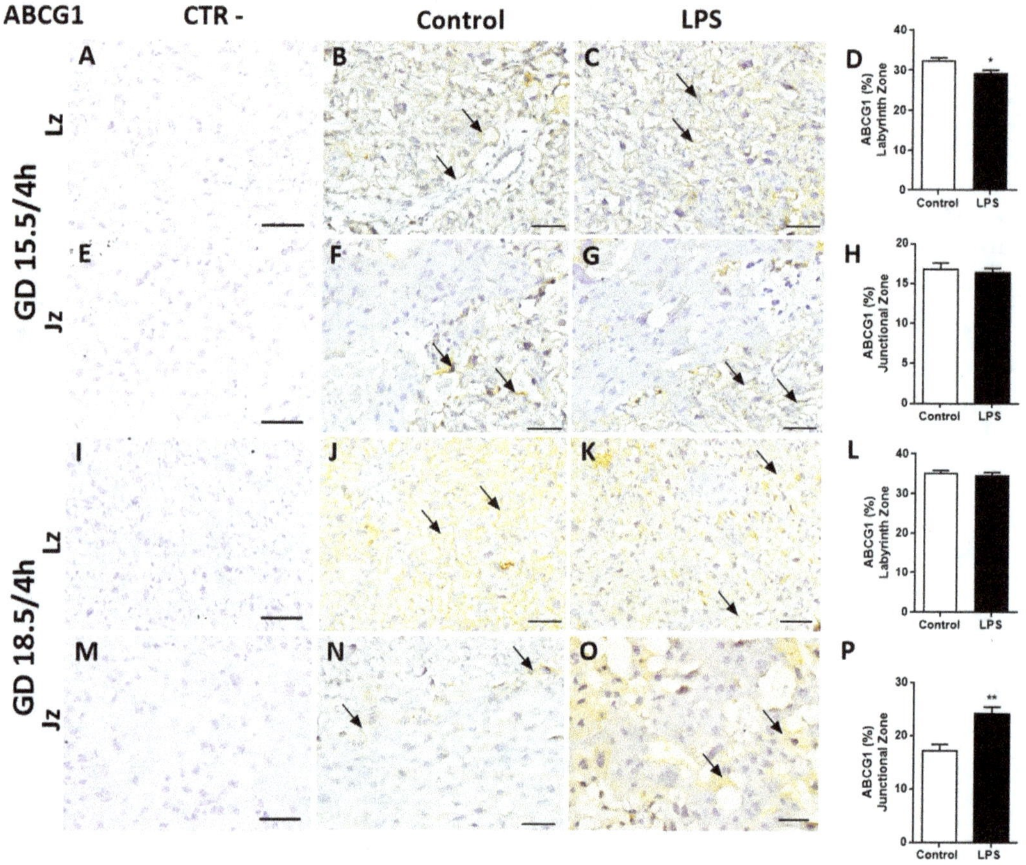

FIGURE 7 | Lipopolysaccharide challenge modulates ABC sub-family G member 1 (Abcg1) protein in the mouse placenta. Representative photomicrographies of immunohistochemistry and semiquantitative analysis of Abcg1 in the labyrinth zone (Lz) and junctional zone (Jz) at GD 15.5/4 h **(A–H)**, GD 18.5/4 h **(I–P)** after LPS administration (4 h). Graphs represent the % of positively stained cells. $n = 5$/group. Scale bar = 50 μm). Statistical analysis: Student's t-test. $^*p < 0.05$; $^{**}p < 0.01$.

TABLE 2 | LPS challenge modulates placental lipid fractions at GD15.5 after LPS administration.

Placental lipid fractions	Groups	Mean ± SEM (μg/mg)	*p*
Triacylglycerol	Control	0.05 ± 0.002	0.0001***
	LPS	0.03 ± 0.002	
Free fatty acids	Control	0.014 ± 0.001	0.0043**
	LPS	0.008 ± 0.001	
Cholesterol ester	Control	0.18 ± 0.02	0.005**
	LPS	0.10 ± 0.01	
Cholesterol	Control	0.05 ± 0.003	0.0043**
	LPS	0.03 ± 0.004	
Monoacylglycerol	Control	0.02 ± 0.0002	0.66
	LPS	0.02 ± 0.002	
Phospholipids	Control	0.073 ± 0.003	0.51
	LPS	0.077 ± 0.005	

*15.5/4 h: n = 6 (control group); n = 5 (LPS group). Statistical analysis: Student's t-test. **p < 0.01; ***p < 0.001.*

TABLE 3 | LPS challenge modulates placental lipid fractions at GD18.5 after LPS administration.

Placental lipid fractions	Groups	Mean ± SEM (μg/mg)	*p*
Triacylglycerol	Control	0.04 ± 0.009	0.03*
	LPS	0.08 ± 0.008	
Free fatty acids	Control	0.004 ± 0.0005	<0.0001****
	LPS	0.03 ± 0.001	
Cholesterol ester	Control	0.23 ± 0.02	0.09
	LPS	0.19 ± 0.01	
Cholesterol	Control	0.026 ± 0.001	<0.0001****
	LPS	0.04 ± 0.0008	
Monoacylglycerol	Control	0.03 ± 0.002	0.0002***
	LPS	0.04 ± 0.003	
Phospholipid	Control	0.065 ± 0.002	0.04*
	LPS	0.071 ± 0.002	

*18.5/4 h: n = 8 (control group); n = 6 (LPS group). Statistical analysis: Student's t-test. *p < 0.05; ***p < 0.001; ****p < 0.0001.*

Labyrinthine Abcg1 expression was also downregulated by LPS at GD15.5. ABC sub-family G member 1 is a cholesterol and phospholipid efflux transporter predominantly localized to the basolateral membrane of the syncytiotrophoblast and in the endothelium of the fetal capillaries of the human placenta, suggesting that it mediates lipid efflux from the maternal compartment to the fetal compartment (Bloise et al., 2016). However, the directionality of Abcg1-mediated lipid exchange in

TABLE 4 | LPS challenge modulates plasma lipid fractions at GD15.5 after LPS administration.

Plasma lipid fractions	Groups	Mean ± SEM (μg/μl)	*p*
Triacylglycerol	Control	0.31 ± 0.02	<0.0001****
	LPS	0.56 ± 0.02	
Free fatty acids	Control	0.14 ± 0.01	<0.0001****
	LPS	0.06 ± 0.003	
Cholesterol ester	Control	0.31 ± 0.02	0.0003***
	LPS	0.19 ± 0.01	
Cholesterol	Control	0.11 ± 0.02	0.59
	LPS	0.13 ± 0.02	
Monoacylglycerol	Control	0.04 ± 0.003	0.095
	LPS	0.06 ± 0.006	
Phospholipid	Control	0.30 ± 0.07	0.26
	LPS	0.38 ± 0.03	

*15.5/4 h: n = 6 (control group); n = 8 (LPS group). Statistical analysis: Student's t-test. ***p < 0.001; ****p < 0.0001.*

TABLE 5 | LPS challenge modulates plasma lipid fractions at GD18.5 after LPS administration.

Plasma lipid fractions	Groups	Mean ± SEM (μg/μl)	*p*
Triacylglycerol	Control	0.76 ± 0.07	0.04*
	LPS	0.57 ± 0.03	
Free fatty acids	Control	0.06 ± 0.01	0.44
	LPS	0.08 ± 0.01	
Cholesterol ester	Control	0.16 ± 0.03	0.4
	LPS	0.22 ± 0.07	
Cholesterol	Control	0.12 ± 0.02	0.23
	LPS	0.15 ± 0.02	
Monoacylglycerol	Control	0.07 ± 0.009	0.26
	LPS	0.06 ± 0.007	
Phospholipid	Control	0.19 ± 0.01	0.19
	LPS	0.20 ± 0.008	

*18.5/4 h: n = 9 (control group); n = 7 (LPS group). Statistical analysis: Student's t-test. *p < 0.05.*

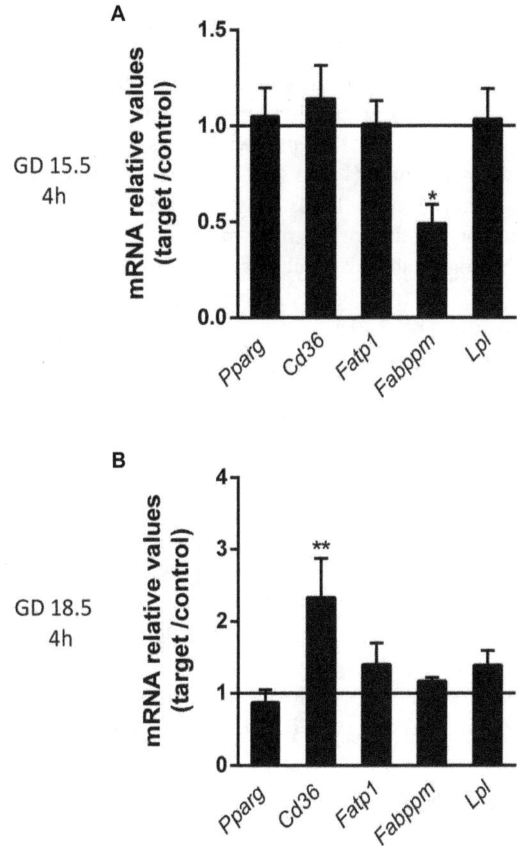

FIGURE 8 | Lipopolysaccharide challenge modulates the mRNA expression of lipid transporters and associated proteins at GDs 15.5 and 18.5, 4 h after the insult. **(A,B)** Quantification of the relative mRNA expression of selected lipid transporters (*Pparg* and *Cd36*) and associated proteins (*Fatp1*, *Fabppm* and *Lpl*) at GD 15.5 and 18.5 4 h after LPS challenge. 15.5/4 h *n* = 8 (control group); *n* = 8 (LPS group). 18.5/4 h: *n* = 9 (control group); *n* = 10 (LPS group). Gene expression was normalized to the levels of the reference genes **(A)** *B2m* and *ß-actin*, or **(B)** *Gapdh* and *Ywhaz*. Statistical analysis: GD 15.5: Student's *t*-test and GD 18.5: Student's *t*-test (*Lpl*, *Fabppm*, *Fatp1*, *Pparg*) and Mann-Whitney nonparametric test (*Cd36*). *$p < 0.05$; **$p < 0.01$. Line shows the expression levels of the control group.

the mouse placenta has yet to be described, preventing us from postulating on the effects of sublethal LPS exposure on placental Abcg1-mediated biodisposition of cholesterol and other lipids.

We did not detect changes in ABC transporter mRNA expression levels at GD 15.5 and 18.5. It is possible that evaluation of placental mRNA extracted from live fetuses at time points different than 4 h, could potentially detect a transcriptional regulation of these transporters. Furthermore, we observed a general disconnection between placental mRNA and protein levels, which has been frequently reported for ABC transporters in the placenta before (Lye et al., 2013; Petrovic et al., 2015; Do Imperio et al., 2018; Connor et al., 2020). This disconnection may indicate post-transcriptional influences of Tlr-4 activation. In fact, there is evidence of miRNAs regulating P-gp in human placenta with chorioamnionitis (Do Imperio et al., 2018). Alternatevly this disconnection may be derived from the fact that we investigated mRNA levels from whole placental tissue, wheres quantification of protein levels was undertaken in the Lz and Jz compartments.

One limitation of the study is that we have not undertaken functional analysis of placental P-gp, Bcrp and Abcg1 activity following sub-lethal LPS exposure. However, as previously discussed, prior work from our group has demonstrated that LPS treatment (150ug/kg for 4), impaired placental P-gp activity at GD15.5 but not later in pregnancy in C57BL/6 mice (Bloise et al., 2013); and that it occurred without changes in placental *Abcb1a* and *Abcb1b* expression. Of importance, LPS challenge in human cerebral microvascular endothelial cells (hCMEC/D3) altered the expression and activity of P-gp and Bcrp in a dose- and time- dependent manner (Eustaquio Do Imperio et al., 2021). In this context, no studies have investigated whether sub-lethal LPS challenge impact placental expression and function of P-gp, Bcrp and Abcg1, simultaneously. This clearly requires further investigation.

Maternal plasma and placental lipid levels were subsequently investigated to better understand how LPS alters lipid homeostasis at the maternal-fetal interface. Maternal levels of triacylglycerol and free fatty acids were altered after LPS exposure at GD15.5. Similar results have been reported in hepatic tissue following LPS exposure (Liu et al., 2015), which occurs in a gestational time-dependent manner. In fact, relevant alterations in plasma lipoproteins occur during injury or infection (Lewis and Desoye, 2017) or in patients with sepsis who occasionally present with hypertriglyceridemia (Lewis and Desoye, 2017). The higher plasma triacylglycerol levels may be directly related to the inflammatory status in pregnant mice and may be associated with the high rates of fetal death at GD15.5. Nevertheless, higher placental triacylglycerol and free fatty acids levels were detected at GD18.5. This later effect may be an attempt to circumvent the lower fetal weight and one possible mechanism responsible for the higher placental weight observed in this group.

Placental fatty acid transport is modulated by different transport systems, including fatty acid transporter family proteins (FATPs), fatty acid binding proteins (FABPs), fatty acid binding protein associated with plasma membrane (*Fabppm*), lipase lipoproteins (LPL) and *Fat/cd36* translocase located on both apical and basolateral membranes of the trophoblast (Cetin et al., 2012; Daniel et al., 2016). We observed decreased placental *Fabppm* at GD15.5 and increased *Fat/cd36* mRNA expression at GD18.5 after LPS exposure (4 h). This finding may at least partially explain the different patterns of free fatty acid accumulation we observed in the present study. Fetuses (and intrauterine tissues) in pregnancies complicated by maternal bacterial infection may be exposed to higher levels of cytokines/chemokines, drugs and environmental toxins present in the maternal circulation. These changes may also be associated with suboptimal placental lipid storage. Combined, these changes may contribute to the inflammatory PTB pathways and lead to the onset of PTB or early labour.

In conclusion, this sublethal LPS model of bacterial infection during pregnancy may induce an increased risk of fetal death or early labour, depending on the gestational age. Pregnancies with increased risk of fetal death and early labour, due to LPS exposure, may exhibit specific maternal and placental inflammatory responses, altered expression of ABC and lipid transporters and altered maternal and placental lipid - homeostasis.

AUTHOR CONTRIBUTIONS

MR, CA, GI, GK, SM, EB, and TO-C: conceptualization of experiments. MR, KF, VM, NS, CA, HG, FB, and GK: formal analysis and performed experiments. EB, SM, and TO-C: funding acquisition. EB, SM, GA, and TO-C: project supervision. MR, EB, SM, and TO-C: manuscript draft. KF, VM, NS, CA, HG, GI, FB, and GA: review and editing. All authors contributed to the article and approved the submitted version.

REFERENCES

Andrade, C. B. V., de Siqueira Monteiro, V. R., Coelho, S. V. A., Gomes, H. R., Sousa, R. P. C., de Oliveira Nascimento, V. M., et al. (2021). ZIKV disrupts placental ultrastructure and drug transporter expression in mice. *Front. Immunol.* 12:680246. doi: 10.3389/fimmu.2021.680246

Aye, I. L. M. H., Jansson, T., and Powell, T. L. (2013). Interleukin-1β inhibits insulin signaling and prevents insulin-stimulated system A amino acid transport in primary human trophoblasts. *Mol. Cell. Endocrinol.* 381, 46–55. doi: 10.1016/j.mce.2013.07.013

Beutler, B., Hoebe, K., Du, X., and Ulevitch, R. J. (2003). How we detect microbes and respond to them: the toll-like receptors and their transducers. *J. Leukoc. Biol.* 74, 479–485. doi: 10.1189/jlb.0203082

Bligh, E. G., and Dyer, B. (1959). A rapid method of total lipid extraction and purification. *Can. J. Biochem. Physiol.* 37, 911–917. doi: 10.1139/o59-099

Bloise, E., Bhuiyan, M., Audette, M. C., Petropoulos, S., Javam, M., Gibb, W., et al. (2013). Prenatal endotoxemia and placental drug transport in the mouse: placental size-specific effects. *PLoS One* 8:e65728. doi: 10.1371/journal.pone.0065728

Bloise, E., Feuer, S. K., and Rinaudo, P. F. (2014). Comparative intrauterine development and placental function of ART concepti: implications for human reproductive medicine and animal breeding. *Hum. Reprod. Update* 20, 822–839. doi: 10.1093/humupd/dmu032

Bloise, E., Lin, W., Liu, X., Simbulan, R., Kolahi, K. S., Petraglia, F., et al. (2012). Impaired placental nutrient transport in mice generated by *in vitro* fertilization. *Endocrinology* 153, 3457–3467. doi: 10.1210/en.2011-1921

Bloise, E., Ortiga-Carvalho, T. M., Reis, F. M., Lye, S. J., Gibb, W., and Matthews, S. G. (2016). ATP-binding cassette transporters in reproduction: a new frontier. *Hum. Reprod. Update* 22, 164–181. doi: 10.1093/humupd/dmv049

Bloise, E., Petropoulos, S., Iqbal, M., Kostaki, A., Ortiga-Carvalho, T. M., Gibb, W., et al. (2017). Acute effects of viral exposure on P-glycoprotein function in the mouse fetal blood-brain barrier. *Cell. Physiol. Biochem.* 41, 1044–1050. doi: 10.1159/000461569

Bloise, E., Torricelli, M., Novembri, R., Borges, L. E., Carrarelli, P., Reis, F. M., et al. (2010). Heat-killed *Lactobacillus rhamnosus* GG modulates urocortin and cytokine release in primary trophoblast cells. *Placenta* 31, 867–872. doi: 10.1016/j.placenta.2010.04.007

Cetin, I., Parisi, F., Berti, C., Mandó, C., and Desoye, G. (2012). Placental fatty acid transport in maternal obesity. *J. Dev. Orig. Health Dis.* 3, 409–414. doi: 10.1017/S2040174412000414

Challis, J. R., Lockwood, C. J., Myatt, L., Norman, J. E., Strauss, J. F., and Petraglia, F. (2009). Inflammation and pregnancy. *Reprod. Sci.* 16, 206–215. doi: 10.1177/1933719108329095

Chen, Z., Liu, Q., Zhu, Z., Xiang, F., Wu, R., and Kang, X. (2020). Toll-like receptor 4 contributes to uterine activation by upregulating pro-inflammatory cytokine and CAP expression via the NF-κB/P38MAPK signaling pathway during pregnancy. *J. Cell. Physiol.* 235, 513–525. doi: 10.1002/jcp.28991

Coan, P. M., Angiolini, E., Sandovici, I., Burton, G. J., Constância, M., and Fowden, A. L. (2008). Adaptations in placental nutrient transfer capacity to meet fetal growth demands depend on placental size in mice. *J. Physiol.* 586, 4567–4576. doi: 10.1113/jphysiol.2008.156133

Connor, K. L., Kibschull, M., Matysiak-Zablocki, E., Nguyen, T. T.-T. N., Matthews, S. G., Lye, S. J., et al. (2020). Maternal malnutrition impacts placental morphology and transporter expression: an origin for poor offspring growth. *J. Nutr. Biochem.* 78:108329. doi: 10.1016/j.jnutbio.2019.108329

Conti, N., Torricelli, M., Voltolini, C., Vannuccini, S., Clifton, V. L., Bloise, E., et al. (2015). Term histologic chorioamnionitis: a heterogeneous condition. *Eur. J. Obstet. Gynecol. Reprod. Biol.* 188, 34–38. doi: 10.1016/j.ejogrb.2015.02.034

Daniel, Z., Swali, A., Emes, R., and Langley-Evans, S. C. (2016). The effect of maternal undernutrition on the rat placental transcriptome: protein restriction up-regulates cholesterol transport. *Genes Nutr.* 11:27. doi: 10.1186/s12263-016-0541-3

Do Imperio, G. E., Bloise, E., Javam, M., Lye, P., Constantinof, A., Dunk, C., et al. (2018). Chorioamnionitis induces a specific signature of placental ABC transporters associated with an increase of miR-331-5p in the human preterm placenta. *Cell. Physiol. Biochem.* 45, 591–604. doi: 10.1159/000487100

Elovitz, M. A., Brown, A. G., Breen, K., Anton, L., Maubert, M., and Burd, I. (2011). Intrauterine inflammation, insufficient to induce parturition, still evokes fetal and neonatal brain injury. *Int. J. Dev. Neurosci.* 29, 663–671. doi: 10.1016/j.ijdevneu.2011.02.011

Eustaquio Do Imperio, G., Lye, P., Bloise, E., and Matthews, S. G. (2021). Function of multidrug resistance transporters is disrupted by infection mimics in human brain endothelial cells. *Tissue Barriers* 9:1860616. doi: 10.1080/21688370.2020.1860616

Festing, M. F. W. (2006). Design and statistical methods in studies using animal models of development. *ILAR J.* 47, 5–14. doi: 10.1093/ilar.47.1.5

Firmal, P., Shah, V. K., and Chattopadhyay, S. (2020). Insight Into TLR4-mediated immunomodulation in normal pregnancy and related disorders. *Front. Immunol.* 11:807. doi: 10.3389/fimmu.2020.00807

Fontes, K. N., Reginatto, M. W., Silva, N. L., Andrade, C. B. V., Bloise, F. F., Monteiro, V. R. S., et al. (2019). Dysregulation of placental ABC transporters in a murine model of malaria-induced preterm labor. *Sci. Rep.* 9:11488. doi: 10.1038/s41598-019-47865-3

Gibb, W. (1998). The role of prostaglandins in human parturition. *Ann. Med.* 30, 235–241. doi: 10.3109/07853899809005850

Goldenberg, R. L., Culhane, J. F., Iams, J. D., and Romero, R. (2009). Preterm birth 1: epidemiology and causes of preterm birth. *Obstet. Anesth. Dig.* 29, 6–7. doi: 10.1097/01.aoa.0000344666.82463.8d

Guo, Y., Ma, Z., Kou, H., Sun, R., Yang, H., Smith, C. V., et al. (2013). Synergistic effects of pyrrolizidine alkaloids and lipopolysaccharide on preterm delivery and intrauterine fetal death in mice. *Toxicol. Lett.* 221, 212–218. doi: 10.1016/j.toxlet.2013.06.238

Harrison, M. S., and Goldenberg, R. L. (2016). Global burden of prematurity. *Semin. Fetal Neonatal Med.* 21, 74–79. doi:10.1016/j.siny.2015.12.007.

Hayward, C. E., Lean, S., Sibley, C. P., Jones, R. L., Wareing, M., Greenwood, S. L., et al. (2016). Placental adaptation: what can we learn from birthweight: placental weight ratio? *Front. Physiol.* 7:28. doi: 10.3389/fphys.2016.00028

Imperio, G. E., Javam, M., Lye, P., Constantinof, A., Dunk, C. E., Reis, F. M., et al. (2018). Gestational age-dependent gene expression profiling of ATP-binding cassette transporters in the healthy human placenta. *J. Cell. Mol. Med.* 23, 610–618. doi: 10.1111/jcmm.13966

Jones, H. N., Jansson, T., and Powell, T. L. (2009). IL-6 stimulates system A amino acid transporter activity in trophoblast cells through STAT3 and increased expression of SNAT2. *Am. J. Phys. Cell Phys.* 297, C1228–C1235. doi: 10.1152/ajpcell.00195.2009

Kalabis, G. M., Kostaki, A., Andrews, M. H., Petropoulos, S., Gibb, W., and Matthews, S. G. (2005). Multidrug resistance phosphoglycoprotein (ABCB1) in the mouse placenta: fetal Protection. *Biol. Reprod.* 73, 591–597. doi: 10.1095/biolreprod.105.042242

Khan, R. N., and Hay, D. P. (2015). A clear and present danger: inflammasomes DAMPing down disorders of pregnancy. *Hum. Reprod. Update* 21, 388–405. doi: 10.1093/humupd/dmu059

Kim, Y. M., Romero, R., Chaiworapongsa, T., Kim, G. J., Kim, M. R., Kuivaniemi, H., et al. (2004). Toll-like receptor-2 and -4 in the chorioamniotic membranes in spontaneous labor at term and in preterm parturition that are associated with chorioamnionitis. *Am. J. Obstet. Gynecol.* 191, 1346–1355. doi: 10.1016/j.ajog.2004.07.009

Leazer, T. M., Barbee, B., Ebron-McCoy, M., Henry-Sam, G. A., and R. J., (2002). Role of the maternal acute phase response and tumor necrosis factor alpha in the developmental toxicity of lipopolysaccharide in the CD-1 mouse. *Reprod. Toxicol.* 16, 173–179. doi: 10.1016/S0890-6238(02)00011-4

Lewis, R. M., and Desoye, G. (2017). Placental lipid and fatty acid transfer in maternal overnutrition. *Ann. Nutr. Metab.* 70, 228–231. doi: 10.1159/000463397

Liong, S., and Lappas, M. (2017). Lipopolysaccharide and double stranded viral RNA mediate insulin resistance and increase system a amino acid transport in human trophoblast cells *in vitro*. *Placenta* 51, 18–27. doi: 10.1016/j.placenta.2017.01.124

Liu, Z., Liu, W., Huang, Y., Guo, J., Zhao, R., and Yang, X. (2015). Lipopolysaccharide significantly influences the hepatic triglyceride metabolism in growing pigs. *Lipids Health Dis.* 14:64. doi: 10.1186/s12944-015-0064-8

Livak, K. J., and Schmittgen, T. D. (2001). Analysis of relative gene expression data using real-time quantitative PCR and the 2(−Delta Delta C(T)) method. *Methods* 25, 402–408. doi: 10.1006/meth.2001.1262

Lye, P., Bloise, E., Dunk, C., Javam, M., Gibb, W., Lye, S. J., et al. (2013). Effect of oxygen on multidrug resistance in the first trimester human placenta. *Placenta* 34, 817–823. doi: 10.1016/j.placenta.2013.05.010

Lye, P., Bloise, E., Javam, M., Gibb, W., Lye, S. J., and Matthews, S. G. (2015). Impact of bacterial and viral challenge on multidrug resistance in first- and third-trimester human placenta. *Am. J. Pathol.* 185, 1666–1675. doi: 10.1016/j.ajpath.2015.02.013

Lye, P., Bloise, E., Nadeem, L., Peng, C., Gibb, W., Ortiga-Carvalho, T. M., et al. (2019). Breast cancer resistance protein (BCRP/ABCG2) inhibits extra villous trophoblast migration: the impact of bacterial and viral infection. *Cell* 8:1150. doi: 10.3390/cells8101150

Martinelli, L. M., Fontes, K. N., Reginatto, M. W., Andrade, C. B. V., Monteiro, V. R. S., Gomes, H. R., et al. (2020a). Malaria in pregnancy regulates P-glycoprotein (P-gp/Abcb1a) and ABCA1 efflux transporters in the mouse visceral yolk sac. *J. Cell. Mol. Med.* 24, 10636–10647. doi: 10.1111/jcmm.15682

Martinelli, L. M., Reginatto, M. W., Fontes, K. N., Andrade, C. B. V., Monteiro, V. R. S., Gomes, H. R., et al. (2020b). Breast cancer resistance protein (Bcrp/Abcg2) is selectively modulated by lipopolysaccharide (LPS) in the mouse yolk sac. *Reprod. Toxicol.* 98, 82–91. doi: 10.1016/j.reprotox.2020.09.001

Mason, C. W., Lee, G. T., Dong, Y., Zhou, H., He, L., and Weiner, C. P. (2014). Effect of prostaglandin E2 on multidrug resistance transporters in human placental cells. *Drug Metab. Dispos.* 42, 2077–2086. doi: 10.1124/dmd.114.059477

McCarthy, R., Martin-Fairey, C., Sojka, D. K., Herzog, E. D., Jungheim, E. S., Stout, M. J., et al. (2018). Mouse models of preterm birth: suggested assessment and reporting guidelines. *Biol. Reprod.* 99, 922–937. doi: 10.1093/biolre/ioy109

Murray, S. A., Morgan, J. L., Kane, C., Sharma, Y., Heffner, C. S., Lake, J., et al. (2010). Mouse gestation length is genetically determined. *PLoS One* 5:e12418. doi: 10.1371/journal.pone.0012418

Nadeau, H. C. G., Subramaniam, A., and Andrews, W. W. (2016). Infection and preterm birth. *Semin Fetal Neonatal Med.* 21, 100–105. doi: 10.1016/j.siny.2015.12.008

Novembri, R., Torricelli, M., Bloise, E., Conti, N., Galeazzi, L. R., Severi, F. M., et al. (2011). Effects of urocortin 2 and urocortin 3 on IL-10 and TNF-α expression and secretion from human trophoblast explants. *Placenta* 32, 969–974. doi: 10.1016/j.placenta.2011.09.013

Ogando, D. G., Paz, D., Cella, M., and Franchi, A. M. (2003). The fundamental role of increased production of nitric oxide in lipopolysaccharide-induced embryonic resorption in mice. *Reproduction* 125, 95–110. doi: 10.1530/rep.0.1250095

Petrovic, V., Kojovic, D., Cressman, A., and Piquette-Miller, M. (2015). Maternal bacterial infections impact expression of drug transporters in human placenta. *Int. Immunopharmacol.* 26, 349–356. doi: 10.1016/j.intimp.2015.04.020

Ruiz, J. I., and Ochoa, B. (1997). Quantification in the subnanomolar range of phospholipids and neutral lipids by monodimensional thin-layer chromatography and image analysis. *J. Lipid Res.* 38, 1482–1489. doi: 10.1016/S0022-2275(20)37430-7

Shynlova, O., Tsui, P., Jaffer, S., and Lye, S. J. (2009). Integration of endocrine and mechanical signals in the regulation of myometrial functions during pregnancy and labour. *Eur. J. Obstet. Gynecol. Reprod. Biol.* 144, S2–S10. doi: 10.1016/j.ejogrb.2009.02.044

Silva, J. F., and Serakides, R. (2016). Intrauterine trophoblast migration: a comparative view of humans and rodents. *Cell Adhes. Migr.* 10, 88–110. doi: 10.1080/19336918.2015.1120397

Toyama, R. P., Xikota, J. C., Schwarzbold, M. L., Frode, T. S., Buss Zda, S., Nunes, J. C., et al. (2015). Dose-dependent sickness behavior, abortion and inflammation induced by systemic LPS injection in pregnant mice. *J. Matern. Fetal Neonatal Med.* 4, 426–430. doi: 10.3109/14767058.2014.918600

Vrachnis, N., Karavolos, S., Iliodromiti, Z., Sifakis, S., Siristatidis, C., Mastorakos, G., et al. (2012). Impact of mediators present in amniotic fluid on preterm labour. *In Vivo* 26, 799–812.

Whittle, W. L., Holloway, A. C., Lye, S. J., Gibb, W., and Challis, J. R. G. (2000). Prostaglandin production at the onset of ovine parturition is regulated by both estrogen-independent and estrogen-dependent pathways. *Endocrinology* 141, 3783–3791. doi: 10.1210/endo.141.10.7703

6

Yellow Fever Vaccination in a Mouse Model is Associated with Uninterrupted Pregnancies and Viable Neonates Except when Administered at Implantation Period

Fernanda C. da Silva[1], *Fernanda M. Magaldi*[1], *Helena K. Sato*[2] *and Estela Bevilacqua*[1*]

[1] *Department of Cell and Developmental Biology, Institute of Biomedical Sciences, University of São Paulo, São Paulo, Brazil,*
[2] *Secretaria do Estado de São Paulo, Epidemiological Surveillance Center, Department of Health, São Paulo, Brazil*

Correspondence:
Estela Bevilacqua
bevilacq@usp.br

The potential risk of yellow fever (YF) infection in unvaccinated pregnant women has aroused serious concerns. In this study, we evaluated the effect of the YF vaccine during gestation using a mouse model, analyzing placental structure, immunolocalization of the virus antigen, and viral activity at the maternal-fetal barrier and in the maternal liver and fetus. The YF vaccine (17DD) was administered subcutaneously at a dose of 2.0 $\log_{10}$ PFU to CD-1 mice on gestational days (gd) 0.5, 5.5, and 11.5 (n = 5–10/group). The control group received sterile saline (n = 5–10/group). Maternal liver, implantation sites with fetus, and placentas were collected on gd18.5. The numbers of implantation sites, reabsorbed embryos, and stillborn fetuses were counted, and placentas and live fetuses were weighed. Tissues (placenta, fetuses, and liver) of vaccinated pregnant mice on gd5.5 (n = 15) were paraffin-embedded in 10% buffered-formalin and collected in TRIzol for immunolocalization of YF vaccine virus and PCR, respectively. PCR products were also subjected to automated sequence analysis. Fetal growth restriction ($p < 0.0001$) and a significant decrease in fetal viability ($p < 0.0001$) occurred only when the vaccine was administered on gd5.5. In stillbirths, the viral antigen was consistently immunolocalized at the maternal-fetal barrier and in fetal organs, suggesting a transplacental transfer. In stillbirths, RNA of the vaccine virus was also detected by reverse transcriptase-PCR indicating viral activity in the maternal liver and fetal tissues. In conclusion, the findings of this study in the mouse suggest that vaccination did not cause adverse outcomes with respect to fetal development except when administered during the early gestational stage, indicating the implantation period as a susceptible period in which the YF vaccine virus might interfere with pregnancy.

Keywords: yellow fever (YF) vaccine, pregnancy, congenital transmission, placenta, fetal losses

INTRODUCTION

Yellow fever (YF) is an acute viral infection associated with hepatitis, jaundice, hemorrhage, and renal failure, and it may progress to death (Monath, 2008; Staples and Monath, 2011). Acute febrile syndrome and hemorrhagic phenomena are the most prominent manifestations of this disease. Vaccination and strategic programs for controlling the main vectors—hematophagous mosquitoes of the genera *Aedes, Haemogogos,* and *Sabethes*—have been successfully implemented in many countries, even though the number of infected persons has increased worldwide over the last two decades (Monath, 2013; Monath and Vasconcelos, 2015). Large outbreaks have been reported in Africa as well as South and Central America, mainly in forested areas infested by the transmission vectors (Staples and Monath, 2011).

In Brazil, no urban outbreak of YF has occurred since the 1940s, when the urban cycle of transmission was eradicated. However, in 1997, YF viral infections were detected in North and Central Brazil, and a new outbreak was registered in 2008 in South and Southeast regions of the country (Monath and Vasconcelos, 2015; Waggoner et al., 2018). In 2017, YF virus (YFV) was detected in non-human primates, and human cases were reported in places where vaccination coverage was low (Leal et al., 2016; Fernandes et al., 2017), a situation that may have been aggravated by public hesitancy toward vaccines.

YF virus are single-stranded RNA viruses of the Flaviviridae family. The direct cytopathic effect of the virus and a potent host immune response are associated with the secretion of TGF-b, TNF-a, and IFN-g, which are believed to play roles in the manifestations and severity of the disease (Quaresma et al., 2006a,b, 2013; Woodson et al., 2011; Engelmann et al., 2014). Transcriptomic analyses of viscerotropic YF in a rhesus macaque model also showed that YF infection correlates with changes in cytokine gene expression before the emergence of clinical symptoms, suggesting these immune factors (cytokines) may influence the disease outcome (Engelmann et al., 2014). The results of *in vitro* studies have suggested that effects of infection on endothelial cells may also contribute to YF pathogenesis (Khaiboullina et al., 2005; Quaresma et al., 2006a). Inoculation of flaviviruses in monkeys indicates that the initial site of replication is the inoculation site in the skin followed by the lymph nodes, where additional replication occurs (Marchette et al., 1973; Monath and Barrett, 2003; Dean et al., 2005). The virus reaches the bloodstream via the lymphatic system and spreads to prevalent organs, such as the liver (Monath and Vasconcelos, 2015). In the liver, the virus infects the Kupffer cells and the hepatocytes, causing severe necrosis (Monath and Barrett, 2003).

The YF vaccine virus is a live attenuated virus, which is prepared and obtained by culturing the 17D strain virus in living chick embryos, and it can induce neutralizing antibodies and T lymphocyte responses. The vaccine differs from YFV by the loss of viscerotropism, despite its replicative activity in cell culture, and by 20 amino acid changes in the envelope protein (Lee and Lobigs, 2008; Monath et al., 2013). In monkeys, the YF 17D vaccine causes a transient low viremia (Monath and Barrett, 2003) accompanied by innate immune responses with detectable levels of cytokines and toll-like receptor-mediated signaling (Monath and Vasconcelos, 2015). Neutralizing antibodies are the principal mediators of protective immunity against flaviviruses (Monath et al., 2013).

After a single dose of the YF 17D vaccine, 80–90% of human subjects become seropositive by day 10 (Monath and Barrett, 2003). A small number of adverse events have been associated with vaccination in humans and monkeys, ranging from severe encephalitis and hepatic failure to neurological symptoms of benign prognosis (Monath and Barrett, 2003; Martins et al., 2015).

In pregnant women, Nishioka et al. (1998) found a relative risk of 2.29 for spontaneous abortions after vaccination. Another study performed on women who inadvertently received YF vaccine during pregnancy reported abortion, stillbirth, and malformation rates similar to those found in the general population (Nasidi et al., 1993; Robert et al., 1999; Suzano et al., 2006; D'Acremont et al., 2008). Nonetheless, due to the theoretical risk of maternal-fetal transmission associated with fetal hepatic and neuronal susceptibility to the YF 17D virus, there is a general recommendation to avoid vaccine administration during pregnancy except when epidemiologically justified (Hagmann et al., 2017). However, the absence of vaccination during pregnancy is a risk to the mother and fetus, thereby increasing the risk of infection to local mosquitoes. Therefore, it is imperative to disseminate knowledge and awareness on gestational vaccination.

A small number of viruses are transmitted from mother to fetus, showing the effectiveness of the hemochorial barrier against these infections (Marinho et al., 2017). However, the mechanisms by which the viruses overcome the placental barrier is still uncertain. Recent studies suggest that maternal immunity, time of gestation, coinfections, and many other factors may be associated with this effectiveness (Marinho et al., 2017).

In this study, we used a mouse model to analyze the effect of YF vaccination during gestation and to identify potential susceptible phases that might compromise embryo/fetal health. This study addressed the birth/mortality rates, as well as the morphology and localization of YF 17D virus in fetuses, placentas, and maternal tissues after vaccination through immunohistochemical reactions and polymerase chain reaction (PCR).

MATERIALS AND METHODS

Animals

Female adult mice (CD-1 mice, 3 months old) were caged overnight with males (1:1) and successful mating was verified the following morning. The presence of a vaginal plug indicated day 0.5 of gestation (gd). All animal care and experimental procedures were carried out according to the Brazilian Society of Science in Laboratory Animals (COBEA) and was approved by the Ethics Committee for Animal Research (CEEA) of Biomedical Sciences Institute of the University of São Paulo, Brazil.

Vaccination

The vaccination protocol was carried out at the Department of Cellular and Developmental Biology in the Biomedical Sciences Institute of the University of São Paulo, under the supervision of the Department of Immunization Center for Epidemiological Surveillance of the State of São Paulo. YF vaccine (17DD, parts 00PVFA028Z; 066VFA061Z; and 082VFB006Z) was obtained from the Oswaldo Cruz Foundation (Bio-Manguinhos, Rio de Janeiro, Brazil). The vaccine was reconstituted with 5 mL of saline and administered subcutaneously at a dose of 2.0 $\log_{10}$ PFU in a final volume of 0.1 mL. In the control group, the vaccine was replaced by sterile saline (PBS, Gibco BRL, Grand Island, NY, United States).

Experimental Design

The experiments were divided into two phases. In the first phase, vaccination was carried out at different stages of pregnancy (0.5, 5.5, and 11.5 gestation days [gd]) for gestational parameter evaluation (n = 5–10 pregnant females/experimental or control group). Day 0.5 of gestation is a period when the zygote is in the lumen of the uterine tube; day 5.5 of gestation represent the onset of implantation, in which the trophoblast giant cells surrounding the blastocyst come into direct contact with the maternal blood; and day 11.5 of pregnancy is the usual time for placenta maturation (Adamson et al., 2002; Cross, 2005; Watson and Cross, 2005; Hu and Cross, 2009; Croy et al., 2014).

In the second phase, immunolocalization of the viral antigen and signals of viral activity were analyzed at periods in which the vaccination had caused relevant changes (gd5.5, n = 15 pregnant females/experimental groups and n = 10/control groups).

Sample Collection for Gestational Performance

Vaccinated and control animals were anesthetized with hydrochloride xylazine (Rompun 2%®, Bayer, São Paulo, Brazil) and ketamine (1:1, v/v, Ketalar, Bayer, São Paulo, Brazil) on gd18.5. Uterine horns were dissected under a stereoscopic microscope, and implantation sites with fetuses and their placentas were exposed. The fetuses were euthanized in a CO_2 chamber. Placentas, resorptions, and living and dead fetuses were counted and weighed. The total number of implantation sites and early reabsorbed embryos was evaluated by incubating the uterine horns in 10% ammonium sulfide for 10 min after the removal of the fetuses, placentas, and late resorptions (Salewsky, 1964).

Birth index (BI) and mortality rate (MR) were respectively calculated as follows:

$$BI = \frac{\text{Total number of implantation sites}-\text{number of stillbirths and resorptions}}{\text{Total number of implantation sites}}$$

$$MR = \frac{\text{Total number of implantation sites}-\text{number of live fetuses}}{\text{Total number of implantation sites}} \times 100$$

Results were expressed as the mean value ± SD, and Student's t-test was used to determine significant differences in comparison with age-control groups. A probability level of less than 5% was considered significant. Statistical analysis was performed using the program Statistical Package for Social Science for Windows.

Collection and Processing of Samples for Morphological Analysis

Under deep anesthesia, fragments of the maternal liver and the uterine horns were obtained. Placentas, fetuses (live fetuses were euthanized by CO_2 inhalation) and material resulting from resorptions were then dissected. Tissues were fixed in 10% buffered formalin and routinely processed for embedding in Histosec® (Merck KGaA, Darmstadt, Germany). Sections were either stained with hematoxylin and eosin or processed for immunoreactions and light microscopy analysis.

Sections of the maternal liver, placenta, and fetus of control females (n = 5) and vaccinated mothers with living (n = 5) and dead (stillbirth, n = 5) fetuses obtained from different mothers were assessed with immunohistochemical (IH) assays. At least three sections from each placenta (three placentas per animal) and of maternal liver and fetus were obtained from each experimental animal for analysis. Deparaffinized and hydrated sections were incubated in the citric acid solution (10 mM, pH 6.0) for 3 min at 60°C and thereafter blocked for 15 min in 3% hydrogen peroxide in distilled water. Sections were incubated for 1 h in M.O.M. mouse IgG blocking reagent (Vector Lab, Burlingame, CA, United States). Next, the samples were immunostained using the polyclonal mouse anti-YF virus antibody (Division of Medical Biology, Department of Virology, Adolfo Lutz Institute, São Paulo, Brazil) diluted at 1:2,000 in TBS containing 1% bovine serum albumin, for 30 min at 37°C, followed by 18 h at 4°C. Labeled polymer-HRP anti-mouse (EnVision + System HRP [DAB], Dako Cytomation) was used as a secondary antibody for 1 h at room temperature. Color development was obtained by incubating with DAB substrate-chromogen solution (0.05% 3,3′- diaminobenzidine in hydrogen peroxide, Sigma-Aldrich, St. Louis, MO, United Ststes) for 5 min. Sections were counterstained with Mayer's hematoxylin and examined using an Axioskop 2 light microscope (Carl Zeiss, Oberkochen, Germany). The images were captured with Axio Vision 4.7 software (Carl Zeiss, Oberkochen, Germany). Negative control was performed by omission of the primary antibody and/or by replacing this antibody with non-immune serum. The sensitivity of the reaction was tested by using immunoreactive liver samples of a patient diagnosed with YF who had a known expression of the viral antigen (positive control).

Detection of Viral RNA by RT-PCR

YF virus envelope protein gene fragments were detected through the PCR assay in maternal liver, placenta, fetal brain, and liver of live fetuses and stillbirths of vaccinated mothers on gd5.5 and in the placenta and liver of mothers vaccinated on gd0.5 and 11.5. Positive control reactions were performed using samples of the YF vaccine. Total RNA was isolated with TRIzol (Invitrogen™, Carlsbad, CA, United States) and suspended again in sterile distilled water according to Chomizynski and Sacchi (1987). All reagents were purchased from Sigma Aldrich (St. Louis, MO, United States), unless otherwise stated. RNA concentration and purity were determined by spectrophotometric measurement of absorbance at 260 nm, and the purity was determined at A260/A280 ratio. The RNA integrity was checked by using

1% agarose gel electrophoresis with 0.4 mol/L Tris-acetate and 0.001 mol/L EDTA buffer. Viral RNA was converted to cDNA using 5.0 μg of RNA, 5.0 μL of specific antisense primer (5′-GCT TTT CCA TAC CCA ATG AA-3′ (MG922934.1), 2.0 μL dNTPs Mix, 0.75 μL M-MLV reverse transcriptase (Invitrogen™), 6.0 μL reaction buffer 5 × and 3.0 μL DTT 0.1 M. The mixture was incubated at 37°C for 90 min and at 95°C for 5 min to inactivate the reverse transcriptase. The viral cDNA (6.0 μL) was amplified by PCR using a 2.5 μL 10 × PCR buffer (Biotools B&M Labs S.A., Madrid, Spain), 2.0 μL $MgCl_2$ (50 mM), 1.0 μL of dNTPs Mix, 0.5 μL DMSO 4%, 0.75 μL DNA polymerase (1 U/μL, Biotools B&M Labs S.A., Madrid, Spain), and 5.0 μL (10 pmol/μL) each of the forward and reverse primers (**1**: 5′-TAC CCT GGA GCA AGA CAA GT-3′; **2**: 5′-GCT TTT CCA TAC CCA ATG AA-3′). The PCR was performed in a Bio-Rad Gene Cycler™ (Bio-Rad Laboratories, Portland, ME, United States). Cycling conditions included denaturation at 94°C for 5 min, 35 PCR cycles of 94°C for 1 min, 58°C for 2 min, 72°C for 3 min and the last step for a final extension at 72°C for 10 min in a thermocycler. PCR was performed using reverse transcripted products from the vaccine's RNA as a template. PCR products were analyzed on 1% agarose gel electrophoresis using a molecular weight marker DNA (100 base pairs, DNA Ladder, Ludwig Biotec, Nova Alvorada, Brazil) as reference. The gel was exposed to a Molecular Imaging screen (G: Box Chemil-R, Syngene, Frederick, MD, United States) for computerized gel documentation (Scion image program, Scion Corp., Frederick, MD, United States). The identity of the 482 bp-amplified products was confirmed by sequence analysis (automated sequence analysis, MegaBACE 1000, GE Healthcare, Buckinghamshire, United Kingdom) at the Center for Human Genome Studies at the University of São Paulo (Brazil). Fluorograms were analyzed using the Cimarron 3.12 base-caller software. A sequence database search was performed using the BLAST network service of the National Center for Biotechnology Information[1].

RESULTS

Vaccination on gd0.5 and 11.5 did not affect the average number of implantation sites and fetal resorption per pregnant female in comparison to controls (**Table 1**). In the group that received vaccination on gd5.5, the mean number of degenerated fetuses and stillbirths and the number of embryo/fetal losses significantly increased (from 0.13 in control group to 1.37 in vaccinated group, $p = 0.01$; and from 0.38 in controls to 3.5 in vaccinated animals, $p = 0.002$, respectively), resulting in an increased mortality rate (from 5.1% in control group to 33.1% in vaccinated group, $p = 0.001$) in comparison to sham controls, as shown in **Table 1**.

Fetal weight gain was significantly lower only when the vaccine was administered in pregnant animals on gd5.5 ($p = 0.004$; **Table 2**). Placental weight was not altered significantly in any vaccinated group compared to the control group. These data indicate the susceptible period to YF vaccination during pregnancy, justifying the subsequent experimental procedures on only day 5.5 of gestation.

Fetuses were macroscopically divided into live fetuses, stillbirths (absence of heartbeat, but no visible degeneration and therefore, considered as late-dead fetuses), early-dead fetuses (with apparent developmental delay and degenerative signals), and post-implantation resorptions (implantation site with no recognizable fetal structures) (**Figure 1**). The subsequent analyses were performed on live fetuses and stillbirths.

In the maternal liver as well as in the liver of live fetuses of the vaccinated females on gd5.5, the viral antigen was rarely immunolocalized (**Figures 2A,B,a,b**). For IH reactions, no immunolabeling was detected in the non-vaccinated group (not shown) in the negative control, which was performed by omitting the primary antibody (**Figures 2G–I**). Biopsies of human liver diagnosed with YF were used as positive control for the IH reactions (**Figure 2J**).

[1] http://www.ncbi.nlm.nih.gov/BLAST/

TABLE 2 | Effect of anti-yellow fever vaccination administered on gestation days 0.5, 5.5, or 11.5 on placental and fetal weights.

	n	Fetal weight (g)	Placental weight (g)
Control gd 0.5	53	0.89 ± 0.17	0.15 ± 0.03
Vaccinated gd 0.5	50	0.87 ± 0.09	0.14 ± 0.02
Control gd 5.5	180	0.95 ± 0.10	0.14 ± 0.04
Vaccinated gd 5.5	158	0.82^a ± 0.12	0.13 ± 0.01
Control gd 11.5	83	0.91 ± 0.11	0.13 ± 0.02
Vaccinated gd 11.5	57	0.88 ± 0.06	0.13 ± 0.02

Values correspond to mean ± SD; values indicated by letters highlight statistical differences in comparison to the respective age-control. Student's t-test ($^a p = 0.004$).

TABLE 1 | Effect of anti-yellow fever vaccination administered on gestation days 0.5, 5.5, and 11.5 on the gestational parameters.

	n	Implantation sites	Number of fetuses	Degenerated fetuses/stillbirths	Embryo/fetal losses	Mortality rate (%)
Control gd 0.5	56	11.2 ± 1.64	10.6 ± 1.95	0.4 ± 0.55	1.0 ± 1.2	9.2 ± 10.3
Vaccinated gd 0.5	53	10.6 ± 3.71	10.0 ± 4.06	0.4 ± 0.89	1.0 ± 1.0	11.6 ± 11.1
Control gd 5.5	96	12.0 ± 2.33	11.7 ± 2.25	0.13 ± 0.35	0.38 ± 0.52	5.1 ± 7.3
Vaccinated gd 5.5	97	12.1 ± 1.89	9.5 ± 1.77	1.37^a ± 1.19	3.5^b ± 1.69	33.1^c ± 17.1
Control gd 11.5	83	10.3 ± 2.38	9.8 ± 2.23	0.25 ± 0.46	0.75 ± 1.16	6.7 ± 9.9
Vaccinated gd11.5	54	10.8 ± 2.17	10.0 ± 2.65	0.4 ± 0.55	1.2 ± 1.10	7.6 ± 9.0

n, Total number of implantation sites. Values correspond to mean number per pregnant female ± SD; $^{a-c}$highlights statistical differences in comparison to the respective age-control. $^a p = 0.01$; $^b p = 0.002$; $^c p = 0.001$ (Student's t-test).

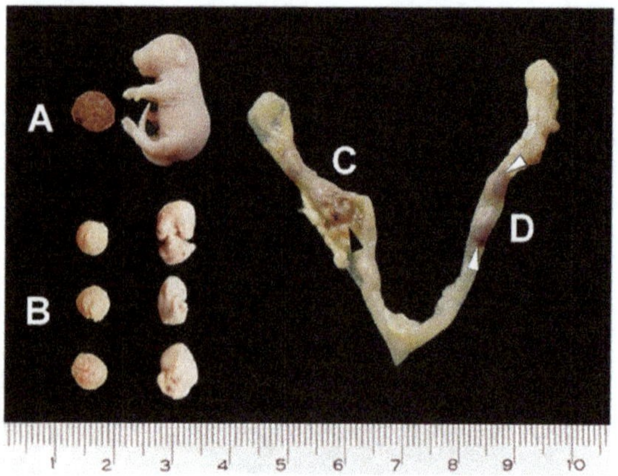

FIGURE 1 | Macroscopic fetal features on gd18.5. Samples from vaccinated pregnant mice present different fetal development, as shown in **(A)** apparently normal (living and stillborn) fetuses, **(B)** early-dead fetuses and **(C,D)** resorptions (black and white arrowheads).

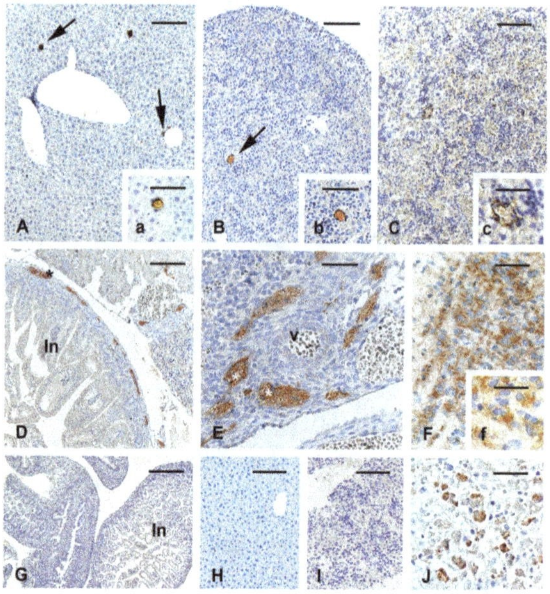

FIGURE 2 | Immunolocalization of the yellow fever (YF) antigen after vaccination on gd 5.5. **(A–C)** In maternal and fetal liver, immunoreactive areas are rare **(A,a)**. Liver of one vaccinated pregnant female **(B,b)**. Liver of a live fetus **(C,c)**. Liver of a stillborn. Reactivity is characterized by a brown colored (arrows) **(D–F)**. Immunolocalization of YF antigen in stillbirths shows reactivity for the virus vaccine in nervous cells in the peripheral area of the developing digestive tract **(D)** and in nerves **(E)** surrounding one arterial vessel (v). Strong reactivity can also be seen in the brain **(F,f)**. Figures **(G–I)** are negative controls of the reaction, in which the primary antibody was replaced by non-immune serum. Figure **(J)** shows the positive control of the IH reaction (liver of a patient with YF). Bars in **(A)** = 150 μm, in **(a,b,E)** = 100 μm, in **(B,C,H,I)** = 200 μm, in **(c,F)** = 60 μm, in **(D)** = 350 μm, in **(f)** = 50 μm, in **(G)** = 600 μm, in **(J)** = 75 μm.

Unlike live fetuses, reactivity to YFV in the stillbirths was intense and distributed in the cells of several organs (**Figures 2C–F**). Reactivity was seen in the liver (**Figures 2C,c**), nervous tissue in the developing intestine (**Figure 2D**), cells surrounding arterial vessels (**Figure 2E**), and in the fetal brain (**Figures 2F,f**).

Histological analysis of placentas from control and viable fetuses of vaccinated animals showed typical morphological features. In live fetuses, immunoreactions revealed the presence of the viral antigen in the trophoblast cells of the junctional zone (trophoblast giant cells, **Figure 3A**) and spongiotrophoblast cells (**Figure 3C**), and only occasionally in the cells of the labyrinthine layers (**Figure 3D**).

In general, placentas from stillbirths showed common characteristics in relation to age-control placentas from vaccinated and control living fetuses. Occasional morphological changes found in this group included the scattering of glycogen cell clusters toward the labyrinthine zone. Viral antigen was seen in the trophoblast giant cells (**Figure 3E**), the spongiotrophoblast cells (**Figure 3F**), and the glycogen cells

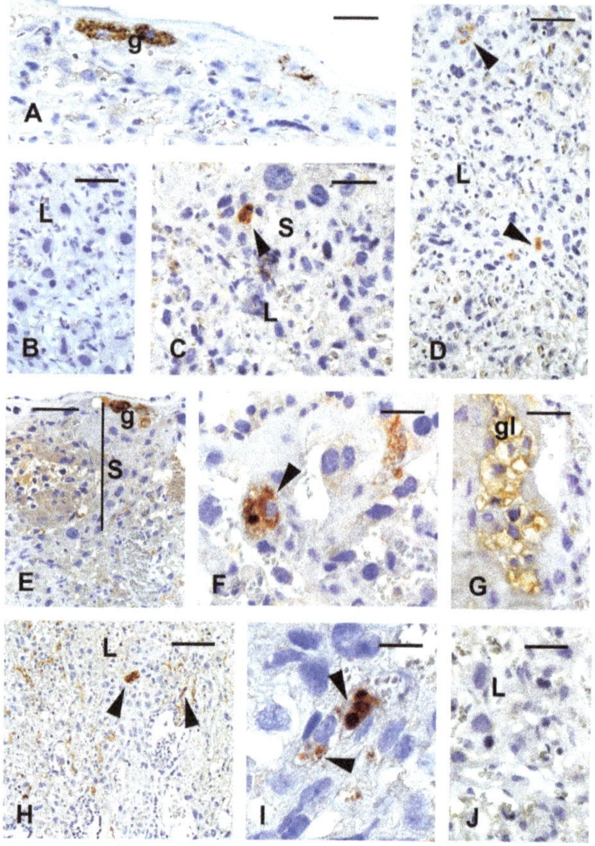

FIGURE 3 | Immunolocalization of the YF antigen after vaccination on gd5.5. Placentas of live fetuses **(A–D)** and stillbirths **(E–J)**. Reactions are characterized by brownish color. The viral antigen is seen at the junctional zone in trophoblast giant cells **(A, g)** and **(C,** arrowhead) in cells of the spongiotrophoblast (S) area. Few cells **(D,** arrowheads) reacted with the antibody against YF virus (YFV) in the labyrinthine region. In stillbirths, the immunoreaction in spongiotrophoblast (S) is intense, in giant cells **(E, g)**, spongiotrophoblast cells **(F,** arrowhead) and in glycogen cells **(G, gl) (H,I)**. Reactivity is also seen in the labyrinth (L, arrowheads). Figures **(B,J)** are negative controls of the reaction. Bars in **(A,D,E)** = 120 μm, in **(B)** = 100 μm, in **(C,G,J)** = 80 μm, in **(F)** = 60 μm, in **(H)** = 240 μm, in **(I)** = 25 μm.

(**Figure 3G**). Reactivity was stronger in the labyrinthine area (**Figures 3H,I**) in different cell types. The negative IH control did not show any reaction in these tissues (**Figures 3B,J**).

The YF vaccine was also detected by RT-PCR using the YFV consensus primer pair. RT-PCR analysis of YFV produced amplicons, as shown in **Figures 4A,B**, in maternal liver, placenta, fetal brain, and liver in stillbirths. In live fetuses, only traces of the amplicons were found in part of the samples (in tissues of 2 fetuses from 7 analyzed). DNA amplification was not observed in the negative control nor in samples from vaccination on gd0.5 and 11.5 (not shown). YFV identity was confirmed by sequencing PCR products obtained from the brain samples of stillbirths ($n = 3$). The sequence was aligned to the YFV strain 17DD-Brazil, and 100% identity was observed (**Figure 4C**).

DISCUSSION

We examined the effect of vaccination against YFV at three different gestational periods in mice and found clear evidence of changes in pregnancy outcomes and fetal infection only when the vaccine was administered during the embryo implantation period (gd 5.5). Vaccination on this particular day of gestation led to increased embryo/fetal losses and growth restriction in live fetuses. The vaccine virus was only occasionally observed in the liver of the live fetuses but consistently found in stillbirths' tissues. Immunolocalization of the vaccine virus was detected in the placenta of both live fetuses and stillbirths, but was more intense in samples of the stillborn fetuses. The presence of the virus in the placenta and fetal organs in the stillbirths indicated that a vertical passage of the vaccine virus may have occurred. In living fetuses, by contrast, the presence of the virus only in the placenta suggests the maternal-fetal interface may assume a protective role. The differences in the fate of individuals belonging to the same litter, however, are not clearly understood.

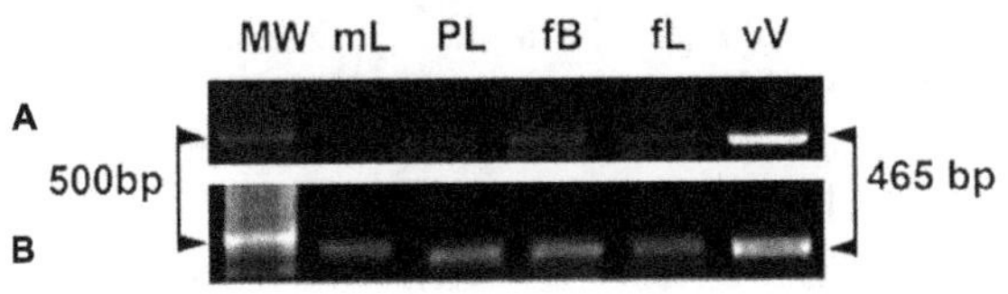

C

```
177p  ACAGCCATTGCCCCAGCCTCTATCAGAATAAGTGCGCTTGCACGCATTGTCCCCTTCGTT  236
      ||||||||||||||||||||||||||||||||||||||||||||||||||||||||||||
1288v ACAGCCATTGCCCCAGCCTCTATCAGAATAAGTGCGCTTGCACGCATTGTCCCCTTCGTT  1229
237p  CTCTTCAGCTAGGTGGGCCTCTCCAGTGCTGGGGCACTTGTCATTAATCTTCACATGAGT  296
      ||||||||||||||||||||||||||||||||||||||||||||||||||||||||||||
1228v CTCTTCAGCTAGGTGGGCCTCTCCAGTGCTGGGGCACTTGTCATTAATCTTCACATGAGT  1169
297p  GAGAACTGCATTGTAACACACTTTCCTCGCCTCAGCAGGTCTATCAATGGCTACTGTCTC  356
      ||||||||||||||||||||||||||||||||||||||||||||||||||||||||||||
1168v GAGAACTGCATTGTAACACACTTTCCTCGCCTCAGCAGGTCTATCAATGGCTACTGTCTC  1109
357p  TAGTGAGATGTCCAATGAAGGCTTGTCAGGGGCCATAACAGTGACACACTTGTCTTGCTC  416
      ||||||||||||||||||||||||||||||||||||||||||||||||||||||||||||
1108v TAGTGAGATGTCCAATGAAGGCTTGTCAGGGGCCATAACAGTGACACACTTGTCTTGCTC  1049
417p  CAGGGTA  423
      |||||||
1048v CAGGGTA  1042
```

FIGURE 4 | Gene expression of the YF viral capsid protein (465 bp) in maternal liver and tissues of viable fetuses **(A)** and stillbirths **(B)**. Maternal liver (mL), placenta (Pl), fetal brain (fB), liver (fL), (Vv) vaccine YF virus (positive control). The first band of each gel corresponds to the DNA weight in which 500 base pairs are highlighted (arrowheads). **(C)** Sequencing of the experimental PCR product obtained from brain of stillbirths. Note the alignment and 100% identity with the yellow fever virus strain 17DD-Brazil.

Genetic background of each individual may be a factor to be considered, as the strain used here is an outbred mouse. In humans, it has been suggested that modulation of susceptibility to the virus may occur as a result of genetic variation, particularly in loci encoding innate immune mediators (Blake and Garcia-Blanco, 2014). In addition, mice generally have an innate resistance to flavivirus-induced mortality/morbidity due to the autosomal dominant *Flvr* allele. When infected, mice exhibit low levels of viral titers in their tissues, which is associated with a low mortality rate (Nathanson and Brinton, 2007). While that might be one contributing factor, there is also evidence suggesting that the transplacental transfer of a flavivirus is a stochastic process (Yuan and Allen, 2011; Björnberg et al., 2014). Stochastic models have been developed to explain the dynamics of viral infection/transmission, which includes random transitions between infection, latent infection, or non-infection in cells, tissues, and organisms (Tuckwell and Le Corfec, 1998; Yuan and Allen, 2011; Björnberg et al., 2014).

A key question in this study is why changes occurred only following the administration of the vaccine on gd5.5. A plausible explanation may be the immaturity of the cells that comprise the maternal-fetal barrier at this stage of gestation. Day 5.5 of gestation marks the beginning of the implantation process. At this time, the trophoblast giant cells assume an invasive phenotype, thereby opening subluminal endometrial capillaries and establishing the first contact with maternal blood (Bevilacqua and Abrahamsohn, 1988, 1989). This process lasts for a few more days until the embryo is fully lodged in the uterine tissue. The placenta then starts the maturation process, which is characterized by the differentiation of the trophoblast cells to assume defensive, endocrine, immune regulatory, and nutritional properties (Adamson et al., 2002; Cross, 2005; Hu and Cross, 2009).

Evidence from a previous study in humans showed that vaccination results in viremia from the second to the sixth day after administration (Reinhardt et al., 1998). In this context, it is possible that in our experiments, maternal viremia had occurred at the phase of trophoblast immaturity soon after implantation. This might foster a condition of viral access to the embryonic tissues, boosting reactions not found when the vaccine is administered in later stages of pregnancy. In summary, on gd5.5 and the subsequent few days, the trophoblast giant cells may not be mature or differentiated enough to act as a barrier to viral passage. Based on this, vaccination in the later stages of gestation (gd11.5) might be related to full placental differentiation and ability for efficient activation of antiviral mechanisms. In contrast, the lack of contact between maternal blood and the embryo during the early stages of development, when the mothers were inoculated on gd0.5 may be the critical factor that prevented adverse fetal outcomes in this group. In both cases, our results over these periods are consistent with the findings of vaccination studies in humans.

The disparity with human vaccination data, however, occurred when vaccine inoculation was performed specifically during embryo implantation (day 5.5 of gestation), which resulted in early and late losses (stillbirths).

Studies assessing YF vaccination during early stages of pregnancy also reported a trend toward increased odds of several adverse events (miscarriages, premature births, and low birth weight) when women inadvertently received the vaccine through mass vaccination programs (Tsai, 1993, 2006; Nishioka et al., 1998). The deleterious effect on gestation outcome and fetal development, however, was considered within the expected population indices (Nasidi et al., 1993; Robert et al., 1999; Suzano et al., 2006; D'Acremont et al., 2008). As mentioned earlier, one possible explanation for this disparity may be the organization of the maternal-fetal barrier in its early stages, as having species-specific functional and structural aspects (Georgiades et al., 2002) may determine the passage of the virus to the fetal organism in rodents, but not in humans. In addition, the discrepancy may in part be due to the impossibility of determining in which gestational phase the vaccine has been administered. Peri-implantation losses in humans are hardly detectable, and hence, they are usually not reported and considered for statistical analysis reported in the literature.

The incidence of growth restriction and stillbirths in mothers vaccinated on gd5.5 may be based on several mechanisms, alone or in association. Viral access and lodgment in the developing mouse placenta may be a major factor. Although, morphologically, we did not see any placental damage or placental maturation defects, the immunoreactivity to the vaccine virus at the spongiotrophoblast and labyrinthine zones (also detected by PCR) may represent early access (gd5.5) and further colonization leading to different degrees of placental function impairment.

Virus immunolocalization graded from placental and fetal tissues with occasional antibody reactions (in the live fetuses) to areas of extensive antibody reactivity (in stillbirths), suggesting that the degree of placental/fetal infection might be related to fetal death.

Another possibility is the commitment of fetal metabolism when the placental barrier has not been able to prevent the passage of the virus. YF infection is characterized by a viral viscerotropism in which the liver and nervous system can be aggressively infected, as reported in humans who have succumbed to the infection post-vaccination (Monath, 2008; Martins et al., 2015; Monath and Vasconcelos, 2015). Our immunolocalization and PCR results also detected the presence of the vaccine virus and activity in the nervous tissues of stillborn fetuses, which may have contributed to the impairment of this system and fetal death as a direct cytopathic effect.

The fetal and maternal immune environment may also be an important factor in determining fetal infection when vaccination occurred on gd5.5. There is a well-orchestrated pro- and anti-inflammatory cytokine network locally produced to modulate the complex process of implantation (Dey et al., 2004; Chaouat et al., 2007). On the other hand, YF vaccination also induces a proinflammatory response, where TNF-α, among other cytokines seems to be a key factor (Monath and Vasconcelos, 2015). This may lead to an immune overreaction with the release of proinflammatory cytokines and other mediators of the innate immune system into the fetal circulation, resulting in outcomes such as early embryo deaths and low birth weight in the surviving fetuses (Chaouat et al., 2007; Chattopadhyay et al., 2010; Kurtis et al., 2011). Recent evidence has also shown that pregnant rat females with Zika virus infection exhibited a robust inflammatory response, including critical cytokines and chemokines, regardless of the mother's response to the virus (Khaiboullina et al., 2019). A similar response is also observed in Zika virus infection in pregnant Rhesus monkeys (Hirsch et al., 2018). From this perspective, the plethora of immune factors that are triggered by viral infections may also have been the cause of the gestational outcomes obtained in this study, a question that deserves further research effort.

This study has no exact answers as to why this does not occur at the same frequency in humans. The greater fragility of the trophoblastic barrier in the early stages of gestation in mice may also be an essential factor. Protective neutralizing antibodies were found 14 days after vaccination in humans (Kohler et al., 2012), which were transferred to the embryo/fetus throughout the term of the human pregnancy, limiting viral growth and its deleterious effects. However, in this study, the short gestational period associated with the interval between vaccination and sacrifice of the mice (gd5.5 to gd18.5) might not be sufficient to transfer appropriate protective IgG to the fetal organism.

In summary, our results showed that mouse vaccination does not change gestational parameters when administered in early or mid-gestation. Adverse outcomes such as fetal growth restriction and increased rate of mortality could be observed only when vaccination occurred during the embryo implantation period. The localization of virus particles in the placenta and fetus indicates that YF vaccine virus may have crossed the placental barrier in a stochastic process. In living fetuses, the presence of the virus was limited or absent, whereas in stillbirths, the immunoreactivity and the viral load were high in the placenta and fetal organs. The heterogeneity of responses suggests that the stage of embryo implantation represents a window of susceptibility in which vaccination and associated immune response may interfere with the course of gestation.

CONCLUSION

The yellow fever vaccine virus passed the placental barrier only when administered during embryo implantation, inducing fetal growth restriction and increased fetal mortality rate.

AUTHOR CONTRIBUTIONS

FS and EB wrote the draft of the manuscript. EB and HS designed the study. All authors except HS participated in data collection. Data analysis was conducted by FS and FM, who vouch for the findings.

ACKNOWLEDGMENTS

The authors thank Rosangela Augusto Oliveira, Helori Vanni Domingos, and Bruna Galves for providing excellent technical assistance, Prof. Charlotte Marianna Harsi for assistance with the YF vaccine doses and, Cristina Takami Kanamura for generous access to the laboratory facilities.

REFERENCES

Adamson, S. L., Lu, Y., Whiteley, K. J., Holmyard, D., Hemberger, M., Pfarrer, C., et al. (2002). Interactions between trophoblast cells and the maternal and fetal circulation in the mouse placenta. *Dev. Biol.* 250, 358–373. doi: 10.1006/dbio.2002.0773

Bevilacqua, E., and Abrahamsohn, P. A. (1988). Ultrastructure of trophoblast giant cell transformation during the invasive stage of implantation of the mouse embryo. *J. Morphol.* 198, 341–345.

Bevilacqua, E., and Abrahamsohn, P. A. (1989). Trophoblast invasion during implantation of the mouse embryo. *Arch. Biol. Med. Exp.* 22, 107–118.

Björnberg, J. E., Britton, T., Broman, E. I., and Natan, E. (2014). A stochastic model for virus growth in a cell population. *J. Applied Prob.* 51, 599–612. doi: 10.1239/jap/1409932661

Blake, L. E., and Garcia-Blanco, M. A. (2014). Human genetic variation and yellow fever mortality during 19th Century U.S. *Epidemics. mBio* 5:e01253-14. doi: 10.1128/mBio.01253-14

Chaouat, G., Dubanchet, S., and Ledée, N. (2007). Cytokines: important for implantation? *J. Assist. Reprod. Genet.* 24, 491–505. doi: 10.1007/s10815-007-9142-9

Chattopadhyay, A., Robinson, N., Sandhu, J. K., Finlay, B. B., Sad, S., and Krishnan, L. (2010). *Salmonella enterica* serovar typhimurium-induced placental inflammation and not bacterial burden correlates with pathology and fatal maternal disease. *Infect. Immun.* 78, 2292–2301. doi: 10.1128/IAI.01186-09

Chomizynski, P., and Sacchi, N. (1987). Single-step method of RNA isolation by acid guanidinium thiocyanate phenol cloroformextration. *Anal. Biochem.* 162, 156–159. doi: 10.1006/abio.1987.9999

Cross, J. C. (2005). How to make a placenta: mechanisms of trophoblast cell differentiation in mice: a review. *Placenta* 26, S3–S9.

Croy, B. A., Yamada, A. T., De Mayo, F. J., and Adamson, S. L. (2014). *The Guide to Investigation of Mouse Pregnancy*. Amsterdam: Elsevier.

D'Acremont, V., Tremblay, S., and Genton, B. (2008). Impact of vaccines given during pregnancy on the offspring of women consulting a travel clinic: a longitudinal study. *J. Travel. Med.* 15, 77–81. doi: 10.1111/j.1708-8305.2007.00175.x

Dean, C. H., Alarcon, J. B., Waterston, A. M., Draper, K., Guirakhoo, F., Monath, T. P., et al. (2005). Cutaneous delivery of a live, attenuated chimeric flavivirus vaccine against Japanese encephalitis (ChimeriVax)-JE) in non-human primates. *Hum. Vaccines.* 1, 106–111. doi: 10.4161/hv.1.3.1797

Dey, S. K., Lim, H., Das, S. K., Reese, J., Paria, B. C., Daikoku, T., et al. (2004). Molecular cues to implantation. *Endocr. Rev.* 25, 341–373. doi: 10.1210/er.2003-0020

Engelmann, F., Josset, L., Girke, T., Park, B., and Barron, A. (2014). Pathophysiologic and transcriptomic analyses of viscerotropic yellow fever in a rhesus macaque model. *PLoS Negl. Trop. Dis.* 8:e3295. doi: 10.1371/journal.pntd.0003295

Fernandes, N., Cunha, M., Guerra, J., Réssio, R. A., Cirqueira, C. S., Iglezias, S. D. A., et al. (2017). Outbreak of yellow fever among nonhuman primates. *Espírito Santo, Brazil. Emerg. Infect. Dis.* 23, 2038–2041. doi: 10.3201/eid2312.170685

Georgiades, P., Ferguson-Smith, A. C., and Burton, G. J. (2002). Comparative developmental anatomy of the murine and human definitive placentae. *Placenta* 23, 3–19. doi: 10.1053/plac.2001.0738

Hagmann, S. H. F., Rao, S. R., LaRocque, R. C., Erskine, S., Jentes, E. S., Walker, A. T., et al. (2017). Travel characteristics and pretravel health care among pregnant or breastfeeding U.S. women preparing for international travel. *Obstet. Gynecol.* 130, 1357–1365. doi: 10.1097/AOG.0000000000002360

Hirsch, A. J., Roberts, V. H. J., Grigsby, P. L., Haese, N., Schabel, M. C., Wang, X., et al. (2018). Zika virus infection in pregnant rhesus macaques causes placental dysfunction and immunopathology. *Nat. Commun.* 9:263. doi: 10.1038/s41467-017-02499-9

Hu, D., and Cross, J. (2009). Development and function of trophoblast giant cells in the rodent placenta. *Int. J. Dev. Biol.* 54, 341–354. doi: 10.1387/ijdb.082768dh

Khaiboullina, S. F., Lopes, P., de Carvalho, T. G., Real, A. L. C. V., Souza, D. G., Costa, V. V., et al. (2019). Host immune response to ZIKV in an immunocompetent embryonic mouse model of intravaginal infection. *Viruses* 11:558. doi: 10.3390/v11060558

Khaiboullina, S. F., Rizvanov, A. A., Holbrook, M. R., and Jeor, S. S. (2005). Yellow fever virus strains Asibi and 17D-204 infect human umbilical cord endothelial cells and induce novel changes in gene expression. *Virology* 342, 167–176. doi: 10.1016/j.virol.2005.07.035

Kohler, S., Bethke, N., Böthe, M., Sommerick, S., Frentsch, M., Romagnani, C., et al. (2012). The early cellular signatures of protective immunity induced by live viral vaccination. *Europ. J. Immunol.* 42, 2363–2373. doi: 10.1002/eji.201142306

Kurtis, J. D., Higashi, A., Wu, H. W., Gundogan, F., McDonald, E. A., Sharma, S., et al. (2011). Maternal Schistosomiasis japonica is associated with maternal, placental, and fetal inflammation. *Infect. Immun.* 79, 1254–1261. doi: 10.1128/IAI.01072-10

Leal, S. G., Romano, A. P., Moreno, R. V., Melo, C. B., Vasconcelos, P. F., and Castro, M. B. (2016). Frequency of histopathological changes in Howler monkeys (Alouatta sp.) naturally infected with yellow fever virus in Brazil. *Rev. Soc. Bras. Med. Trop.* 49, 29–33. doi: 10.1590/0037-8682-0363-2015

Lee, E., and Lobigs, M. (2008). E Protein domain III determinants of yellow fever virus 17D vaccine strain enhance binding to glycosaminoglycans, impede virus spread, and attenuate virulence. *J. Virol.* 82, 6024–6033. doi: 10.1128/JVI.02509-07

Marchette, N. J., Halstead, S. B., Falkler, R., Stenhouse, A., and Nash, D. (1973). Studies on the pathogenesis of dengue infection in monkeys. 3. sequential distribution of virus in primary and heterologous infections. *J. Infect. Dis.* 128, 23–30. doi: 10.1093/infdis/128.1.23

Marinho, P. S., Cunha, A. J., Amim Junior, J., and Prata-Barbosa, A. (2017). A review of selected arboviruses during pregnancy. *Matern. Health Neonatol. Perinatol.* 3:17. doi: 10.1186/s40748-017-0054-0

Martins, R., Fernandes, M. L. L., and Homma, A. (2015). Serious adverse events associated with yellow fever vaccine. *Hum. Vaccin. Immunother.* 11, 2183–2187. doi: 10.1080/21645515.2015.1022700

Monath, T. P. (2008). Treatment of yellow fever. *Antiviral Res.* 78, 116–124.

Monath, T. P. (2013). 17D yellow fever virus vaccine. *Am. J. Trop. Med. Hyg.* 89:1225. doi: 10.4269/ajtmh.13-0443a

Monath, T. P., and Barrett, A. D. T. (2003). Pathogenesis and pathophysiology of yellow fever. *Adv. Virus Res.* 60, 343–395. doi: 10.1016/s0065-3527(03)60009-6

Monath, T. P., Gershman, M., Staples, E. J., and Barrett, A. D. T. (2013). "Yellow fever vaccine," in *Vaccines*, 6th Edn, eds S. A. Plotkin, W. A. Orenstein, and P. A. Offit, (Philadelphia, PA: Saunders), 870–896.

Monath, T. P., and Vasconcelos, P. F. (2015). Yellow fever. *J. Clin. Virol.* 64, 160–173. doi: 10.1016/j.jcv.2014.08.030

Nasidi, A., Monath, T. P., Vanderberg, J., Tomori, O., Calosher, C. H., Hunrtgen, X., et al. (1993). Yellow fever vaccination and pregnancy: a four-year prospective study. *Trans. R. Soc. Trop. Med. Hyg.* 87, 337–339. doi: 10.1016/0035-9203(93)90156-k

Nathanson, N., and Brinton, M. A. (2007). "Host susceptibility to viral diseases," in *Viral Pathogenesis and Immunity*, 2nd Edn, eds N. Nathanson, R. Ahmed, C. A.

Biron, M. Brinton, F. Gonzales-Scarano, D. E. Griffin, et al. (London: Academic Press:), 174–183.

Nishioka, S., Nunes-Araújo, F. R., Pires, W. P., Silva, F. A., and Costa, H. L. (1998). Yellow fever vaccination during pregnancy and spontaneous abortion: a case control study. *Trop. Med. Int. Health* 3, 29–33. doi: 10.1046/j.1365-3156.1998.00164.x

Quaresma, J. A., Barros, V. L., Pagliari, C., Fernandes, E. R., Guedes, F., Takakura, C. F., et al. (2006a). Revisiting the liver in human yellow fever: virus-induced apoptosis in hepatocytes associated with TGF-β. TNF-α and NK cells activity. *Virology* 345, 22–30. doi: 10.1016/j.virol.2005.09.058

Quaresma, J. A., Duarte, M. I. S., and Vasconcelos, P. F. C. (2006b). Midzonal lesions in yellow fever: a specific pattern of liver injury caused by direct virus action and in situ inflammatory response. *Med. Hypotheses* 67, 618–621. doi: 10.1016/j.mehy.2006.01.060

Quaresma, J. A., Pagliari, C., Medeiros, D. B. A., Duarte, M. I. S., and Vasconcelos, P. F. C. (2013). Immunity and immune response, pathology and pathologic changes: progress and challenges in the immunopathology of yellow fever. *Rev. Med. Virol.* 23, 305–318. doi: 10.1002/rmv.1752

Reinhardt, B., Jaspert, R., Niedrig, M., Kostner, C., and L'age-Stehr, J. (1998). Development of viremia and humoral and cellular parameters of immune activation after vaccination with yellow fever virus strain 17D: a model of human flavivirus infection. *J. Med. Virol.* 56, 159–167. doi: 10.1002/(sici)1096-9071(199810)56:2<159::aid-jmv10>3.0.co;2-b

Robert, E., Vial, T., Schaefer, C., Arnon, J., and Reuvers, M. (1999). Exposure to yellow fever vaccine in early pregnancy. *Vaccine* 17, 283–285. doi: 10.1016/s0264-410x(98)00051-6

Salewsky, E. (1964). *Färbemethode* zum *makroskopschen* nachweis von implantationsstellen am uterus der ratte. *Arch. Exp. Path. Pharm.* 247:367. doi: 10.1007/bf02308461

Staples, E. J., and Monath, T. P. (2011). "Yellow Fever," in *Tropical Infectious Diseases: Principles, Pathogens and Practice*, 3rd Edn, eds R. L. Guerrant, D. H. Walker, and P. F. Weller, (Philadelphia, PA: Saunders), 492–503.

Suzano, C. E. S., Amaral, E., Sato, H. K., and Papaiordanou, P. M. (2006). The effects of yellow fever immunization (17DD) inadvertently used in early pregnancy during a mass campaign in Brazil. *Vaccine* 24, 1421–1426. doi: 10.1016/j.vaccine.2005.09.033

Tsai, T. F. (1993). Congenital yellow fever virus infection after immunization in pregnancy. *J. Infect. Dis.* 168, 1520–1523. doi: 10.1093/infdis/168.6.1520

Tsai, T. F. (2006). Congenital arboviral infections: something new, something old. *Pediatrics* 117, 537–545.

Tuckwell, H. C., and Le Corfec, E. (1998). A stochastic model for early HIV-1 population dynamics. *J. Theor. Biol.* 195, 451–463. doi: 10.1006/jtbi.1998.0806

Waggoner, J. J., Rojas, A., and Pinsky, B. A. (2018). Yellow fever virus: diagnostics for a persistent arboviral threat. *J. Clin. Microbiol.* 56:e00827-18. doi: 10.1128/JCM.00827-18

Watson, E. D., and Cross, J. C. (2005). Development of structures and transport functions in the mouse placenta. *Physiology* 20, 180–193. doi: 10.1152/physiol.00001.2005

Woodson, S. E., Freiberg, A. N., and Holbrook, M. R. (2011). Differential cytokine responses from primary human Kupffer cells following infection with wild-type or vaccine strain yellow fever virus. *Virology* 412, 188–195. doi: 10.1016/j.virol.2011.01.012

Yuan, Y., and Allen, L. J. (2011). Stochastic models for virus and immune system dynamics. *Math. Biosci.* 234, 84–94. doi: 10.1016/j.mbs.2011.08.007

7

Toll-Like Receptor 2 is Involved in Abnormal Pregnancy in Mice Infected with *Toxoplasma gondii* during Late Pregnancy

Rina Ikeda[1], Nanako Ushio[1], Ahmed M. Abdou[1,2], Hidefumi Furuoka[3] and Yoshifumi Nishikawa[1]*

[1]National Research Center for Protozoan Diseases, Obihiro University of Agriculture and Veterinary Medicine, Obihiro, Japan, [2]Department of Forensic Medicine and Toxicology, Faculty of Veterinary Medicine, South Valley University, Qena, Egypt, [3]Division of Pathobiological Science, Department of Basic Veterinary Medicine, Obihiro University of Agriculture and Veterinary Medicine, Obihiro, Japan

***Correspondence:**
Yoshifumi Nishikawa
nisikawa@obihiro.ac.jp

Infection with *Toxoplasma gondii* during pregnancy causes failure of pregnancy maintenance, resulting in fetal death, abortion, stillbirth, or premature birth, but the mechanism of disease onset remains unclear. Although Toll-like receptor 2 (TLR2) is expressed on antigen-presenting cells and trophoblasts, the role of TLR2 in *T. gondii* infection during pregnancy is unknown. In this study, we investigated the role of TLR2 in congenital toxoplasmosis using TLR2-deficient ($TLR2^{-/-}$) mice. *T. gondii* infection on gestational day 12.5 (Gd12.5) induced more abnormal pregnancy, including premature birth and stillbirth, in wild-type mice than in $TLR2^{-/-}$ mice. Multiple calcifications were observed in the placentas of the infected wild-type mice. At Gd18.5 (6 days postinfection), the parasite numbers in the placenta and uterus and the histological changes did not differ significantly between the wild-type and $TLR2^{-/-}$ mice. However, *T. gondii* infection reduced the mRNA expression of interleukin-12p40 (IL-12p40) and increased IL-4 and IL-10 mRNAs in the placentas of the wild-type mice. In contrast, the placentas of the $TLR2^{-/-}$ mice showed no changes in the expression of these cytokines, including IL-6 and tumor necrosis factor α, in response to *T. gondii* infection. Serum interferon-γ levels were significantly lower in the infected $TLR2^{-/-}$ mice than in the infected wild-type mice on Gd18.5. Thus, the $TLR2^{-/-}$ mice were less susceptible to the induction of immune responses by *T. gondii* infection during late pregnancy. Therefore, TLR2 signaling may play a role in the development of disease states during pregnancy, specifically placental hypofunction.

Keywords: *Toxoplasma gondii*, congenital toxoplasmosis, TLR2, mouse, multiple calcifications, pregnancy

INTRODUCTION

Toxoplasma gondii is an obligate intracellular eukaryotic parasite of the phylum Apicomplexa, which is thought to infect about 30% of the world's population (Montoya and Liesenfeld, 2004). It infects humans and homothermic animals, causing toxoplasmosis. In humans, first infection with *T. gondii* during pregnancy can cause a wide variety of morbidities, including abortion, stillbirth, and premature birth, depending upon the stage of pregnancy (Hill and Dubey, 2002; Givens and Marley, 2008). The development of preventive and therapeutic measures against *T. gondii* infections during pregnancy is an important issue, but the mechanism of disease onset remains unclear.

The dynamics of the immune system during pregnancy are associated with the maintenance of pregnancy. Pathogen infection during early pregnancy stimulates inflammatory responses at the fetal–maternal interface, resulting in embryo resorption and abortion (Entrican, 2002). During *T. gondii* infection, the proinflammatory T-helper 1 (Th1)-type cytokines, such as tumor necrosis factor α (TNF-α), interferon γ (IFN-γ), interleukin 2 (IL2) and migration inhibitory factor, can be detrimental to pregnancy and fetal survival, whereas such inflammatory responses play an important role in the host defenses (Chaouat et al., 1990; Coutinho et al., 2012; Gomes et al., 2018). In particular, excessive IFN-γ released during pregnancy can cause the apoptosis of mouse decidual cells at the fetal–maternal interface (Senegas et al., 2009; Coutinho et al., 2012) and of human trophoblast cells (Angeloni et al., 2013; Zhang et al., 2015). In previous studies, we showed that chemokine receptors are involved in the host defenses, the apoptosis of embryos, and fetal resorption during early pregnancy. The C-X-C motif chemokine receptor 3 (CXCR3)-dependent immune response reduces the embryo resorption and fetal loss caused by *T. gondii* infection (Nishida et al., 2021), whereas C-C chemokine receptor type 5 triggers the apoptosis of embryos and fetal resorption in mice infected with *T. gondii* (Nishimura et al., 2017). These findings suggest that the maternal immune response is associated with the maintenance or the failure of early pregnancy dependent on the host receptor.

Microbes infect trophoblasts and other placental cells, resulting in pregnancy complications such as abortion and stillbirth (Gibbs, 2002; Goldenberg et al., 2010; Robbins and Bakardjiev, 2012). Placental immune tolerance is required to prevent fetal rejection and maintain pregnancy. The trophoblast expresses pattern recognition receptors (PRRs) and constitutively secretes cytokines to regulate the immune balance at the maternal–fetal borders and to maintain pregnancy. *T. gondii* infection disrupts the balance of PRR-mediated cytokine secretion in the placenta and induces an inflammatory response at the maternal–fetal interface, making the maintenance of pregnancy difficult (Abrahams et al., 2005; Costello et al., 2007). Furthermore, primary trophoblast cells express all the 10 types of TLR, TLR1-10, while choriocarcinoma cell lines possess broad TLR gene expression, but lacked functional cytokine response to TLR ligand activation (Gierman et al., 2015). Toll-like receptor 2 (TLR2) is an important PRR that controls *T. gondii* infection. During *T. gondii* infection in nonpregnant mice, TLR2 induces a Th1 immune response, with the production of IFN-γ, IL-12, and nitric oxide, and plays an important role in the elimination of the parasite (Mun et al., 2003; Umeda et al., 2017; Ihara et al., 2019). TLR2 is also involved in the production of cytokines and prostaglandin E_2 by brain cells, astrocytes, and microglia (Umeda et al., 2017). It is reported to recognize glycosylphosphatidylinositol from *T. gondii* (Debierre-Grockiego et al., 2003), and is one of the PRRs expressed on antigen-presenting cells and trophoblasts in early and late gestation (Abrahams et al., 2004; Rindsjö et al., 2007). TLR2 tends to be highly expressed in the placentas of pregnant women with chorioamnionitis, suggesting a relationship between TLR2 and pregnancy failure (Kim et al., 2004; Riley and Nelson, 2010; Thaxton et al., 2010).

Significant immunomodulation of the Th1 immune response occurs at mid-gestation, resulting in a Th2 cytokine environment at the maternal–fetal interface (Reinhard et al., 1998). Because *T. gondii* cannot be controlled by Th2 cytokines, the consequence of infection will be the death of the fetus or the offspring may be born and show adverse symptoms at birth (Wang et al., 2011). However, the role of TLR2 in the maintenance of late gestation during *T. gondii* infection remains unknown. In this study, we investigated the disease status of *T. gondii* infection during late gestation using TLR2-deficient ($TLR2^{-/-}$) mice to clarify the TLR2-dependent immunological mechanism of pregnancy failure.

MATERIALS AND METHODS

Ethics Statement

This study was performed in strict accordance with the recommendations of the Guide for the Care and Use of Laboratory Animals of the Ministry of Education, Culture, Sports, Science and Technology, Japan. The protocol was approved by the Committee on the Ethics of Animal Experiments at Obihiro University of Agriculture and Veterinary Medicine, Obihiro, Japan (permit numbers 18–50, 19–56, 20–27). All surgeries were performed under isoflurane anesthesia, and every effort was made to minimize animal suffering.

Mice

C57BL/6 mice (wild-type) were obtained from CLEA Japan (Tokyo, Japan). Homozygous *TLR2*-knockout ($TLR2^{-/-}$) mice were a kind gift from Dr. Satoshi Uematsu and Dr. Shizuo Akira of Osaka University (Osaka, Japan; Takeuchi et al., 2000). The mice shown in **Supplementary Tables S1–S3** were maintained under specific-pathogen-free conditions on a 12-h light/dark cycle with free access to water and food in the animal facility of the National Research Center for Protozoan Diseases at the Obihiro University of Agriculture and Veterinary Medicine.

Preparation of *T. gondii* Tachyzoites

Kidney epithelial cells extracted from an African green monkey (Vero cells) cultured in Eagle's minimum essential medium (Sigma, St. Louis, MO, United States) containing 8% heat-inactivated fetal bovine serum and 1% penicillin–streptomycin were used as the host cells for the passage of *T. gondii* (strain PLK; type II) tachyzoites. To purify the tachyzoites, *T. gondii*-infected Vero cells were washed with sterile phosphate-buffered saline detached, suspended in RPMI 1640 medium (Sigma), passed several times through a syringe with a 27G needle, and then passed through a 5.0-mm pore-size filter (Millipore, Bedford, MA, United States).

Comparison of Abnormal Pregnancies Due to Infection

Virgin female wild-type and TLR2$^{-/-}$ mice, aged 8–12 weeks, were mated with males of the same strain. The vulvas of the female mice were observed at 08:00, and a visible vaginal plug was deemed to indicate day 0.5 of pregnancy [gestational day 0.5 (Gd0.5)]. The female mice were weighed daily, and mice with abdominal distension at Gd12.5 were deemed to be pregnant. The pregnant mice were inoculated intraperitoneally with *T. gondii* tachyzoites (1.0×10^4/0.4 ml RPMI-1640 medium) on Gd12.5. Uninfected pregnant mice from both groups were inoculated intraperitoneally with 0.4 ml of RPMI-1640 medium on Gd12.5. A normal birth was defined as "when the weight of the pregnant mouse increased day by day and birth occurred between Gd19.5 and Gd20.5," and all other pregnancies were considered abnormal. Abnormal pregnancies included premature births and stillbirths.

The definition of premature birth was "when delivery occurred earlier than the scheduled date" (McCarthy et al., 2018), and the definition of stillbirth was "when weight loss was observed in the pregnant mouse for two consecutive days and the pups died *in utero*, detected with laparotomy" (Rahman et al., 2017). The information on the mice used in the experiment and the outcomes of the births is shown in **Supplementary Table S1**. Samples were collected immediately after birth in cases of normal and premature births. In cases of stillbirth, samples were collected at the time of confirmation of the death of the pups with laparotomy. For the sampling, live animals were euthanized. Blood samples were collected for the quantitative analysis of serum cytokines. Uteri were collected for the quantitative analysis of parasite numbers. Half the placentas were used for histopathological analysis, and the other half were used to quantify the numbers of parasites and for reverse transcription–real-time quantitative PCR (RT–qPCR) analysis. Information on the samples collected in the postpartum period, including at stillbirth and at Gd18.5 [6 days postinfection (dpi)], is shown in **Supplementary Tables S2 and S3**, respectively.

Quantitative PCR Analysis of Parasite Numbers

The numbers of parasites in the tissues collected from the wild-type and TLR2$^{-/-}$ mice were quantified with a qPCR analysis of *T. gondii* DNA per 50 ng of tissue DNA. For DNA preparation, the tissues were lysed with 10 times the weight of the tissue in extraction buffer (0.1 M Tris–HCl [pH 9.0], 1% SDS, 0.1 M NaCl, and 1 mM EDTA) and 100 µg/ml of proteinase K (Sigma) and incubated at 50°C. DNA was extracted from the tissues with phenol–chloroform–isoamyl alcohol (25:24:1; Sigma), followed by DNA purification by ethanol. Quantitative PCR was performed with the ABI Prism 7900HT Sequence Detection System (Applied Biosystems, Bedford, MA, United States), with Power SYBR™ Green PCR Master Mix (Applied Biosystems), according to the product protocol. The parasite DNA was amplified with primers specific for the *T. gondii B1* gene: forward primer B1-B22 (5'-AACGGGCGAGTAGCACCTGAGGAGA-3') and reverse primer B1-B23 (5'-TGGGTCTACGTCGATGGCATGACAAC-3'; Contini et al., 2005). The parasite numbers were calculated with standard curve interpolation on a plot of the cycle threshold (CT) values against known concentrations of the parasite (serially diluted samples ranging from 10,000 to 0.01 parasites; Tanaka et al., 2013).

Histopathological Analysis

The placental tissues were fixed in 10% neutral-buffered formalin solution for 1–2 weeks at room temperature, dehydrated, and embedded in paraffin, according to the standard method, using a sealed automatic fixation and embedding system (Tissue-Tek VIP 5 Jr., Sakura, Tokyo, Japan). Paraffin blocks were prepared with a paraffin-embedded block preparation system (Tissue-Tek TEC™, Sakura). The paraffin blocks were sliced to 3-µm thickness to prepare the tissue sections, which were stained with hematoxylin and eosin (HE). The tissues were observed with an all-in-one fluorescence microscope (BZ-9000; Keyence, Osaka, Japan) and the BZ-II analysis software (Keyence). All sections were analyzed in a blinded manner. The resultant slides were observed by two veterinary pathologists (N.U. and H.F.).

Immunohistochemistry for Caspase-3 and Image Analysis

Immunohistochemistry for caspase-3 was performed to examine apoptosis in the placentas at Gd18.5. After deparaffinization, antigen was retrieved by microwave oven with citrate buffer (pH 6.0) at 98°C for 15 min. In order to inactivate endogenous peroxidase, the sections were immersed in 3% hydrogen peroxide in methanol for 5 min. Subsequently, the sections were washed with Tris-buffered saline (TBS) and then blocked with 8% skim milk in TBS at 37°C for 40 min. After incubation with the primary antibodies for caspase-3 (Cat# ab13847, Abcam, Cambridge, United Kingdom) at 4°C overnight, the sections were incubated with the DAKO EnVision+ system horseradish peroxidase-labeled polymer anti-rabbit secondary antibody (Dako, Tokyo, Japan) at 37°C for 40 min. Immunolabeled antigens were visualized using 0.05% 3,3'-diaminobenzidine plus 0.03% hydrogen peroxide in a Tris-hydrochloric acid buffer and then counterstained with hematoxylin. The severity of apoptosis in the placenta was quantified using an image-processing method. Immunopositive areas were measured using ImageJ software (National Institutes of Health, Bethesda, MD). Briefly, immunopositive pixels were counted in five randomly selected fields in the placenta.

Real-Time PCR Analysis

To measure mRNA expression, placental tissues were collected from the pregnant mice in the following groups: infected wild-type mice, uninfected wild-type mice, infected TLR2$^{-/-}$ mice, and uninfected TLR2$^{-/-}$ mice. The tissues were crushed with a Bio Masher (Nippi, Tokyo, Japan). The total RNA was extracted with Tri Reagent (Sigma) and then washed with ethanol. cDNA was synthesized from 500 ng of total RNA with Prime Script™ RT Master Mix (Takara, Kusatsu, Japan), according to the product protocol. Real-time PCR was performed with the ABI Prism 7900HT Sequence Detection System (Applied Biosystems), with Power SYBR™ Green PCR Master Mix (Applied Biosystems), according to the product protocol. The relative amounts of mRNA were calculated with the ddCt method, according to the manufacturer's instructions (User Bulletin no. 2; PerkinElmer, Boston, MA, United States). The primer sequences, designed with the Primer Express software (Applied Biosystems), were: β-actin sense primer 5'-GCTCTGGCTCCTAGCACCAT-3', β-actin antisense primer 5'-GCCACCGATCCACACAGAGT-3'; glyceraldehyde 3-phosphate dehydrogenase (GAPDH) sense primer 5'-TGTGTCCGTCGTGGATCTGA-3', GAPDH antisense primer 5'-CCTGCTTCACCACCTTCTTGAT-3'; IL-12p40 sense primer 5'-CGCAGCAAAGCAAGATGTGT-3', IL-12p40 antisense primer 5'-TGGCAAACCAGGAGATGGTT-3'; IL-6 sense primer 5'-TTCCATCCAGTTGCCTTCTTG-3', IL-6 antisense primer 5'-GAAGGCCGTGGTTGTCACC- 3'; TNF-α sense primer 5'-GGCAGGTCTACTTTGGAGTCATTGC-3', TNF-α antisense primer 5'-ACATTCGAGGCTCCAGTGAA-3'; IL-4 sense primer 5'-CACGGATGCGACAAAAATCA-3', IL-4 antisense primer 5'-CTCGTTCAAAATGCCGATGA-3'; and IL-10 sense primer 5'-AAGGGTTACTTGGGTTGC-3', IL-10 antisense primer 5'-AAGGAGTTGTTTCCGTTA-3'. Foxp3 sense primer 5'-GAGAAAGCGGATACCAAA-3', antisense primer 5'-TGTGAGGACTACCGAGCC-3'. The β-actin mRNA was used as the internal control gene after comparison with GAPDH mRNA using RefFinder (Xie et al., 2012). Gene-specific expression was normalized to the expression of the mouse β-actin mRNA.

Analyses of Cytokine and Prostaglandin E2

Blood samples were collected from the mice, and the serum concentrations of IFN-γ and IL4 were measured with enzyme-linked immunosorbent assays (ELISAs; BD Bioscience, San Jose, CA, United States), according to the manufacturers' protocol. The concentration of prostaglandin E2 in sera was also tested with an enzyme immunoassay kit (Cayman Chemical Co., MI, United States).

Statistical Analysis

The analysis software used was GraphPad Prism software (GraphPad Software Inc., La Jolla, CA, United States). Data are presented as means ± standard deviations (SD). Statistical analyses were performed with Fisher's exact test, one-way analysis of variance (ANOVA), two-way ANOVA, F-test, Student's t test, or the Mann–Whitney U test. The levels of statistical significance are shown with asterisks and are defined in each figure legend, together with the name of the statistical test used. p values of <0.05 were considered statistically significant.

RESULT

Abnormal Pregnancy Caused by *T. gondii* Infection

Although there was no significant difference in the bodyweight gain between the uninfected TLR2$^{-/-}$ mice and the infected TLR2$^{-/-}$ mice, the mean bodyweight of the infected wild-type mice at Gd18.5 was lower than that of the uninfected wild-type mice (**Figure 1**). Among the mice infected with *T. gondii*, some animals had abnormal pregnancies, including premature births and stillbirths (**Figure 2A**). The abnormal pregnancy rate was 75% (9/12) in the infected wild-type mice and 12.5% (1/8) in the infected TLR2$^{-/-}$ mice. This result indicates significantly higher abnormal pregnancy rates in the infected wild-type mice, whereas both types of uninfected mice also had normal pregnancies and births (**Figure 2B, Supplementary Table S1**).

Impact of *T. gondii* Infection on Pups and Placentas

We examined the pups and placentas in the postpartum period, including stillbirths, because fetal and placental dysfunction are common causes of pregnancy failure. The number of parasites in the livers of the pups from the infected wild-type and infected TLR2$^{-/-}$ mice was quantified (**Figure 3A**). A small number of *T. gondii* (<4.0 parasites) were detected in the infected wild-type mice (2/48), but not in the infected TLR2$^{-/-}$ mice (0/14), indicating little vertical transmission of *T. gondii* in either type of mouse (**Figure 3A**). In the wild-type mice, relatively higher numbers of parasites were detected in the placentas associated with stillbirths and the uteri associated with premature births, but they did not differ significantly from the samples associated with normal pregnancies

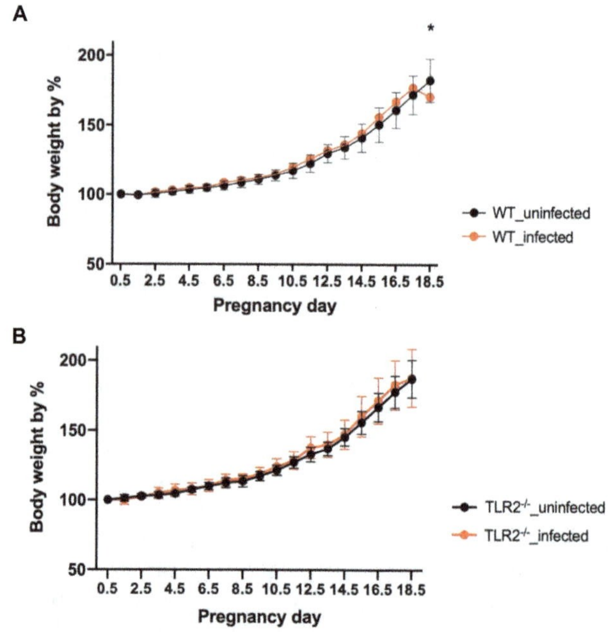

FIGURE 1 | Bodyweight changes in uninfected mice and mice infected with *T. gondii*. Values presented are the means ± standard deviations of each group. **(A)** Bodyweight changes in uninfected wild-type (WT) and *T. gondii*-infected WT mice. **(B)** Bodyweight changes in uninfected TLR2$^{-/-}$ and *T. gondii*-infected TLR2$^{-/-}$ mice. The statistical analysis was performed with two-way ANOVA and Bonferroni's multiple-comparison test. $^{*}p<0.05$.

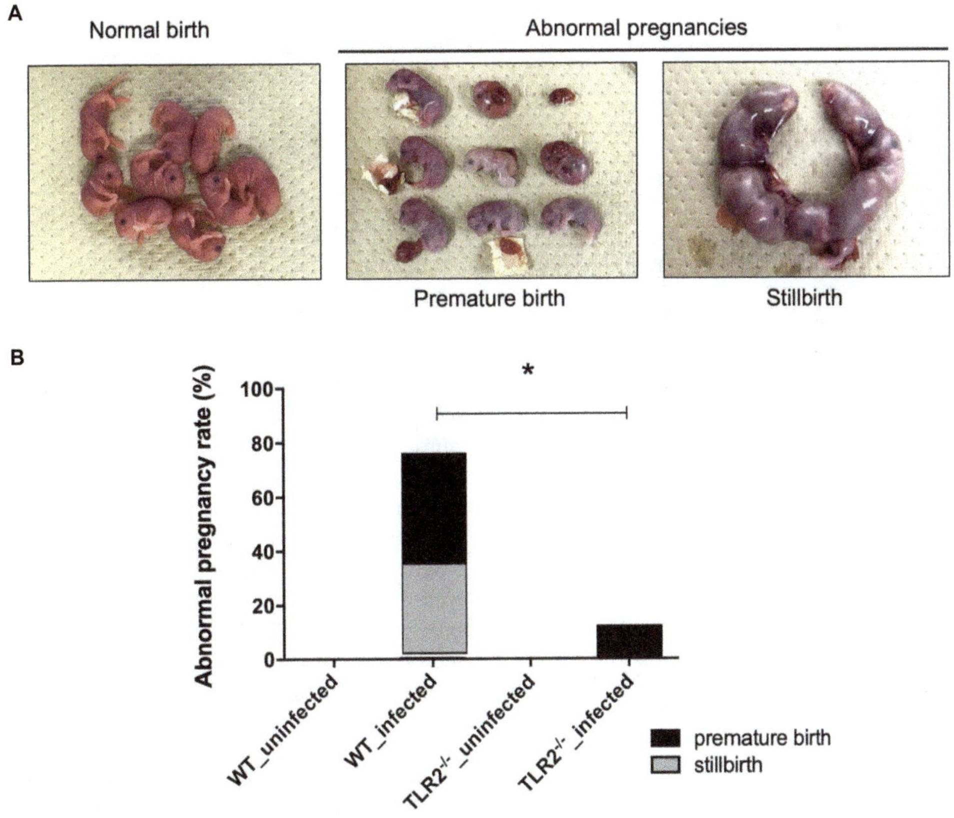

FIGURE 2 | Abnormal pregnancy rates in mice uninfected and infected with *T. gondii*. **(A)** Pups from normal births and dead pups from abnormal pregnancies, such as premature births and stillbirths. Representative photographs are shown. **(B)** Abnormal pregnancy rates in uninfected and infected mice. Abnormal pregnancy rates in each group are shown in a bar graph (uninfected wild-type [WT] mice, 0/12, 0%; infected WT mice, 9/12, 75%; uninfected $TLR2^{-/-}$ mice, 0/5, 0%; infected $TLR2^{-/-}$ mice, 1/8, 12.5%). Statistical analysis was performed with Fisher's exact test. $^{*}p<0.05$.

(**Figures 3B,C**). A histological comparison of the brains and livers of the wild-type and $TLR2^{-/-}$ pups in the uninfected and infected groups showed no histological changes attributable to infection (**Supplementary Figure S1**). The placentas of the infected wild-type mice with abnormal pregnancies were analyzed histologically, and multiple calcifications were observed in seven of the eight mice (**Figure 4** and **Supplementary Figure S2**). We confirmed one case of premature birth in the infected $TLR2^{-/-}$ mice, but we could not collect the placenta.

Immunological Response to *T. gondii* Infection

To confirm the inflammatory response in terms of pathological changes in the placenta, histological and molecular analyses were performed at Gd18.5 (6 dpi). Although higher parasite numbers were detected in the placentas and uteri of some $TLR2^{-/-}$ mice, there was no significant difference in the parasite numbers between the wild-type and $TLR2^{-/-}$ mice (**Supplementary Figure S3**). A histological comparison of the placentas of the uninfected and infected groups showed no histological changes attributable to infection in either the wild-type or $TLR2^{-/-}$ mice (**Supplementary Figure S3**). Immunohistochemistry, however, revealed that trophoblasts and endothelial cells of the placenta were strongly positive for caspase-3 in the infected wild-type mice (**Figure 5B**), compared with the uninfected wild-type and $TLR2^{-/-}$ mice (**Figures 5A,C**) and the infected $TLR2^{-/-}$ mice (**Figure 5D**). Image analysis revealed that caspase-3-positive area was significantly increased in the infected wild-type mice than the infected $TLR2^{-/-}$ mice (**Figure 5E**).

The levels of IL-12p40, IL-6, TNF-α, IL-4, and IL-10 mRNAs in the placenta were measured with qPCR (**Figure 6**). In the wild-type mice, *T. gondii* infection increased IL-4 and IL-10 mRNA expression and reduced IL-12p40 mRNA expression compared with that in the uninfected mice. The level of IL-12p40 mRNA in the uninfected $TLR2^{-/-}$ mice was significantly lower than that in the uninfected wild-type mice and was similar to that in the infected $TLR2^{-/-}$ mice. The levels of IL-6, TNF-α, IL-4, and IL-10 mRNAs were significantly lower in the infected $TLR2^{-/-}$ mice than in the infected wild-type mice. However, statistically significant difference was not seen in Foxp3 expression among the groups.

The IFN-γ and IL-4 levels in the mouse sera were measured with ELISAs as indicators of their systemic immune status. Serum IFN-γ levels were increased significantly by *T. gondii*

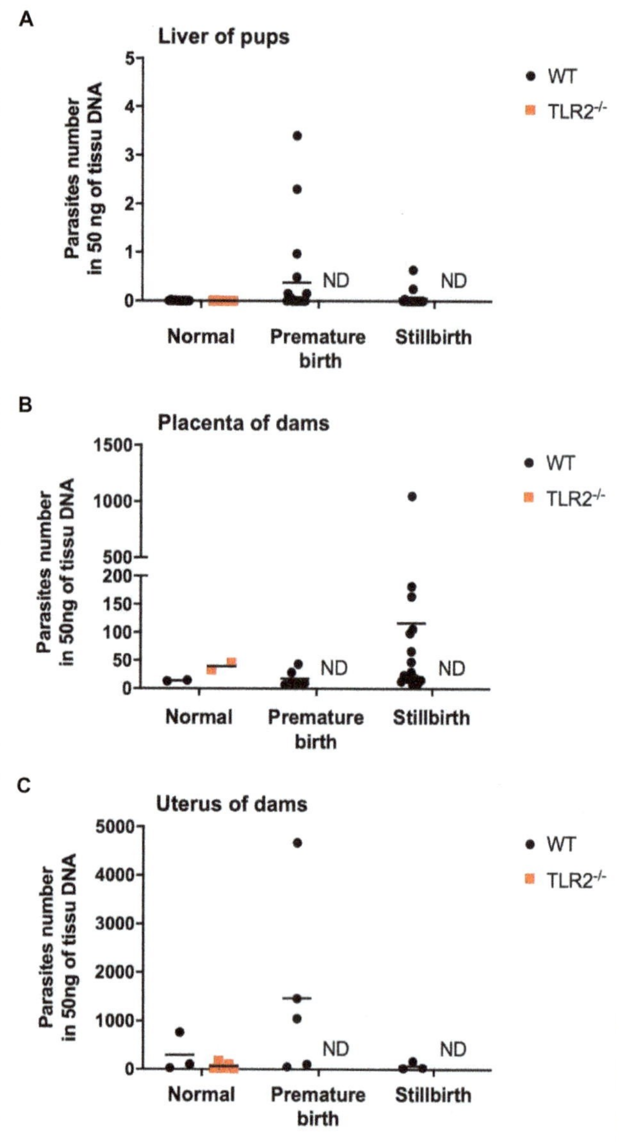

FIGURE 3 | Quantification of the numbers of parasites in the livers of pups and the placentas and uteri of dams. Numbers of parasites in the livers of pups **(A)**, placentas of dams **(B)**, and uteri of dams **(C)** from infected wild-type (WT) and TLR2$^{-/-}$ mice were analyzed with quantitative PCR. Each point on the graph represents one tissue, and the horizontal lines indicate the mean values for each group. **(A)** Normal birth: WT (n = 11), TLR2$^{-/-}$ (n = 14); premature birth: WT (n = 20), TLR2$^{-/-}$ (n = 0); stillbirth: WT (n = 15), TLR2$^{-/-}$ (n = 0). **(B)** Normal: WT (n = 2), TLR2$^{-/-}$ (n = 2); premature birth: WT (n = 6), TLR2$^{-/-}$ (n = 0); stillbirth: WT (n = 16), TLR2$^{-/-}$ (n = 0). **(C)** Normal: WT (n = 3), TLR2$^{-/-}$ (n = 5); premature birth: WT (n = 5), TLR2$^{-/-}$ (n = 0); stillbirth: WT (n = 3), TLR2$^{-/-}$ (n = 0). Statistical analysis of normal birth samples was performed with the Mann-Whitney U test or t test, but no differences were detected. ND: not done because no sample was available.

infection in both the wild-type mice and TLR2$^{-/-}$ mice, but the IFN-γ levels were significantly lower in the infected TLR2$^{-/-}$ mice than in the infected wild-type mice (**Figure 7**). Serum IL4 was not detectable in this study. Additionally, serum prostaglandin E_2 was measured because TLR2 is important to trigger prostaglandin E_2 production (Umeda et al., 2017) and prostaglandin E_2 can favor the parasite proliferation in trophoblast cells (Barbosa et al., 2014). As shown in **Figure 7C**, *T. gondii* infection showed a tendency to increase serum prostaglandin E_2 in wild-type mice, not in TLR2$^{-/-}$ mice, while there was no statistically significant difference among the experimental groups.

DISCUSSION

The maternal immune system plays two major roles against pathogen infection during pregnancy: It maintains the pregnancy and combats the pathogen (Robinson and Klein, 2012; Rowe et al., 2013). However, immunomodulation in the placenta is strongly affected by pathogens, resulting in a high pathogen burden at the fetal–maternal interface, which causes pregnancy complications such as abortion and stillbirth (Gibbs, 2002; Goldenberg et al., 2010; Robbins and Bakardjiev, 2012). The infection of pregnant animals with *T. gondii* can cause embryonic death, fetal resorption, fetal death, abortion, and congenital transmission (Dubey, 2009). Furthermore, infection with *T. gondii* during early pregnancy has more severe consequences (e.g., fetal resorption, reduced offspring survival rates, and increased parasite transmission rates) than infection during late pregnancy (Shirahata et al., 1992; Montoya and Liesenfeld, 2004; Wang et al., 2011). Although the effects of *T. gondii* infection during late pregnancy are poorly understood, changes in the immune response and interactions with PRRs may be associated with pregnancy complications. Because TLR2 is expressed in trophoblast cells in late gestation (Abrahams et al., 2004; Rindsjö et al., 2007), in the present study, we examined the roles of TLR2 in late pregnancy after *T. gondii* infection.

The rate of bodyweight gain at Gd18.5 was significantly lower in the infected wild-type mice than in the uninfected wild-type mice (**Figure 1A**), suggesting that some mice lost bodyweight through premature birth or stillbirth triggered by *T. gondii* infection. In contrast, the infected TLR2$^{-/-}$ mice showed no reduction in bodyweight gain (**Figure 1B**). In this study, the pregnant mice were inoculated intraperitoneally with *T. gondii* tachyzoites (1.0×10^4/0.4 ml RPMI-1640 medium) on Gd12.5. So, Gd 18.5 is 6 days post-infection. Generally, clinical symptoms in *T. gondii*-infected C57BL/6 mice are seen after 5–7 days postinfection. Therefore, despite the fact that C57BL/6 is known to be highly susceptible to *T. gondii* infection, there was almost no difference between groups on body weight. Moreover, the TLR2$^{-/-}$ mice had significantly fewer abnormal pregnancies in response to *T. gondii* infection than the infected wild-type mice (**Figure 2B, Supplementary Table S1**). These results suggest that TLR2 is involved in disease exacerbation during *T. gondii* infection in late pregnancy.

The damage to the placenta and pups caused by *T. gondii* infection is a factor causing pregnancy failure in mice (Coutinho et al., 2012; Zhang et al., 2015; Vargas-Villavicencio et al., 2016). Moreover, infection of the placenta and pups has been detected in *Calomys callosus* (a South American rodent of the family Cricetidae, often used in experiments involving acute *T. gondii* infection; Ferro et al., 2002). In the present study,

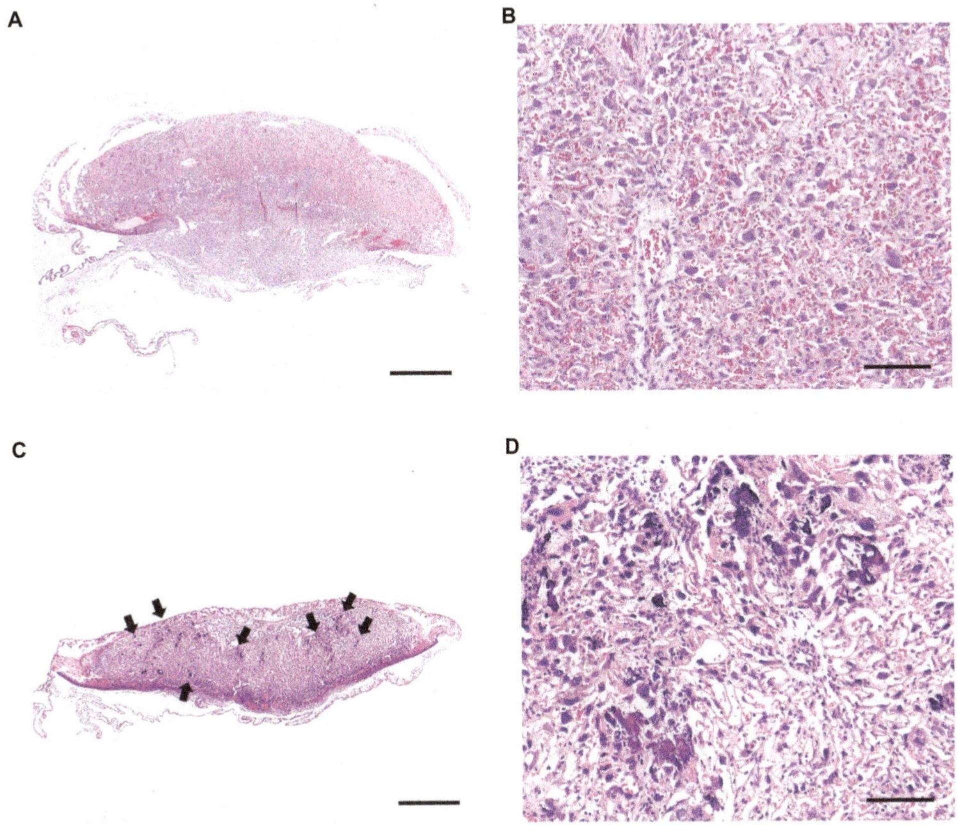

FIGURE 4 | Histological changes in the placentas of *T. gondii*-infected wild-type mice with abnormal pregnancies. Tissue sections from the placentas of infected wild-type mice with abnormal pregnancies showed multiple calcifications in 19 of 25 samples. Representative photographs are shown. **(A)** Normal placenta on day 18.5 of pregnancy (Gd18.5). Bar = 1.0 mm. **(B)** High magnification of the labyrinth of the normal placenta. A large number of mature erythrocytes were observed in the vascular spaces of the labyrinth. Bar = 100 μm. **(C)** Placenta of a stillbirth mouse at Gd19.5. Bar = 1.0 mm. Multifocal calcification (arrows) were observed at the labyrinth of the placenta. A few of mature erythrocytes were observed in the vascular spaces of the labyrinth. **(D)** High magnification of the labyrinth. Bar = 100 μm.

few parasites were detected in the pups from the infected dams, suggesting the low vertical transmission of *T. gondii* under our experimental conditions. Previous study also showed that placental infection of *T. gondii* was seen in C57BL/6 mice infected with 30 cysts of *T. gondii* (type II strain) at Gd11.0, while no vertical transmission was observed (Shiono et al., 2007). A histopathological analysis of sheep neonates experimentally infected with *T. gondii* during pregnancy showed leukomalacia, glial cell infiltration in the brain, and the necrosis of multiple tissues throughout the whole body (Castaño et al., 2016). However, our histopathological analysis of the brains and livers of mouse pups indicated that no histological changes were caused by *T. gondii* infection during late pregnancy. However, the *T. gondii B1* gene was detected in placentas and uteri of the infected dams. These results suggest that *T. gondii* infection does not cause pathological changes in the pups because the placenta is a barrier to its vertical transmission when infection occurs during late pregnancy (Robbins and Bakardjiev, 2012).

Human, rats and mice have hemochorial type of placentas, characterized by a limited cellular barrier without the maternal tissue layer (Furukawa et al., 2014). Cellular barrier is composed of one to three layers of cytotrophoblasts and syncytiotrophoblasts (Soares et al., 2018). An *in vitro* analysis of human placenta suggested that the placenta is a barrier to *T. gondii* infection and indicated the particular importance of syncytiotrophoblasts (Robbins et al., 2012). Although there are some differences in the structures of human and mouse placentas, syncytiotrophoblasts may also act as a barrier in mice (Maltepe et al., 2010). A histopathological analysis of the placentas from the infected mice with abnormal pregnancies showed multiple calcifications in seven of the eight mice (**Figures 4C,D**). Because calcinosis occurs when calcium salts are deposited at the site of cell or tissue death (dystrophic calcification), an inflammatory response occurs in the placenta, resulting in cell death. The results of placental infection with *T. gondii* and calcification suggest that *T. gondii* infection during late pregnancy is involved in the deterioration of placental function. The death of pups in a dam (stillbirth) is presumed to be caused by a lack of oxygen and the nutrients required by the pups, arising from the deterioration of the placenta. No histological changes were observed in the pups because histological lesions rarely appear in cases of rapid death due to lack of oxygen. Because multiple calcifications were not seen in the placentas of the

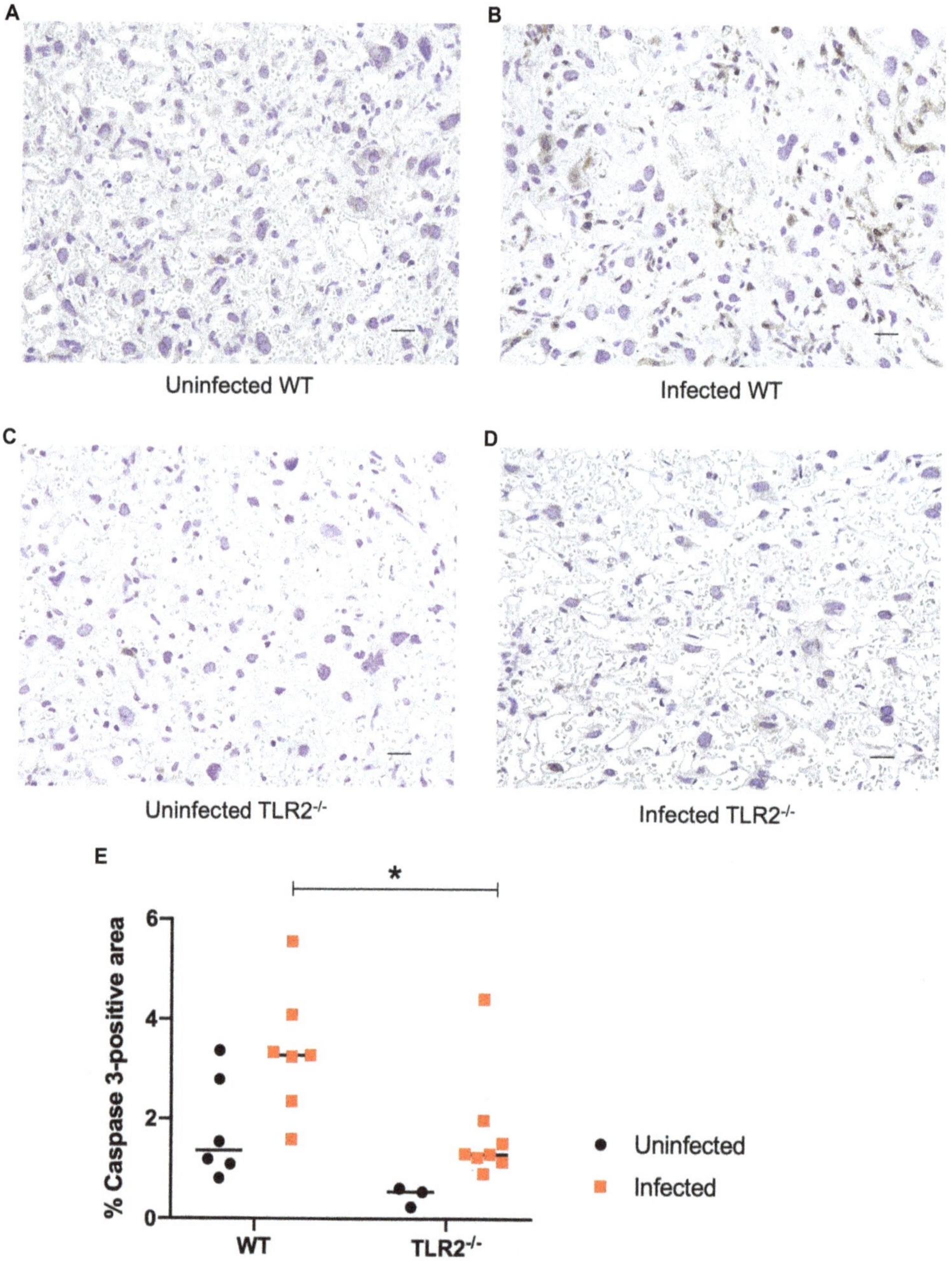

FIGURE 5 | Immunohistochemistry and image analysis for caspase-3 in the placenta on day 18.5 of pregnancy. Trophoblasts and endothelial cells were positive for caspase-3 in the placenta of the infected wild-type mice. Representative photographs are shown. **(A)** The placenta of an uninfected wild-type mouse. **(B)** The placenta of an infected wild-type mouse. **(C)** The placenta of an infected TLR2$^{-/-}$ mouse. **(D)** The placenta of an infected TLR2$^{-/-}$ mouse. Bar = 20 μm. Trophoblasts and endothelial cells were positive for caspase-3 in an infected wild-type mice. **(E)** Image analysis of immunihistochemistry for caspase-3. Positive areas were compared between WT and TLR2$^{-/-}$ mice. Horizontal bars represent the mean value. Data were analyzed with two-way ANOVA followed by the Tukey–Kramer multiple-comparison test. $^*p < 0.05$.

TLR2$^{-/-}$ mice, TLR2 signaling during late pregnancy may be involved in this placental damage.

To investigate the immune changes caused by *T. gondii* infection during pregnancy, we analyzed the parasite burden and the immune response at Gd18.5 (6 dpi). Unexpectedly, there were no significant differences in the parasite numbers in the placentas and uteri of the wild-type and TLR2$^{-/-}$ mice (**Supplementary Figure S3**). We found higher parasite numbers in the placentas and uteri of some TLR2$^{-/-}$ mice, possibly because TLR2 plays an important role in the elimination of the parasite by inducing a Th1 immune response. In addition, prostaglandin E_2 induced by *T. gondii* infection might support the parasite proliferation in trophoblast of wild-type mice, not TLR2$^{-/-}$ mice (**Figure 7C**; Barbosa et al., 2014). Furthermore, no histopathological changes were seen in the placentas of either group of animals (**Supplementary Figure S4**). However,

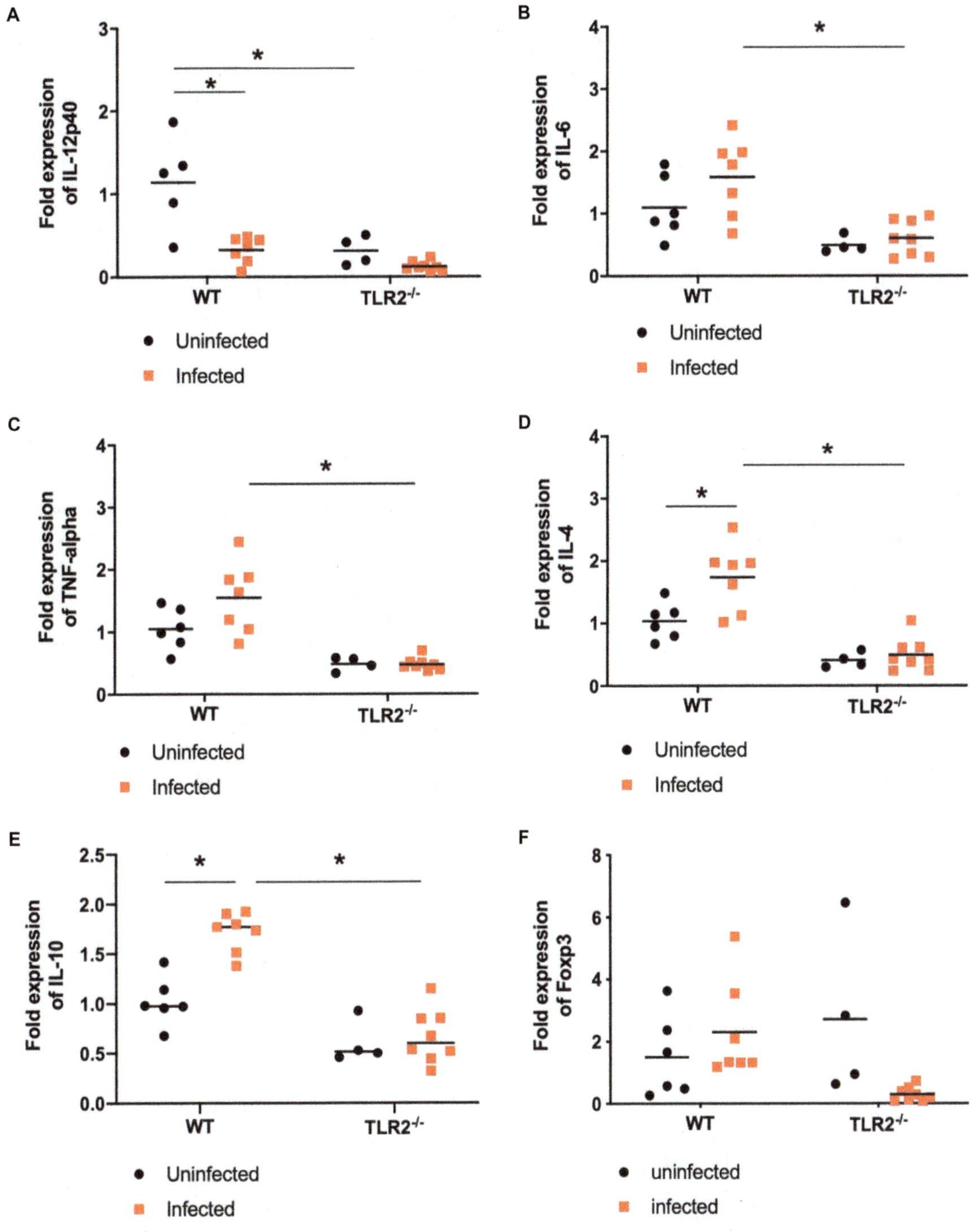

FIGURE 6 | Relative mRNA expression of cytokines in placenta on day 18.5 of pregnancy. Levels of IL-12p40 **(A)**, IL-6 **(B)**, TNF-a **(C)** IL-4 **(D)**, IL-10 **(E)** and Foxp3 **(F)** mRNAs in the placentas of each group were measured with RT PCR. Using synthesized cDNA, the mRNA expression levels of cytokines relative to those in uninfected wild-type (WT) mice were quantified with RT qPCR. Because embryos and placentas collected from one mouse were pooled into one sample, each symbol indicates the data from a single mouse. Uninfected WT mice ($n=6$), infected WT mice ($n=7$), uninfected TLR2$^{-/-}$ mice ($n=4$), infected TLR2$^{-/-}$ mice ($n=8$). The horizontal lines show the mean values for each group. Data were analyzed with two-way ANOVA followed by the Tukey–Kramer multiple-comparison test. $^{*}p<0.05$.

some differences in cytokine mRNA expression were detected in the placentas (**Figure 6**). *T. gondii* infection downregulated the IL-12p40 mRNA expression and upregulated the mRNA expression of IL-4 and IL-10 in the placenta at Gd18.5 (6 dpi). These results contradict a report that *T. gondii* type II strains, including PLK, stimulate IL-12 production in an MYD88-dependent manner in nonpregnant animals (Robben et al., 2004; Kim et al., 2006). *In vitro* studies with the human placental

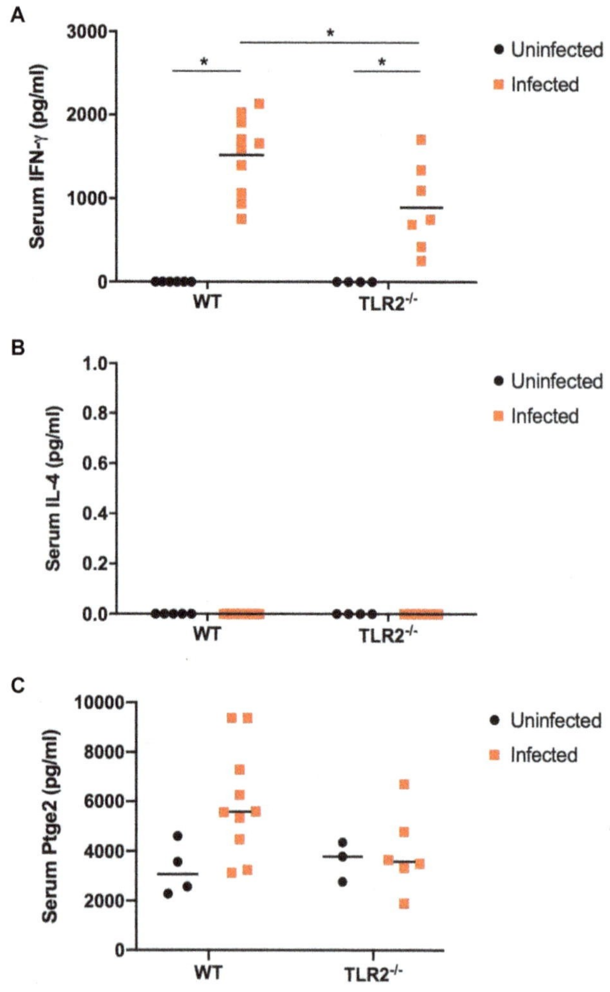

FIGURE 7 | Serum levels of IFN-γ **(A)**, IL4 **(B)** and prostaglandin E2 **(C)** on day 18.5 of pregnancy. Serum levels of IFN-γ, IL4 and prostaglandin E2 in each group were measured. Each point on the graph represents a single mouse, and the horizontal lines indicate the mean values for each group. Uninfected WT mice ($n=6$), infected WT mice ($n=10$), uninfected TLR2$^{-/-}$ mice ($n=4$), infected TLR2$^{-/-}$ mice ($n=7$). Data were analyzed with two-way ANOVA followed by the Tukey–Kramer multiple-comparison test. $^*p<0.05$.

cell line BeWo showed that the expression of the proinflammatory cytokines IL-6 and TNF-α is downregulated by high concentrations of IFN-γ (Barbosa et al., 2015). In the present study, *T. gondii* infection significantly increased the serum levels of IFN-γ, a known proinflammatory cytokine (**Figure 7**). Therefore, in the placenta, high levels of IFN-γ may downregulate the expression of the Th1 cytokine IL-12p40, resulting in the upregulation of the Th2 cytokines IL-4 and IL-10, to maintain the Th1/Th2 balance.

Macrophages at the maternal–fetal interface characterized by alternative activation (M2 polarization) exhibit immunosuppressive functions for the maintenance of pregnancy. However, *T. gondii* infection changes the bias of M2 decidual macrophages toward M1, resulting in the immunosuppressive microenvironment at the maternal–fetal interface and the adverse pregnancy outcomes (Liu et al., 2018). IL-4 plays an important role in the maintenance of pregnancy by reducing the inflammatory response. IL-4 induces M2 macrophages, which are responsible for the production of the growth factors and anti-inflammatory cytokines that promote wound healing and tissue remodeling, and improves the metabolism and endocrine signaling in tissues (Murray and Wynn, 2011). Like IL-4, IL-10 is a cytokine involved in the Th2 response. In nonpregnant mice infected with *T. gondii*, IL-4 deficiency increased mortality, but reduced the brain tissue cyst burden (Roberts et al., 1996; Alexander et al., 1998). In contrast, significant mortality occurred immediately postpartum in wild-type dams, whereas all IL-4-deficient dams survived (Alexander et al., 1998). These results and our present data suggest a role for IL4 in pregnancy-induced immunomodulation and the associated increased susceptibility to *T. gondii* infection. According to a report by Gazzinelli et al. (1996), nonpregnant mice lacking IL-10 produced excessive amounts of IL-12, IFN-γ, and TNF-α in response to *T. gondii* infection, resulting in a lethal immune response, with severe cellular infiltration and necrosis in the liver (Gazzinelli et al., 1996). In contrast to IL-4, IL-10 reduces the apoptosis of decidual regulatory T cells (Treg cells), improving adverse pregnancy outcomes after *T. gondii* infection (Lao et al., 2015). The higher levels of IL-10 mRNA expression seen in the placentas of the infected wild-type dams in the present study require further research. Together, the changes in cytokine expression in the placenta after *T. gondii* infection during pregnancy may affect the parasite burden and calcinosis in the placenta. Moreover, TLR2 is involved in this disease outcome because no changes in the expression levels of IL-12p40, IL-6, TNF-α, or IL-4 were observed in the TLR2$^{-/-}$ mice during *T. gondii* infection (**Figure 6**).

Several kinds of immune cells should be considered for maintenance of pregnancy. Worse pregnancy outcomes observed in mice were associated with higher TNF-α and IL-6 at the maternal–fetal interface, with lower Foxp3 expression (Sousa et al., 2021). Because Foxp3 is an essential molecular marker of regulatory T cell (Treg) development (Kim and Rudensky, 2006), Treg plays an important role on maintenance of pregnancy. *T. gondii* infection significantly downregulates the number of whole decidual Treg cell population by upregulating the suppressive function of programmed cell death protein 1 (PD-1)$^+$ Treg cell population (Zhang H et al., 2019) and apoptosis (Qiu et al., 2018), resulting in adverse pregnancy outcomes. On the other hand, Treg cell population and transforming growth factor-beta (TGF-β) level contribute to pregnancy outcomes (Xu et al., 2017; Zhao et al., 2017). Thus, immune inhibitory activity is one of the important factors. However, mRNA expression of Foxp3 in placenta on day 18.5 of pregnancy did not show significant difference among the experimental groups in our study (**Figure 6F**).

Immune inhibitory molecules such as T cell immunoglobulin and mucin domain-containing protein 3 (Tim-3) and leukocyte immunoglobulin-like receptor subfamily B member 4 (LILRB$_4$) contribute on the pregnancy outcome. The Tim-3 is discovered to be expressed on some decidual immune cells and participates in the maintenance of maternal–fetal tolerance. Dysregulation of

Tim-3 expression on decidual NK (dNK) cells and decidual macrophages was observed in several cases of pregnancy complications. Tim-$3^{-/-}$ pregnant mice displayed more worse pregnancy outcomes with *T. gondii* infection (Zhang D et al., 2019; Li et al., 2021). $LILRB_4$ expressed by macrophages and dendritic cells plays an important immune-regulatory role at the maternal–fetal interface. *T. gondii* infection strengthens M1 activation functions and weakened M2 tolerance functions by downregulation of LILRB4 on decidual macrophages (Li et al., 2017). Moreover, LILRB4 expression on uterine dendritic cells subsets from mid-gestation is obviously downregulated after *T. gondii* infection (Zhan et al., 2018). Contribution of Tim-3 and $LILRB_4$ should be clarified in our experimental models for future study.

We consider that the calcification of the placenta observed in the infected wild-type mice was due to cell death *via* a caspase-3 pathway caused by increased levels of IFN-γ in the blood. IFN-γ is a well-known cytokine that is important for the elimination of *T. gondii* in nonpregnant animals (Sturge and Yarovinsky, 2014). However, an *in vitro* study reported that IFN-γ did not prevent the growth of *T. gondii* in BeWo cells (Barbosa et al., 2015), suggesting that the primary role of IFN-γ in the placenta may be other than the inhibition of parasite growth. One mechanism of pregnancy failure involving TLR2 involves the apoptosis of trophoblast cells. An *in vitro* study using human placentas showed that the administration of peptidoglycan, a ligand of TLR2, caused the apoptosis of trophoblast cells (Abrahams et al., 2004), and an *in vivo* study of pregnant mice showed that the intrauterine administration of peptidoglycan induced preterm delivery, mainly characterized by apoptosis (Ilievski et al., 2007). IFN-γ is associated with the apoptosis of trophoblasts *via* a caspase-3- and caspase-8-dependent pathway (Zhang et al., 2015). Senegas et al. reported that the IFN-γ-dependent apoptosis of placental cells is involved in embryo resorption in *T. gondii*-infected mice during early pregnancy (Senegas et al., 2009). In the present study of late pregnancy, the apoptosis and dystrophic calcification of trophoblast cells in the infected wild-type mice may have been induced by the production of IFN-γ *via* the activation of TLR2. However, the production of IFN-γ was lower in the infected TLR$2^{-/-}$ mice than in the infected wild-type mice, resulting in less induction of trophoblast apoptosis and fewer dams with abnormal pregnancies.

Cell death in the placenta reduces its ability to act as a physical barrier to infection by *T. gondii* and may promote the transmission of the parasite to the fetus. An *in vitro* study using human placenta by Robbins et al. (2012) reported that *T. gondii* was abundant at sites of syncytiotrophoblast disruption, suggesting that placental damage and the vertical transmission of *T. gondii* are related. In the present study, fewer parasites were detected in the livers of pups from infected TLR$2^{-/-}$ mice than in the pups from the infected wild-type mice (**Figure 3A**). Our results suggest that the infected TLR$2^{-/-}$ mice were less likely to experience apoptosis of the placenta caused by IFN-γ and that the physical barrier function of the placenta against *T. gondii* was not compromised. Therefore, TLR$2^{-/-}$ mice may be more resistant to the vertical transmission of *T. gondii*.

Our results indicate that TLR2 signaling makes a major contribution to abnormal pregnancies after *T. gondii* infection. Notably, TLR2 signaling is important because glycosylphosphatidylinositol is a parasite ligand of TLR2 and TLR4 (Debierre-Grockiego et al., 2007). Therefore, the regulation of TLR2 signaling may be a potential target in controlling congenital toxoplasmosis.

AUTHOR CONTRIBUTIONS

RI was involved in data curation, formal analysis, investigation, and writing—original draft. NU contributed to investigation and writing—review and editing. AA performed investigation. HF done data curation, investigation, methodology, and writing—review and editing. YN was involved in data curation, formal analysis, investigation, writing—review and editing, conceptualization, project administration, funding acquisition, and supervision. All authors contributed to the article and approved the submitted version.

ACKNOWLEDGMENTS

We thank the members of the Research Unit for Host Defense (National Research Center for Protozoan Diseases, Obihiro University of Agriculture and Veterinary Medicine) for their technical support with the mouse experiments.

REFERENCES

Abrahams, V. M., Bole-Aldo, P., Kim, Y. M., Straszewski-Chavez, S. L., Chaiworapongsa, T., Romero, R., et al. (2004). Divergent trophoblast responses to bacterial products mediated by TLRs. *J. Immunol.* 173, 4286–4296. doi: 10.4049/jimmunol.173.7.4286

Abrahams, V. M., Visintin, I., Aldo, P. B., Guller, S., Romero, R., and Mor, G. (2005). A role for TLRs in the regulation of immune cell migration by first trimester trophoblast cells. *J. Immunol.* 175, 8096–8104. doi: 10.4049/jimmunol.175.12.8096

Alexander, J., Jebbari, H., Bluethmann, H., Brombacher, F., and Roberts, C. W. (1998). The role of IL-4 in adult acquired and congenital toxoplasmosis. *Int. J. Parasitol.* 28, 113–120. doi: 10.1016/S0020-7519(97)00168-9

Angeloni, M. B., Guirelli, P. M., Franco, P. S., Barbosa, B. F., Gomes, A. O., Castro, A. S., et al. (2013). Differential apoptosis in BeWo cells after infection with highly (RH) or moderately (ME49) virulent strains of *toxoplasma gondii* is related to the cytokine profile secreted, the death receptor Fas expression and phosphorylated ERK1/2 expression. *Placenta* 34, 973–982. doi: 10.1016/j.placenta.2013.09.005

Barbosa, B. F., Lopes-Maria, J. B., Gomes, A. O., Angeloni, M. B., Castro, A. S., Franco, P. S., et al. (2015). IL10, TGF beta1, and IFN gamma modulate intracellular signaling pathways and cytokine production to control *toxoplasma gondii* infection in BeWo trophoblast cells. *Biol. Reprod.* 92:82. doi: 10.1095/biolreprod.114.124115

Barbosa, B. F., Paulesu, L., Ietta, F., Bechi, N., Romagnoli, R., Gomes, A. O., et al. (2014). Susceptibility to *toxoplasma gondii* proliferation in BeWo human trophoblast cells is dose-dependent of macrophage migration inhibitory factor (MIF), via ERK1/2 phosphorylation and prostaglandin E2 production. *Placenta* 35, 152–162. doi: 10.1016/j.placenta.2013.12.013

Castaño, P., Fuertes, M., Regidor-Cerrillo, J., Ferre, I., Fernández, M., Ferreras, M. C., et al. (2016). Experimental ovine toxoplasmosis: influence of the gestational stage on the clinical course, lesion development and parasite distribution. *Vet. Res.* 47:43. doi: 10.1186/s13567-016-0327-z

Chaouat, G., Menu, E., Clark, D. A., Dy, M., Minkowski, M., and Wegmann, T. G. (1990). Control of fetal survival in CBA x DBA/2 mice by lymphokine therapy. *J. Reprod. Fertil.* 89, 447–458. doi: 10.1530/jrf.0.0890447

Contini, C., Seraceni, S., Cultrera, R., Incorvaia, C., Sebastiani, A., and Picot, S. (2005). Evaluation of a real-time PCR-based assay using the lightcycler system for detection of *toxoplasma gondii* bradyzoite genes in blood specimens from patients with toxoplasmic retinochoroiditis. *Int. J. Parasitol.* 35, 275–283. doi: 10.1016/j.ijpara.2004.11.016

Costello, M. J., Joyce, S. K., and Abrahams, V. M. (2007). NOD protein expression and function in first trimester trophoblast cells. *Am. J. Reprod. Immunol.* 57, 67–80. doi: 10.1111/j.1600-0897.2006.00447.x

Coutinho, L. B., Gomes, A. O., Araújo, E. C., Barenco, P. V., Santos, J. L., Caixeta, D. R., et al. (2012). The impaired pregnancy outcome in murine congenital toxoplasmosis is associated with a pro-inflammatory immune response, but not correlated with decidual inducible nitric oxide synthase expression. *Int. J. Parasitol.* 42, 341–352. doi: 10.1016/j.ijpara.2012.01.006

Debierre-Grockiego, F., Azzouz, N., Schmidt, J., Dubremetz, J. F., Geyer, H., Geyer, R., et al. (2003). Roles of glycosylphosphatidylinositols of *toxoplasma gondii*. Induction of tumor necrosis factor-alpha production in macrophages. *J. Biol. Chem.* 278, 32987–32993. doi: 10.1074/jbc.M304791200

Debierre-Grockiego, F., Campos, M. A., Azzouz, N., Schmidt, J., Bieker, U., Resende, M. G., et al. (2007). Activation of TLR2 and TLR4 by glycosylphosphatidylinositols derived from Toxoplasma gondii. *J. Immunol.* 15, 1129–1137. doi: 10.4049/jimmunol.179.2.1129

Dubey, J. P. (2009). Toxoplasmosis in sheep--the last 20 years. *Vet. Parasitol.* 163, 1–14. doi: 10.1016/j.vetpar.2009.02.026

Entrican, G. (2002). Immune regulation during pregnancy and host-pathogen interactions in infectious abortion. *J. Comp. Pathol.* 126, 79–94. doi: 10.1053/jcpa.2001.0539

Ferro, E. A., Silva, D. A., Bevilacqua, E., and Mineo, J. R. (2002). Effect of *toxoplasma gondii* infection kinetics on trophoblast cell population in *Calomys callosus*, a model of congenital toxoplasmosis. *Infect. Immun.* 70, 7089–7094. doi: 10.1128/IAI.70.12.7089-7094.2002

Furukawa, S., Kuroda, Y., and Sugiyama, A. (2014). A comparison of the histological structure of the placenta in experimental animals. *J. Toxicol. Pathol.* 27, 11–18. doi: 10.1293/tox.2013-0060

Gazzinelli, R. T., Wysocka, M., Hieny, S., Scharton-Kersten, T., Cheever, A., Kühn, R., et al. (1996). In the absence of endogenous IL-10, mice acutely infected with *toxoplasma gondii* succumb to a lethal immune response dependent on CD4+ T cells and accompanied by overproduction of IL-12, IFN-gamma and TNF-alpha. *J. Immunol.* 157, 798–805

Gibbs, R. S. (2002). The origins of stillbirth: infectious diseases. *Semin. Perinatol.* 26, 75–78. doi: 10.1053/sper.2002.29839

Gierman, L. M., Stødle, G. S., Tangerås, L. H., Austdal, M., Olsen, G. D., Follestad, T., et al. (2015). Toll-like receptor profiling of seven trophoblast cell lines warrants caution for translation to primary trophoblasts. *Placenta* 36, 1246–1253. doi: 10.1016/j.placenta.2015.09.004

Givens, M. D., and Marley, M. S. (2008). Infectious causes of embryonic and fetal mortality. *Theriogenology* 70, 270–285. doi: 10.1016/j.theriogenology.2008.04.018

Goldenberg, R. L., McClure, E. M., Saleem, S., and Reddy, U. M. (2010). Infection-related stillbirths. *Lancet* 375, 1482–1490. doi: 10.1016/S0140-6736(09)61712-8

Gomes, A. O., Barbosa, B. F., Franco, P. S., Ribeiro, M., Silva, R. J., Gois, P. S. G., et al. (2018). Macrophage migration inhibitory factor (MIF) prevents maternal death, but contributes to poor Fetal outcome during congenital toxoplasmosis. *Front. Microbiol.* 9:906. doi: 10.3389/fmicb.2018.00906

Hill, D., and Dubey, J. P. (2002). *Toxoplasma gondii*: transmission, diagnosis and prevention. *Clin. Microbiol. Infect.* 8, 634–640. doi: 10.1046/j.1469-0691.2002.00485.x

Ihara, F., Tanaka, S., Fereig, R. M., Nishimura, M., and Nishikawa, Y. (2019). Involvement of toll-like receptor 2 in the cerebral immune response and behavioral changes caused by latent *toxoplasma infection* in mice. *PLoS One* 14:e0220560. doi: 10.1371/journal.pone.0220560

Ilievski, V., Lu, S. J., and Hirsch, E. (2007). Activation of toll-like receptors 2 or 3 and preterm delivery in the mouse. *Reprod. Sci.* 14, 315–320. doi: 10.1177/1933719107302959

Kim, L., Butcher, B. A., Lee, C. W., Uematsu, S., Akira, S., and Denkers, E. Y. (2006). *Toxoplasma gondii* genotype determines MyD88-dependent signaling in infected macrophages. *J. Immunol.* 177, 2584–2591. doi: 10.4049/jimmunol.177.4.2584

Kim, Y. M., Romero, R., Chaiworapongsa, T., Kim, G. J., Kim, M. R., Kuivaniemi, H., et al. (2004). Toll-like receptor-2 and -4 in the chorioamniotic membranes in spontaneous labor at term and in preterm parturition that are associated with chorioamnionitis. *Am. J. Obstet. Gynecol.* 191, 1346–1355. doi: 10.1016/j.ajog.2004.07.009

Kim, J. M., and Rudensky, A. (2006). The role of the transcription factor Foxp3 in the development of regulatory T cells. *Immunol. Rev.* 212, 86–98. doi: 10.1111/j.0105-2896.2006.00426.x

Lao, K., Zhao, M., Li, Z., Liu, X., Zhang, H., Jiang, Y., et al. (2015). IL-10 regulate decidual Tregs apoptosis contributing to the abnormal pregnancy with *toxoplasma gondii* infection. *Microb. Pathog.* 89, 210–216. doi: 10.1016/j.micpath.2015.10.002

Li, T., Cui, L., Xu, X., Zhang, H., Jiang, Y., Ren, L., et al. (2021). The role of Tim-3 on dNK cells dysfunction during abnormal pregnancy with *toxoplasma gondii* infection. *Front. Cell. Infect. Microbiol.* 11:587150. doi: 10.3389/fcimb.2021.587150

Li, Z., Zhao, M., Li, T., Zheng, J., Liu, X., Jiang, Y., et al. (2017). Decidual macrophage functional polarization during abnormal pregnancy due to *toxoplasma gondii*: role for LILRB4. *Front. Immunol.* 8:1013. doi: 10.3389/fimmu.2017.01013

Liu, X., Jiang, M., Ren, L., Zhang, A., Zhao, M., Zhang, H., et al. (2018). Decidual macrophage M1 polarization contributes to adverse pregnancy induced by *toxoplasma gondii* PRU strain infection. *Microb. Pathog.* 124, 183–190. doi: 10.1016/j.micpath.2018.08.043

Maltepe, E., Bakardjiev, A. I., and Fisher, S. J. (2010). The placenta: transcriptional, epigenetic, and physiological integration during development. *J. Clin. Invest.* 120, 1016–1025. doi: 10.1172/JCI41211

McCarthy, R., Martin-Fairey, C., Sojka, D. K., Herzog, E. D., Jungheim, E. S., Stout, M. J., et al. (2018). Mouse models of preterm birth: suggested assessment and reporting guidelines. *Biol. Reprod.* 99, 922–937. doi: 10.1093/biolre/ioy109

Montoya, J. G., and Liesenfeld, O. (2004). Toxoplasmosis. *Lancet* 363, 1965–1976. doi: 10.1016/S0140-6736(04)16412-X

Mun, H. S., Aosai, F., Norose, K., Chen, M., Piao, L. X., Takeuchi, O., et al. (2003). TLR2 as an essential molecule for protective immunity against *toxoplasma gondii* infection. *Int. Immunol.* 15, 1081–1087. doi: 10.1093/intimm/dxg108

Murray, P. J., and Wynn, T. A. (2011). Protective and pathogenic functions of macrophage subsets. *Nat. Rev. Immunol.* 11, 723–737. doi: 10.1038/nri3073

Nishida, A., Ikeda, R., Furuoka, H., and Nishikawa, Y. (2021). CXCR3-dependent immune pathology in mice following infection with *toxoplasma gondii* during early pregnancy. *Infect. Immun.* 89:e00253-20. doi: 10.1128/IAI.00253-20

Nishimura, M., Umeda, K., Suwa, M., Furuoka, H., and Nishikawa, Y. (2017). CCR5 is involved in interruption of pregnancy in mice infected with *toxoplasma gondii* during early pregnancy. *Infect. Immun.* 85:e00257-17. doi: 10.1128/IAI.00257-17

Qiu, J., Zhang, R., Xie, Y., Wang, L., Ge, K., Chen, H., et al. (2018). Estradiol attenuates the severity of primary *toxoplasma gondii* infection-induced adverse pregnancy outcomes through the regulation of Tregs in a dose-dependent manner. *Front. Immunol.* 9:1102. doi: 10.3389/fimmu.2018.01102

Rahman, A., Cahill, L. S., Zhou, Y. Q., Hoggarth, J., Rennie, M. Y., Seed, M., et al. (2017). A mouse model of antepartum stillbirth. *Am. J. Obstet. Gynecol.* 217, 443.e1–443.e11. doi: 10.1016/j.ajog.2017.06.009

Reinhard, G., Noll, A., Schlebusch, H., Mallmann, P., and Ruecker, A. V. (1998). Shifts in the TH1/TH2 balance during human pregnancy correlate with apoptotic changes. *Biochem. Biophys. Res. Commun.* 245, 933–938. doi: 10.1006/bbrc.1998.8549

Riley, J. K., and Nelson, D. M. (2010). Toll-like receptors in pregnancy disorders and placental dysfunction. *Clin. Rev. Allergy Immunol.* 39, 185–193. doi: 10.1007/s12016-009-8178-2

Rindsjö, E., Holmlund, U., Sverremark-Ekström, E., Papadogiannakis, N., and Scheynius, A. (2007). Toll-like receptor-2 expression in normal and pathologic human placenta. *Hum. Pathol.* 38, 468–473. doi: 10.1016/j.humpath.2006.09.009

Robben, P. M., Mordue, D. G., Truscott, S. M., Takeda, K., Akira, S., and Sibley, L. D. (2004). Production of IL-12 by macrophages infected with *toxoplasma gondii* depends on the parasite genotype. *J. Immunol.* 172, 3686–3694. doi: 10.4049/jimmunol.172.6.3686

Robbins, J. R., and Bakardjiev, A. I. (2012). Pathogens and the placental fortress. *Curr. Opin. Microbiol.* 15, 36–43. doi: 10.1016/j.mib.2011.11.006

Robbins, J. R., Zeldovich, V. B., Poukchanski, A., Boothroyd, J. C., and Bakardjiev, A. I. (2012). Tissue barriers of the human placenta to infection with *toxoplasma gondii*. *Infect. Immun.* 80, 418–428. doi: 10.1128/IAI.05899-11

Roberts, C. W., Ferguson, D. J., Jebbari, H., Satoskar, A., Bluethmann, H., and Alexander, J. (1996). Different roles for interleukin-4 during the course of *toxoplasma gondii* infection. *Infect. Immun.* 64, 897–904. doi: 10.1128/iai.64.3.897-904.1996

Robinson, D. P., and Klein, S. L. (2012). Pregnancy and pregnancy-associated hormones alter immune responses and disease pathogenesis. *Horm. Behav.* 62, 263–271. doi: 10.1016/j.yhbeh.2012.02.023

Rowe, J. H., Ertelt, J. M., Xin, L., and Way, S. S. (2013). Regulatory T cells and the immune pathogenesis of prenatal infection. *Reproduction* 146, R191–R203. doi: 10.1530/REP-13-0262

Senegas, A., Villard, O., Neuville, A., Marcellin, L., Pfaff, A. W., Steinmetz, T., et al. (2009). *Toxoplasma gondii*-induced foetal resorption in mice involves interferon-gamma-induced apoptosis and spiral artery dilation at the maternofoetal interface. *Int. J. Parasitol.* 39, 481–487. doi: 10.1016/j.ijpara.2008.08.009

Shiono, Y., Mun, H. S., He, N., Nakazaki, Y., Fang, M., Aosai, F., et al. (2007). Maternal-fetal transmission of *toxoplasma gondii* in interferon-gamma deficient pregnant mice. *Parasitol. Int.* 56, 141–148. doi: 10.1016/j.parint.2007.01.008

Shirahata, T., Muroya, N., Ohta, C., Goto, H., and Nakane, A. (1992). Correlation between increased susceptibility to primary *toxoplasma gondii* infection and depressed production of gamma interferon in pregnant mice. *Microbiol. Immunol.* 36, 81–91. doi: 10.1111/j.1348-0421.1992.tb01644.x

Soares, M. J., Varberg, K. M., and Iqbal, K. (2018). Hemochorial placentation: development, function, and adaptations. *Biol. Reprod.* 99, 196–211. doi: 10.1093/biolre/ioy049

Sousa, R. O., Cariaco, Y., Almeida, M. P. O., Nascimento, L. A. C., Coutinho, L. B., Ferreira-Júnior, A. A., et al. (2021). The imbalance of TNF and IL-6 levels and FOXP3 expression at the maternal-fetal interface is involved in adverse pregnancy outcomes in a susceptible murine model of congenital toxoplasmosis. *Cytokine* 143:155517. doi: 10.1016/j.cyto.2021.155517

Sturge, C. R., and Yarovinsky, F. (2014). Complex immune cell interplay in the gamma interferon response during *toxoplasma gondii* infection. *Infect. Immun.* 82, 3090–3097. doi: 10.1128/IAI.01722-14

Takeuchi, O., Hoshino, K., and Akira, S. (2000). Cutting edge: TLR2-deficient and MyD88-deficient mice are highly susceptible to *Staphylococcus aureus* infection. *J. Immunol.* 165, 5392–5396. doi: 10.4049/jimmunol.165.10.5392

Tanaka, S., Nishimura, M., Ihara, F., Yamagishi, J., Suzuki, Y., and Nishikawa, Y. (2013). Transcriptome analysis of mouse brain infected with *toxoplasma gondii*. *Infect. Immun.* 81, 3609–3619. doi: 10.1128/IAI.00439-13

Thaxton, J. E., Nevers, T. A., and Sharma, S. (2010). TLR-mediated preterm birth in response to pathogenic agents. *Infect. Dis. Obstet. Gynecol.* 2010:378472. doi: 10.1155/2010/378472

Umeda, K., Tanaka, S., Ihara, F., Yamagishi, J., Suzuki, Y., and Nishikawa, Y. (2017). Transcriptional profiling of toll-like receptor 2-deficient primary murine brain cells during *toxoplasma gondii* infection. *PLoS One* 12:e0187703. doi: 10.1371/journal.pone.0187703

Vargas-Villavicencio, J. A., Cedillo-Peláez, C., Rico-Torres, C. P., Besné-Mérida, A., García-Vázquez, F., Saldaña, J. I., et al. (2016). Mouse model of congenital infection with a non-virulent *toxoplasma gondii* strain: vertical transmission, "sterile" fetal damage, or both? *Exp. Parasitol.* 166, 116–123. doi: 10.1016/j.exppara.2016.04.002

Wang, T., Liu, M., Gao, X. J., Zhao, Z. J., Chen, X. G., and Lun, Z. R. (2011). *Toxoplasma gondii*: the effects of infection at different stages of pregnancy on the offspring of mice. *Exp. Parasitol.* 127, 107–112. doi: 10.1016/j.exppara.2010.07.003

Xie, F., Xiao, P., Chen, D., Xu, L., and Zhang, B. (2012). miRDeepFinder: a miRNA analysis tool for deep sequencing of plant small RNAs. *Plant Mol. Biol.* 80, 75–84. doi: 10.1007/s11103-012-9885-2

Xu, X., Zhang, J., Zhan, S., Li, Z., Liu, X., Zhang, H., et al. (2017). TGF-β1 improving abnormal pregnancy outcomes induced by *toxoplasma gondii* infection: regulating NKG2D/DAP10 and killer subset of decidual NK cells. *Cell. Immunol.* 317, 9–17. doi: 10.1016/j.cellimm.2017.04.004

Zhan, S., Zheng, J., Zhang, H., Zhao, M., Liu, X., Jiang, Y., et al. (2018). LILRB4 decrease on uDCs exacerbate abnormal pregnancy outcomes following *toxoplasma gondii* infection. *Front. Microbiol.* 9:588. doi: 10.3389/fmicb.2018.00588

Zhang, H., Cui, L., Ren, L., Liu, X., Jiang, Y., Yang, C., et al. (2019). The role of Decidual PD-1+ Treg cells in adverse pregnancy outcomes due to *toxoplasma gondii* infection. *Inflammation* 42, 2119–2128. doi: 10.1007/s10753-019-01075-1

Zhang, D., Ren, L., Zhao, M., Yang, C., Liu, X., Zhang, H., et al. (2019). Role of Tim-3 in decidual macrophage functional polarization during abnormal pregnancy with *toxoplasma gondii* infection. *Front. Immunol.* 10:1550. doi: 10.3389/fimmu.2019.01550

Zhang, L., Zhao, M., Jiao, F., Xu, X., Liu, X., Jiang, Y., et al. (2015). Interferon gamma is involved in apoptosis of trophoblast cells at the maternal-fetal interface following *toxoplasma gondii* infection. *Int. J. Infect. Dis.* 30, 10–16. doi: 10.1016/j.ijid.2014.10.027

Zhao, M., Zhang, H., Liu, X., Jiang, Y., Ren, L., and Hu, X. (2017). The effect of TGF-β on Treg cells in adverse pregnancy outcome upon *toxoplasma gondii* infection. *Front. Microbiol.* 8:901. doi: 10.3389/fmicb.2017.00901

8

Fetal-Derived MyD88 Signaling Contributes to Poor Pregnancy Outcomes during Gestational Malaria

Renato Barboza[1], Lutero Hasenkamp[2], André Barateiro[2], Oscar Murillo[2], Erika Paula Machado Peixoto[2], Flávia Afonso Lima[2], Aramys Silva Reis[2], Lígia Antunes Gonçalves[2], Sabrina Epiphanio[3] and Claudio R. F. Marinho[2]*

[1] Departamento de Ciências Biológicas, Universidade Federal de São Paulo, Diadema, Brazil, [2] Departamento de Parasitologia, Instituto de Ciências Biomédicas, Universidade de São Paulo, São Paulo, Brazil, [3] Departamento de Análises Clínicas e Toxicológicas, Faculdade de Ciências Farmacêuticas, Universidade de São Paulo, São Paulo, Brazil

***Correspondence:**
Claudio R. F. Marinho
marinho@usp.br

Placental malaria (PM) remains a severe public health problem in areas of high malaria transmission. Despite the efforts to prevent infection poor outcomes in *Plasmodium* endemic areas, there is still a considerable number of preterm births and newborns with low birth weight resulting from PM. Although local inflammation triggered in response to malaria is considered crucial in inducing placental damage, little is known about the differential influence of maternal and fetal immune responses to the disease progression. Therefore, using a PM mouse model, we sought to determine the contribution of maternal and fetal innate immune responses to PM development. For this, we conducted a series of cross-breeding experiments between mice that had differential expression of the MyD88 adaptor protein to obtain mother and correspondent fetuses with distinct genetic backgrounds. By evaluating fetal weight and placental vascular spaces, we have shown that the expression of MyD88 in fetal tissue has a significant impact on PM outcomes. Our results highlighted the existence of a distinct contribution of maternal and fetal immune responses to PM onset. Thus, contributing to the understanding of how inflammatory processes lead to the dysregulation of placental homeostasis ultimately impairing fetal development.

Keywords: mouse model, pregnancy, placenta, malaria, MyD88, *Plasmodium berghei*

INTRODUCTION

Placental malaria (PM) constitutes a serious public health issue in areas of high malaria transmission as pregnant women are particularly susceptible to *Plasmodium* infection (Fried and Duffy, 2017). Despite the significant efforts that have been done to prevent and treat malaria, every year a considerable number of newborns with low birth weight are still reported as a result of PM (Rogerson et al., 2018). In addition, malaria during pregnancy can affect the transplacental transfer of nutrients, which contributes to the impaired development of the fetus (Rogerson et al., 2007).

The negative consequences of PM are related to the accumulation of infected red blood cells (iRBCs) in the intervillous space of the placenta. During *P. falciparum* infections, this accumulation is mediated by the protein VAR2CSA (Doritchamou et al., 2012), a member of the *P. falciparum* erythrocyte membrane protein 1 (PfEMP1) that promotes the binding of iRBCs to the chondroitin sulfate A (CSA) (Fried and Duffy, 1996; Beeson et al., 2000). The adhesion of iRBCs to the placenta is sufficient to induce an inflammatory process mainly through the recruitment of inflammatory cells and the production of pro-inflammatory mediators. Also, the immune response can disrupt a normal angiogenic process that can progress and culminate in low birth weight and preterm birth (Brabin et al., 2004; Desai et al., 2007; Umbers et al., 2011).

The trigger of pro-inflammatory mediators could be induced by the activation of the innate immune system via Pattern Recognition Receptors (PRRs) that recognize the Pathogen-associated molecular pattern (PAMPs). One of the most relevant PRRs family are the Toll-like receptors (TLRs). These receptors act as immune sensors for microorganisms and internal danger signals (Kawai and Akira, 2010). It is known that *Plasmodium* components can activate the TLR pathway (Franklin et al., 2009). As an example, *Plasmodium* glycosylphosphatidylinositol (GPI) is recognized by TLR2 and TLR4 (Krishnegowda et al., 2005), cytosolic RNA by TLR7 (Baccarella et al., 2013; Wu et al., 2014), and hemozoin and DNA by TLR9 (Parroche et al., 2007; Pichyangkul et al., 2004; Coban et al., 2010). Additionally, several TLRs polymorphisms have been associated with increased susceptibility to PM (Mockenhaupt et al., 2006; Leoratti et al., 2008; Hamann et al., 2010). All TLRs, except the TLR3, use as adaptor molecule the Myeloid differentiation primary response 88 (MyD88) protein. Upon activation of a TLR, the MyD88 allows the recruitment of several other proteins, which lead to a signaling pathway downstream that culminate in the production of pro-inflammatory proteins via MAPK and the NF-κB pathway (Kawai and Akira, 2010). The MyD88 protein was discovered in 1990 (Lord et al., 1990) and since then has been widely studied. MyD88, together with TLR7 or TLR9, has been associated as a protective factor for immunity to malaria (Gowda et al., 2012; Spaulding et al., 2016). Gowda et al. showed that MyD88$^{-/-}$ mice lacked cell-mediated immunity to malaria due to a reduction of pro-inflammatory proteins production. Additionally, the study shows that the MyD88 and TLR9 deficiency impaired NK and CD8^{+} T cell cytotoxic activity. Furthermore, other report showed that NK cell production of IFN-γ in response to *P. falciparum* infection is dependent of MyD88, which its expression in macrophages is crucial for an efficient response (Baratin et al., 2005). Accordingly, we have described that MyD88 and TLR4 signaling are fundamental to the placental inflammatory process induced by *Plasmodium* infection (Barboza et al., 2014, 2017).

Albeit the studies which agree that local inflammation in response to *Plasmodium* infection is crucial for the development of PM, little is known about the differential influence of maternal and fetal tissue to local immune response. Recently, Rodrigues-Duarte et al. (2018) presented results showing that fetal-derived TLR4 contributes to the iRBCs uptake by trophoblasts and to placental innate immune responses triggered in response to *P. berghei* infection.

Herein, we used an experimental mouse model that manifests several clinical features of the human disease in order to determine the contribution of maternal and fetal innate immune activation on PM pathogenesis. Therefore, we conducted a series of cross-breeding between mice with different MyD88 genotypes to generate several fetal genotypes born from mothers with distinct MyD88 backgrounds. Our findings have shown that the expression of fetal-derived MyD88 is detrimental for illness-induced complications of PM. These results extend and complete our previous observations showing the crucial role of MyD88 for local inflammation and consequent disease onset (Barboza et al., 2014).

MATERIALS AND METHODS

Animals

C57Bl/6 WT, MyD88$^{+/-}$, and MyD88$^{-/-}$ mice with 8- to 10-weeks were bred and maintained in conventional housing with constant light-dark cycle (12 h:12 h) at the Animal Facility of the Department of Parasitology from the Institute of Biomedical Sciences at the University of São Paulo (ICB/USP). Mice received water and were fed *ad libitum* with commercial NUVILAB CR-1 ration (Nuvital®, Brazil). All experiments were performed in accordance with the ethical guidelines for experiments with mice, and the protocols were approved by the Animal Health Committee of the Institute of Biomedical Sciences of the University of São Paulo (CEUA No. 015fls82livro2). The guidelines for animal use and care were based on the standards established by the National Council for Control of Animal Experimentation (CONCEA).

Cross-Breeding Experiments

To study the contribution of maternal and fetal MyD88 expression to PM development, heterogenic litters from females with heterozygous (**Figure 1A**) or null (**Figure 1B**) MyD88 expression were generated and then compared to WT and MyD88 full knockout fetuses/mothers. The generation of knockout (MyD88$^{-/-}$) and heterozygous (MyD88$^{+/-}$) fetuses from heterozygous mothers started by mating MyD88$^{-/-}$ males with C57Bl/6 WT females (I from **Figure 1A**) to obtain a heterozygous progeny (II from **Figure 1A**). From these offspring, MyD88$^{+/-}$ females were backcrossed with MyD88$^{-/-}$ males (II from **Figure 1A**) and the fetuses and placentas (diamonds, sex not defined) from generation III were evaluated. Additionally, to obtain MyD88$^{+/-}$ fetuses from MyD88$^{-/-}$ mothers, we crossed C57Bl/6 WT males with MyD88$^{-/-}$ females (I from **Figure 1B**), and the fetuses and placentas (diamonds, sex not defined) from generation II were evaluated.

MyD88 Genotyping

To determine the genetic background of the generated offspring, tail genomic DNA was isolated, and genotyping was performed through conventional PCR using the following set of primers: Forward – 5′ TGG CAT GCC TCC ATC ATA GTT AAC C 3′; Reverse – 5′ GTC AGA AAC AAC CAC CAC CAT GC 3′; and, MyD88 neo – 5′ ATC GCC TTC TAT CGC CTT CTT GAC G 3′ (Leadbetter et al., 2002). The forward primer is common for both PCR reactions, while the reverse is specific for the wild-type gene and the neo is specific for the deficient gene. The PCR products

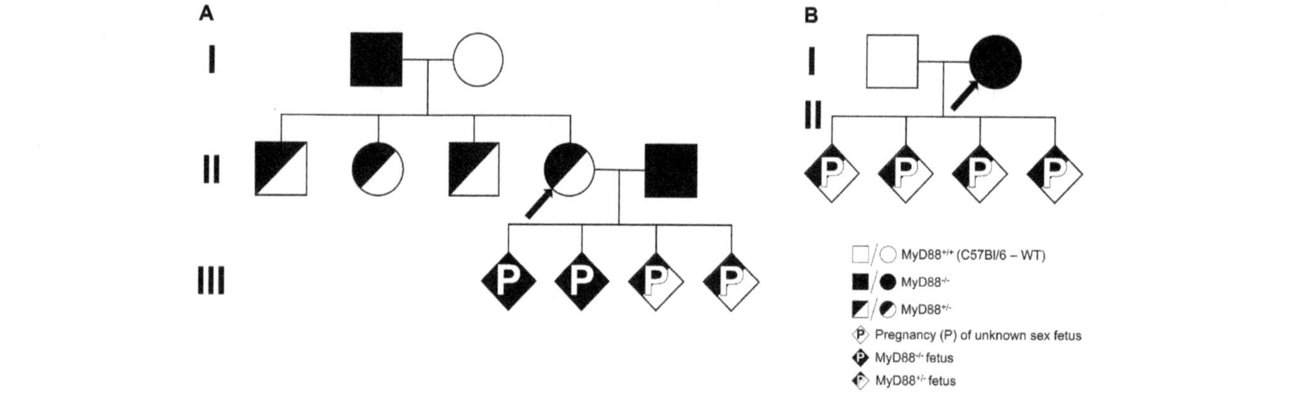

FIGURE 1 | Breeding scheme. A schematic of the breeding strategy used to generate mice containing combinations of the maternal and fetal MyD88 genotypes. **(A)** MyD88 deficient (MyD88$^{-/-}$) males (black square) mated with C57Bl/6 (MyD88$^{+/+}$) females (white circle), generation **I**, to produce a heterozygous progeny (MyD88$^{+/-}$, half-shaded symbols). MyD88$^{+/-}$ females (half-shaded circle) from generation **II** were backcrossed with MyD88$^{-/-}$ males (black square) to obtain fetus with MyD88$^{+/-}$ (half-shaded diamond) and MyD88$^{-/-}$ (black diamond) genotypes, generation **III**. **(B)** C57Bl/6 (MyD88$^{+/+}$) males (white square) mated with MyD88 deficient (MyD88$^{-/-}$) females (black circle), generation **I**, to obtain fetus with MyD88$^{+/-}$ (half-shaded diamond) genetic background, generation **II**. Diamond represents pregnancy (P) of a fetus with unknown sex. The arrows depict the MyD88 maternal genotype for each MyD88 fetal genotype (**IIIA, IIB**).

were subjected to 1% agarose gel electrophoresis to verify the presence of a MyD88 allele (**Supplementary Figure 1**).

Pregnancy Monitoring and Experimental Infection

Pregnancy was monitored as described elsewhere (Freyre et al., 2006). Briefly, we combine the detection of a vaginal plug and body weight measurement to determine the gestation time. The day in which a vaginal plug was detected was considered gestational day 1 (G1) and, from there on, pregnancy progression was monitored every day by regularly controlling weight variation. Successful fecundation was confirmed between G10 and G13 when females exhibited an average increase of 3–4 g in their body weight. Therefore, weight gain was taken as an indication of pregnancy, whereas unexpected weight loss was interpreted as an indicator of pregnancy complications or interruption. As such, pregnant mice were intravenously inoculated at G13 with 10^5 *P. berghei* NK65^{GFP} iRBCs stored in frozen vials, and parasitemia was assessed. G13 was determined as the optimal time point for the infection, allowing to analyze the pathological features of malaria along the course of pregnancy and in the developing fetus. The infection at an earlier stage would not allow reaching the pregnancy term, which is consistent with previous reports (Neres et al., 2008; Marinho et al., 2009). Parasitemia was assessed by Giemsa-stained thin blood smears until G19, gestational day that cesarean section was performed. Fetal weight was measured, and placentas were used for histopathological analysis and RNA extraction. Non-pregnant infected and non-infected pregnant mice were used as controls whenever appropriate.

Placenta Collection and Morphometric Analysis

Placentas from infected and non-infected pregnant mice were processed similarly. Briefly, placentas were divided into halves: one-half was fixed in 1.6% paraformaldehyde supplemented with 20% sucrose for further processing, and the other half was collected into an RNA stabilizer (RNAlater^{TM}, Invitrogen^{TM}, CA) for subsequent RNA extraction. Non-consecutive paraffin-embedded placentas were sectioned and stained with hematoxylin-eosin (H&E) for further microscope examination.

The placental morphometric analysis was performed as previously described (Marinho et al., 2009; Rodrigues-Duarte et al., 2012). In short, vascular spaces were quantified by analyzing the hematoxylin-eosin (H&E) stained sections. For each section, three areas of intervillous space were randomly selected for image acquisition (200× magnification) using a Zeiss color camera (Axio Cam HRc) connected to a Zeiss light microscope (Axio Imager M2). Images were analyzed using an Image J software[1]. Briefly, images were subjected to an automated light analysis procedure in which noise removal was applied to ensure color and image quality standardization across sections and specimens. Images were given a color threshold to cover the area corresponding to blood space lumen. Percentage of coverage was calculated as the ratio between the number of pixels covered by the threshold-defined area and the total amount of pixels in the image. Blood vascular area in each placenta was assessed from the analysis of three non-consecutive sections. Reported results correspond to individual pregnant mice, representing the average result from 3–9 placentas.

Gene Expression Analysis by qPCR

Total RNA was extracted from each placenta obtained at G19 using the RNeasy Minikit (Qiagen) in accordance with manufacturer's protocol for animal tissue (Animal Cell 1). One microgram of mRNA was converted into cDNA using First Strand cDNA Synthesis Transcriptor kit (Roche, Penzberg, Germany). The expression of *Il6*, *Il10*, *Tnf*, *Cxcl1* (KC),

[1] http://rsbweb.nih.gov/ij/

Ccl3 (MIP-1α) and *Ccl4* (MIP-1β) was quantified by using the following TaqMan® probes: *Il6* (Mm00446190_m1), *Il10* (Mm01288386_m1), *Tnf* (Mm00443258_m1), *Cxcl1* (Mm04207460_m1), *Ccl3* (Mm00441259_g1) and *Ccl4* (Mm00443111_m1). Gene expression quantifications were performed according to the manufacturer's instructions on Applied Biosystems 7500 Fast Real-Time PCR System. All results were obtained through the comparative ΔΔCT method after normalization to the constitutive expression of the GAPDH gene (*gpdh*: Mm99999915_g1).

Statistical Analysis

Statistical analysis was performed using the GraphPad Prism version 7.0 software (GraphPad Software, San Diego, CA, United States). To evaluate survival curves, the Long-rank test was used, the differences between groups were evaluated using the One or Two-way analysis of variance (ANOVA) as indicated at the figure's legends. *P*-values < 0.05 were considered statistically significant.

RESULTS

MyD88 Expression Influences the Progression of Murine Malaria Infection

In a previous study, we have shown that the MyD88 pathway is essential for the development of PM (Barboza et al., 2014). However, the results did not allow for individualizing the fetal-

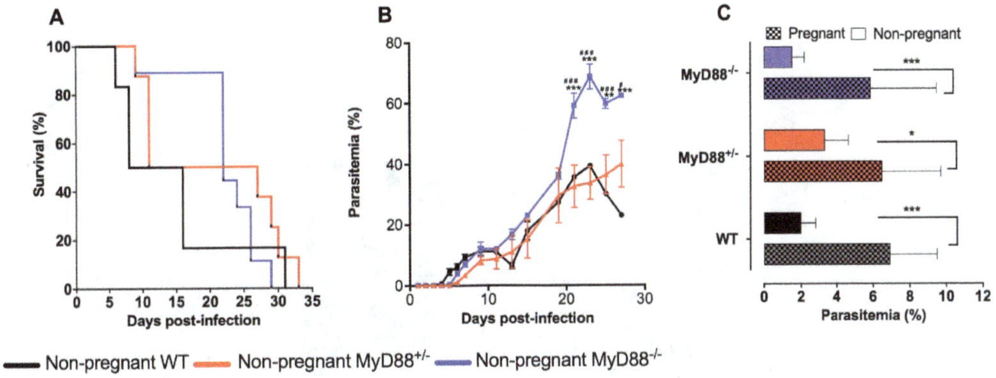

FIGURE 2 | MyD88 expression influences disease progression in mice infected with *P. berghei* NK65. **(A,B)** Non-pregnant C57Bl/6 (WT), MyD88 deficient (MyD88$^{-/-}$) and heterozygous (MyD88$^{-/-}$) mice were infected intravenously with 10^5 *P. berghei* NK65^{GFP} iRBCs. Evaluation of Kaplan-Meier survival curves **(A)** and parasitemia levels **(B)**. **(C)** Pregnant WT, MyD88$^{+/-}$ and MyD88$^{-/-}$ mice were intravenously infected at gestational day 13 (G13) with 10^5 *P. berghei* NK65^{GFP} iRBCs. Parasitemia was measured at G19 before C-section and compared with non-pregnant mice, also with 6 days of infection. Plain bars represent non-pregnant mice, and square-patterned bars represent pregnant mice. In B and C data are presented as mean ± SD. The statistical differences were achieved by a Long-rank (Mantel-Cox) test **(A)** and Two-way analysis of variance (ANOVA) with the Bonferroni's *post hoc* test **(B,C)**. $^{**}P$-value <0.01 and $^{***}P$-value < 0.001 when compared with WT **(B)** or non-pregnant mice **(C)**; $^{\#}P$-value < 0.05 and $^{\#\#\#}P$-value < 0.001 when compared with MyD88$^{+/-}$ mice **(B)**.

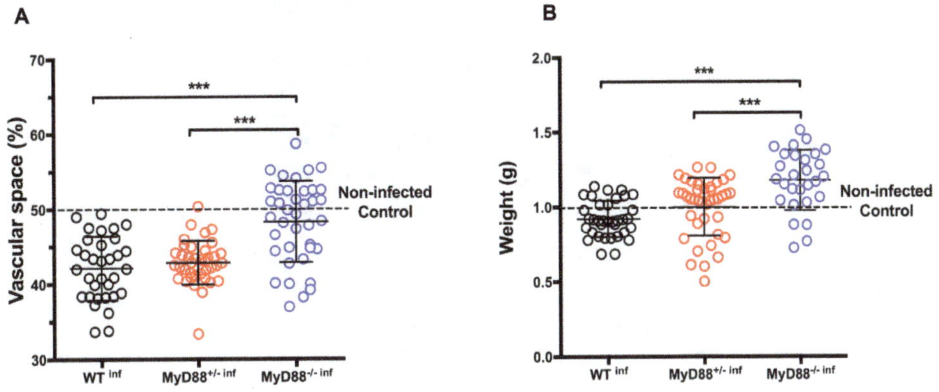

FIGURE 3 | MyD88 expression is associated with reduced placental vascular space and fetal weight in mice infected with *P. berghei* NK65. Pregnant C57Bl/6 (WT), and MyD88 deficient (MyD88$^{-/-}$) and heterozygous (MyD88$^{-/-}$) mice were intravenously infected (^{inf}) with 10^5 *P. berghei* NK65^{GFP} iRBCs at gestational day 13 (G13) and C-section performed at G19. The placenta/fetus share the same maternal MyD88 genotype. **(A)** Placental vascular spaces (n: WT^{inf} – 33; MyD88$^{+/-inf}$ – 38; MyD88$^{-/-inf}$ – 39) and **(B)** fetal weight (n: WT^{inf} – 35; MyD88$^{+/-inf}$ – 40; MyD88$^{-/-inf}$ – 28) measures. Data are presented as scatter plot with indication of the median ± SD; each dot represents an independent measurement. Dotted line represents mean values of the control group (non-infected pregnant WT mice; n: 34, vascular space, and 32, fetal weight). The statistical differences were achieved by a One-way analysis of variance (ANOVA) with *post hoc* Tukey's test. $^{***}P$-value < 0.001.

and maternal-derived MyD88 specific role in PM pathogenesis. To ascertain this, a series of experiments were conducted using C57Bl/6 (MyD88$^{+/+}$ – WT), MyD88$^{+/-}$ and MyD88$^{-/-}$ mice, evaluating their survival and parasitemia progression upon infection with *P. berghei* NK65-iRBCs. The distinct groups of mice did not present significant differences regarding the survival rates when compared among each other (**Figure 2A**). However, it was possible to note that the MyD88$^{-/-}$ group started to die later, probability due to the augment of parasitemia levels observed from the twentieth day post-infection onward (**Figure 2B**).

The evaluation of parasitemia did not show significant differences, with MyD88$^{+/-}$ mice behaving similarly to the WT group (**Figure 2B**). Moreover, our data corroborate previous studies showing that pregnancy increases mice susceptibility to infection, irrespective of the maternal genotype (**Figure 2C**).

Although there were no differences between peripheral parasitemia of pregnant mice with different genotypes, we hypothesized that heterozygous and null MyD88 expression might be involved in placental damage and poor pregnancy outcomes. Therefore, we evaluated the placental vascular spaces as an indicator for placental abnormalities. The expression of only one MyD88 allele is sufficient to induce placental structural changes as similarly to WT infected mice (WT^{inf}), MyD88$^{+/-}$ infected mice (MyD88$^{+/-inf}$) presented reduced vascular spaces (**Figure 3A**). On the other hand, the absence of the two MyD88 alleles (MyD88$^{-/-inf}$) showed no infection deleterious impact in the placental vasculature, identical to the non-infected controls (dashed line). Moreover, fetal weight exhibited a similar pattern. Like fetuses born from WT^{inf}, the progeny from heterozygous MyD88 pregnant mice (MyD88$^{+/-inf}$) also presented reduced

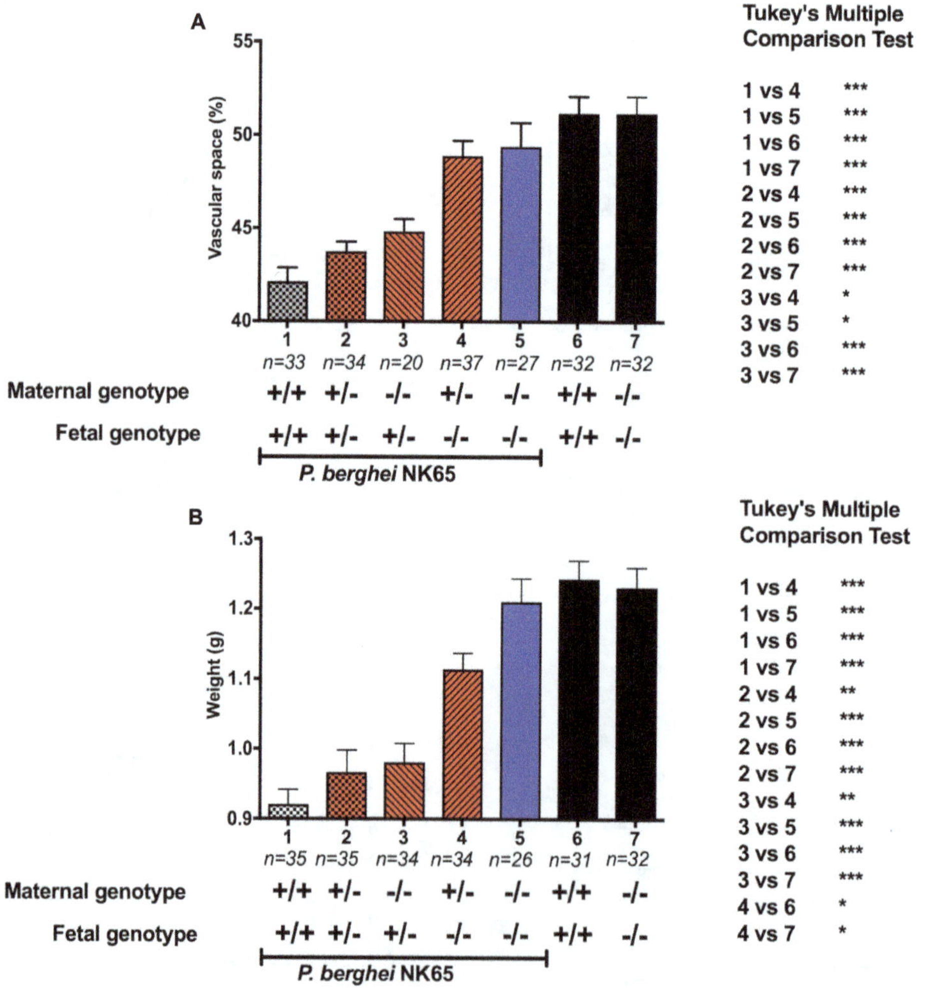

FIGURE 4 | Fetal MyD88 expression is detrimental to disease development in an experimental mouse model of PM. To ascertain the differential contribution of the maternal- and fetal-derived MyD88 expression different combinations of maternal/fetal genotypes were evaluated. Pregnant mice were intravenously infected with 10^5 *P. berghei* NK65^{GFP} iRBCs at gestational day (G13), with the following maternal-fetus pairs: WT/WT (1), MyD88$^{+/-}$/MyD88$^{+/-}$ (2), MyD88$^{-/-}$/MyD88$^{+/-}$ (3), MyD88$^{+/-}$/MyD88$^{-/-}$ (4), and MyD88$^{-/-}$/MyD88$^{-/-}$ (5). C-section was performed at G19 and fetus were genotyped and evaluated. **(A)** Placental vascular spaces and **(B)** fetal weight measures. Infected WT maternal-fetus pair is a positive control (1) and non-infected WT and MyD88$^{-/-}$ maternal-fetus pairs are negative controls (6 and 7, respectively). Data are presented as mean ± sem. The statistical differences were achieved by a One-way analysis of variance (ANOVA) with Tukey's *post hoc* test. *P-value < 0.05; **P-value < 0.01; ***P-value < 0.001.

fetal weight upon infection. Notably, in the fetuses born from MyD88$^{-/-}$ infected mice malaria did not impair their weight when compared to WT^{inf} and MyD88$^{+/-inf}$ mice (**Figure 3B**). The fetal weight in these fetuses reached values resembling those from healthy WT mice.

MyD88 Expression on Fetal-Derived Tissue Is Detrimental for Pregnancy Outcomes

To investigate the role of maternal- and fetal-derived MyD88 in PM-associated pregnancy outcomes. We performed a comparative analysis between placental vascular spaces (**Figure 4A**) and fetal weight (**Figure 4B**) associated with different MyD88 genotypes, pairing maternal and fetal genetic backgrounds. Including an infected WT maternal-fetus pair as a positive control (group 1) and as negative controls a non-infected WT and MyD88$^{-/-}$ maternal-fetus pairs (group 6 and 7, respectively). The results demonstrate that the presence of only one fetal-derived MyD88 allele is sufficient to contribute to a prominent reduction of placental vascular spaces (**Figure 4A**, groups 2 and 3) and fetal weight (**Figure 4B**, groups 2 and 3) upon *P. berghei* NK65 infection when comparing to full knockout fetuses (**Figure 4**, group 4 and 5). Also, these results show that there are no influence of maternal MyD88 genotype since MyD88$^{-/-}$ fetuses from infected MyD88$^{+/-}$ did not have a negative impact on either vascular spaces or fetal weight (**Figure 4**, group 4).

To validate our results, we performed a second multivariable statistical analysis, excluding the control groups (1, 6, and 7) from the analysis. The new analysis reinforced the idea that the fetuses genotype has a significant effect on both fetuses' weight and the placental vascular space while the maternal genotype does not (**Supplementary Figure 2** and **Supplementary Table 1**). Together, our results support the idea that fetal-derived MyD88 is associated with local parasite sensing, triggering inflammation and, consequently leading to poor pregnancy outcomes and PM development. Interestingly, the deletion of one maternal MyD88 allele was sufficient to negatively modulate the expression of placental inflammatory cytokines mRNA, except for the *Il10* (**Supplementary Figure 3**), indicating the possible involvement of other mechanisms.

DISCUSSION

Innate immune activation during pregnancy represents a substantial problem for the mother and the growing fetus. Regarding *Plasmodium* infection, it has been shown that innate immune activation in response to parasite accumulation results in placental injuries, which ultimately leads to impaired fetal development. Previously, we have demonstrated that MyD88 signaling is associated with poor pregnancy outcomes (Barboza et al., 2014, 2017). Other studies also have unveiled that the MyD88 protein plays an important role in inducing immune protection to *Plasmodium* infection (Baratin et al., 2005; Gowda et al., 2012; Spaulding et al., 2016). Herein, using mice cross-breeding strategies, we managed to obtain distinct MyD88 genetic backgrounds and determine the maternal- and fetal-derived MyD88 contribution to PM. Our results extend previous observations, showing that fetal-derived MyD88 is markedly associated with murine PM development.

Since the placenta is constituted by cells from at least two different individuals, one can argue that those cellular components can differentially influence placental physiology. The results presented here evidence the contribution of fetal-derived MyD88 expression in the disease onset, highlighting the influence of fetal components in detriment of the maternal components. Such impact is perceived when we evaluate placental vascular spaces of infected pregnant mice. Our work revealed that placental vascular spaces reduction upon infection is mediated by fetal-derived MyD88, even when only one allele is carried (**Figure 4A** group 2 and 3 and **Supplementary Figure 2**). Of note, the importance of this observation is supported by the minor impact of maternal MyD88 expression (**Figure 4A** group 4 and **Supplementary Figure 2**). Previously, it was described that in murine PM the reduction of placental vascular spaces is correlated with low birth weight (Neres et al., 2008; Marinho et al., 2009; Medeiros et al., 2013; Barboza et al., 2014). In fact, we also observed a parallel reduction of fetal weight, which was equally determined by fetal-derived MyD88 expression (**Figure 4B** group 2 and 3). We should emphasize that the deletion of the MyD88 gene does not impact the mice growth nor produces abnormalities (Adachi et al., 1998), as well as have no influence in pregnancy in general, as non-infected MyD88$^{-/-}$ and MyD88$^{+/-}$ have no differences in the pregnancy outcome.

In line with our observation, Rodrigues-Duarte et al. (2018) have recently reported that maternal and fetal counterparts act in opposite directions during murine PM. This study showed that TLR4 and IFNAR1 expression in the maternal tissue has a deleterious effect on fetal development, which is counteracted by fetal tissue. The role of these family of innate immune receptors on PM has been extensively studied in humans and murine malaria models (Adegnika et al., 2008; McDonald et al., 2015; Odorizzi and Feeney, 2016; Barboza et al., 2017; Rodrigues-Duarte et al., 2018). These studies have shown that local immune activation via innate immune receptors is correlated with placental damage, which results in impaired fetal development.

The negative impact of innate immune activation observed in the fetuses is correlated with a rupture of maternal-fetal interactions during pregnancy. For instance, to achieve a successful pregnancy it is necessary that trophoblasts (fetal-derived cells which populate most of the placenta) and maternal decidual immune cells interact, allowing the development of the embryo in the uterus (Prabhudas et al., 2015). One way of promoting this rupture is through the activation of MyD88-dependent pathways induced by TLR activation in trophoblasts, which are known to broadly express TLRs (Abrahams et al., 2004; Mitsunari et al., 2006; Lucchi and Moore, 2007; Aldo et al., 2010; Tangerås et al., 2014). Moreover, TLR activation has been associated with pregnancy complications (Mockenhaupt et al., 2006; Rindsjö et al., 2007; Leoratti et al., 2008; Hamann et al., 2010; Pineda et al., 2011; Koga et al., 2014). Thus, TLR activation by the parasite components can lead to NF-κB activation and, as a consequence, to the production of pro-inflammatory mediators such as chemokines and cytokines, contributing to tissue damage and PM development.

Nevertheless, our work may present some limitations. The PM murine models recapitulate many features observed in the human's disease, which represent numerous advantages in the research and acquisition of knowledge of this disease (Hviid et al., 2010). Though, human and mouse pregnancy differences do not allow us to make direct assumptions, such as the placental architecture or the immunological responses (Moffett and Loke, 2006; Carter, 2007). Hence, it would be of crucial relevance the validation of murine results with human samples, whenever is possible. Following our results in murine models, it would be interesting to ascertain the correlation of the maternal and fetal genetic interplay with pregnancy outcomes upon *Plasmodium* infection.

Our results on the placental vasculature and fetal weight obtained using heterogenic mice progeny from different maternal MyD88 genetic backgrounds have evidenced a marked impact of the fetal immune system in the PM onset. In summary, this study highlights the importance of maternal and fetal immune response in the context of pregnancy-associated malaria, which ultimately contributes to the placental pathology and poor pregnancy outcomes.

AUTHOR CONTRIBUTIONS

RB and CM designed the study. LH, RB, OM, AB, EP, FL, AR, LG, SE, and CM were involved in data acquisition and scientific input. RB, LH, LG, SE, and CM contributed to the analysis and/or interpretation of the data. RB, LG, and CM wrote the manuscript. SE revised the manuscript. CM, SE, and RB were the main funders of this work. CM has full access to all the data in the study and takes responsibility for the integrity of the data and the accuracy of the data analysis. All authors reviewed and approved the definitive version of this manuscript.

ACKNOWLEDGMENTS

We thank Bernardo Paulo Albe for his technical support.

REFERENCES

Abrahams, V. M., Bole-Aldo, P., Kim, Y. M., Straszewski-Chavez, S. L., Chaiworapongsa, T., Romero, R., et al. (2004). Divergent trophoblast responses to bacterial products mediated by TLRs. *J. Immunol.* 173, 4286–4296. doi: 10.4049/jimmunol.173.7.4286

Adachi, O., Kawai, T., Takeda, K., Matsumoto, M., Tsutsui, H., Sakagami, M., et al. (1998). Targeted disruption of the MyD88 gene results in loss of IL-1- and IL-18-mediated function. *Immunity* 9, 143–150.

Adegnika, A. A., Köhler, C., Agnandji, S. T., Chai, S. K., Labuda, L., Breitling, L. P., et al. (2008). Pregnancy-associated malaria affects toll-like receptor ligand-induced cytokine responses in cord blood. *J. Infect. Dis.* 198, 928–936. doi: 10.1086/591057

Aldo, P. B., Mulla, M. J., Romero, R., Mor, G., and Abrahams, V. M. (2010). Viral ssRNA induces first trimester trophoblast apoptosis through an inflammatory mechanism. *Am. J. Reprod. Immunol.* 64, 27–37. doi: 10.1111/j.1600-0897.2010.00817.x

Baccarella, A., Fontana, M. F., Chen, E. C., and Kim, C. C. (2013). Toll-like receptor 7 mediates early innate immune responses to Malaria. *Infect. Immun.* 81, 4431–4442. doi: 10.1128/IAI.00923-13

Baratin, M., Roetynck, S., Lépolard, C., Falk, C., Sawadogo, S., Uematsu, S., et al. (2005). Natural killer cell and macrophage cooperation in MyD88-dependent innate responses to *Plasmodium falciparum*. *Proc. Natl. Acad. Sci. U.S.A.* 102, 14747–14752. doi: 10.1073/pnas.0507355102

Barboza, R., Lima, F. A., Reis, A. S., Murillo, O. J., Peixoto, E. P. M., Bandeira, C. L., et al. (2017). TLR4-mediated placental pathology and pregnancy outcome in experimental Malaria. *Sci. Rep.* 7:8623. doi: 10.1038/s41598-017-08299-x

Barboza, R., Reis, A. S., da Silva, L. G., Hasenkamp, L., Pereira, K. R. B., Camara, N. O. S., et al. (2014). MyD88 signaling is directly involved in the development of murine placental Malaria. *Infect. Immun.* 82, 830–838. doi: 10.1128/IAI.01288-13

Beeson, J. G., Rogerson, S. J., Cooke, B. M., Reeder, J. C., Chai, W., Lawson, A. M., et al. (2000). Adhesion of *Plasmodium falciparum*-infected erythrocytes to hyaluronic acid in placental malaria. *Nat. Med.* 6, 86–90. doi: 10.1038/71582

Brabin, B. J., Romagosa, C., Abdelgalil, S., Menéndez, C., Verhoeff, F. H., McGready, R., et al. (2004). The sick placenta—the role of Malaria. *Placenta* 25, 359–378. doi: 10.1016/j.placenta.2003.10.019

Carter, A. M. (2007). Animal models of human placentation - a review. *Placenta* 28(Suppl. A), S41–S47. doi: 10.1016/j.placenta.2006.11.002

Coban, C., Igari, Y., Yagi, M., Reimer, T., Koyama, S., Aoshi, T., et al. (2010). Immunogenicity of whole-parasite vaccines against *Plasmodium falciparum* involves malarial hemozoin and host TLR9. *Cell Host Microbe* 7, 50–61. doi: 10.1016/j.chom.2009.12.003

Desai, M., ter Kuile, F. O., Nosten, F., McGready, R., Asamoa, K., Brabin, B., et al. (2007). Epidemiology and burden of malaria in pregnancy. *Lancet Infect. Dis.* 7, 93–104. doi: 10.1016/S1473-3099(07)70021-X

Doritchamou, J., Bertin, G., Moussiliou, A., Bigey, P., Viwami, F., Ezinmegnon, S., et al. (2012). First-trimester *Plasmodium falciparum* infections display a typical placental phenotype. *J. Infect. Dis.* 206, 1911–1919. doi: 10.1093/infdis/jis629

Franklin, B. S., Parroche, P., Ataíde, M. A., Lauw, F., Ropert, C., de Oliveira, R. B., et al. (2009). Malaria primes the innate immune response due to interferon-gamma induced enhancement of toll-like receptor expression and function. *Proc. Natl. Acad. Sci. U.S.A.* 106, 5789–5794. doi: 10.1073/pnas.0809742106

Freyre, A., Falcon, J., Mendez, J., Rodriguez, A., Correa, L., Gonzalez, M., et al. (2006). Refinement of the mouse model of congenital toxoplasmosis. *Exp. Parasitol.* 113, 154–160. doi: 10.1016/j.exppara.2005.12.019

Fried, M., and Duffy, P. E. (1996). Adherence of *Plasmodium falciparum* to Chondroitin sulfate A in the human placenta. *Science* 272, 502–504.

Fried, M., and Duffy, P. E. (2017). Malaria during pregnancy. *Cold Spring Harb. Perspect. Med.* 7:a025551. doi: 10.1101/cshperspect.a025551

Gowda, N. M., Wu, X., and Gowda, D. C. (2012). TLR9 and MyD88 are crucial for the development of protective immunity to Malaria. *J. Immunol.* 188, 5073–5085. doi: 10.4049/jimmunol.1102143

Hamann, L., Bedu-Addo, G., Eggelte, T. A., Schumann, R. R., and Mockenhaupt, F. P. (2010). The toll-like receptor 1 variant S248N influences placental malaria. *Infect. Genet. Evol.* 10, 785–789. doi: 10.1016/j.meegid.2010.05.005

Hviid, L., Marinho, C. R. F., Staalsoe, T., and Penha-Gonçalves, C. (2010). Of mice and women: rodent models of placental malaria. *Trends Parasitol.* 26, 412–419. doi: 10.1016/j.pt.2010.04.010

Kawai, T., and Akira, S. (2010). The role of pattern-recognition receptors in innate immunity: update on toll-like receptors. *Nat. Immunol.* 11, 373–384. doi: 10.1038/ni.1863

Koga, K., Izumi, G., Mor, G., Fujii, T., and Osuga, Y. (2014). Toll-like receptors at the maternal-fetal interface in normal pregnancy and pregnancy complications. *Am. J. Reprod. Immunol.* 72, 192–205. doi: 10.1111/j.1600-0897.2010.00848.x

Krishnegowda, G., Hajjar, A. M., Zhu, J., Douglass, E. J., Uematsu, S., Akira, S., et al. (2005). Induction of proinflammatory responses in macrophages by the glycosylphosphatidylinositols of *Plasmodium falciparum*: cell signaling receptors, glycosylphosphatidylinositol (GPI) structural requirement, and regulation of GPI activity. *J. Biol. Chem.* 280, 8606–8616. doi: 10.1074/jbc.M413541200

Leadbetter, E. A., Rifkin, I. R., Hohlbaum, A. M., Beaudette, B. C., Shlomchik, M. J., and Marshak-rothstein, A. (2002). Chromatin - IgG complexes activate B cells by dual engagement of IgM and Toll-like receptors. *Nature* 416, 603–607.

Leoratti, F. M. S., Farias, L., Alves, F. P., Suarez-Mútis, M. C., Coura, J. R., Kalil, J., et al. (2008). Variants in the toll-like receptor signaling pathway and clinical outcomes of Malaria. *J. Infect. Dis.* 198, 772–780.

Lord, K. A., Hoffman-Liebermann, B., and Liebermann, D. A. (1990). Nucleotide sequence and expression of a cDNA encoding MyD88, a novel myeloid differentiation primary response gene induced by IL6. *Oncogene* 5, 1095–1097. doi: 10.1093/nar/18.9.2823

Lucchi, N. W., and Moore, J. M. (2007). LPS induces secretion of chemokines by human syncytiotrophoblast cells in a MAPK-dependent manner. *J. Reprod. Immunol.* 73, 20–27. doi: 10.1016/j.jri.2006.05.005

Marinho, C. R. F., Neres, R., Epiphanio, S., Gonçalves, L. A., Catarino, M. B., and Penha-Gonçalves, C. (2009). Recrudescent *Plasmodium berghei* from pregnant mice displays enhanced binding to the placenta and induces protection in multigravida. *PLoS One* 4:e5630. doi: 10.1371/journal.pone.0005630

McDonald, C. R., Tran, V., and Kain, K. C. (2015). Complement activation in placental Malaria. *Front. Microbiol.* 6:1460. doi: 10.3389/fmicb.2015.01460

Medeiros, M. M., Da Silva, H. B., Reis, A. S., Barboza, R., Thompson, J., Lima, M. R. D. I., et al. (2013). Liver accumulation of *Plasmodium chabaudi*-infected red blood cells and modulation of regulatory T cell and dendritic cell responses. *PLoS One* 8:e81409. doi: 10.1371/journal.pone.0081409

Mitsunari, M., Yoshida, S., Shoji, T., Tsukihara, S., Iwabe, T., Harada, T., et al. (2006). Macrophage-activating lipopeptide-2 induces cyclooxygenase-2 and prostaglandin E2 via toll-like receptor 2 in human placental trophoblast cells. *J. Reprod. Immunol.* 72, 46–59. doi: 10.1016/j.jri.2006.02.003

Mockenhaupt, F. P., Cramer, J. P., Hamann, L., Stegemann, M. S., Eckert, J., Oh, N. R., et al. (2006). Toll-Like Receptor (TLR) polymorphisms in African children: common TLR-4 variants predispose to severe malaria. *J. Commun. Dis.* 38, 230–245. doi: 10.1073/pnas.0506803102

Moffett, A., and Loke, C. (2006). Immunology of placentation in eutherian mammals. *Nat. Rev. Immunol.* 6, 584–594. doi: 10.1038/nri1897

Neres, R., Marinho, C. R. F., Gonçalves, L. A., Catarino, M. B., and Penha-Gonçalves, C. (2008). Pregnancy outcome and placenta pathology in *Plasmodium berghei* ANKA infected mice reproduce the pathogenesis of severe malaria in pregnant women. *PLoS One* 3:e1608. doi: 10.1371/journal.pone.0001608

Odorizzi, P. M., and Feeney, M. E. (2016). Impact of In utero exposure to Malaria on fetal T cell immunity. *Trends Mol. Med.* 22, 877–888. doi: 10.1016/j.molmed.2016.08.005

Parroche, P., Lauw, F. N., Goutagny, N., Latz, E., Monks, B. G., Visintin, A., et al. (2007). Malaria hemozoin is immunologically inert but radically enhances innate responses by presenting malaria DNA to Toll-like receptor 9. *Proc. Natl. Acad. Sci. U.S.A.* 104, 1919–1924. doi: 10.1073/pnas.0608745104

Pichyangkul, S., Yongvanitchit, K., Kum-arb, U., Hemmi, H., Akira, S., Krieg, A. M., et al. (2004). Malaria blood stage parasites activate human plasmacytoid dendritic cells and murine dendritic cells through a toll-like receptor 9-dependent pathway. *J. Immunol.* 172, 4926–4933. doi: 10.4049/jimmunol.172.8.4926

Pineda, A., Verdin-Terán, S. L., Camacho, A., and Moreno-Fierros, L. (2011). Expression of toll-like receptor TLR-2, TLR-3, TLR-4 and TLR-9 is increased in placentas from patients with Preeclampsia. *Arch. Med. Res.* 42, 382–391. doi: 10.1016/j.arcmed.2011.08.003

Prabhudas, M., Bonney, E., Caron, K., Dey, S., Erlebacher, A., Fazleabas, A., et al. (2015). Commentary Immune mechanisms at the maternal-fetal interface: perspectives and challenges. *Nat. Immunol.* 16, 328–334. doi: 10.1038/ni.3131

Rindsjö, E., Holmlund, U., Sverremark-Ekström, E., Papadogiannakis, N., and Scheynius, A. (2007). Toll-like receptor-2 expression in normal and pathologic human placenta. *Hum. Pathol.* 38, 468–473. doi: 10.1016/j.humpath.2006.09.009

Rodrigues-Duarte, L., de Moraes, L. V., Barboza, R., Marinho, C. R. F., Franke-Fayard, B., Janse, C. J., et al. (2012). Distinct placental malaria pathology caused by different *Plasmodium berghei* lines that fail to induce cerebral malaria in the C57BL/6 mouse. *Malar. J.* 11:231. doi: 10.1186/1475-2875-11-231

Rodrigues-Duarte, L., Pandya, Y., Neres, R., and Penha-Gonçalves, C. (2018). Fetal and maternal innate immunity receptors have opposing effects in severity of experimental malaria in pregnancy: beneficial roles for fetal-derived TLR4 and IFNAR1. *Infect. Immun.* 86, e708–e717. doi: 10.1128/IAI.00708-17

Rogerson, S. J., Desai, M., Mayor, A., Sicuri, E., Taylor, S. M., and van Eijk, A. M. (2018). Burden, pathology, and costs of malaria in pregnancy: new developments for an old problem. *Lancet Infect. Dis.* 18, e107–e118. doi: 10.1016/S1473-3099(18)30066-5

Rogerson, S. J., Hviid, L., Duffy, P. E., Leke, R. F. G., and Taylor, D. W. (2007). Malaria in pregnancy: pathogenesis and immunity. *Lancet Infect. Dis.* 7, 105–117. doi: 10.1016/S1473-3099(07)70022-1

Spaulding, E., Fooksman, D., Moore, J. M., Saidi, A., Feintuch, C. M., Reizis, B., et al. (2016). STING-licensed macrophages prime type I IFN production by Plasmacytoid dendritic cells in the bone marrow during severe *Plasmodium yoelii* Malaria. *PLoS Pathog.* 12:e1005975. doi: 10.1371/journal.ppat.1005975

Tangerås, L. H., Stødle, G. S., Olsen, G. D., Leknes, A. H., Gundersen, A. S., Skei, B., et al. (2014). Functional toll-like receptors in primary first-trimester trophoblasts. *J. Reprod. Immunol.* 106, 89–99. doi: 10.1016/j.jri.2014.04.004

Umbers, A. J., Aitken, E. H., and Rogerson, S. J. (2011). Malaria in pregnancy: small babies, big problem. *Trends Parasitol.* 27, 168–175. doi: 10.1016/j.pt.2011.01.007

Wu, J., Tian, L., Yu, X., Pattaradilokrat, S., Li, J., Wang, M., et al. (2014). Strain-specific innate immune signaling pathways determine malaria parasitemia dynamics and host mortality. *Proc. Natl. Acad. Sci. U.S.A.* 111, E511–E520. doi: 10.1073/pnas.1316467111

9

Congenital Transmission of *Trypanosoma cruzi*: A Review about the Interactions between the Parasite, the Placenta, the Maternal and the Fetal/Neonatal Immune Responses

Ulrike Kemmerling[1], Antonio Osuna[2]*, Alejandro Gabriel Schijman[3]* and Carine Truyens[4]**

[1] Programa de Anatomía y Biología del Desarrollo, Instituto de Ciencias Biomédicas, Facultad de Medicina, Universidad de Chile, Santiago, Chile, [2] Grupo de Bioquímica y Parasitología Molecular, Departamento de Parasitología, Instituto de Biotecnología, Universidad de Granada, Granada, Spain, [3] Molecular Biology of Chagas Disease Laboratory, Genetic Engineering and Molecular Biology Research Institute Dr. Héctor Torres (INGEBI-CONICET), Buenos Aires, Argentina, [4] Laboratory of Parasitology, Faculty of Medicine, Université Libre de Bruxelles, Brussels, Belgium

***Correspondence:**
Ulrike Kemmerling
ukemmerling@uchile.cl
Antonio Osuna
aosuna@ugr.es
Alejandro Gabriel Schijman
schijman@dna.uba.ar
Carine Truyens
ctruyens@ulb.ac.be

Chagas disease (CD), caused by the protozoan parasite *Trypanosoma cruzi*, is considered a neglected tropical disease by the World Health Organization. Congenital transmission of CD is an increasingly relevant public health problem. It progressively becomes the main transmission route over others and can occur in both endemic and non-endemic countries. Though most congenitally infected newborns are asymptomatic at birth, they display higher frequencies of prematurity, low birth weight, and lower Apgar scores compared to uninfected ones, and some suffer from severe symptoms. If not diagnosed and treated, infected newborns are at risk of developing disabling and life-threatening chronic pathologies later in life. The success or failure of congenital transmission depends on interactions between the parasite, the placenta, the mother, and the fetus. We review and discuss here the current knowledge about these parameters, including parasite virulence factors such as exovesicles, placental tropism, potential placental defense mechanisms, the placental transcriptome of infected women, gene polymorphism, and the maternal and fetal/neonatal immune responses, that might modulate the risk of *T. cruzi* congenital transmission.

Keywords: *Trypanosoma cruzi*, infection, maternal-fetal interactions, placenta, congenital chagas disease

CHAGAS DISEASE

Trypanosoma cruzi, a protozoan parasite, is the etiological agent of CD, a neglected tropical disease (WHO, 2015; Lenk et al., 2018) endemic to Latin American countries. Affected countries extend from the United States to Argentina and Chile (Pérez-Molina and Molina, 2018). The parasite is primarily transmitted by insect vectors, but can also be transmitted through blood transfusion, organ transplantation, consumption of parasite-contaminated food, and vertically from mother to child. In Latin America, CD is an important cause of cardiovascular morbidity and premature death (Rassi et al., 2012; WHO, 2015).

The disease evolves in two phases. The acute phase, defined by high parasitemia, lasts 2–3 months. It is often asymptomatic or involves non-specific flu-like symptoms. However, 2–12% of the infected individuals, mostly children under 3 years, die from acute myocardiopathy at times associated with a meningoencephalic compromise (Carlier and Truyens, 2015). The immune response eliminates most but not all parasites. As a consequence, the individual enters the chronic phase and remains infected for the rest of their lives. Although most patients remain asymptomatic for periods ranging in length from several months to decades, 30 - 40% of the infected people develop cardiac (mostly) and/or digestive tract (less frequent) pathologies that may lead to premature death (Rassi et al., 2012; de Oliveira et al., 2018).

CONGENITAL CHAGAS DISEASE

Most women of gestational age are chronically infected, having acquired the infection during infancy. Around 5% of them transmit the parasite to their fetus, and thus approximately 9000 newborns infected with CD in Latin America are born every year. Cases of congenital CD have also been reported outside of the naturally endemic area (WHO, 2015; Antinori et al., 2017). Congenital infection is gaining importance as a route of *T. cruzi* transmission in endemic countries, due to control programs of vectorial and transfusional transmission routes, and is now estimated to account for 22% of new cases (WHO, 2015; Picado et al., 2018). In non-endemic countries, most of the new cases result from congenital transmission (Howard et al., 2014; WHO, 2015). Importantly, since *T. cruzi* maternal-fetal transmission can be repeated at each pregnancy and observed from one generation to another, this way of transmission can easily expand in time (Messenger et al., 2017).

Congenital CD is characteristically an acute parasite infection. Though most (around 60%) congenitally infected newborns are asymptomatic at birth, they display higher frequencies of low birth weight, prematurity, and lower Apgar scores at birth compared to uninfected newborns, while some infected newborns suffer from severe symptoms that can rapidly lead to death (Torrico et al., 2004; Liempi et al., 2016). Moreover, congenitally infected infants are at risk of disabling and life-threatening chronic pathologies later in life (Cardoso et al., 2012; Requena-Méndez et al., 2014; Carlier et al., 2015; Antinori et al., 2017). It is therefore essential to prevent congenital transmission and to rapidly diagnose and treat congenitally infected newborns.

Importantly, the occurrence of congenital transmission depends on interactions between *T. cruzi*, the placenta, the maternal immune system, and the developing fetal/neonatal immune response (Carlier and Truyens, 2015; Liempi et al., 2016). Here we will discuss the factors mentioned above that modulate the risk and probability of *T. cruzi* maternal-fetal transmission.

THE PARASITE DIVERSITY

Trypanosoma cruzi belongs to the Kinetoplastida order, Trypanosomatidae family and presents a complex life cycle involving invertebrate triatomine hosts. Four main cellular forms can be identified during its life cycle: (i) the blood trypomastigote is the infective extracellular non-replicative form of the parasite, which is found in the bloodstream of the mammalian host, (ii) the metacyclic trypomastigote, also non-replicative, is present in the terminal portion of the digestive and urinary tracts of the vectors, (iii) the epimastigote is the replicative extracellular form of the parasite present in the triatomin insect vector, and (iv) the amastigote is the intracellular replicative form of the parasite in the vertebrate host (Rodrigues et al., 2014).

Trypanosoma cruzi is a paradigmatic case of predominantly clonal evolution (Tibayrenc et al., 1986) with "unequivocal evidence of genetic recombination" (Gaunt et al., 2003). Actually, the different known strains and clones of the parasite are classified into seven discrete typing units (DTUs), that are defined as a "sets of stocks that are genetically closer to each other than to any other stock and are identifiable by common molecular, genetic, biochemical, or immunological markers" (Tibayrenc, 1998). The DTUs ranged from *T. cruzi* I to *T. cruzi* VI, and lately, *T. cruzi* bat was also added (Zingales et al., 2012; Lima et al., 2015). Parasites from these DTUs are distributed differentially among insect and mammalian host species and therefore lives in different geographical areas (Zingales et al., 2012; Brenière et al., 2016). All *T. cruzi* parasites, regardless of the DTUs or where they belong, can cause CD. However, epidemiological studies suggest that *T. cruzi* I is associated with anthroponotic as well as sylvatic environments. On the other hand, *T. cruzi* II, V, and VI are mainly related to human environments and particularly chronic CD patients contrarily to *T. cruzi* III and IV which are found to be present in sylvatic habitats (Yeo et al., 2005). An association between DTUs and clinical outcomes is suspected (Messenger et al., 2015). These host and geographic specificities have been proposed to determine the probability of transmission and are related to the pathogenesis of CD. Parasites belonging to diverse DTUs have different biological properties, including growth rates in cultures, tropisms to tissue and organs, antigenicity, capacity to infect potential insect vectors, drug susceptibility, number of chromosomes, and DNA content (Macedo and Pena, 1998; Macedo et al., 2004). Characterization of the gene content and genome architecture of *T. cruzi*, as well as a whole-organism proteomic analysis of its four life cycle stages, has been reported (El-Sayed et al., 2005). Further, comparative genomics of different strains using different sequencing strategies and technologies provide data for the identification of genes associated with host tropism, pathogenicity, and modes of transmission (Berná et al., 2018; Callejas-Hernández et al., 2018; Reis-Cunha et al., 2018).

Whether all *T. cruzi* DTUs can be congenitally transmitted *in utero* is a matter of debate. There is presently no clear evidence that particular *T. cruzi* DTUs, as defined by the currently used molecular markers, would preferentially be transmitted congenitally [reviewed in Carlier and Truyens (2015), Truyens and Carlier (2017)]. We however, recently observed that congenital transmissions in Argentina and Mexico were associated with a maternal portage of "non-TcI" parasites (we did not detect congenital cases harboring TcI DTU) (Buekens et al., 2018). Concordantly, higher congenital transmission rates were reported in Brazilian regions where *T. cruzi* DTU V predominantly circulates as compared to a country where Tc II predominates (Luquetti et al., 2015).

PARASITE TROPISM FOR PLACENTA

Tissue tropism to the placenta of different *T. cruzi* strains has been described previously, particularly in the murine model (Andrade, 1982). *T. cruzi* I (Colombiana strain) parasites present a high incidence of placental parasitism (98%) compared to *T. cruzi* II (Y strain) parasites that only infect 17% of the placentas. The same strains also present differences regarding the localization of the amastigotes in the placenta; only the Colombian strain could be observed consistently in the vascular part of the placenta. In a more recent work, chronic infected mice with two different *T. cruzi* strains, one obtained from a congenital CD patient [VD: Tc VI (Risso et al., 2004)] and the other one previously characterized as non-transmissible in mice [K98,Tc I (Solana et al., 2002)] showed, by means of DNA amplification and 18s ribosomal RNA expression studies, that VD displayed stronger placental tropism and lower parasitic loads in peripheral blood than the K98 strain (Juiz et al., 2017). On the other hand, female mice infected with the K98 strain present higher parasitemia than the ones infected with the RA strain (DTU VI). However, in RA infected females, the infected mice produced parasite-infected newborns, while K98 did not.

We also showed recently in human placental explants (HPE), as well as in a placenta-derived epithelial cell line (BeWo), that VD parasites present a higher infection capacity compared to the Y strain (Medina et al., 2018). These studies suggest that the parasite genotype plays a role in tissue tropism toward the placenta and might contribute to the probability of congenital transmission.

PARASITE EXOVESICLES AS VIRULENCE FACTORS

The persistence of *T. cruzi* parasites at a low level within specific tissues causes chronic pathogenic inflammation in some patients. How *T. cruzi* manages to persist and what factors released by the parasite influence its dynamics in tissue during chronic infection, remains poorly known (Teixeira et al., 2011). Nearly all cells can release extracellular vesicles, or exovesicles (EVs), which have been recognized as a mode of communication between cells. EVs may also participate in pathogenic processes (van Niel et al., 2006; Trocoli Torrecilhas et al., 2009; Cestari et al., 2012; de Pablos Torró et al., 2018). EVs are small membrane vesicles that are classified according to size, biogenesis, and composition, into exosomes and microvesicles (MVs). Exosomes, of 30 to 100 nm in size, are of endocytic origin, have a lipid bilayer, and are released into the extracellular compartment through the fusion of the multivesicular body (MVB) with the plasma membrane of the cell (Raposo and Stoorvogel, 2013). MVs are also referred to as ectosomes; are more heterogeneous in shape; and can vary between 100 and 300 nm in diameter. They are released as a result of the evagination toward the extracellular space from the plasma membrane. EVs differ not only in origin and size but also in lipid and protein composition. They have been identified in all biological fluids (Villagrasa et al., 2014), and their functions include intercellular communication, host-pathogen interactions, as well as the modulation of the immune response against infectious diseases or afflictions such as cancer (Schorey and Bhatnagar, 2008; Webber et al., 2015). We recently published reviews on the existence of EVs in protozoa and parasitic helminths and on the role of *T. cruzi* EVs (Marcilla et al., 2014; de Pablos Torró et al., 2018). Moreover, the induction of physiological modifications in cells by EVs derived from *T. cruzi* trypomastigotes has been recently demonstrated. These alterations involve the blocking of the cell cycle of the host cell, the permeabilization of the cells, and the disorganization of the cytoskeleton, among others (Retana Moreira et al., 2019).

EVs in *T. cruzi* were first described in 1970 (da Silveira et al., 1979) and found to be rich in glycoconjugates. Surface glycoconjugates are formed from glycoproteins (mucins) (de Lederkremer and Colli, 1995; Acosta-Serrano et al., 2001; Buscaglia et al., 2006; Mendonça-Previato et al., 2013), glycolipids (lipopeptidophosphoglycan-LPPG or glycoinosytolphospholipids-GIPL), and glycopeptides (NETNES) (Macrae et al., 2005). Electron microscopy and cryo-fracture have demonstrated that the vesicles come from the plasma membrane of the protozoan and the flagellar pocket. Recently, several surface proteins of the trans-sialidase, the cruzipain and the mucin-associated surface proteins (MASPs) families have been described in EVs, whose activity had previously been related to the modulation of the immune response by means of activating B cells and inducing a Th17 response or processes of adherence and cell invasion (Bermejo et al., 2011, 2013). Interestingly, MASPs are strongly expressed in the parasite and present a high variability between the different strains (Seco-Hidalgo et al., 2015). In recent works, we demonstrated that EVs, circulating in patients with CD, contained immature MASPs, with the presence of the C-proximal and N-terminal regions (peptide signal) (De Pablos et al., 2016; Díaz Lozano et al., 2017). MASPs are linked to the membrane through glycosylphosphatidylinositol (GPI) anchors. GPI participates in the inflammation processes that characterize CD (Almeida and Gazzinelli, 2001). The immature MASPs present in EVs (De Pablos et al., 2016; Díaz Lozano et al., 2017) are recognized by antibodies from CD patients. They help the parasite, in the presence of anti-*T. cruzi* antibodies, to evade the immune response by inhibiting the activity of C3 convertase and thereby impairing complement activation (Cestari et al., 2012). Similarly, the EVs isolated from the sera of CD patients are recognized both by the antibodies of the patients as well as by the serum of mice infected with the parasite. Therefore, it has been proposed that the immature MASPs in the outer side of the membrane of these EVs can form immunocomplexes with the IgGs of the patients (Díaz Lozano et al., 2017). In these studies, we demonstrate the involvement of EVs in the inhibition of the complement pathway, in which the terminal regions C- and N- of the immature MASPs participate. We also show how the antigens of the C- and N- immature regions of these MASPs inhibit the complement by antigen competition, in the presence of antibodies from CD patients. Besides, we identified differences in antigen recognition of the EVs by sera from the patients, depending on the pathology manifested by those affected by CD (De Pablos et al., 2016; Díaz Lozano et al., 2017). These results allowed us to consider *T. cruzi* EVs as markers of pathology, suggesting that they play a role in the pathogeny of CD. Their role in modulating the interactions between the parasite and the placenta and the congenital transmission is under investigation. However, preliminary results show that the parasite increases placenta-derived exosomes in HPE (Castillo et al., 2017a). The placenta is a rich source of exosomes which are related to fetal-placental-maternal communication, fetal allograft survival, and resistance to specific infections, among other functions (Ouyang et al., 2014; Schorey and Harding, 2016). Therefore, it is highly probable that placenta-derived exosomes play essential roles during *T. cruzi*-host interplay.

PLACENTAL RESPONSES TO *T. cruzi*

The placenta is a temporary organ that separates the maternal and fetal compartments throughout pregnancy (Arora et al., 2017). The placenta is responsible for the metabolic exchange between mother and fetus, and fulfills endocrine and immune functions that ensure normal prenatal development of the fetus and pregnancy-related changes in the mother (Liempi et al., 2016; Arora et al., 2017). Mainly due to its regulatory role in the maternal/fetal immune response, this organ is able to protect the fetus against several pathogens (Delorme-Axford et al., 2014; Mor et al., 2017) (see below).

The human placenta is a highly invasive (hemochorial) chorioallantoic placenta. The functional units, where the placental barrier is located, are the free-floating chorionic villi formed by the trophoblast and the villous stroma. Maternal blood surrounds and contacts the trophoblast in the placental intervillous space (IVS). The trophoblast is a bi-stratified covering epithelium composed of a superficial non-proliferative syncytiotrophoblast (ST) and a proliferative germinal layer, the cytotrophoblast (CT). The trophoblast is connected to and separated from the villous stroma (VS), the fetal connective tissue by a basal lamina, a specialized structure of extracellular matrix (ECM) (Benirschke et al., 2012). Therefore, trophoblast, basal *laminae* and VS, the latter containing fetal capillaries, form the placental barrier that must be crossed by *T. cruzi* in order to infect the fetus during trans-placental transmission (**Figure 1**; Duaso et al., 2010; Carlier et al., 2012; Liempi et al., 2016). Of note, *T. cruzi* displays a high tropism for the decidual part of the placenta as compared to the heart, that is likely related to the local immune environment [see further and (Mjihdi et al., 2002)]. Also, in the placenta of mothers of congenitally infected infants, only a few amastigotes can be found in stromal cells such as macrophages, fibroblasts, and giant cells while they are not or scarcely found in the trophoblast, except in case of severe mortal cases of congenital infection (Carlier and Truyens, 2015).

Since the trophoblast is the first placental tissue in contact with the maternal blood, the ST is the first fetal cell layer exposed to the parasite. It has been demonstrated that a high concentration of *T. cruzi* trypomastigotes induces the destruction of the trophoblast in *ex vivo* infected HPE (Duaso et al., 2010). However, low parasite concentration induces cellular proliferation (Liempi et al., 2016; Droguett et al., 2017) and differentiation (Liempi et al., 2014, 2016) in the same placental tissue (see below). The basal *laminae*, located between trophoblast and the fetal connective tissue and around the fetal vessels are other structures that *T. cruzi* needs to overcome (Duaso et al., 2010). *T. cruzi* can bind to ECM molecules such as glycosaminoglycans, fibronectin, and laminin (Lima et al., 2002) using surface molecules such as gp85 (Maeda et al., 2014) and gp83 (Nde et al., 2006). The VS, the placental fetal connective tissue, is also an important obstacle for the parasite. The parasite presents several proteases, among which the cruzipain has been proposed to be responsible for collagen I destruction and disorganization in placentas from mothers with chronic CD or in *ex vivo* infected HPE (Scharfstein and Morrot, 1999; Castillo et al., 2012; Duaso et al., 2012; Maeda et al., 2014). Matrix metalloproteinases (MMPs) such as MMP-2 and MMP-9 are activated, and their expression levels are increased in the presence of the parasite. Interestingly, if these MMPs are inhibited, the parasite-induced damage in the placental tissue is prevented, and the presence of parasite DNA is decreased in *ex vivo* infected HPE (Castillo et al., 2012). Importantly, the ECM forms a complex tridimensional network with different types of elastic fibers and collagen molecules including collagen I fibers, glycoproteins, and proteoglycans (Duaso et al., 2010; Theocharis et al., 2019). Collagen I fibers are the main components of the ECM, and if these molecules are disorganized or destroyed, the 3D network of the ECM is also disrupted, a fact that could facilitate the parasite's motility in the tissue, and its entrance into cells (Duaso et al., 2010). Moreover, *in vitro* studies have shown that during parasite-ECM interactions, the parasite changes its cytoskeletal conformation, the state of protease activation and adapts its metabolism (Mattos et al., 2019). In addition, parasite-induced ECM changes modulate the presence of cytokines and chemokines, allowing *T. cruzi* to manipulate and escape the innate and adaptive immune responses (Marino et al., 2003). Studies performed in CD patients with cardiac alteration have shown that *T. cruzi* derived-antigens promote a differential expression of MMP-2 and MMP-9. There is a positive correlation between MMP-2 and the immunomodulating cytokine IL-10, and a negative one with the pro-inflammatory cytokine IL-1β, whereas MMP-9 showed a negative correlation with IL-10. Therefore, it has been suggested that MMPs and cytokines produced in the myocardium in patients with CD are essential contributors to cardiac remodeling (Medeiros et al., 2017). It would be interesting to study the interactions between parasite-modulated MMPs and cytokines in the placenta.

Another placental response to the parasite is the trophoblast epithelial turnover. The epithelial turnover is part of the innate immune system. Pathogens adhere to the plasma membrane

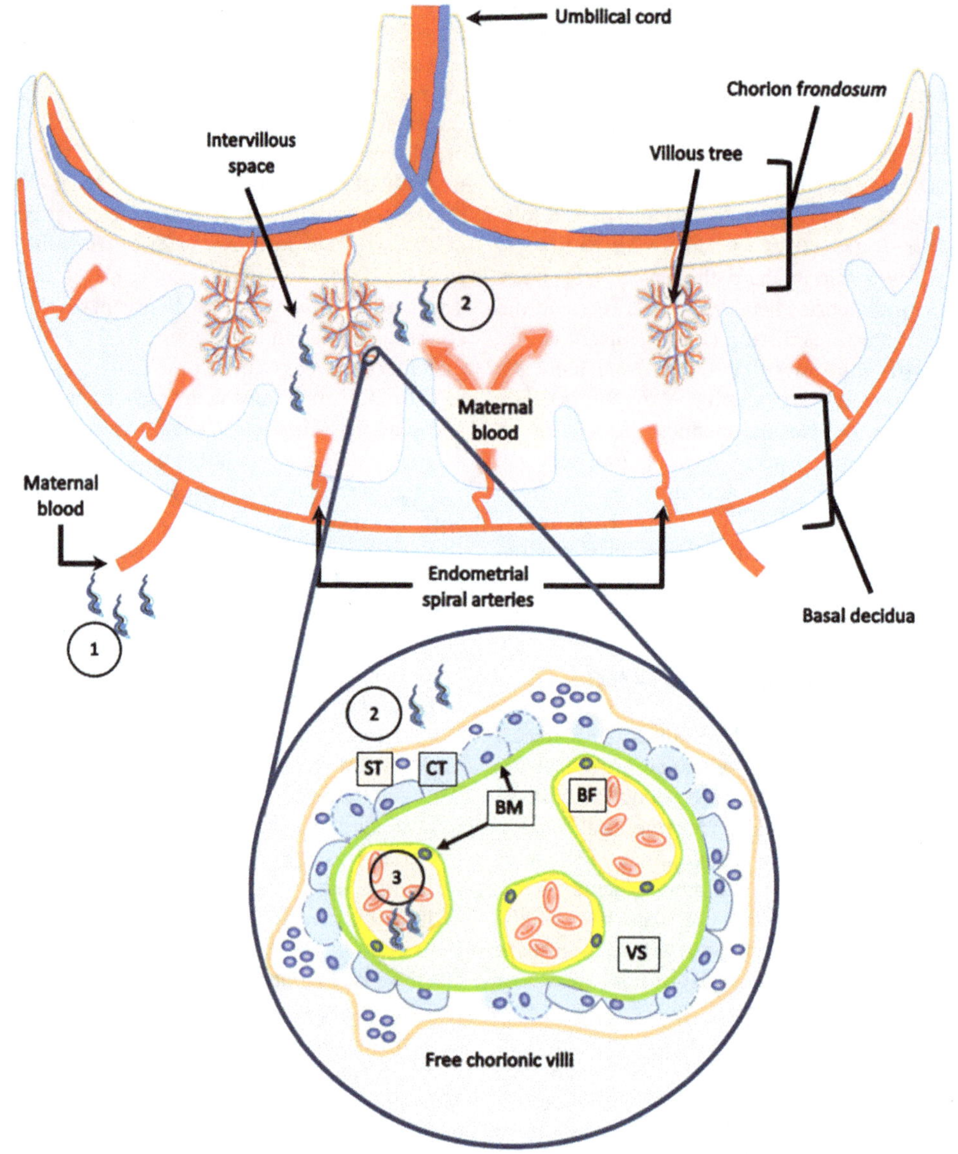

FIGURE 1 | Human placental barrier. The human placenta is classified as a hemochorial chorioallantoic placenta. The placenta is composed of a fetal portion, developed from the chorion frondosum, and a maternal portion, or basal decidua, which originates from the endometrium. The functional units, were the placental barrier is located, are the free-floating chorionic villi formed by the trophoblast, and the villous stroma. Maternal blood surrounds and contacts the trophoblast in the placental intervillous space. The trophoblast is a bi-stratified covering epithelium composed of a superficial non-proliferative syncytiotrophoblast (ST), and a proliferate germinal layer, the cytotrophoblast (CT). The trophoblast is connected to and separated from the villous stroma (VS), the fetal connective tissue, and by a basal lamina. The parasite present in the maternal blood (1), that comes in contact with the trophoblast in the intervillous space (2), must cross the placental barrier in order to reach the fetal capillaries (3), and infect the fetus during transplacental transmission.

before invading host cells and, in case of a lining epithelium, they adhere to the cells of the superficial cell layer which is continuously removed. Therefore, the attached pathogens are removed with the superficial epithelial cells (Liempi et al., 2016).

The trophoblast turnover implies precise orchestration of different cellular processes: (i) cell proliferation of the CT, (ii) cellular differentiation (referring to the incorporation of CT cells into a non-replicative ST), and (iii) cell death by forming apoptotic bodies (knots) in the ST that counterbalance the proliferation of the CT cells. The apoptotic knots are released into the IVS where the maternal blood circulates (Benirschke et al., 2012; Mayhew, 2014; Liempi et al., 2016).

We have previously shown that *T. cruzi* induces the above-mentioned cellular processes related to the epithelial turnover in the trophoblast in both *ex vivo* infected HPE and *in vitro* infected BeWo cells (trophoblastic cell line) (Duaso et al., 2011; Liempi et al., 2014, 2016; Carrillo et al., 2016; Droguett et al., 2017). Thus, *T. cruzi* increases DNA synthesis as well as cellular proliferation markers such as PCNA (proliferating cell nuclear antigen) (Liempi et al., 2016). In BeWo cells, the parasite also increases the percentage of cells in the S and G_2/M cell cycle phases and other commonly used proliferation markers (AgNORs and Ki67) (Droguett et al., 2017). It is noteworthy that PCNA modulates other cellular processes including DNA repair, cell cycle, survival, and gene expression (Wang, 2014), and that an increase of PCNA expression might occur in response to *T. cruzi*-induced damage. Regarding trophoblast differentiation, the parasite increases, in HPE and BeWo cells, the expression and or secretion of the main biochemical markers, including β-human chorionic gonadotropin (β-hCG) and syncytin (Liempi et al., 2014, 2016). Additionally, in BeWo cells *T. cruzi* induces cell fusion as demonstrated by the analysis of the re-distribution of desmoplakin (intercellular adhesion protein) and by a two-color fusion assay (Liempi et al., 2014). The parasite also activates the ERK1/2 MAPK pathway (Castillo et al., 2013b), one of the MAPK signaling pathways that mediate trophoblast differentiation (Forbes and Westwood, 2010). Finally, the parasite induces apoptotic cell death as part of trophoblast turnover (Liempi et al., 2016). Indeed, *T. cruzi* activates in HPE a caspase 3 like activity, followed by DNA fragmentation and pyknosis (Duaso et al., 2011). These data indicate that *T. cruzi* can boost all steps of the turnover of chorionic trophoblasts. Interestingly, a relation exists in trophoblasts between the cellular processes related to apoptosis and their differentiation (Gauster et al., 2009a,b). This is through caspase 8, a caspase operating upstream the pro-apoptotic caspase 3. Caspase 8 is transiently activated in CT cells just before their fusion into ST and is an essential protein in the process of formation of the ST barrier (Huppertz and Borges, 2008). We observed that *T. cruzi* infection increases the expression and activation of caspase 8 in BeWo cells as well as in HPE (Duaso et al., 2011; Carrillo et al., 2016). This fact might favor the integrity of the ST barrier as well as limit parasite entrance into ST (by favoring its turnover). Also, we showed that caspase 8 can slow down intracellular parasite multiplication (Carrillo et al., 2016), pinpointing caspase-8 activity as part of the trophoblast cell defense mechanisms against *T. cruzi* infection. Altogether, these results suggest that the trophoblastic response to *T. cruzi* may be a mechanism that reduces the risk of congenital transmission of the parasite. On the other hand, caspase 8 has recently been disclosed to display pro-inflammatory effects, by optimizing the cytokinic response to TLRs and by being able to activate the cytokine IL-1β (Lawlor et al., 2017). We speculate that such pro-inflammatory action causes placental lesions, favoring the trans-placental passage of *T. cruzi*.

As mentioned above, the placenta is an immune regulatory organ that modulates fetal as well as maternal immune responses (Mor et al., 2017). Pathogens are recognized by pattern recognition receptors (PRRs), including *Toll*-like receptors (TLRs). Activation of those PPRs results in the secretion of cytokines and chemokines aiming to fight infections (Janeway and Medzhitov, 2002). The human trophoblast expresses all ten of the known functional TLRs (Koga et al., 2009). *T. cruzi* is recognized by TLR-2 and TLR-4 (present at the cell surface) as well as the endosomal TLR-7 and TLR-9 (Tarleton, 2007; Gravina et al., 2013; Castillo et al., 2017b). We have shown, in HPE, that *T. cruzi* infection induces protein expression and activation of TLR-2, but not of TLR-4 and TLR-9 (Castillo et al., 2017b). *T. cruzi* induces the secretion of IL-1β, IL-6, IL-8, IL-10, and TNF-α in HPE (Castillo et al., 2017b). Of note is that secretion of IL-1β, IL-6, and TNF-α have been associated, within the trophoblast, with cellular proliferation, and differentiation (Haider and Knöfler, 2009; Hamilton et al., 2012). Interestingly, the inhibition of TLR-2 impairs trophoblast turnover and increases parasite infection (Castillo et al., 2017c). However, to date we do not know if cells other than trophoblasts, such as macrophages in the VS, are also involved in TLR activation. However, our results allow us to propose TLR-2 initiated cytokine profile as a local placental defense mechanism.

TRANSCRIPTOMIC STUDIES IN PLACENTAS IN RESPONSE TO *T. cruzi* INFECTION

The global placental transcriptomic response to *T. cruzi* infection has also been studied. This approach allows us to study the gene expression profiles during infection, allowing the identification of new genes and/or pathways implicated in the establishment of the infection and pathogenesis. The RNA-seq study has been carried out in placentas obtained from term deliveries in *T. cruzi*-infected and non-infected women. Forty-two differentially expressed genes (DEGs) were identified, and gene-set association analysis was performed to detect pathways linked to parasite infection. It showed, not surprisingly, that the inflammatory and the immune responses were upregulated in infected placentas while the anti-inflammatory cytokine IL-38 (formerly IL-1 family member 10-IL1F10) (Garraud et al., 2018) was under-represented (Juiz et al., 2018). Placental inflammation is in line with other reports showing that: (i) newborns of *T. cruzi*-infected mothers are prone to produce higher levels of pro-inflammatory cytokines in comparison to those born to non-infected mothers (Vekemans et al., 2000), (ii) *T. cruzi* infection of pregnant women affects the developing immune system of fetuses independently of congenital infection (Dauby et al., 2009), which might be related to placental inflammation (Jennewein et al., 2017), and (iii) the parasite induces, as mentioned above, in *ex vivo* infected HPE, a highly significant increase of pro-inflammatory and immunomodulatory cytokines (Castillo et al., 2017b,c).

Analysis of DEGs also suggests that the placental inflammation might be counter-regulated in infected mothers. For instance, placentas from infected women displayed lower expression of genes related to exocytosis pathways and neutrophil degranulation, probably limiting damages associated with inflammation. Moreover, the expression of the immunomodulatory HLA-G was increased (Juiz et al., 2018). HLA-G is responsible for the generation of immunological tolerance during gestation by inducing regulatory T cells and tolerogenic dendritic cells (Carosella, 2011; Ferreira et al., 2017) and might increase susceptibility to infections. Hence, in malaria, increased levels of HLA-G in infected mothers are associated with an increased risk to acquire malaria during infancy (Sadissou et al., 2014). S100A14 is another interesting parasite-modulated gene, that is downregulated in placentas from women with CD. This gene codes for a member of the S100 protein family that regulates cell cycle progression, cellular differentiation, and triggers an inflammatory response by engaging the receptor for advanced glycation end products (RAGE) (Jin et al., 2011). Interestingly, this same protein, S100A14, is reported to increase the expression of the collagenase MMP2 (Chen et al., 2012; Qian et al., 2016), which as explained above regulates parasite infection. This might be in line with the observation that mutations on the MMP2 gene favor congenital *T. cruzi* transmission (see hereunder). On the other hand, PRG2 a gene that encodes the precursor form of the eosinophil major basic protein (proMBP) is an upregulated DEG in *T. cruzi*-infected placentas. MBP can participate in the extracellular killing of parasites in the absence of antibodies (Nakhle et al., 2018). Another important function of MBP in the placenta is the inhibition of the pregnancy-associated plasma protein A (PAPPA) (Weyer and Glerup, 2011), whose low levels are associated with intrauterine growth restriction (Albu et al., 2014). Therefore, overexpression of the PAPPA inhibitor in the placenta of women with CD might also play a role in the congenital transmission of *T. cruzi*.

Other, DEGs observed in placentas from seropositive women and related to pregnancy were the genes CGB5 and KISS1, which encode for hCG and kisspeptin, respectively. Both genes were downregulated, and low serum levels of both proteins have been proposed as markers of miscarriage (Jayasena et al., 2014). Low KISS1 expression is associated with recurrent pregnancy loss as well as preeclampsia and intrauterine growth restriction (Armstrong et al., 2009; Park et al., 2012). In contrast, the DEG TAC3 gene [encoding neurokinin B (NKB)] was upregulated in placentas from seropositive women. NKB overexpression in the trophoblast is associated with a decreased blood flow to the placenta and increased vasoconstriction in the endometrium and therefore related to preeclampsia (Familari et al., 2017). Interestingly, NKB and kisspeptin have a role in hCG placental expression in response to estradiol (Oride et al., 2015) and hCG, as described above, is induced by *T. cruzi* in HPE and BeWo cells (Liempi et al., 2014).

A microarray-based transcriptomics study carried out in *ex vivo* infected HPE (Castillo et al., 2018), corroborates most data obtained by RNA-seq in whole placentas (Juiz et al., 2017, 2018) as well as the *T. cruzi*-invasion mechanisms in HPE. Genes that are involved with ECM remodeling are upregulated, in concordance with our previous findings that demonstrate the parasite-induced expression and activation of MMP-2 and MMP-9 (Castillo et al., 2012). The changes in gene expression regarding signal transduction pathways were also confirmed (Castillo et al., 2013b, 2017b). Genes involved in innate immunity were overexpressed, including CD46 and C1q that regulate or form part of the complement system. Upregulation of C1q might have an impact since it binds the *T. cruzi* calreticulin, thereby enhancing the infection (Castillo et al., 2013a). On the other hand, TLR-7 and TLR-8 are mainly increased while TLR-2, whose inhibition favors infection and tissue damage (Castillo et al., 2017c), appeared not to be upregulated in the microarray analysis. Another contradictory observation was that a high *T. cruzi* concentration decreased IL-6 expression more than 60-fold as compared to control non-infected explants, whereas no changes were observed when HPE were infected with a low parasite concentration. On the other hand, mRNA expression analysis showed a higher level of transcription, suggesting that regulation of IL-6 could occur at post-transcriptional stages (Castillo et al., 2017c).

Furthermore, similar to the study in whole placentas, the majority of overexpressed genes were related to fetal development and pregnancy-related processes, particularly *GH2*, *CSH1*, and *CSH2* genes that encode the pregnancy-specific beta-1-glycoproteins growth hormone 2, chorionic somatomammotropin hormone 1 and 2, respectively.

Another microarray-based study was done in placental tissues from C57Bl/6J mice chronically infected with two distinct *T. cruzi* strains (VD and K98, see above) (Juiz et al., 2017) A total of 247 DEGs were identified between infected and non-infected mice: 140 and 107 genes were up- and genes downregulated, respectively, compared to non-infected mice. Placentas infected with the VD parasites showed a higher number of DEGs compared to the K98 infected ones (211 vs. 89 DEGs). There were DEGs common to both infected groups and specific ones for each infected group; while 69% (59/89) of genes were downregulated by K98 infection, VD infection produced this response only in 39% (83/211) of genes. Analysis of DEG networks by GeneMANIA showed that the "Secretory Granule" pathway was downregulated in both infected groups, whereas "Response to Interferon-gamma" as well as "Innate Immune Response" pathways were upregulated only in placental tissues infected with VD. This is interesting since, as said above, the K98 strain displays poor placental tropism and no congenital transmissibility, contrary to the VD strain. It suggests the role of placental inflammation in the process of congenital transmission. Another analysis that detects small changes in predetermined gene sets (Gene-Set Enrichment Analysis algorithm) showed downregulation of genes involved in transcription, macromolecular transport, and metabolism in infected placentas and upregulation of genes regulating signal transduction pathways. Genes regulating apoptotic cell death were downregulated in the murine placentas infected with both parasite strain.

These transcriptomic analyses identify a gene expression profile in the placentas from *T. cruzi*- seropositive mothers that are different from those from seronegative women. It globally shows that affected genes are involved in cell adhesion, cellular proliferation and differentiation, apoptosis, vesicle transport processes, ECM organization, lipid and protein metabolism, and the inflammatory/immune responses.

FAMILY CLUSTERING OF CONGENITAL TRANSMISSION OF *T. cruzi* INFECTION AND SNPs

It is still unknown why some infected mothers transmit the infection in successive gestations to their babies while others do not, leading to family clustering of congenital transmission. A case-control study of single-nucleotide polymorphisms (SNPs) located within human loci encoding different proteins expressed in placental tissues was performed using genomic DNA from clinical samples of 116 non-infected children born to seropositive women and children with congenital *T. cruzi* infection. Logistic regression analysis showed that susceptibility of congenital infection was associated with SNPs in sites rs243866, rs17859821, and rs2285053from MMP2 gene and rs11244787 and rs1871054 sites from the ADAM 12 locus. In case of MMP2 rs243866 and rs17859821 positions, one or both copies of the mutant allele (Adenine) increased the likelihood of congenital infection, whereas, for rs2285053, both T alleles are needed for susceptibility to infection. Mutation in rs2285053 interrupts a CCACC box promoter site (Sp1-type) causing a weaker activity of the promotor. The rs243866 position is located upstream of a half-palindromic potential estrogen receptor binding site (Harendza et al., 2003). Both rs243866 and rs2285053 mutant alleles reduce the transcription activity of MMP2, which in turn modulate the ECM-remodeling and immune responses, and thus the susceptibility to infection. ADAM12 belongs to the ADAM protein family; it is a membrane-bound MMP-protease with a role in cell-cell and cell-matrix interactions that are associated with muscle development, fertilization, neurogenesis inflammatory, and immune responses. In preeclampsia (Grill et al., 2009) and ectopic pregnancy (Rausch and Barnhart, 2012), among other disorders related to pregnancy, ADAM 12 plasmatic concentrations are altered. Also, ADAM 12 promotes the transforming growth factor β (TGF-β) signaling activation leading to transcriptional activation. Importantly, TGF-β activation increases host cell susceptibility to *T. cruzi* infection (Ming et al., 1995; Hall and Pereira, 2000).

Various other SNPs have been related to the susceptibility to *T. cruzi* infection and progression of CD. Particularly, genes encoding cytokines/chemokines involved in inflammatory and immune response have been proposed as biomarkers (Calzada et al., 2009; Torres et al., 2010; Pissetti et al., 2011; Flórez et al., 2012; Nogueira et al., 2015; Furini et al., 2016; Ferreira et al., 2018). Thus, TGF-β1 polymorphism, mainly CT and TT genotypes at position - 509 of the TGFB1 gene have been associated with the susceptibility of acquiring CD in a Brazilian population (Ferreira et al., 2018). The same genotype, in addition to the genotypes −988 C/A; −800 G/A; −10 T/C; and 263 C/T has been studied in the Colombian and Peruvian populations. In this study, the genotype 10 C/C was increased in the group of CD patients of both populations and has been proposed to be involved in differential susceptibility to *T. cruzi* infection (Torres et al., 2010). Another important pro-inflammatory cytokine involved in CD is TNF-α. The TNF- α gene is located in the MHC locus, and its polymorphism is associated with many infectious diseases, including parasitic ones. TNF-α is increased in the hearts of patients with chronic chagasic cardiomyopathy and is associated with tissue damage. An association was observed between the absence of the TNF-238A allele and negative serology for CD. Seropositive individuals carrying the TNF-238A allele produced significantly higher TNF-alpha levels than healthy ones and therefore the TNF-α polymorphism at position −238 has also been associated to the susceptibility to *T. cruzi* infection and CD progression (Pissetti et al., 2011). Other SNPs in genes encoding for cytokines and molecules involved in the immune response has been related to CD, including interferon (IFN)-γ (-874 T/A) (Torres et al., 2010) and IL-18 (rs2043055 polymorphism) (Flórez et al., 2012; Nogueira et al., 2015), RANTES, and chemokine receptors CCR2 and CCR5 (Flórez et al., 2012). It would thus be worthwhile to also investigate such polymorphisms in the context of congenital transmission of *T. cruzi*.

MATERNAL *T. cruzi* SYSTEMIC IMMUNE RESPONSE, GESTATION, AND CONGENITAL INFECTION

The immune system during pregnancy is characterized by a subtle balance between immune tolerance and activation. Regulatory T cells are increased during pregnancy in order to avoid fetal rejection. Indeed, the maternal immune cells recognize paternal antigens expressed by the trophoblast and other fetal cells crossing the placenta to the maternal circulation. The mechanisms leading to this regulatory environment have been largely described elsewhere (Aluvihare et al., 2004; Racicot et al., 2014). Maternal immune tolerance is fundamental to a successful pregnancy. It does, however, not mean that the pregnant women are unable to mount immune responses, and trophoblasts possess multiple ways to escape immune attack (Straszewski-Chavez et al., 2004). Besides, immune responses during gestation are, except for the periods of implantation, placentation, and parturition, physiologically oriented toward a Th2-type. It likely aims to protect the uteroplacental unit and the fetus against harmful inflammation (Mor et al., 2017). Whereas the regulatory and Th2-biased environments are particularly pronounced at the level of the UPU, it may also impact peripheral, and systemic immune responses (Reinhard et al., 1998).

Trypanosoma cruzi infection induces a complex immune response. The control of *T. cruzi* infection relies on diverse effector mechanisms needed to fight both extracellular trypomastigotes and intracellular amastigotes. Therefore, IFN-γ, cytotoxic cells, and antibodies (Abs) all play a role in the control of the infection [reviewed in Truyens and Carlier (2017)]. Antibodies potentially participate in extracellular parasite elimination mainly by inducing complement-dependent and independent lysis of parasites and phagocytosis of opsonized parasites. IFN-γ, initially produced by NK cells, then by both CD4 + Th1 and CD8 + T cells, is a significant player in the immune responses against intracellular pathogens (Kak et al., 2018). It activates among other the microbicidal properties of phagocytes, mainly macrophages, allowing them to limit and/or kill the intracellular parasites. Infected cells can be killed by cytotoxic CD8 + T cells while the cytotoxic action of NK cell on *T. cruzi*-infected cells is likely not significant (Truyens and Carlier, 2017). The cellular response to *T. cruzi* is thus mainly Th1-oriented. Our studies in mice show that this inflammatory immune response has serious harmful effects on gestation when the host is in the acute phase of infection. Indeed, acute infection impedes reproduction, related to either infertility induced by the infection (inhibition of cell division of the embryo before implantation) or fetal loss occurring along gestation, due to massive placental invasion by parasites. Chronic maternal infection does not affect reproductive capacity but induces reversible fetal growth retardation (Carlier et al., 1987). Such deleterious effects did not rely on congenital infection but were associated with increased production of TNF-α (Rivera et al., 1995; Mjihdi et al., 2002). In humans, most women of gestational age have a chronic infection (see above). We have similarly observed that *T. cruzi*-infected women give birth to newborns with low birth weight, in the absence of congenital infection more frequently (Torrico et al., 2004).

Besides, in the absence of congenital transmission, several data indicate bidirectional and opposite interactions between the immune response to *T. cruzi* and the immune environment of gestation. On one side, pregnancy dampens and modifies the immune response to *T. cruzi*. Indeed, we found that blood cells from chronically infected pregnant women released, on average, two to threefold less IFN-γ and IL-2 in response to non-specific lymphocyte stimulants (PHA and LPS) than non-pregnant women (Hermann et al., 2004). They also produced, on average, sevenfold less IL-10. Accordingly, lower levels of IL-10 and IFN-γ were detected in the serum of pregnant infected women than in non-pregnant infected ones (Cardoni et al., 2004). This shows that pregnancy reduces the global capacity of their lymphocytes to be activated (though it is not completely inhibited), likely as a result of the relative immunosuppression associated with gestation. Also, the cytokine profile moved toward a more inflammatory environment in infected pregnant women, since the capacity to produce the inflammatory cytokine IFN-γ was less inhibited during pregnancy than the capacity to produce IL-10 (an anti-inflammatory cytokine), being in line with the inflammatory transcriptome detected in the placenta of *T. cruzi*-infected women [see above (Juiz et al., 2018)]. On the other hand, Egui et al. recently observed in a murine experimental *T. cruzi* infection model that chronic infection reduced the expression of gestation-induced inhibitory receptors on T cells (CTLA4 on CD4 + and CD8 + T cells and CD160 on CD8 + T cells), suggesting that *T. cruzi* chronic infection counteracts the immunosuppression associated with gestation but does not impact the gestation outcome (Egui et al., 2017).

Our previous studies in pregnant chronically infected women showed that gestation also reduced the specific IFN-γ response to parasite antigens as compared to the response of non-pregnant infected ones (Hermann et al., 2004). This was the case for women that transmitted (T mothers) as well as those that did not transmit (NT mothers) the parasite to their fetus. Strikingly, this specific IFN-γ response was markedly lower in T than NT mothers and was associated with less activated monocytes (Hermann et al., 2004). On the other hand, we and others have reported that the circulating parasite load is slightly increased during the second and third trimester of pregnancy (Brutus et al., 2010; Siriano et al., 2011). Moreover, T mothers displayed higher parasitemia than NT ones (Hermann et al., 2004; Kaplinski et al., 2015). IFN-γ is well known as a key factor in the control of *T. cruzi* infection (Truyens and Carlier, 2017). These data strongly suggest that the increase of parasite burden in T mothers results from a reduced control of the infection and points to a central role of parasite burden as a risk factor of congenital transmission. In line with this, several studies underline that congenital transmission occurs mostly in mothers displaying blood parasites amounts that are detectable by PCR (i.e., PCRs are generally negative in NT mothers). The microbial burden is also a key factor of congenital transmission of other pathogens (Lilleri and Gerna, 2017).

The increase of parasite burden during gestation likely results from the relative immunosuppression associated with gestation, while the increased parasite load in T mothers probably relates to their more depressed IFN-γ response. The question is, thus, why T mothers display such feature? Several factors may be considered, concerning the parasite, the host, or epidemiological parameters. Living in endemic countries where vectorial transmission occurs may lead to frequent reinfections. Multiple infections, though leading to transiently increased parasite levels, result in lower parasitemia in the long term, the hypothesis being that repeated antigen exposure reinforces the Th1 response that controls the parasite (Machado et al., 2001; Bustamante et al., 2007; Kaplinski et al., 2015). In line with this, it was observed that higher vector exposure of women living in endemic countries decreases the risk of congenital transmission (Sánchez Negrette et al., 2005; Kaplinski et al., 2015). Congenital transmission rates are also lower in non-endemic countries (2.7%), free of vectorial reinfections, than in endemic countries [2.7% vs. 5%, respectively (Howard et al., 2014)]. Parasite load may also vary according to the parasite genotype/strain (Moreira et al., 2013).

Our data also suggest that host factors modulate the risk of congenital transmission of *T. cruzi*. Genetic and epigenetic factors may influence the efficacy of immune responses against pathogens and consequently modulate the microbial load (Möller et al., 2018). For instance, polymorphism of genes encoding proteins of the axis IL-12-IFN-γ and genetic variations affecting the modulatory action of long non-coding RNAs or micro-RNAs are reported to impact diseases (Vannberg et al., 2011; Duval et al., 2017; Gao and Wei, 2017; Ellwanger et al., 2018). We compared the ability of T and NT women to produce IFN-γ to *T. cruzi* and mitogens several months after they had given birth, i.e., in the absence of the immunosuppression of pregnancy (Hermann et al., 2004). We found that T women still displayed a more depressed ability to produce this cytokine than NT women, suggesting that inherent host factors involved might be genetic. Likewise, we have recently reported that several genes related to the immune system were differentially expressed in the placenta of T and NT mothers as well as an association between congenital *T. cruzi* transmission and the presence of polymorphism among some gene expressed in the placenta (see above) (Juiz et al., 2016, 2018). Of note, differential immune responses associated with the congenital transmission of other pathogens have also been recently reported (Lilleri and Gerna, 2017; Wujcicka et al., 2018). Besides, epigenetic modulation may also have occurred in some women in relation either with the *T. cruzi* strains present in the host or to their history of infections with other pathogens (Gomez et al., 2013; Smith and Denning, 2014).

Finally, we and others noticed that T mothers were younger and had a lower mean number of previous pregnancies than the NT mothers (Hermann et al., 2004; Kaplinski et al., 2015), which might be related to the immuno-enhancing effect of multiparity on the maternal immune system (Skowron-Cendrzak et al., 1999).

NEONATAL IMMUNE RESPONSE TO *T. cruzi*

Immune responses in early life are physiologically different from adult responses. Similarly, to what occurs during pregnancy, the neonatal immune system is characterized by a certain degree of immunodeficiency and weak Th1 but excessive Th2 responses, contributing to high susceptibility to pathogens and the development of suboptimal immune responses to vaccines administered in early life. However, the mechanisms leading to immunodeficiency and Th2 bias are completely different from those activated during pregnancy and have been reviewed elsewhere (Levy, 2007; PrabhuDas et al., 2011; Elahi et al., 2013). Mechanisms responsible for the regulatory environment comprises, among others, impaired signaling pathways downstream of *Toll-like* receptors 3 and 4, the presence of higher circulating levels of adenosine, the presence of higher numbers of regulatory T cells, and the presence of particular inhibitory "erythroid cells." The Th2 bias results from the hypermethylation of the *IFNG* gene, while the Th2 locus is hypomethylated. Also, the proliferation of Th1 T cells in early life is strongly hindered due to the expression of a particular receptor for IL-4 produced by Th2 T cells. Engagement of this receptor induces apoptosis of Th1 cells.

Our studies in humans, performed in infants from chagasic mothers, point out that *T. cruzi* infection triggers neonatal type 1 immune responses, overcoming the physiological immune deficiency associated with early life (Hermann et al., 2002). Indeed, CD8 + T cells, and CD4 + T cells to a lesser extent, were activated in *T. cruzi* congenitally infected new-borns to an adult-like level and produced IFN-γ. Besides, their NK cells display phenotypic and functional alterations suggestive of a previous *in utero* activation when parasites were transmitted from the mother (Hermann et al., 2006). It also pinpoints the imprinting of the maternal *T. cruzi* infection on the neonatal immune system, revealing an immuno-stimulatory/adjuvant property of the parasite, as both congenitally infected and uninfected infants from chagasic mothers responded more strongly to vaccines directly administered during the first 6 months of life, like those against BCG, hepatitis B, tetanus, and diphtheria (Dauby et al., 2009). In trying to decipher the mechanisms allowing the parasite to induce type 1 immune responses in early life, we showed that the parasite could strongly activate neonatal NK cells to produce IFN-γ, known to drive Th1 type responses rapidly. NK cell activation by *T. cruzi* is indirect and depends on cross-talk with monocytes (and not with dendritic cells), on IL-12 synthesis and engagement of TLR2, 4, 7, and 9 (Guilmot et al., 2013). The parasite also very efficiently licensed neonatal dendritic cells to activate CD4 + and CD8 + T cells. Interestingly, DC and monocyte activation by *T. cruzi* is reinforced in the presence of maternal IgG isolated from cord blood samples from neonates born to NT infected mothers, i.e., carrying *T. cruzi*-specific IgG (Rodriguez et al., 2012). These observations allow us to make the hypothesis that monocytes, likely activated in fetuses from infected mothers combined with the maternally transmitted *T. cruzi* - specific antibodies might allow the fetus to fight parasites and maybe in some cases to eliminate them if only a few parasites were transmitted.

FINAL REMARKS

Some relevant questions regarding the role of parasite diversity, host genetic response, and host immune responses deserve further investigations. The study of gene expression profiles during infection constitutes a powerful tool to analyze global responses of several kinds of cells and tissues, allowing the identification of new genes and/or pathways implicated in the establishment of the infection and pathogenesis as well as possible local tissue responses. Other aspects such as the role of maternal microbiomes in the likelihood of vertical transmission of *T. cruzi* have not been investigated yet.

AUTHOR CONTRIBUTIONS

All authors listed have made a substantial, direct and intellectual contribution to the work, and approved it for publication.

REFERENCES

Acosta-Serrano, A., Almeida, I. C., Freitas-Junior, L. H., Yoshida, N., and Schenkman, S. (2001). The mucin-like glycoprotein super-family of *Trypanosoma cruzi*: structure and biological roles. *Mol. Biochem. Parasitol.* 114, 143–150. doi: 10.1016/s0166-6851(01)00245-6

Albu, A. R., Anca, A. F., Horhoianu, V. V., and Horhoianu, I. A. (2014). Predictive factors for intrauterine growth restriction. *J. Med. Life* 7, 165–171.

Almeida, I. C., and Gazzinelli, R. T. (2001). Proinflammatory activity of glycosylphosphatidylinositol anchors derived from *Trypanosoma cruzi*: structural and functional analyses. *J. Leukoc. Biol.* 70, 467–477.

Aluvihare, V. R., Kallikourdis, M., and Betz, A. G. (2004). Regulatory T cells mediate maternal tolerance to the fetus. *Nat. Immunol.* 5, 266–271. doi: 10.1038/ni1037

Andrade, S. G. (1982). The influence of the strain of *Trypanosoma cruzi* in placental infections in mice. *Trans. R. Soc. Trop. Med. Hyg.* 76, 123–128. doi: 10.1016/0035-9203(82)90036-0

Antinori, S., Galimberti, L., Bianco, R., Grande, R., Galli, M., and Corbellino, M. (2017). Chagas disease in Europe: a review for the internist in the globalized world. *Eur. J. Intern. Med.* 43, 6–15. doi: 10.1016/j.ejim.2017.05.001

Armstrong, R. A., Reynolds, R. M., Leask, R., Shearing, C. H., Calder, A. A., and Riley, S. C. (2009). Decreased serum levels of kisspeptin in early pregnancy are associated with intra-uterine growth restriction and pre-eclampsia. *Prenat. Diagn.* 29, 982–985. doi: 10.1002/pd.2328

Arora, N., Sadovsky, Y., Dermody, T. S., and Coyne, C. B. (2017). Microbial vertical transmission during human pregnancy. *Cell Host Microbe* 21, 561–567. doi: 10.1016/j.chom.2017.04.007

Benirschke, K., Kaufmann, P., and Baergen, P. (2012). *Pathology of the Human Placenta*, 6 th Edn. New York, NY: Springer Link.

Bermejo, D. A., Amezcua Vesely, M. C., Khan, M., Acosta Rodríguez, E. V., Montes, C. L., Merino, M. C., et al. (2011). *Trypanosoma cruzi* infection induces a massive extrafollicular and follicular splenic B-cell response which is a high source of non-parasite-specific antibodies. *Immunology* 132, 123–133. doi: 10.1111/j.1365-2567.2010.03347.x

Bermejo, D. A., Jackson, S. W., Gorosito-Serran, M., Acosta-Rodriguez, E. V., Amezcua-Vesely, M. C., Sather, B. D., et al. (2013). Trypanosoma cruzi trans-sialidase initiates a program independent of the transcription factors RORγt and Ahr that leads to IL-17 production by activated B cells. *Nat. Immunol.* 14, 514–522. doi: 10.1038/ni.2569

Berná, L., Rodriguez, M., Chiribao, M. L., Parodi-Talice, A., Pita, S., Rijo, G., et al. (2018). Expanding an expanded genome: long-read sequencing of *Trypanosoma cruzi*. *Microb. Genomics* 4:e000177. doi: 10.1099/mgen.0.000177

Brenière, S. F., Waleckx, E., and Barnabé, C. (2016). Over six thousand *Trypanosoma cruzi* strains classified into discrete typing units (DTUs): attempt at an inventory. *PLoS Negl. Trop. Dis.* 10:e0004792. doi: 10.1371/journal.pntd.0004792

Brutus, L., Castillo, H., Bernal, C., Salas, N. A., Schneider, D., Santalla, J.-A., et al. (2010). Detectable *Trypanosoma cruzi* parasitemia during pregnancy and delivery as a risk factor for congenital Chagas disease. *Am. J. Trop. Med. Hyg.* 83, 1044–1047. doi: 10.4269/ajtmh.2010.10-0326

Buekens, P., Cafferata, M. L., Alger, J., Althabe, F., Belizán, J. M., Bustamante, N., et al. (2018). Congenital transmission of *Trypanosoma cruzi* in Argentina, Honduras, and Mexico: an observational prospective study. *Am. J. Trop. Med. Hyg.* 98, 478–485. doi: 10.4269/ajtmh.17-0516

Buscaglia, C. A., Campo, V. A., Frasch, A. C. C., and Di Noia, J. M. (2006). *Trypanosoma cruzi* surface mucins: host-dependent coat diversity. *Nat. Rev. Microbiol.* 4, 229–236. doi: 10.1038/nrmicro1351

Bustamante, J. M., Novarese, M., Rivarola, H. W., Lo Presti, M. S., Fernández, A. R., Enders, J. E., et al. (2007). Reinfections and *Trypanosoma cruzi* strains can determine the prognosis of the chronic chagasic cardiopathy in mice. *Parasitol. Res.* 100, 1407–1410. doi: 10.1007/s00436-006-0425-3

Callejas-Hernández, F., Rastrojo, A., Poveda, C., Gironès, N., and Fresno, M. (2018). Genomic assemblies of newly sequenced *Trypanosoma cruzi* strains reveal new genomic expansion and greater complexity. *Sci. Rep.* 8:14631. doi: 10.1038/s41598-018-32877-2

Calzada, J. E., Beraún, Y., González, C. I., and Martín, J. (2009). Transforming growth factor beta 1 (TGFβ1) gene polymorphisms and Chagas disease susceptibility in Peruvian and Colombian patients. *Cytokine* 45, 149–153. doi: 10.1016/j.cyto.2008.11.013

Cardoni, R. L., García, M. M., and De Rissio, A. M. (2004). Proinflammatory and anti-inflammatory cytokines in pregnant women chronically infected with Trypanosoma cruzi. *Acta Trop.* 90, 65–72. doi: 10.1016/j.actatropica.2003.09.020

Cardoso, E. J., Valdéz, G. C., Campos, A. C., Sanchez, R., de la, L., Mendoza, C. R., et al. (2012). Maternal fetal transmission of *Trypanosoma cruzi*: a problem of public health little studied in Mexico. *Exp. Parasitol.* 131, 425–432. doi: 10.1016/j.exppara.2012.05.013

Carlier, Y., Rivera, M. T., Truyens, C., Puissant, F., and Milaire, J. (1987). Interactions between chronic murine *Trypanosoma cruzi* infection and pregnancy: fetal growth retardation. *Am. J. Trop. Med. Hyg.* 37, 534–540. doi: 10.4269/ajtmh.1987.37.534

Carlier, Y., Sosa-Estani, S., Luquetti, A. O., and Buekens, P. (2015). Congenital Chagas disease: an update. *Mem. Inst. Oswaldo Cruz* 110, 363–368. doi: 10.1590/0074-02760140405

Carlier, Y., and Truyens, C. (2015). Congenital Chagas disease as an ecological model of interactions between *Trypanosoma cruzi* parasites, pregnant women, placenta and fetuses. *Acta Trop.* 151, 103–115. doi: 10.1016/j.actatropica.2015.07.016

Carlier, Y., Truyens, C., Deloron, P., and Peyron, F. (2012). Congenital parasitic infections: a review. *Acta Trop.* 121, 55–70. doi: 10.1016/j.actatropica.2011.10.018

Carosella, E. D. (2011). The tolerogenic molecule HLA-G. *Immunol. Lett.* 138, 22–24. doi: 10.1016/j.imlet.2011.02.011

Carrillo, I., Droguett, D., Castillo, C., Liempi, A., Muñoz, L., Maya, J. D., et al. (2016). Caspase-8 activity is part of the BeWo trophoblast cell defense mechanisms against *Trypanosoma cruzi* infection. *Exp. Parasitol.* 168, 9–15. doi: 10.1016/j.exppara.2016.06.008

Castillo, C., Carrillo, I., Libisch, G., Juiz, N., Schijman, A. G., Robello, C., et al. (2018). Host-parasite interaction: changes in human placental gene expression induced by Trypanosoma cruzi. *Parasit. Vectors* 11, 1–13. doi: 10.1186/s13071-018-2988-0

Castillo, C., Carrillo, I., Liempi, A., Medina, L., Navarrete, A., López, P., et al. (2017a). *Trypanosoma cruzi* exosomes increases susceptibility to parasite infection in human placental chorionic villi explants. *Placenta* 51, 123–124. doi: 10.1016/J.PLACENTA.2017.01.086

Castillo, C., Muñoz, L., Carrillo, I., Liempi, A., Gallardo, C., Galanti, N., et al. (2017b). Ex vivo infection of human placental chorionic villi explants with *Trypanosoma cruzi* and *Toxoplasma gondii* induces different Toll-like receptor expression and cytokine/chemokine profiles. *Am. J. Reprod. Immunol.* 78, 1–8. doi: 10.1111/aji.12660

Castillo, C., Muñoz, L., Carrillo, I., Liempi, A., Medina, L., Galanti, N., et al. (2017c). Toll-like receptor-2 mediates local innate immune response against *Trypanosoma cruzi* in ex vivo infected human placental chorionic villi explants. *Placenta* 60, 40–46. doi: 10.1016/j.placenta.2017.10.005

Castillo, C., López-Muñoz, R. A., Duaso, J., Galanti, N., Jaña, F., Ferreira, J., et al. (2012). Role of matrix metalloproteinases 2 and 9 in ex vivo *Trypanosoma cruzi* infection of human placental chorionic villi. *Placenta* 33, 991–997. doi: 10.1016/j.placenta.2012.10.004

Castillo, C., Ramírez, G., Valck, C., Aguilar, L., Maldonado, I., Rosas, C., et al. (2013a). The interaction of classical complement component C1 with parasite and host calreticulin mediates *Trypanosoma cruzi* infection of human placenta. *PLoS Negl. Trop. Dis.* 7:e2376. doi: 10.1371/journal.pntd.0002376

Castillo, C., Villarroel, A., Duaso, J., Galanti, N., Cabrera, G., Maya, J. D. J. D., et al. (2013b). Phospholipase C gamma and ERK1/2 Mitogen Activated Kinase Pathways are differentially modulated by *Trypanosoma cruzi* during tissue invasion in human placenta. *Exp. Parasitol.* 133, 12–17. doi: 10.1016/j.exppara.2012.10.012

Cestari, I., Ansa-Addo, E., Deolindo, P., Inal, J. M., and Ramirez, M. I. (2012). *Trypanosoma cruzi* immune evasion mediated by host cell-derived microvesicles. *J. Immunol.* 188, 1942–1952. doi: 10.4049/jimmunol.1102053

Chen, H., Yuan, Y., Zhang, C., Luo, A., Ding, F., Ma, J., et al. (2012). Involvement of S100A14 protein in cell invasion by affecting expression and function of matrix metalloproteinase (MMP)-2 via p53-dependent transcriptional regulation. *J. Biol. Chem.* 287, 17109–17119. doi: 10.1074/jbc.M111.326975

da Silveira, J. F., Abrahamsohn, P. A., and Colli, W. (1979). Plasma membrane vesicles isolated from epimastigote forms of *Trypanosoma cruzi*. *Biochim. Biophys. Acta* 550, 222–232. doi: 10.1016/0005-2736(79)90209-8

Dauby, N., Alonso-Vega, C., Suarez, E., Flores, A., Hermann, E., Córdova, M., et al. (2009). Maternal infection with *Trypanosoma cruzi* and congenital Chagas disease induce a trend to a type 1 polarization of infant immune responses to vaccines. *PLoS Negl. Trop. Dis.* 3:e571. doi: 10.1371/journal.pntd.0000571

de Lederkremer, R. M., and Colli, W. (1995). Galactofuranose-containing glycoconjugates in trypanosomatids. *Glycobiology* 5, 547–552. doi: 10.1093/glycob/5.6.547

de Oliveira, A. B. B., Alevi, K. C. C., Imperador, C. H. L., Madeira, F. F., and de Azeredo-Oliveira, M. T. V. (2018). Parasite-vector interaction of chagas disease: a mini-review. *Am. J. Trop. Med. Hyg.* 98, 653–655. doi: 10.4269/ajtmh.17-0657

De Pablos, L. M., Díaz Lozano, I. M., Jercic, M. I., Quinzada, M., Giménez, M. J., Calabuig, E., et al. (2016). The C-terminal region of *Trypanosoma cruzi* MASPs is antigenic and secreted via exovesicles. *Sci. Rep.* 6:27293. doi: 10.1038/srep27293

de Pablos Torró, L. M., Retana Moreira, L., and Osuna, A. (2018). Extracellular vesicles in Chagas disease: a new passenger for an old disease. *Front. Microbiol.* 9:1190. doi: 10.3389/fmicb.2018.01190

Delorme-Axford, E., Sadovsky, Y., and Coyne, C. B. (2014). The placenta as a barrier to viral infections. *Annu. Rev. Virol.* 1, 133–146. doi: 10.1146/annurev-virology-031413-085524

Díaz Lozano, I. M., De Pablos, L. M., Longhi, S. A., Zago, M. P., Schijman, A. G., and Osuna, A. (2017). Immune complexes in chronic Chagas disease patients are formed by exovesicles from *Trypanosoma cruzi* carrying the conserved MASP N-terminal region. *Sci. Rep.* 7:44451. doi: 10.1038/srep44451

Droguett, D., Carrillo, I., Castillo, C., Gómez, F., Negrete, M., Liempi, A., et al. (2017). *Trypanosoma cruzi* induces cellular proliferation in the trophoblastic cell line BeWo. *Exp. Parasitol.* 173, 9–17. doi: 10.1016/j.exppara.2016.12.005

Duaso, J., Rojo, G., Cabrera, G., Galanti, N., Bosco, C., Maya, J. D. J. D., et al. (2010). Trypanosoma cruzi induces tissue disorganization and destruction of chorionic villi in an ex vivo infection model of human placenta. *Placenta* 31, 705–711. doi: 10.1016/j.placenta.2010.05.007

Duaso, J., Rojo, G., Jaña, F., Galanti, N., Cabrera, G., Bosco, C., et al. (2011). Trypanosoma cruzi induces apoptosis in ex vivo infected human chorionic villi. *Placenta* 32, 356–361. doi: 10.1016/j.placenta.2011.02.005

Duaso, J., Yanez, E., Castillo, C., Galanti, N., Cabrera, G., Corral, G., et al. (2012). Reorganization of extracellular matrix in placentas from women with asymptomatic chagas disease: mechanism of parasite invasion or local placental defense? *J. Trop. Med.* 2012:758357. doi: 10.1155/2012/758357

Duval, M., Cossart, P., and Lebreton, A. (2017). Mammalian microRNAs and long noncoding RNAs in the host-bacterial pathogen crosstalk. *Semin. Cell Dev. Biol.* 65, 11–19. doi: 10.1016/j.semcdb.2016.06.016

Egui, A., Lasso, P., Thomas, M. C., Carrilero, B., González, J. M., Cuéllar, A., et al. (2017). Expression of inhibitory receptors and polyfunctional responses of T cells are linked to the risk of congenital transmission of *T. cruzi*. *PLoS Negl. Trop. Dis.* 11:e0005627. doi: 10.1371/journal.pntd.0005627

Elahi, S., Ertelt, J. M., Kinder, J. M., Jiang, T. T., Zhang, X., Xin, L., et al. (2013). Immunosuppressive CD71+ erythroid cells compromise neonatal host defence against infection. *Nature* 504, 158–162. doi: 10.1038/nature12675

Ellwanger, J. H., Zambra, F. M. B., Guimarães, R. L., and Chies, J. A. B. (2018). MicroRNA-related polymorphisms in infectious diseases-tiny changes with a huge impact on viral infections and potential clinical applications. *Front. Immunol.* 9:1316. doi: 10.3389/fimmu.2018.01316

El-Sayed, N. M., Myler, P. J., Bartholomeu, D. C., Nilsson, D., Aggarwal, G., Tran, A.-N., et al. (2005). The genome sequence of *Trypanosoma cruzi*, etiologic agent of Chagas disease. *Science* 309, 409–415. doi: 10.1126/science.1112631

Familari, M., Cronqvist, T., Masoumi, Z., and Hansson, S. R. (2017). Placenta-derived extracellular vesicles: their cargo and possible functions. *Reprod. Fertil. Dev.* 29, 433–447. doi: 10.1071/RD15143

Ferreira, L. M. R., Meissner, T. B., Tilburgs, T., and Strominger, J. L. (2017). HLA-G: at the interface of maternal–fetal tolerance. *Trends Immunol.* 38, 272–286. doi: 10.1016/j.it.2017.01.009

Ferreira, R. R., Madeira, F., da, S., Alves, G. F., Chambela, M., da, C., et al. (2018). TGF- β polymorphisms are a risk factor for Chagas disease. *Dis. Markers* 2018, 1–10. doi: 10.1155/2018/4579198

Flórez, O., Martín, J., and González, C. I. (2012). Genetic variants in the chemokines and chemokine receptors in Chagas disease. *Hum. Immunol.* 73, 852–858. doi: 10.1016/j.humimm.2012.04.005

Forbes, K., and Westwood, M. (2010). Maternal growth factor regulation of human placental development and fetal growth. *J. Endocrinol.* 207, 1–16. doi: 10.1677/JOE-10-0174

Furini, A. A., da, C., Cassiano, G. C., Petrolini Capobianco, M., Dos Santos, S. E. B., and Dantas Machado, R. L. (2016). Frequency of TNFA, INFG, and IL10 gene polymorphisms and their association with malaria vivax and genomic ancestry. *Mediat. Inflamm.* 2016:5168363. doi: 10.1155/2016/5168363

Gao, P., and Wei, G.-H. (2017). Genomic insight into the role of lncRNA in cancer susceptibility. *Int. J. Mol. Sci.* 18:E1239. doi: 10.3390/ijms18061239

Garraud, T., Harel, M., Boutet, M.-A., Le Goff, B., and Blanchard, F. (2018). The enigmatic role of IL-38 in inflammatory diseases. *Cytokine Growth Factor Rev.* 39, 26–35. doi: 10.1016/j.cytogfr.2018.01.001

Gaunt, M. W., Yeo, M., Frame, I. A., Stothard, J. R., Carrasco, H. J., Taylor, M. C., et al. (2003). Mechanism of genetic exchange in American trypanosomes. *Nature* 421, 936–939. doi: 10.1038/nature01438

Gauster, M., Moser, G., Orendi, K., and Huppertz, B. (2009a). Factors involved in regulating trophoblast fusion: potential role in the development of preeclampsia. *Placenta* 30(Suppl. A), S49–S54. doi: 10.1016/j.placenta.2008.10.011

Gauster, M., Siwetz, M., and Huppertz, B. (2009b). Fusion of villous trophoblast can be visualized by localizing active caspase 8. *Placenta* 30, 547–550. doi: 10.1016/j.placenta.2009.03.007

Gomez, J. A., Wapinski, O. L., Yang, Y. W., Bureau, J.-F., Gopinath, S., Monack, D. M., et al. (2013). The NeST long ncRNA controls microbial susceptibility and epigenetic activation of the interferon-γ locus. *Cell* 152, 743–754. doi: 10.1016/j.cell.2013.01.015

Gravina, H. D., Antonelli, L., Gazzinelli, R. T., and Ropert, C. (2013). Differential use of TLR2 and TLR9 in the regulation of immune responses during the infection with *Trypanosoma cruzi*. *PLoS One* 8:e63100. doi: 10.1371/journal.pone.0063100

Grill, S., Rusterholz, C., Zanetti-Dällenbach, R., Tercanli, S., Holzgreve, W., Hahn, S., et al. (2009). Potential markers of preeclampsia – a review. *Reprod. Biol. Endocrinol.* 7:70. doi: 10.1186/1477-7827-7-70

Guilmot, A., Bosse, J., Carlier, Y., and Truyens, C. (2013). Monocytes play an IL-12-dependent crucial role in driving cord blood NK cells to produce IFN-g in response to *Trypanosoma cruzi*. *PLoS Negl. Trop. Dis.* 7:e2291. doi: 10.1371/journal.pntd.0002291

Haider, S., and Knöfler, M. (2009). Human tumour necrosis factor: physiological and pathological roles in placenta and endometrium. *Placenta* 30, 111–123. doi: 10.1016/j.placenta.2008.10.012

Hall, B. S., and Pereira, M. A. (2000). Dual role for transforming growth factor beta-dependent signaling in *Trypanosoma cruzi* infection of mammalian cells. *Infect. Immun.* 68, 2077–2081. doi: 10.1128/iai.68.4.2077-2081.2000

Hamilton, S. T., Scott, G., Naing, Z., Iwasenko, J., Hall, B., Graf, N., et al. (2012). Human cytomegalovirus-induces cytokine changes in the placenta with implications for adverse pregnancy outcomes. *PLoS One* 7:e52899. doi: 10.1371/journal.pone.0052899

Harendza, S., Lovett, D. H., Panzer, U., Lukacs, Z., Kuhnl, P., and Stahl, R. A. K. (2003). Linked common polymorphisms in the gelatinase a promoter are associated with diminished transcriptional response to estrogen and genetic fitness. *J. Biol. Chem.* 278, 20490–20499. doi: 10.1074/jbc.M211536200

Hermann, E., Alonso-Vega, C., Berthe, A., Truyens, C., Flores, A., Cordova, M., et al. (2006). Human congenital infection with *Trypanosoma cruzi* induces phenotypic and functional modifications of cord blood NK cells. *Pediatr. Res.* 60, 38–43. doi: 10.1203/01.pdr.0000220335.05588.ea

Hermann, E., Truyens, C., Alonso-Vega, C., Even, J., Rodriguez, P., Berthe, A., et al. (2002). Human fetuses are able to mount an adultlike CD8 T-cell response. *Blood* 100, 2153–2158.

Hermann, E., Truyens, C., Alonso-Vega, C., Rodriguez, P., Berthe, A., Torrico, F., et al. (2004). Congenital transmission of *Trypanosoma cruzi* is associated with maternal enhanced parasitemia and decreased production of interferon-gamma in response to parasite antigens. *J. Infect. Dis.* 189, 1274–1281. doi: 10.1086/382511

Howard, E., Xiong, X., Carlier, Y., Sosa-Estani, S., and Buekens, P. (2014). Frequency of the congenital transmission of *Trypanosoma cruzi*: a systematic review and meta-analysis. *BJOG* 121, 22–33. doi: 10.1111/1471-0528.12396

Huppertz, B., and Borges, M. (2008). "Placenta trophoblast fusion," in *Methods in molecular biology*, ed. E. H. Chen (Totowa, NJ: Humana press), 135–147. doi: 10.1007/978-1-59745-250-2_8

Janeway, C. A., and Medzhitov, R. (2002). Innate immune recognition. *Annu. Rev. Immunol.* 20, 197–216. doi: 10.1146/annurev.immunol.20.083001.084359

Jayasena, C. N., Abbara, A., Izzi-Engbeaya, C., Comninos, A. N., Harvey, R. A., Gonzalez Maffe, J., et al. (2014). Reduced levels of plasma Kisspeptin during the antenatal booking visit are associated with increased risk of miscarriage. *J. Clin. Endocrinol. Metab.* 99, E2652–E2660. doi: 10.1210/jc.2014-1953

Jennewein, M. F., Abu-Raya, B., Jiang, Y., Alter, G., and Marchant, A. (2017). Transfer of maternal immunity and programming of the newborn immune system. *Semin. Immunopathol.* 39, 605–613. doi: 10.1007/s00281-017-0653-x

Jin, Q., Chen, H., Luo, A., Ding, F., and Liu, Z. (2011). S100A14 stimulates cell proliferation and induces cell apoptosis at different concentrations via receptor for advanced glycation end products (RAGE). *PLoS One* 6:e19375. doi: 10.1371/journal.pone.0019375

Juiz, N. A., Cayo, N. M., Burgos, M., Salvo, M. E., Nasser, J. R., Búa, J., et al. (2016). Human polymorphisms in placentally expressed genes and their association with susceptibility to congenital *Trypanosoma cruzi* infection. *J. Infect. Dis.* 213, 1299–1306. doi: 10.1093/infdis/jiv561

Juiz, N. A., Solana, M. E., Acevedo, G. R., Benatar, A. F., Ramirez, J. C., da Costa, P. A., et al. (2017). Different genotypes of *Trypanosoma cruzi* produce distinctive placental environment genetic response in chronic experimental infection. *PLoS Negl. Trop. Dis.* 11:e0005436. doi: 10.1371/journal.pntd.0005436

Juiz, N. A., Torrejón, I., Burgos, M., Torres, A. M. F., Duffy, T., Cayo, N. M., et al. (2018). Alterations in placental gene expression of pregnant women with chronic Chagas disease. *Am. J. Pathol.* 188, 1345–1353. doi: 10.1016/j.ajpath.2018.02.011

Kak, G., Raza, M., and Tiwari, B. K. (2018). Interferon-gamma (IFN-γ): exploring its implications in infectious diseases. *Biomol. Concepts* 9, 64–79. doi: 10.1515/bmc-2018-0007

Kaplinski, M., Jois, M., Galdos-Cardenas, G., Rendell, V. R., Shah, V., Do, R. Q., et al. (2015). Sustained domestic vector exposure is associated with increased Chagas Cardiomyopathy risk but decreased parasitemia and congenital transmission risk among young women in Bolivia. *Clin. Infect. Dis.* 61, 918–926. doi: 10.1093/cid/civ446

Koga, K., Aldo, P. B., and Mor, G. (2009). Toll-like receptors and pregnancy: trophoblast as modulators of the immune response. *J. Obstet. Gynaecol. Res.* 35, 191–202. doi: 10.1111/j.1447-0756.2008.00963.x

Lawlor, K. E., Feltham, R., Yabal, M., Conos, S. A., Chen, K. W., Ziehe, S., et al. (2017). XIAP Loss Triggers RIPK3- and Caspase-8-Driven IL-1β activation and cell death as a consequence of TLR-MyD88-Induced cIAP1-TRAF2 degradation. *Cell Rep.* 20, 668–682. doi: 10.1016/j.celrep.2017.06.073

Lenk, E. J., Redekop, W. K., Luyendijk, M., Fitzpatrick, C., Niessen, L., Stolk, W. A., et al. (2018). Socioeconomic benefit to individuals of achieving 2020 targets for four neglected tropical diseases controlled/eliminated by innovative and intensified disease management: human African trypanosomiasis, leprosy, visceral leishmaniasis, Chagas disease. *PLoS Negl. Trop. Dis.* 12:e0006250. doi: 10.1371/journal.pntd.0006250

Levy, O. (2007). Innate immunity of the newborn: basic mechanisms and clinical correlates. *Nat. Rev. Immunol.* 7, 379–390. doi: 10.1038/nri2075

Liempi, A., Castillo, C., Carrillo, I., Muñoz, L., Droguett, D., Galanti, N., et al. (2016). A local innate immune response against *Trypanosoma cruzi* in the human placenta: the epithelial turnover of the trophoblast. *Microb. Pathog.* 99, 123–129. doi: 10.1016/j.micpath.2016.08.022

Liempi, A., Castillo, C., Duaso, J., Droguett, D., Sandoval, A., Barahona, K., et al. (2014). *Trypanosoma cruzi* induces trophoblast differentiation: a potential local antiparasitic mechanism of the human placenta? *Placenta* 35, 1035–1042. doi: 10.1016/j.placenta.2014.09.017

Lilleri, D., and Gerna, G. (2017). Maternal immune correlates of protection from human cytomegalovirus transmission to the fetus after primary infection in pregnancy. *Rev. Med. Virol.* 27:e1921. doi: 10.1002/rmv.1921

Lima, A. P. C. A., Almeida, P. C., Tersariol, I. L. S., Schmitz, V., Schmaier, A. H., Juliano, L., et al. (2002). Heparan sulfate modulates kinin release by *Trypanosoma cruzi* through the activity of cruzipain. *J. Biol. Chem.* 277, 5875–5881. doi: 10.1074/jbc.M108518200

Lima, L., Espinosa-Álvarez, O., Ortiz, P. A., Trejo-Varón, J. A., Carranza, J. C., Pinto, C. M., et al. (2015). Genetic diversity of *Trypanosoma cruzi* in bats, and multilocus phylogenetic and phylogeographical analyses supporting Tcbat as an independent DTU (discrete typing unit). *Acta Trop.* 151, 166–177. doi: 10.1016/j.actatropica.2015.07.015

Luquetti, A. O., Tavares, S. B., Siriano Lda, R., Oliveira, R. A., Campos, D. E., de Morais, C. A., et al. (2015). Congenital transmission of *Trypanosoma cruzi* in central Brazil. A study of 1,211 individuals born to infected mothers. *Mem. Inst. Oswaldo Cruz* 110, 369–376. doi: 10.1590/0074-02760140410

Macedo, A. M., Machado, C. R., Oliveira, R. P., and Pena, S. D. J. (2004). *Trypanosoma cruzi*: genetic structure of populations and relevance of genetic variability to the pathogenesis of chagas disease. *Mem. Inst. Oswaldo Cruz* 99, 1–12. doi: 10.1590/s0074-02762004000100001

Macedo, A. M., and Pena, S. D. (1998). Genetic variability of *Trypanosoma cruzi*: implications for the pathogenesis of Chagas disease. *Parasitol. Today* 14, 119–124. doi: 10.1016/s0169-4758(97)01179-4

Machado, E. M., Fernandes, A. J., Murta, S. M., Vitor, R. W., Camilo, D. J., Pinheiro, S. W., et al. (2001). A study of experimental reinfection by *Trypanosoma cruzi* in dogs. *Am. J. Trop. Med. Hyg.* 65, 958–965. doi: 10.4269/ajtmh.2001.65.958

Macrae, J. I., Acosta-Serrano, A., Morrice, N. A., Mehlert, A., and Ferguson, M. A. J. (2005). Structural characterization of NETNES, a novel glycoconjugate in *Trypanosoma cruzi* epimastigotes. *J. Biol. Chem.* 280, 12201–12211. doi: 10.1074/jbc.M412939200

Maeda, F. Y., Cortez, C., Izidoro, M. A., Juliano, L., and Yoshida, N. (2014). Fibronectin-degrading activity of *Trypanosoma cruzi* cysteine proteinase plays a role in host cell invasion. *Infect. Immun.* 82, 5166–5174. doi: 10.1128/IAI.02022-14

Marcilla, A., Martin-Jaular, L., Trelis, M., de Menezes-Neto, A., Osuna, A., Bernal, D., et al. (2014). Extracellular vesicles in parasitic diseases. *J. Extracell. Vesicles* 3:25040. doi: 10.3402/jev.v3.25040

Marino, A. P. M. P., Silva, A. A., Pinho, R. T., and Lannes-Vieira, J. (2003). *Trypanosoma cruzi* infection: a continuous invader-host cell cross talk with participation of extracellular matrix and adhesion and chemoattractant molecules. *Braz. J. Med. Biol. Res.* 36, 1121–1133. doi: 10.1590/s0100-879x2003000800020

Mattos, E. C., Canuto, G., Manchola, N. C., Magalhães, R. D. M., Crozier, T. W. M., Lamont, D. J., et al. (2019). Reprogramming of *Trypanosoma cruzi* metabolism triggered by parasite interaction with the host cell extracellular matrix. *PLoS Negl. Trop. Dis.* 13:e0007103. doi: 10.1371/journal.pntd.0007103

Mayhew, T. M. (2014). Turnover of human villous trophoblast in normal pregnancy: What do we know and what do we need to know? *Placenta* 35, 229–240. doi: 10.1016/j.placenta.2014.01.011

Medeiros, N. I., Fares, R. C. G., Franco, E. P., Sousa, G. R., Mattos, R. T., Chaves, A. T., et al. (2017). Differential expression of matrix metalloproteinases 2, 9 and cytokines by neutrophils and monocytes in the clinical forms of Chagas disease. *PLoS Negl. Trop. Dis.* 11:e0005284. doi: 10.1371/journal.pntd.0005284

Medina, L., Castillo, C., Liempi, A., Herbach, M., Cabrera, G., Valenzuela, L., et al. (2018). Differential infectivity of two *Trypanosoma cruzi* strains in placental cells and tissue. *Acta Trop.* 186, 35–40. doi: 10.1016/j.actatropica.2018.07.001

Mendonça-Previato, L., Penha, L., Garcez, T. C., Jones, C., and Previato, J. O. (2013). Addition of α-O-GlcNAc to threonine residues define the post-translational modification of mucin-like molecules in *Trypanosoma cruzi*. *Glycoconj. J.* 30, 659–666. doi: 10.1007/s10719-013-9469-7

Messenger, L. A., Gilman, R. H., Verastegui, M., Galdos-Cardenas, G., Sanchez, G., Valencia, E., et al. (2017). Toward improving early diagnosis of congenital Chagas disease in an endemic setting. *Clin. Infect. Dis.* 65, 268–275. doi: 10.1093/cid/cix277

Messenger, L. A., Miles, M. A., and Bern, C. (2015). Between a bug and a hard place: *Trypanosoma cruzi* genetic diversity and the clinical outcomes of Chagas disease. *Expert Rev. Anti. Infect. Ther.* 13, 995–1029. doi: 10.1586/14787210.2015.1056158

Ming, M., Ewen, M. E., and Pereira, M. E. (1995). Trypanosome invasion of mammalian cells requires activation of the TGF beta signaling pathway. *Cell* 82, 287–296. doi: 10.1016/0092-8674(95)90316-x

Mjihdi, A., Lambot, M.-A., Stewart, I. J., Detournay, O., Noël, J.-C., Carlier, Y., et al. (2002). Acute *Trypanosoma cruzi* infection in mouse induces infertility or placental parasite invasion and ischemic necrosis associated with massive fetal loss. *Am. J. Pathol.* 161, 673–680. doi: 10.1016/S0002-9440(10)64223-X

Möller, M., Kinnear, C. J., Orlova, M., Kroon, E. E., van Helden, P. D., Schurr, E., et al. (2018). Genetic resistance to *Mycobacterium tuberculosis* infection and disease. *Front. Immunol.* 9:2219. doi: 10.3389/fimmu.2018.02219

Mor, G., Aldo, P., and Alvero, A. B. (2017). The unique immunological and microbial aspects of pregnancy. *Nat. Rev. Immunol.* 17, 469–482. doi: 10.1038/nri.2017.64

Moreira, O. C., Ramírez, J. D., Velázquez, E., Melo, M. F. A. D., Lima-Ferreira, C., Guhl, F., et al. (2013). Towards the establishment of a consensus real-time qPCR to monitor *Trypanosoma cruzi* parasitemia in patients with chronic Chagas disease cardiomyopathy: a substudy from the BENEFIT trial. *Acta Trop.* 125, 23–31. doi: 10.1016/j.actatropica.2012.08.020

Nakhle, M. C., de Menezes M da, C., and Irulegui, I. (2018). Eosinophil levels in the acute phase of experimental Chagas' disease. *Rev. Inst. Med. Trop. Sao Paulo* 31, 384–391. doi: 10.1590/s0036-46651989000600004

Nde, P. N., Simmons, K. J., Kleshchenko, Y. Y., Pratap, S., Lima, M. F., and Villalta, F. (2006). Silencing of the laminin gamma-1 gene blocks *Trypanosoma cruzi* infection. *Infect. Immun.* 74, 1643–1648. doi: 10.1128/IAI.74.3.1643-1648.2006

Nogueira, L. G., Frade, A. F., Ianni, B. M., Laugier, L., Pissetti, C. W., Cabantous, S., et al. (2015). Functional IL18 polymorphism and susceptibility to chronic Chagas disease. *Cytokine* 73, 79–83. doi: 10.1016/j.cyto.2015.01.037

Oride, A., Kanasaki, H., Mijiddorj, T., Sukhbaatar, U., Ishihara, T., and Kyo, S. (2015). Regulation of kisspeptin and gonadotropin-releasing hormone expression in rat placenta: study using primary cultures of rat placental cells. *Reprod. Biol. Endocrinol.* 13:90. doi: 10.1186/s12958-015-0083-3

Ouyang, Y., Mouillet, J. F., Coyne, C. B., and Sadovsky, Y. (2014). Review: placenta-specific microRNAs in exosomes - good things come in nano-packages. *Placenta* 35, S69–S73. doi: 10.1016/j.placenta.2013.11.002

Park, D.-W., Lee, S.-K., Hong, S. R., Han, A.-R., Kwak-Kim, J., and Yang, K. M. (2012). Expression of Kisspeptin and its receptor GPR54 in the first trimester trophoblast of women with recurrent pregnancy loss. *Am. J. Reprod. Immunol.* 67, 132–139. doi: 10.1111/j.1600-0897.2011.01073.x

Pérez-Molina, J. A., and Molina, I. (2018). Chagas disease. *Lancet* 391, 82–94. doi: 10.1016/S0140-6736(17)31612-4

Picado, A., Cruz, I., Redard-Jacot, M., Schijman, A. G., Torrico, F., Sosa-Estani, S., et al. (2018). The burden of congenital Chagas disease and implementation of molecular diagnostic tools in Latin America. *BMJ Glob. Heal.* 3:e001069. doi: 10.1136/bmjgh-2018-001069

Pissetti, C. W., Correia, D., de Oliveira, R. F., Llaguno, M. M., Balarin, M. A. S., Silva-Grecco, R. L., et al. (2011). Genetic and functional role of TNF-alpha in the development *Trypanosoma cruzi* infection. *PLoS Negl. Trop. Dis.* 5:e976. doi: 10.1371/journal.pntd.0000976

PrabhuDas, M., Adkins, B., Gans, H., King, C., Levy, O., Ramilo, O., et al. (2011). Challenges in infant immunity: implications for responses to infection and vaccines. *Nat. Immunol.* 12, 189–194. doi: 10.1038/ni0311-189

Qian, J., Ding, F., Luo, A., Liu, Z., and Cui, Z. (2016). Overexpression of S100A14 in human serous ovarian carcinoma. *Oncol. Lett.* 11, 1113–1119. doi: 10.3892/ol.2015.3984

Racicot, K., Kwon, J.-Y., Aldo, P., Silasi, M., and Mor, G. (2014). Understanding the complexity of the immune system during pregnancy. *Am. J. Reprod. Immunol.* 72, 107–116. doi: 10.1111/aji.12289

Raposo, G., and Stoorvogel, W. (2013). Extracellular vesicles: exosomes, microvesicles, and friends. *J. Cell Biol.* 200, 373–383. doi: 10.1083/jcb.201211138

Rassi, A., Rassi, A., and Marcondes de Rezende, J. (2012). American trypanosomiasis (Chagas disease). *Infect. Dis. Clin. North Am.* 26, 275–291. doi: 10.1016/j.idc.2012.03.002

Rausch, M. E., and Barnhart, K. T. (2012). Serum biomarkers for detecting ectopic pregnancy. *Clin. Obstet. Gynecol.* 55, 418–423. doi: 10.1097/GRF.0b013e31825109f6

Reinhard, G., Noll, A., Schlebusch, H., Mallmann, P., and Ruecker, A. V. (1998). Shifts in the TH1/TH2 balance during human pregnancy correlate with apoptotic changes. *Biochem. Biophys. Res. Commun.* 245, 933–938. doi: 10.1006/bbrc.1998.8549

Reis-Cunha, J. L., Baptista, R. P., Rodrigues-Luiz, G. F., Coqueiro-dos-Santos, A., Valdivia, H. O., de Almeida, L. V., et al. (2018). Whole genome sequencing of *Trypanosoma cruzi* field isolates reveals extensive genomic variability and complex aneuploidy patterns within TcII DTU. *BMC Genomics* 19:816. doi: 10.1186/s12864-018-5198-4

Requena-Méndez, A., Albajar-Viñas, P., Angheben, A., Chiodini, P., Gascón, J., and Muñoz, J. (2014). Health policies to control Chagas disease transmission in European countries. *PLoS Negl. Trop. Dis.* 8:e3245. doi: 10.1371/journal.pntd.0003245

Retana Moreira, L., Rodríguez Serrano, F., and Osuna, A. (2019). Extracellular vesicles of *Trypanosoma cruzi* tissue-culture cell-derived trypomastigotes: induction of physiological changes in non-parasitized culture cells. *PLoS Negl. Trop. Dis.* 13:e0007163. doi: 10.1371/journal.pntd.0007163

Risso, M. G., Garbarino, G. B., Mocetti, E., Campetella, O., Gonzalez Cappa, S. M., Buscaglia, C. A., et al. (2004). Differential expression of a virulence factor, the trans-sialidase, by the main *Trypanosoma cruzi* phylogenetic lineages. *J. Infect. Dis.* 189, 2250–2259. doi: 10.1086/420831

Rivera, M. T., Marques de Araujo, S., Lucas, R., Deman, J., Truyens, C., Defresne, M. P., et al. (1995). High tumor necrosis factor alpha (TNF-alpha) production in *Trypanosoma cruzi*-infected pregnant mice and increased TNF-alpha gene transcription in their offspring. *Infect. Immun.* 63, 591–595.

Rodrigues, J. C. F., Godinho, J. L. P., and de Souza, W. (2014). Biology of human pathogenic trypanosomatids: epidemiology, lifecycle and ultrastructure. *Sub Cell. Biochem.* 74, 1–42. doi: 10.1007/978-94-007-7305-9_1

Rodriguez, P., Carlier, Y., and Truyens, C. (2012). Activation of cord blood myeloid dendritic cells by *Trypanosoma cruzi* and parasite-specific antibodies, proliferation of CD8+ T cells, and production of IFN-γ. *Med. Microbiol. Immunol.* 201, 157–169. doi: 10.1007/s00430-011-0217-y

Sadissou, I., d'Almeida, T., Cottrell, G., Luty, A., Krawice-Radanne, I., Massougbodji, A., et al. (2014). High plasma levels of HLA-G are associated with low birth weight and with an increased risk of malaria in infancy. *Malar. J.* 13, 312. doi: 10.1186/1475-2875-13-312

Sánchez Negrette, O., Mora, M. C., and Basombrío, M. A. (2005). High prevalence of congenital *Trypanosoma cruzi* infection and family clustering in Salta, Argentina. *Pediatrics* 115, e668–e672. doi: 10.1542/peds.2004-1732

Scharfstein, J., and Morrot, A. (1999). A role for extracellular amastigotes in the immunopathology of Chagas disease. *Mem. Inst. Oswaldo Cruz* 94(Suppl. 1), 51–63. doi: 10.1590/s0074-02761999000700005

Schorey, J. S., and Bhatnagar, S. (2008). Exosome function: from tumor immunology to pathogen biology. *Traffic* 9, 871–881. doi: 10.1111/j.1600-0854.2008.00734.x

Schorey, J. S., and Harding, C. V. (2016). Extracellular vesicles and infectious diseases: new complexity to an old story. *J. Clin. Invest.* 126, 1181–1189. doi: 10.1172/JCI81132

Seco-Hidalgo, V., De Pablos, L. M., and Osuna, A. (2015). Transcriptional and phenotypical heterogeneity of *Trypanosoma cruzi* cell populations. *Open Biol.* 5:150190. doi: 10.1098/rsob.150190

Siriano, L., da, R., Luquetti, A. O., Avelar, J. B., Marra, N. L., and de Castro, A. M. (2011). Chagas disease: increased parasitemia during pregnancy detected by hemoculture. *Am. J. Trop. Med. Hyg.* 84, 569–574. doi: 10.4269/ajtmh.2011.10-0015

Skowron-Cendrzak, A., Rudek, Z., Sajak, A., Kubera, M., Basta-Kaim, A., and Shani, J. (1999). Effect of multiparity on T-cell proliferation response to mitogen stimulation in elderly women. *Int. J. Immunopharmacol.* 21, 177–183. doi: 10.1016/s0192-0561(98)00078-2

Smith, N. L. D., and Denning, D. W. (2014). Clinical implications of interferon-γ genetic and epigenetic variants. *Immunology* 143, 499–511. doi: 10.1111/imm.12362

Solana, M. E., Celentano, A. M., Tekiel, V., Jones, M., and González Cappa, S. M. (2002). *Trypanosoma cruzi*: effect of parasite subpopulation on murine pregnancy outcome. *J. Parasitol.* 88, 102–106. doi: 10.1645/0022-3395(2002)088%5B0102:tceops%5D2.0.co;2

Straszewski-Chavez, S. L., Abrahams, V. M., Funai, E. F., and Mor, G. (2004). X-linked inhibitor of apoptosis (XIAP) confers human trophoblast cell resistance to Fas-mediated apoptosis. *Mol. Hum. Reprod.* 10, 33–41. doi: 10.1093/molehr/gah001

Tarleton, R. L. (2007). Immune system recognition of *Trypanosoma cruzi*. *Curr. Opin. Immunol.* 19, 430–434. doi: 10.1016/j.coi.2007.06.003

Teixeira, A. R. L., Hecht, M. M., Guimaro, M. C., Sousa, A. O., and Nitz, N. (2011). Pathogenesis of Chagas' disease: parasite persistence and autoimmunity. *Clin. Microbiol. Rev.* 24, 592–630. doi: 10.1128/CMR.00063-10

Theocharis, A. D., Manou, D., and Karamanos, N. K. (2019). The extracellular matrix as a multitasking player in disease. *FEBS J.* doi: 10.1111/febs.14818 [Epub ahead of print].

Tibayrenc, M. (1998). Genetic epidemiology of parasitic protozoa and other infectious agents: the need for an integrated approach. *Int. J. Parasitol.* 28, 85–104. doi: 10.1016/s0020-7519(97)00180-x

Tibayrenc, M., Ward, P., Moya, A., and Ayala, F. J. (1986). Natural populations of *Trypanosoma cruzi*, the agent of Chagas disease, have a complex multiclonal structure. *Proc. Natl. Acad. Sci. U.S.A.* 83, 115–119. doi: 10.1073/pnas.83.1.115

Torres, O. A., Calzada, J. E., Beraún, Y., Morillo, C. A., González, A., González, C. I., et al. (2010). Role of the IFNG +874T/A polymorphism in Chagas disease in a Colombian population. *Infect. Genet. Evol.* 10, 682–685. doi: 10.1016/j.meegid.2010.03.009

Torrico, F., Alonso-Vega, C., Suarez, E., Rodriguez, P., Torrico, M.-C., Dramaix, M., et al. (2004). Maternal *Trypanosoma cruzi* infection, pregnancy outcome, morbidity, and mortality of congenitally infected and non-infected newborns in Bolivia. *Am. J. Trop. Med. Hyg.* 70, 201–209. doi: 10.4269/ajtmh.2004.70.201

Trocoli Torrecilhas, A. C., Tonelli, R. R., Pavanelli, W. R., da Silva, S., Schumacher, R. I., de Souza, W., et al. (2009). *Trypanosoma cruzi*: parasite shed vesicles increase heart parasitism and generate an intense inflammatory response. *Microbes Infect.* 11, 29–39. doi: 10.1016/j.micinf.2008.10.003

Truyens, C., and Carlier, Y. (2017). "Protective host response to *Trypanosoma cruzi* and its limitations", in *American Trypanosomiasis Chagas Disease*, 2nd Edn, eds J. Telleria and M. Tibayrenc (London: Elsevier), 579–604. doi: 10.1016/B978-0-12-801029-7.00026-5

van Niel, G., Porto-Carreiro, I., Simoes, S., and Raposo, G. (2006). Exosomes: a common pathway for a specialized function. *J. Biochem.* 140, 13–21. doi: 10.1093/jb/mvj128

Vannberg, F. O., Chapman, S. J., and Hill, A. V. S. (2011). Human genetic susceptibility to intracellular pathogens. *Immunol. Rev.* 240, 105–116. doi: 10.1111/j.1600-065X.2010.00996.x

Vekemans, J., Truyens, C., Torrico, F., Solano, M., Torrico, M. C., Rodriguez, P., et al. (2000). Maternal *Trypanosoma cruzi* infection upregulates capacity of uninfected neonate cells To produce pro- and anti-inflammatory cytokines. *Infect. Immun.* 68, 5430–5434. doi: 10.1128/iai.68.9.5430-5434.2000

Villagrasa, A., Álvarez, P. J., Osuna, A., Garrido, J. M., Aránega, A., and Rodríguez-Serrano, F. (2014). Exosomes derived from breast cancer cells, small Trojan Horses? *J. Mammary Gland Biol. Neoplasia* 19, 303–313. doi: 10.1007/s10911-015-9332-5

Wang, S.-C. (2014). PCNA: a silent housekeeper or a potential therapeutic target? *Trends Pharmacol. Sci.* 35, 178–186. doi: 10.1016/j.tips.2014.02.004

Webber, J., Yeung, V., and Clayton, A. (2015). Extracellular vesicles as modulators of the cancer microenvironment. *Semin. Cell Dev. Biol.* 40, 27–34. doi: 10.1016/j.semcdb.2015.01.013

Weyer, K., and Glerup, S. (2011). Placental regulation of peptide hormone and growth factor activity by proMBP. *Biol. Reprod.* 84, 1077–1086. doi: 10.1095/biolreprod.110.090209

WHO (2015). Chagas disease in Latin America: an epidemiological update based on 2010 estimates. *Relev. Epidemiol. Hebd.* 90, 33–43.

Wujcicka, W., Wilczyński, J., Śpiewak, E., and Nowakowska, D. (2018). Genetic modifications of cytokine genes and *Toxoplasma gondii* infections in pregnant women. *Microb. Pathog.* 121, 283–292. doi: 10.1016/j.micpath.2018.05.048

Yeo, M., Acosta, N., Llewellyn, M., Sánchez, H., Adamson, S., Miles, G. A. J., et al. (2005). Origins of Chagas disease: *Didelphis* species are natural hosts of *Trypanosoma cruzi* I and armadillos hosts of *Trypanosoma cruzi* II, including hybrids. *Int. J. Parasitol.* 35, 225–233. doi: 10.1016/j.ijpara.2004.10.024

Zingales, B., Miles, M. A., Campbell, D. A., Tibayrenc, M., Macedo, A. M., Teixeira, M. M. G., et al. (2012). The revised *Trypanosoma cruzi* subspecific nomenclature: rationale, epidemiological relevance and research applications. *Infect. Genet. Evol.* 12, 240–253. doi: 10.1016/j.meegid.2011.12.009

10

Congenital Transmission of Apicomplexan Parasites

*Maura Rojas-Pirela[1,2,3], Lisvaneth Medina[1], Maria Verónica Rojas[2], Ana Isabel Liempi[1], Christian Castillo[1,4], Elizabeth Pérez-Pérez[3], Jesús Guerrero-Muñoz[1], Sebastian Araneda[1,5] and Ulrike Kemmerling[1]**

[1] Instituto de Ciencias Biomédicas, Facultad de Medicina, Universidad de Chile, Santiago, Chile, [2] Instituto de Biología, Pontificia Universidad Católica de Valparaíso, Valparaíso, Chile, [3] Facultad de Farmacia y Bioanálisis, Universidad de Los Andes, Mérida, Venezuela, [4] Núcleo de Investigación Aplicada en Ciencias Veterinarias y Agronómicas, Facultad de Medicina Veterinaria y Agronomía, Universidad de Las Américas, Santiago, Chile, [5] Facultad de Salud y Odontología, Universidad Diego Portales, Santiago, Chile

***Correspondence:**
Ulrike Kemmerling
ukemmerling@uchile.cl

Apicomplexans are a group of pathogenic protists that cause various diseases in humans and animals that cause economic losses worldwide. These unicellular eukaryotes are characterized by having a complex life cycle and the ability to evade the immune system of their host organism. Infections caused by some of these parasites affect millions of pregnant women worldwide, leading to various adverse maternal and fetal/placental effects. Unfortunately, the exact pathogenesis of congenital apicomplexan diseases is far from being understood, including the mechanisms of how they cross the placental barrier. In this review, we highlight important aspects of the diseases caused by species of *Plasmodium, Babesia, Toxoplasma*, and *Neospora*, their infection during pregnancy, emphasizing the possible role played by the placenta in the host-pathogen interaction.

Keywords: Apicomplexa, congenital transmission, placenta, infection-immunology, host–parasite interactions

INTRODUCTION

The phylum Apicomplexa constitutes a broad group of parasitic protists that include more than 6000 species (Votýpka et al., 2017), distributed in a wide diversity of environments, including soil, freshwater, and marine habitats (del Campo et al., 2019). Many of these parasites have significant clinical and economic relevance since they cause important human and veterinary diseases worldwide. In this context, malaria (*Plasmodium* species), babesiosis (*Babesia* sp.), toxoplasmosis (*Toxoplasma gondii*), neosporosis (*Neospora* sp.), and cryptosporidiosis (*Cryptosporidium parvum*) are diseases caused by apicomplexan parasites (Chakraborty et al., 2017; Martínez-Ocampo, 2018).

All those parasites present complex life cycles, infecting one or more hosts and undergoing multiple morphological and metabolic differentiation (Martínez-Ocampo, 2018; Jeninga et al., 2019). Additionally, in the life cycles of most of the apicomplexan, an alternation between asexual and sexual reproduction can be observed. Thus, in the different life cycles, three different states can be observed: sporozoite (infective stage), merozoite (a result of asexual reproduction), and gametocyte (germ cells) (Votýpka et al., 2017).

Apicomplexan parasites are characterized by having a complex of apical secretory organelles composed of micronemes, rhoptries, and dense granules. These organelles vary between species and are involved in host cell attachment, motility, invasion, and intracellular parasitophorous vacuole formation (Votýpka et al., 2017). In addition, all apicomplexan examined so far (except

Cryptosporidium and *Gregarine*) possess an apicoplast (Salomaki and Kolisko, 2019), a relict plastid involved in several essential metabolic pathways, such as fatty acid, isoprenoid, and heme biosynthesis, that are crucial for parasite replication and establishment of infection (Ralph et al., 2004; Chakraborty, 2016).

Apicomplexan presents different transmission routes (Votýpka et al., 2017). However, for some species such as *Neospora, Babesia microti* (*B. microti*), and *Toxoplasma gondii (T. gondii)*, the infection from mother to fetus constitutes an important transmission route (Joseph et al., 2012; Hide, 2016; Khan et al., 2020). The incidence of congenital malaria, caused by *Plasmodium*, is relatively low in endemic regions. However, some reports have documented that the incidence can reach 37% (Ouédraogo et al., 2012; Olupot-Olupot et al., 2018). Regarding *T. gondii*, when primo-infection occurs during pregnancy, the congenital transmission rates are high (Hide, 2016), increasing from the first to the third trimester of pregnancy (McAuley, 2014). Importantly, these congenital infections can be detrimental to maternal and child health (Maldonado et al., 2017; Tegegne et al., 2019). The frequency of the transplacental transmission of these parasites is associated with different factors such as maternal and developing fetus immune systems and genetic background (Ortiz-Alegría et al., 2010; Ouédraogo et al., 2012; Gómez-Chávez et al., 2019), the passive transfer of maternal antibodies (Ortiz-Alegría et al., 2010; Dobbs and Dent, 2016) characteristics of the fetal environment (De Silva et al., 1982), and the functioning of the placenta as a physical barrier and immune organ (Robbins et al., 2012; Sharma and Shukla, 2017). Thus, the placenta is a crucial organ determining the probability of infection (Castillo et al., 2018).

The present review is focused on the congenital transmission of *Plasmodium, Babesia, T. gondii, Neospora* and the role of the placenta.

DISEASES CAUSED BY APICOMPLEXAN PARASITES: SOCIAL AND ECONOMIC IMPACT

Diseases caused by apicomplexan parasites affect millions of people, mainly in low- and middle-income countries located in the tropical and subtropical regions (Votýpka et al., 2017). Moreover, some of those infections have been included in the group of Neglected Tropical Diseases (NTD) (PLoS Neglected Tropical Disease, 2020), implying a significant social and economic impact that can reach millions of dollars each year (Laha et al., 2015; Ozawa et al., 2019; Stelzer et al., 2019).

Malaria is caused by five members of the genus *Plasmodium*, where *P. falciparum* and *P. vivax* species represent the most significant threat (Geleta and Ketema, 2016). Malaria is an important public health problem; it was estimated in 2018 that 228 million people were infected worldwide, and 405,000 malaria deaths were reported (WHO, 2019). Children aged under 5 years and pregnant women constitute the most vulnerable population (Gabrielli et al., 2016; WHO, 2019). The attempts to control and eradicate malaria present an estimated economic impact of 2.7 billion dollars (WHO, 2019).

Babesiosis is a globally distributed disease with malaria-like symptoms that affects elderly and immunocompromised patients (Kim et al., 2016), caused by erythrocytic parasites of the genus *Babesia*. Many of the 100 species of *Babesia* constitute a significant threat to humans, domestic animals, and livestock (Young et al., 2019), being in humans, *B. microti, B. divergens, B. duncani,* and *B. venatorum* the causal agents (Sun et al., 2014; Young et al., 2019). The mortality rate of this disease is approximately 5%; however, in case of infection through blood transfusion, the mortality rate increases to 19% (Katz and Dodd, 2019). In addition to human health effects, some *Babesia* species cause a significant loss to the cattle industry due to death, a loss of beef production of infected animals, and death (Mosqueda et al., 2012).

Toxoplasmosis is a zoonotic disease that affects approximately one-third of the world population (Ngô et al., 2017; Stelzer et al., 2019). The infection in immunocompetent individuals is generally asymptomatic; however, severe symptoms are observed in newborns (i.e., mental retardation, ocular disease) when the primoinfection occurs in the pregnant mother. Additionally, infection during pregnancy can cause abortion (Tegegne et al., 2016). Toxoplasmosis can be fatal in immunosuppressed patients since the reactivation of latent infection can lead to the development of encephalitis and, in some cases, reactivation of malignancies (Maciel et al., 2000; Wang Z.D. et al., 2017). In the case of animals, it is considered one of the leading causes of reproductive losses in small ruminants worldwide, which also play an important role in transmitting the parasite to humans. In some countries, such as Australia, the losses attributed to this disease can be up to 70 million dollars (Stelzer et al., 2019).

Neosporosis is a devastating worldwide disease responsible for abortions, neonatal mortality, and central nervous system diseases in animals. It is mainly caused by the species *Neospora caninum* (*N. caninum*) and *Neospora hughesi* (*N. hughesi*) and is transmitted by horizontal and vertical routes (Dubey, 2003; Donahoe et al., 2015). *N. caninum* affects dogs and cattle but occasionally infects horses, sheep, and deer, while *N. hughesi* only infects horses causing Equine Protozoal Myeloencephalitis (Dubey, 2003; Wobeser et al., 2009).

Neosporosis is associated with sporadic abortions (between 10 and 12.5%) in cattle herds with a frequent congenital transmission. However, the percentage of abortions increases (30–57%) in herds when the parasite is acquired by the pregnant mother (Dubey et al., 2007). *N. caninum* infections have a significant global economic impact; for instance, in New Zealand, the losses attributed to this disease exceed US$ 35.7 million (Reichel et al., 2013).

HOST–APICOMPLEXAN INTERACTIONS AT THE MAMMALIAN PLACENTA

As mentioned above, apicomplexan parasites can be transmitted congenitally. Within this group *Plasmodium* spp. and *T. gondii* are the most documented (Carlier et al., 2012). The placenta is a transitory organ that acts as the interface between the mother and fetus, which mediates nutrition and gas exchange between the fetus and the mother, ensuring growth and normal embryo-fetal development and supporting the maternal changes associated with pregnancy (Griffiths and Campbell, 2015; Castillo et al., 2018). The chorioallantoic is the main placenta in mammals during middle to late gestation and develops from the endometrium of the uterus and the trophoblast of the embryo. According to the extent of trophoblast invasion into the uterus, placentation is classified into hemochorial (highly invasive), endotheliochorial (moderate invasive) or epitheliochorial (low invasive) (Liempi et al., 2020). In the case of the human placenta, it is classified as discoidal, villous, and hemochorial, made up of a fetal portion that (originates from the *Chorion frondosum*) and a maternal portion or decidua basalis (originates from the endometrium) (Castillo et al., 2018).

The functional units in the human placenta are the chorionic villi, formed by the trophoblast a lining epithelium formed by two types of cell populations, undifferentiated cytotrophoblasts (CT) and fully differentiated syncythiotrophoblasts (ST), and the villous stroma (VS) (Gude et al., 2004; Castillo et al., 2018). The trophoblast is connected to and separated from the villous stroma (VS), the fetal connective tissue by a basal lamina, a specialized structure of extracellular matrix (ECM) (Benirschke et al., 2012). Therefore, trophoblast, basal *laminae,* and VS, the latter containing fetal capillaries, form the placental barrier that pathogens must cross to infect the fetus during transplacental transmission (Kemmerling et al., 2019). However, the placenta can protect the developing fetus from some kind of pathogens (Zeldovich et al., 2013). That is the case of the kinetoplastid *Trypanosoma cruzi* (*T. cruzi*), where only a few parasite antigens and DNA can be identified in human chorionic villi (Duaso et al., 2010). Additionally, the presence of *T. cruzi* activates local placental defense mechanisms such as the epithelial turnover of the BLT and secretion of pro-inflammatory cytokines through Toll-like receptors (TLR) activation and NFkB signaling (Liempi et al., 2016, 2019; Castillo et al., 2017a,b).

The ovine and bovine placenta are of cotyledonary shape, villous and epitheliochorial. The fetal component is formed by the fusion of the avascular chorion and the vascular allantois. The placental barrier is composed by six tissue layers: maternal capillary endothelium, maternal endometrial connective tissue, maternal endometrial epithelium, trophoblast, chorionic connective tissue, and fetal endothelium (Benirschke et al., 2012; Liempi et al., 2020).

The type of placental barrier has been associated with the probability of transmission of pathogens. Thus, it has been proposed that in the hemochorial placenta, where the trophoblast is in direct contact with maternal blood, the placental infection and, therefore, the transmission to the fetus is facilitated. Moreover, considering that the complexity of the placental barriers increases from hemochorial (human) to epitheliochorial (ovine), it could be assumed that the parasites cross the hemochorial barrier more easily. However, the same hemochorial barrier favors the transfer of maternal antibodies to the fetus, and in less invasive placentas, a greater variety of pathogens is observed (Capellini et al., 2015; Liempi et al., 2020).

Unfortunately, most pathogens, including apicomplexan, can surpass the placental barrier and infect the fetus. As we will see in the following sections, these parasites use very similar adhesion mechanisms to the placenta, based on the modulation of the expression of adhesion molecules on the surface of placental cells. Additionally, the presence of these pathogens induces alterations in the immune response and a change in the Th1/Th2 balance, favoring the activation of defense mechanisms based on cellular immunity, which harms placental function and fetal growth.

CONGENITAL MALARIA

Malaria represents a high risk to the pregnant woman, fetus, and newborn. In some endemic areas, the prevalence of exposure to infection during pregnancy is 35%. Globally, malaria causes each year over 10,000 maternal and 75.000–200,000 neonatal deaths (Dombrowski et al., 2018; WHO, 2019). Congenital malaria is characterized by the sequestration of erythrocytes infected with *Plasmodium* parasites and the infiltration of immune cells within the intervillous space (IVS) of the placenta (**Figure 1A**), and the acquisition of a dark color of the basal plate, the fetal membranes (FM), fetal capillaries (FC), and monocytes (Mo) in the IVS, due to the deposition of the hemozoin malarial pigment (Parekh et al., 2010; Sharma and Shukla, 2017). The presence of parasites causes a pro-inflammatory environment in the placenta, leading to structural and functional alterations (**Figure 1B**). Placental damage, in turn, alters the nutrient exchange system between mother and fetus, leading to pregnancy-related complications including abortion, stillbirth, intrauterine growth retardation (IUGR), and low birth weight (LBW) (Briand et al., 2016; Sharma and Shukla, 2017). It has been proposed that due to hormonal and immunological changes in pregnancy (McLean et al., 2015), together with the fact that the parasite is localized inside red blood cells, it can more easily evade the maternal immune response (Sharma and Shukla, 2017). Interestingly, first-time pregnant women are more susceptible to malaria infection than women conceived a second or third time. This resistance to malaria infection in multigravida women is attributed to the development of placental parasite-specific immunity (Soulard et al., 2011).

Any of the Plasmodium species can cause congenital malaria; however, depending on the geographic region, infection by a specific species may predominate. Thus, in endemic regions of the Indian and African subcontinent, most congenital malaria cases are due to *P. falciparum* and *P. vivax* (Bhatia et al., 2016), while in European countries, *P. malariae* and *P. vivax* are predominate (Vottier et al., 2008). In South America, *P. vivax* accounts for the majority of malaria cases (Recht et al., 2017). In addition, *P. ovale* is a rare causative agent of congenital malaria (Jenkins, 1957; Penazzato et al., 2007), is limited to specific areas of tropical Africa and islands in the Western Pacific (Collins and Jeffery, 2005).

Adhesion of *Plasmodium* to the Placenta

Plasmodium parasites invade red blood cells and induce the expression of parasite-derived proteins on the cell surface

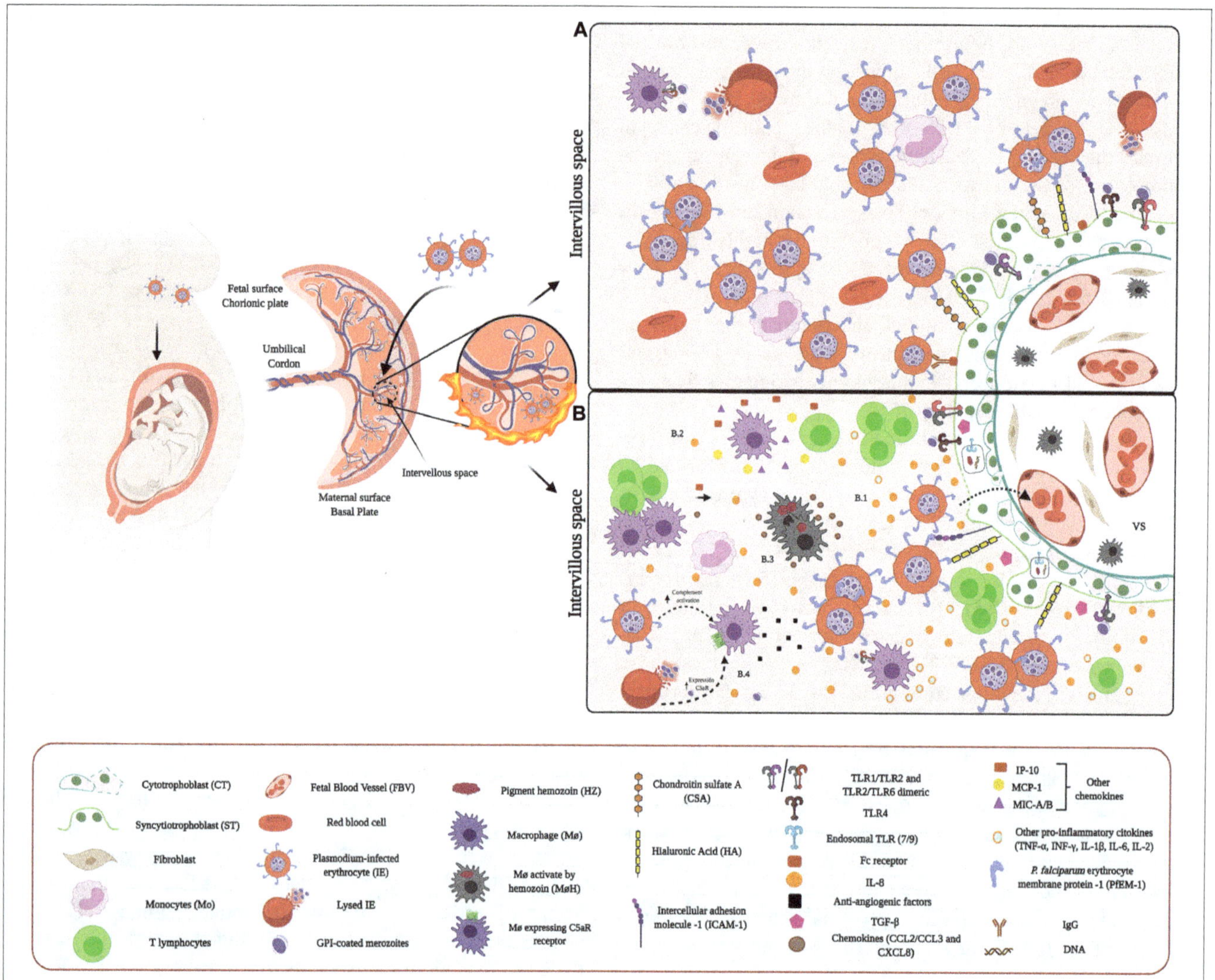

FIGURE 1 | Host–pathogen interaction between *Plasmodium* and placenta: **(A)** Adhesion and sequestration of parasite-IEs. IEs express parasite-derived proteins on their surface. For example, the PfEMP1 protein family is highly expressed in placental IEs and acts as a surface antigen and ligand for their adhesion and sequestration. PfEMP1 selectively binds to specific placental receptors such as CSA. Other receptor molecules such as HI and ICAM-1, expressed in ST, participate as key molecules in the adhesion process. **(B)** Microenvironment and inflammatory response **(B.1,B.2)** Inflammation in the IVS is attributed to chemokines and cytokines secreted by maternal Mo, T cells, and ST. **(B.3)** Parasite's hemozoin induces activation of MΦ, and subsequent release of chemokines. **(B.4)** Schizonts activate C5 and rupture releasing parasite components containing GPI that induce expression of C5aR and activate MΦ.

of the infected erythrocyte (IEs) (Chan et al., 2014). These parasite-derived proteins, known as variant surface antigens (VSAs), enable the IEs to adhere to the endothelium and subsequently infect different organs, including the placenta (Autino et al., 2012). In addition, VSAs bind to serum proteins forming red blood cell aggregates (rosetting), allowing the evasion of the host immune response, and establish chronic infection (Wahlgren et al., 2017). Among, VSAs *P. falciparum* erythrocyte membrane protein 1 (PfEMP1) is a major surface antigen involved in vascular adhesion and sequestration of IEs (Chan et al., 2014). Notably, fEMP1 proteins are encoded by a polymorphic *var* multigene family (approximately 60 copies per genome), characterized by expression through allelic exclusion, allowing switching between PfEMP1 proteins and subsequent modification of the antigenic and binding properties of IEs (Wahlgren et al., 2017).

PfEMP1 proteins mediate the adhesion of IEs to different receptors and surface molecules including integrins (Chesnokov et al., 2018), endothelial protein C receptor (EPCR) (Gillrie et al., 2015), CD36 (Hsieh et al., 2016), intercellular adhesion molecule-1 and 2 (ICAM-1/2) (Lennartz et al., 2019), proteoglycans, such as chondroitin sulphate A (CSA) (Pehrson et al., 2016), glycosaminoglycans (GAGs), such as hyaluronic acid (HA) (Beeson and Brown, 2004), *P*-selectin, *E*-Selectin (Metwally et al., 2017) and Platelet/endothelial cell adhesion molecule-1 (PECAM-1) (Berger et al., 2013). In the placenta, the PfEMP1 variant VAR2CSA is predominantly expressed in IEs (Tuikue Ndam et al., 2005) and is the main VSA responsible for parasite-binding tropism (Nunes and Scherf, 2007; Smith, 2014) in this organ (Benavente et al., 2018). Notably, a selective accumulation of mature asexual stages of *P. falciparum*- IEs occurs in the IVS and chorionic villi surface (Beeson et al., 2002; Muthusamy et al., 2004; **Figure 1A**). The accumulation of IEs is mediated by receptors and molecules on the ST surface, macrophages (MΦ) monocytes (Mo), the fibrinoid deposits, and blood vessels in the VS (Beeson et al., 1999; Matejevic et al., 2001; Sugiyama et al., 2001).

Chondroitin sulphate A is the principal placental IEs receptor (Fried et al., 2006; Chishti, 2015). However, other molecules such as HA, non-immune immunoglobulins (IgG/IgM), and ICAM-1, present on the ST, can act as adhesion receptors (Maubert et al., 1997; Sartelet et al., 2000; Flick et al., 2001; Beeson and Brown, 2004; Barfod et al., 2011; **Figure 1A**). CD38 is only localized in the cytoplasm of stromal cells, fibroblasts, and MΦ, where the presence of IEs might influence its expression without being directly implicated in the sequestration of these (Sartelet et al., 2000). On the other side, HA is associated mainly with the aggregation or clumping of IEs (Beeson and Brown, 2004). Importantly, the expression of the different receptors is influenced by *P. falciparum*-induced proinflammatory cytokines (Vásquez et al., 2013).

In addition, other factors determine the accumulation and the sequestration of IEs in the placenta, including the low placental blood flow associated with trophoblast conformational changes, for the formation of cytotrophoblastic prolongations, known as "Coan-Burton bridges" (Moraes et al., 2013), IEs cell deformability (Safeukui et al., 2018), and the presence of Mo (Sugiyama et al., 2001). The adhesion and invasion of IEs also depend on the type of *Plasmodium* species. Thus, *P. vivax* and *P. falciparum* can bind to placental CSA and HA. However, *P. vivax* cannot bind to CD36 and ICAM-1 (Chotivanich et al., 2012), ligands widely used by *P. falciparum*.

So far, the *Plasmodium* mechanisms of adhesion to the placenta are the best known among apicomplexan parasites. However, as we will see in the following sections, these mechanisms are preserved in related apicomplexan parasites such *Babesia*, *Toxoplasma*, and *Neospora*. In these organisms, the parasite proteins expressed in the infected cells, or the proteins present on the parasite's surface play fundamental roles in the adhesion and infection processes in the placenta.

Immune Response Against *Plasmodium*

The development of severe malaria during pregnancy depends on parasite and host factors, including the immune response (Clark, 2019). During pregnancy, an increase of hormones, including cortisol, progesterone, estradiol, and testosterone, polarize the immune response toward a Th2-type one, characterized by an increase of regulatory T cells (Tregs) and anti-inflammatory cytokines (Robinson and Klein, 2012). The presence of the parasite alters this response causing infiltration of immune cells and a strong inflammatory response (Suguitan et al., 2003; Chêne et al., 2014).

Toll-like receptors, particularly TLRs-2 -4 -7-and -9, expressed on the trophoblast and cells of the VS, play a key role in the immune response against *Plasmodium* (Lucchi et al., 2011; Zhu et al., 2011; Barboza et al., 2014, 2017; Reis et al., 2020). TLR-2 and -4 recognize glycosylphosphatidylinositol (GPI) anchors (Krishnegowda et al., 2005), while nucleic acids and hemozoin are recognized by TLR7 and TLR9 (Coban et al., 2005; Parroche et al., 2007; **Figure 1B**). The expression of TLR-4 and -9 is regulated by *Plasmodium* (Barboza et al., 2017) and polymorphisms of the TLRs have been associated with the susceptibility to infection (Hamann et al., 2010).

The binding of IEs and parasite antigens to TLR expressed on the trophoblast promotes the activation of MAPK pathways leading to the secretion of pro-inflammatory cytokines, including TNF-α, IFN-γ, TGF-β, and IL-8, and consequent activation of immune cell (Lucchi et al., 2008; Reis et al., 2020; **Figure 1B**). Concomitantly, the chemokines interferon γ–induced protein-10 (IP-10), monocyte chemoattractant protein-1 (MCP-1), and macrophage inflammatory protein (MIP)-1a/b expressed in maternal white blood cells (WBCs) contribute to the accumulation of Mo and MΦ in the IVS (Suguitan et al., 2003). Then, the presence of the immune cells and cyto/chemokines leads to a Th1-type immune response, where in addition to the cytokines mentioned above, IL1β, IL-2, IL-6, (Dobaño et al., 2018) and IL-8 (Fried et al., 1998) are secreted (**Figure 1B**). Thus, T cells proliferation is induced, and MΦ phagocytosis is enhanced, aiming to limit the parasite's replication (Ozarslan et al., 2019).

Overproduction of cytokine IL-10, an immunoregulating cytokine, is associated with response to placental malaria infections (Suguitan et al., 2003; Chêne et al., 2014) attenuating the detrimental effects on the placental barrier exerted by the exacerbated inflammatory response (Okamgba et al., 2018). Alternatively, the increase in IL-10 could modulate lymphoid dendritic cell (DC) subpopulations shifting the Th1/Th2 balance toward a TH1 response and consequently promote infection (Diallo et al., 2008).

Mo-secreted IL-1β in response to IEs alters the amino acid transport system in the trophoblast impairing their transfer to the fetus and contributes to PM-associated FGR's pathogenesis. Moreover, the accumulation of Mo in the malarial placenta promotes the decrease of insulin-like growth factor-1, one of the most influential factors in fetal growth and life (Umbers et al., 2011).

Different MΦ populations are related to functional modification of the placenta and maternal-fetal tolerance (Ordi et al., 1998; Gaw et al., 2019). Thus, maternal-intervillous monocytes (MIM) are associated with massive chronic villositis and placental damage (Ordi et al., 1998). Likewise, a decrease in the anti-inflammatory M2-type Hofbauer cells (HBC), located in the VS, is associated with LBW in placental malaria (Gaw et al., 2019).

Plasmodium also activates the complement cascade (C) and subsequently modulates the release of the anti-angiogenic factors (Conroy et al., 2011; Chau et al., 2017; **Figure 1B**). Together, an excessive mononuclear cells activation, such as MΦ, and an increase of soluble vascular endothelial growth factor (VEGF) receptor-1 (sFlt-1), which reduce the bioavailability of the pro-angiogenic VEGF and placental growth factor (PGF), impair normal angiogenesis (Azimi-Nezhad, 2014; Chau et al., 2017) and trigger functional placental insufficiency, and ultimately, FGR (Conroy et al., 2011).

The presence of Hemozoin (Hz) is another determining factor in the placental malaria immune environment. Hz can stimulate the trophoblast, MΦ, and DCs to secrete chemokines and cytokines [CCL2, CCL3, and CXCL8 and tumor necrosis factor (TNF)], contributing to the recruitment of peripheral blood mononuclear cells, especially Mo (Lucchi et al., 2011) and inflammatory response (Moormann et al., 1999; Abrams et al., 2003; **Figure 1B**). In addition, phagocytosis of this pigment increases the expression of matrix metalloproteinase (MMPs), particularly MMP-9, in the trophoblast (Clark, 2019) inducing cleavage and liberation of the extracellular domain of Syndecan-1; therefore allowing the adherence of IEs and promote their accumulation in the placenta (Clark, 2019).

CONGENITAL BABESIOSIS

Congenital babesiosis, caused by *B. microti* and *Babesia* sp., is considered a rare disease; to date, a total of 10 cases have been reported in the United States (Esernio-Jenssen et al., 1987; New et al., 1997; Sethi et al., 2009; Aderinboye and Syed, 2010; Cornett et al., 2012; Joseph et al., 2012; Yager et al., 2014; Surra and Jesus, 2015; Saetre et al., 2018). Although transplacental babesiosis has been reported, so far, no histological studies have been conducted in *Babesia*-infected placentas. However, it has been proposed that *B. microti* sporozoites can invade red blood cells and cross the placental barrier and infect the fetus (**Figure 2A**). On the other side, the presence of the parasite in amniotic fluid has been demonstrated (Cornett et al., 2012). During gestational babesiosis, clinical manifestations similar to the HELLP syndrome (hemolysis, elevated liver enzymes, and low platelets) may develop, causing significant maternal and neonatal morbidity and mortality (Khangura et al., 2019). In infants, in addition to presenting hemolytic anemia, thrombocytopenia, and fever, hepatosplenomegaly is one of the most common symptoms (Saetre et al., 2018).

Babesiosis has also been documented in other mammals such as canines, felines, cattle, and rodents (Schoeman, 2009; Tołkacz et al., 2017). In these animals, babesiosis is caused by several species of babesia, which are relatively host-specific. However, all *Babesia* species can be transferred to other hosts through infected blood (Cox, 1982). Interestingly, in rodents, the placental transmission of *B. microti* is higher than in other mammals, including humans (Tołkacz et al., 2017; Tufts and Diuk-Wasser, 2018).

Adhesion of *Babesia* to the Placenta

The pathogenesis of Babesia is strikingly similar to that of malaria (**Figure 2A**). Thus, alterations in the adhesive properties of IEs due to antigenic modifications of their membrane (Cooke et al., 2005; Hutchings et al., 2007), caused by the expression of a variant of the parasite-derived erythrocyte surface antigen protein (VESA), can be observed (Jackson et al., 2014). VESAs are proteins encoded by various families of ves1α and ves1β genes and secreted by the parasite (Allred et al., 2000; Allred, 2019). In addition, VESAs appear to play essential roles in pathogenicity (Pedroni et al., 2013), immune evasion (Jackson et al., 2014), persistence, and survival of the parasites (Allred, 2019). VESAs, variant erythrocyte surface antigenic- 1 (VESA1) protein, is one of the most studied in *B. bovis*. This protein acts as an endothelial cell ligand and mediator of antigenic variation in *B. bovis*-IEs (O'Connor and Allred, 2000; Wang et al., 2012). The host cell adhesion receptors for VESA have not yet been identified (Gallego-Lopez et al., 2019). However, structural similarities between fEMP1 and VESA1 suggest that the latter could bind to equivalent host cell receptors of PfEMP1 such as CD36 (Hutchings et al., 2007), ICAM-1, *P*-selectin, CSA, and CD31 (Gallego-Lopez et al., 2019; **Figure 2A**). Furthermore, studies performed with *B. bigemina* and *B. ridhaini* have demonstrated the adhesion IEs to thrombospondin (PST) (Parrodi et al., 1990) present in endothelial cells (Baruch et al., 1996).

Importantly, the severity of babesiosis is highly dependent on the babesia species (Cooke et al., 2005). For example, babesiosis caused by *Babesia microti, B. bovis, B. Lengua,* and *B. canis* is associated with the development of severe syndromes such as brain babesiosis and multi-organ failure due to the sequestration of IEs in the organ's microvasculature (Wright et al., 1979; Aikawa et al., 1992; Bosman et al., 2013; Sondgeroth et al., 2013; Ripoll et al., 2018; Schetters, 2019).

Immune Response Against *Babesia*

There are few reports related to the placental immune response against *Babesia*. However, it has been suggested that pro-inflammatory cytokine activation and erythrocyte adhesion in babesiosis are similar to malaria (Krause et al., 2007; **Figure 2B**). Some studies have even documented that prior infection with *B. microti* protects against fatal malaria in mice and primates through a mechanism of cross-protection (van Duivenvoorde et al., 2010; Efstratiou et al., 2020).

Toll-like receptors also recognize *Babesia* through the presence of its surface of GPI-linked molecules. The main TLRs studied regarding *Babesia* species are TLR-3 and -4, which can signal downstream through MyD88 independent pathways (Skariah et al., 2017). Similarly, TLR2 could play a role in this inflammatory response, mediating MΦ activation in the placenta. Previous studies have shown that lipid extracts from *B. bovis* stimulate TLR-2-mediated MΦ activation (Gimenez et al., 2010; **Figure 2B**) and consequently induces the secretion of pro-inflammatory cytokines, including TNF-α, IL-1, IL-12, and the immunomodulating IL-8 and nitric oxide (NO) (Shoda et al., 2000; Terkawi et al., 2015). In addition, T lymphocytes and natural killer (NK) cells, responsible for INF-γ production, and B lymphocytes are essential elements in the immune response against this parasite (Krause et al., 2007; Vannier and Krause, 2012; Yi et al., 2018; **Figure 2B**). Notably, the DNA of this parasite also has immunomodulatory effects on both B cells and MΦ, through the induction of IL-12, TNF-α, and NO production (Shoda et al., 2001).

Babesia, like *Plasmodium*, increases in the expression of MCP-1 and MIP-1a chemokines, contributing to the accumulation of Mo and MΦ in the IVS (Skariah et al., 2017; Zhao et al., 2020). Also, other chemokines such as CCL4 (MIP-1β) and CCL5

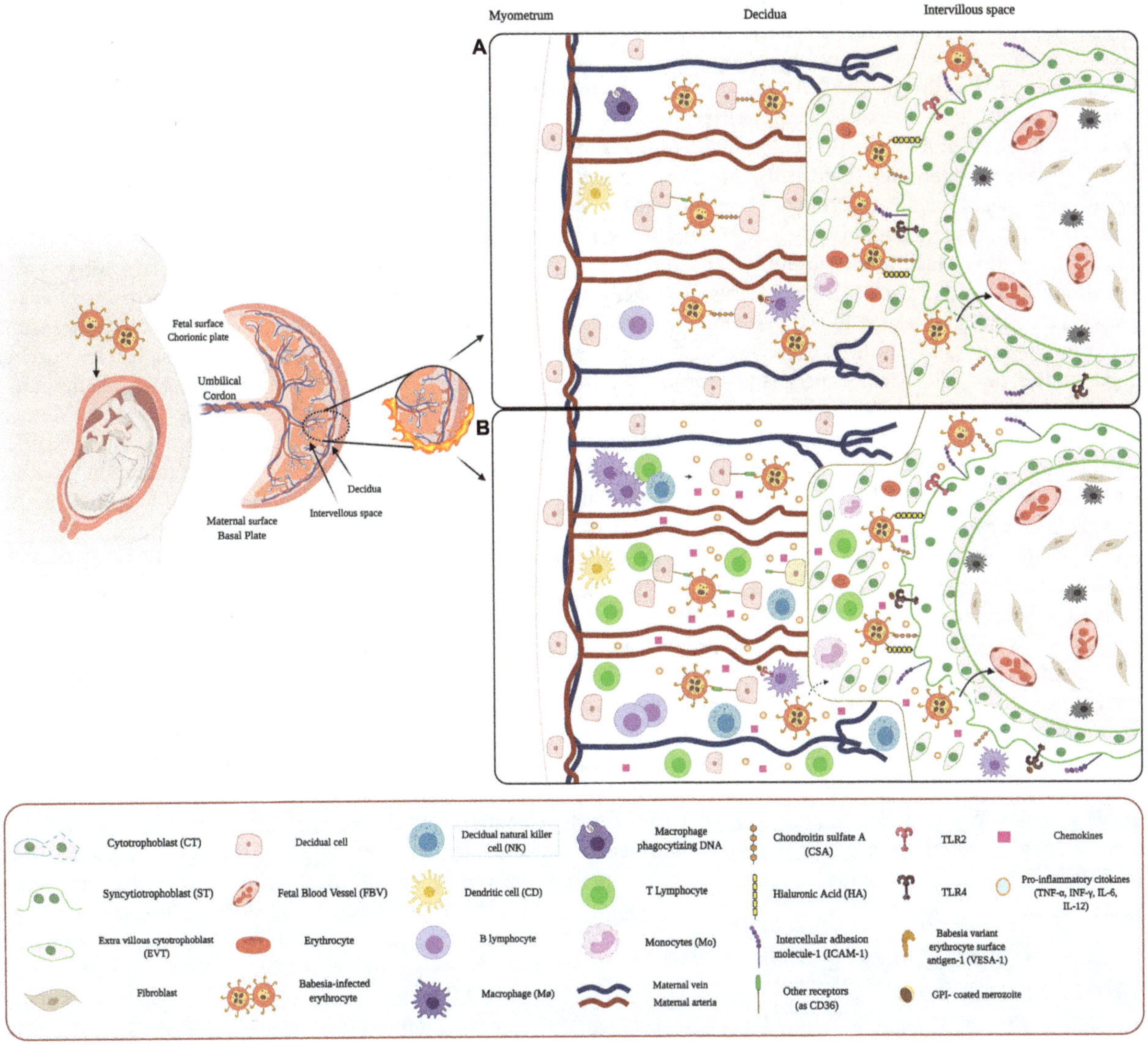

FIGURE 2 | Host–pathogen interaction between *Babesia* and placenta: **(A)** Adhesion and sequestration of *Babesia*-IEs Infection of erythrocytes by the parasite induces expression of parasite-derived proteins on the surface of the IEs. Babesia-infected IEs highly express the VESA1 family and possibly act as a surface antigen and ligand for adhesion and sequestration of IEs in the placenta. VESA1 selectively binds to specific placental receptors, such as CSA, HA, and ICAM-1, expressed by ST, participate as key molecules in this adhesion process. In addition, some receptors such as CD36 could also facilitate the adhesion of IEs in other regions of the placenta, such as the decidua. **(B)** Microenvironment and inflammatory response against *Babesia*. Inflammation in the IVS and decidua could be attributed to chemokines and cytokines secreted by maternal MΦ, Mo, B cell, and T cells, as well as ST.

(RANTEs) have been associated with an inflammatory process in response to this parasite (Skariah et al., 2017).

CONGENITAL TOXOPLASMOSIS

Congenital toxoplasmosis is one of the leading causes of infant morbidity and mortality (Melamed et al., 2010). Although it is a disease with global distribution, its prevalence is markedly variable from one region to another (Melamed et al., 2010; Torgerson and Mastroiacovo, 2013), with a global estimated incidence of 190100 annual cases (Torgerson and Mastroiacovo, 2013). Congenital toxoplasmosis occurs predominantly after primary infection in pregnant women (Pappas et al., 2009). However, congenital transmission has been reported in pregnant women infected before pregnancy (Pons et al., 1995; Vogel et al., 1996), chronically infected women, in whom the *T. gondii* infection was reactivated due to immunosuppression by HIV or by drug treatment for underlying diseases (Marty et al., 1994; Bachmeyer et al., 2006), and in women previously infected with one serotype who developed a new infection with a second serotype acquired during pregnancy (Fortier et al., 1991; Valdès et al., 2011).

During congenital transmission, the parasite crosses the placenta directly or with the help of infected immune cells, Mo, and DCs, using them as "Trojan horses" (**Figure 3A**;

Robert-Gangneux et al., 2011; Arranz-Solís et al., 2021), inducing phenotypic and functional alterations in infected cells, including overexpression of adhesion molecules and receptors, hypermotility, and downregulation of cytokine expression (Lachenmaier et al., 2011; Masocha and Kristensson, 2012; Sanecka and Frickel, 2012; Arranz-Solís et al., 2021). The parasite induces an inflammatory response (**Figure 3B**) that compromises mother and child health and the success of pregnancy (Robert-Gangneux et al., 2011). In addition, *T. gondii* causes severe neuro-ocular alterations such as chorioretinitis and the worst-case fetal death (Melamed et al., 2010). The severity of congenital Toxoplasmosis is inversely related to the gestational age at the time of primary maternal infection, implying that maternal infections in the first trimester of pregnancy lead to more serious clinical manifestations (McAuley, 2014). Besides, the clinical outcome of congenital Toxoplasmosis also is related to the *T. gondii* genotypes (Gilbert et al., 2008; McAuley, 2014), being the type I and II isolates related to more severe congenital Toxoplasmosis (Fuentes et al., 2001; Hutson et al., 2015; Rico-Torres et al., 2016; Lahmar et al., 2020; Arranz-Solís et al., 2021).

Toxoplasma gondii infects warm-blooded animals, including birds, cats, sheep, dogs, cows, goats, and pigs (Mondragon et al., 1998; Dubey et al., 2003; Stelzer et al., 2019); being isolates type II III the most frequent genotypes (Lachkhem et al., 2021). In some animals, the congenital transmission frequency is also high (Duncanson et al., 2001; Dos Santos et al., 2016) and is associated with fetal loss and economic losses (Stelzer et al., 2019). Interestingly, the potential risk of parasite transmission in animals through ingestion of contaminated milk has been suggested (Dubey et al., 2014; Ossani et al., 2017), increasing, therefore, the risk of zoonotic infection.

Adhesion of *Toxoplasma gondii* to the Placenta

Toxoplasma gondii cell invasion is a multi-step process that depends on the parasite's motility, surface antigens, and the sequential secretion of proteins present in the apical secretory organelles (Carruthers and Boothroyd, 2007; Robert-Gangneux and Dardé, 2012).

The invasion process starts with low-affinity interaction between *T. gondii* surface molecules, including glycosylphosphatidylinositol (GPI)-attached surface antigens (SAG), SAG-related sequence proteins (SRS), and non-SAG-related surface antigens (SUSA) and the cell membrane of the host cell (Pollard et al., 2008; Blader and Saeij, 2009). The SAGs multigenic family comprises more than 150 genes distributed and tandemly arrayed throughout the genome (Lekutis et al., 2001; Jung et al., 2004). SAG and SRS1 proteins are predominantly expressed on the tachyzoite (rapidly dividing parasites) surface cells (Tomavo, 1996; Manger et al., 1998). Regarding the SUSA molecules, 31 genes have been identified, and the proteins are highly expressed in bradyzoites (slow dividing parasites) (Pollard et al., 2008). Significantly, all these surface antigens are also involved in immune modulation, virulence, and protection of the parasite to survive in the environment (Lekutis et al., 2001; Crawford et al., 2009), for what they are considered redundant systems of adhesion to the host cell (Manger et al., 1998). The host cell surface molecules include GAGs, proteoglycans, and glycosaminoglycan-like carbohydrates (Jacquet et al., 2001; He et al., 2002; Azzouz et al., 2013). In addition, proteins of apical secretory organelles also play a key role in parasite-cell adhesion. For example, rhoptry proteins (ROP 2, ROP 4) and dense granules protein (GRA2) are lectins that bind to sulfated GAGs and then participate in the moving junction complex (MJ complex) (Azzouz et al., 2013).

Additionally, *T. gondii* is recognized and adheres to ICAM-1 on the host cell surface. Thus, micronemal proteins (MICs), such as MIC2, binds to ICAM-1 and facilitate the transmigration of the parasite through the blood-brain barrier (Lachenmaier et al., 2011). Also, interactions with ECM laminin (Furtado et al., 1992) and sialylated oligosaccharides (Blumenschein et al., 2007) have been reported. In the placenta, *T. gondii* infects different cell types, including decidual cells, extravillous trophoblasts (EVT), and the trophoblast (Abbasi et al., 2003; Robbins et al., 2012). The parasite's binding to these cells is mediated by sulfated proteoglycan and ICAM-1 (Abbasi et al., 2003; Barragan et al., 2005; **Figure 3A.1**). ICAM-1 is abundantly expressed at intercellular junctions and the surface of in human trophoblast cell line (BeWo) (Barragan et al., 2005). Also, *T. gondii* induces syncytial expression of this adhesion molecule (Juliano et al., 2006) increasing the adhesion of *T. gondii*-infected immune cells to the trophoblast (Pfaff et al., 2005). Thus, parasite infection of Mo and maternal leukocytes promotes their adhesion to trophoblasts through the upregulation of ICAM-1, contributing to placental and ultimately fetal infection (Xiao et al., 1997; Pfaff et al., 2005). Moreover, decidual DCs could serve as a vehicle for *T. gondii* to travel across the placenta and infect the fetus (Sanecka and Frickel, 2012; Arranz-Solís et al., 2021; **Figure 3A.2**). In addition, *T. gondii* can exploit natural routes for leukocyte extravasation to cross the placental barrier (**Figure 3A.3**). In vascular endothelium, CD162 is recognized by the vascular adhesion molecule-1 (VCAM-1) and E-selectin of infected cells mediating their attachment (Harker et al., 2013). Interestingly, CD162 has been identified in trophoblast cell lines (Multhaup et al., 2018).

The adhesion of infected immune cells to the endothelium serves as a signal to the parasite, allowing to schedule its leukocyte output at the target organ and minimizing the attack by the immune system (Baba et al., 2017). Thus *T. gondii* reaches the placenta inside maternal leukocytes and adheres to the trophoblast (**Figure 3A.3**). In the case of Mo, the presence *T. gondii* antigens, such as soluble tachyzoite antigen (STAg), induces the overexpression of macrophage migration inhibitory factor (MIF), allowing the adhesion to the trophoblast (Ferro et al., 2008). Moreover, the adhesion of infected immune cells can also induce local destruction of the trophoblast (Juliano et al., 2006) through the induction of pro-inflammatory cytokine-dependent apoptosis (Garcia-Lloret et al., 2000; Juliano et al., 2006). It has also been proposed that the accumulation of leukocytes is responsible for placental villitis (Yavuz et al., 2006).

The ECM degradation is another strategy used by *T. gondii* to cross and damage the placental barrier (Wang and Lai, 2013; Liempi et al., 2020; **Figure 3A.4**). Placental infections increase

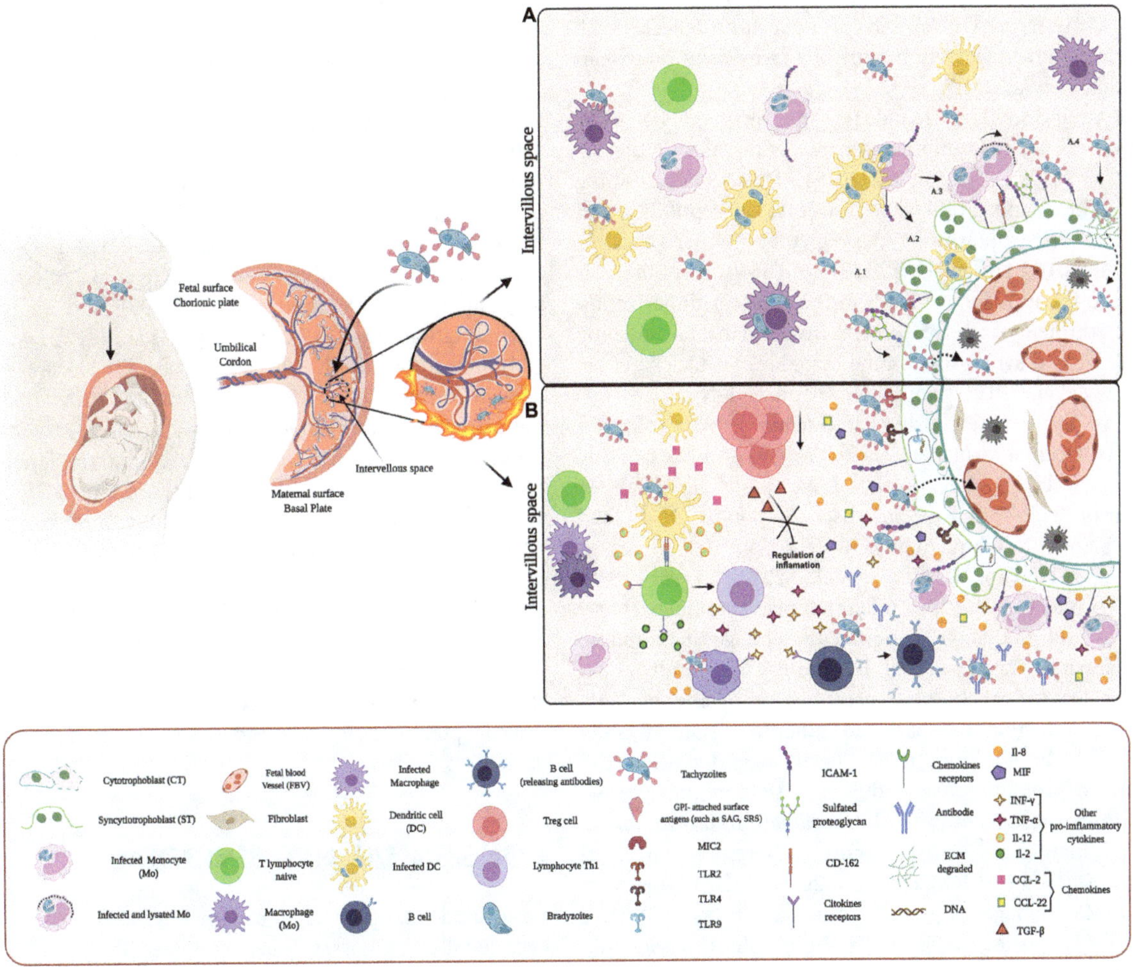

FIGURE 3 | Host–pathogen interaction between *Toxoplasma* and placenta: **(A)** Adhesion of *T. gondii* in the placenta. *Toxoplasma* adhesion to the placenta can occur through proteins belonging to the SAG, SRS, and MIC families. These proteins expressed on the surface of the parasite act as surface antigens and ligands for molecules present on the surface of placental cells. These surface antigens could bind to GAGs, glycoproteins, adhesion molecules, and some extracellular matrix components. Once attached to the placenta, *T. gondii* crosses the placenta by different mechanisms: (i) without altering the integrity of the barrier **(A.1)**; (ii) infecting immune cells (such as CDs) and using them as Trojan horses **(A.2)**; (iii) exploiting the natural routes of leukocytes extravasation and coordinating its exit with the arrival at the target organ, thus minimizing attack by the immune system during the vehicle transition to target cells **(A.3)**; and (iv) and promoting EMC degradation, through modulation of MMP expression and secretion **(A.4)**. **(B)** Microenvironment and inflammatory response against *T. gondii*. Recognition of *T. gondii* by TLR (TLR2/4/9) induces IL-8 expression and secretion. Additionally, infection by this parasite promotes the expression of MIF and CCL-2. Recognition of the parasite by immune cells (such as CDs and MΦ) activates an inflammatory response characterized by cytokine and chemokine production such as IL-12, CCL-2, and CCL-22, which activate naive T cells. Subsequently, these cells differentiate to Th1 and produce cytokines (such as IL-2, INF-γ, and TNF-α) that promote an exacerbated pro-inflammatory environment, which stimulates the recruitment and activation of other immune cells at the site of infection. Additionally, infection by *T. gondii* promotes a decrease in Tregs, contributing to the exacerbated inflammatory reaction.

the expression and secretion of MMPs, MMP-2, MMP-9, and MMP-12 in the VS, causing ECM degradation (Wang and Lai, 2013) particularly of fibronectin, collagen I and IV, and laminin (Chen and Aplin, 2003).

Immune Response Against *Toxoplasma gondii*

Toxoplasma gondii infection in the placenta induces an inflammatory response characterized by a robust production of pro-inflammatory cytokines and chemokines (Sasai et al., 2018; Sasai and Yamamoto, 2019).

Toll-like receptors are critical in initiating defense against *T. gondii*; they recognize in the parasite glycosylphosphatidylinositol (GPI) anchored proteins and lipid anchors, heat shock protein 70 (TgHSP70), and profilin-like protein (TgPF) (Yarovinsky and Sher, 2006; Denkers, 2010; Yarovinsky, 2014; Sasai et al., 2018). GPI, are recognized primarily by TLR-2, TL-4 and TL2/TL1/6 heterodimers (Debierre-Grockiego et al., 2007) while TgPF is recognized by the TLR-5, 11 and -12 (Andrade et al., 2013; Salazar Gonzalez et al., 2014; Yarovinsky et al., 2005). On the other hand, parasite's RNA and DNA are recognized by the endosomal TLR-7 and -9 (Yarovinsky, 2014). TLR activation leads to an increase of IL-12,

IL-6, IL-8, and TNF-α cytokines, chemokines (CCL5, CCL12, and XCL1), interferons (IFNs), and other effector molecules such as NO, which favors infection control (Yarovinsky and Sher, 2006; Wujcicka et al., 2013).

Haplotype and single nucleotide polymorphisms (SNPs) of *tlr* genes can influence susceptibility to parasitic diseases (Wujcicka et al., 2013, 2017; Turkey et al., 2019). Thus, SNPs residing in TLR2, TLR4, and TLR9 genes increase susceptibility and development of toxoplasmosis in pregnancy (Wujcicka et al., 2013, 2014, 2017; Turkey et al., 2019). This susceptibility is attributed to the influence of SNPs in the receptor dimerization and the recruitment of adapter proteins involved in TLR signaling and the decreased synthesis of some cytokines (Wujcicka et al., 2017; Turkey et al., 2019), such as INF-γ and TNF-α.

We have shown previously that during *ex vivo* infection of human placental explants (HPE), *T. gondii* increases the expression of TLR-9, but not of TLR-2 and -4. However, inhibition of TLR-4 and -9 increases *T. gondii* DNA load in the explants. Notably, only IL-8 secretion was increased (Muñoz et al., 2016; Castillo et al., 2017a; **Figure 3B**); even the protective and pro-inflammatory cytokines INF-γ and TNF-α did not show a significant change in response to the parasite (Castillo et al., 2017a). This result could explain, at least partially, the susceptibility of the placenta to *T. gondii* infection compared to other parasites (Castillo et al., 2017a). In addition, it has been suggested that IL-8 promotes the proliferation and differentiation of the infected host cell, and subsequently, the intracellular multiplication of parasites (Milian et al., 2019), promoting, therefore, congenital transmission (Gómez-Chávez et al., 2019, 2020). Moreover, *T. gondii* Macrophage Migration Inhibitory Factor (TgMIF) cytokine-like, an analog to the host MIF, promotes IL-8 secretion and subsequent recruitment of immune cells to the site of infection (Sommerville et al., 2013) causing the above-described effects (Lambert et al., 2006).

On the other hand, the low INF-γ expression (Muñoz et al., 2016; Castillo et al., 2017a) could also be a placental mechanism to limit infection. Both INF-γ and TNF-α promote the adhesion of infected immune cells to the trophoblast through surface overexpression of ICAM-1 (Pfaff et al., 2005; Ferro et al., 2008). Therefore, it is possible that the downregulation of these pro-inflammatory cytokines, in addition to benefiting the maintenance of pregnancy, also limits the transfer of the parasite through the placental barrier. Furthermore, this could be related to the production of CCL22 chemoattractant in response to *T. gondii* (Ander et al., 2018) since CCL22 can replace the effect of IFN-γ and recruit Tregs modulating the inflammatory response. However, this increased T-reg recruitment may also be a parasite strategy to promote its persistence (Rowe et al., 2011). Furthermore, MIF is also overexpressed in responses to *T. gondii* infection (de Oliveira Gomes et al., 2011; **Figure 3B**), promoting the adhesion of infected immune cells to the trophoblast, activating the ERK1/2 MAPK pathway and subsequent production of prostaglandin E, favoring parasite proliferation and persistence through inhibition of IL-6, IL17, and TNF-α production (Kelly et al., 2005; Passos et al., 2010; Barbosa et al., 2014; Qiu et al., 2016).

The presence of *T. gondii* causes an imbalance of the Treg/T-helper type 17 (Th17) cells response inducing deleterious alterations in the placenta that can lead to abortion (Zhang et al., 2012). *T. gondii*, as mentioned above, promotes the production of IL-12, CCL-2, and CCL-22 activating naïve T cells. In addition, activated T cells secrete IL-2, INF-γ, and TNF-α, developing a pro-inflammatory environment that stimulates MΦ and B cells (Gómez-Chávez et al., 2020) and decreases Tregs and TGF-β levels (**Figure 3B**). The decrease of Tregs may be due to various factors, including apoptosis (Ge et al., 2008), limitation of proliferation (Oldenhove et al., 2009), and an increase in differentiation into Th17 cells (Zhang et al., 2012).

Importantly, all the factors involved in decreasing Tregs have in common the activation of multiple pathways, including the pro-inflammatory ones (Ge et al., 2008; Oldenhove et al., 2009; Zhang et al., 2012). The increased differentiation of TH17 cells is associated with altered expression of TGF-β, IL-17A, and IL-6 cytokines, transcription factors [i.e., Forkhead box-p3 (Foxp3)], and receptors [i.e., Retinoic acid-related orphan receptor γt (RORγt)], keys in cell differentiation and regulating Treg/Th17 balance (Zhang et al., 2012). Although it is unclear how *T. gondii* regulates the expression of TFG-B and Foxp3, it influences suppressive functions of Tregs in the placenta (Zhang et al., 2012), resulting in an exacerbated inflammatory reaction, causing placental damage and favors the transmission of the parasite to the fetus.

CONGENITAL NEOSPOROSIS

Congenital neosporosis affects mainly dogs and cattle, but occasionally also horses, sheep, and deer (Dubey, 2003), leading to abortion, stillbirth, and weak offspring (Mesquita et al., 2018). In sheep, congenital transmission rates are high, reaching values between 66.7 and 93% (González-Warleta et al., 2018). Transplacental transmission can be exogenous or endogenous. Exogenous transmission occurs following ingestion of sporulated oocysts by pregnant females, while endogenous one occurs as the reactivation of a pre-existent infection. The latter is the primary mechanism responsible for maintaining the parasite within livestock populations. The presence of the parasite induces an inflammatory response leading to placental damage and consequent abortion (Cantón et al., 2014b; Al-Shaeli et al., 2020).

Thus, multiple necrotic lesions, thickening of the chorionic plate, and mineralization of necrotic foci can be observed in the infected ovine placenta. Notably, both the oocysts (sexual state) and tachyzoites (rapidly dividing parasite stage) of *N. caninum* can be detected in placental tissue (Mesquita et al., 2018; Al-Shaeli et al., 2020; **Figure 4A**). In the fetus, *N. caninum* causes severe damage to the brain, heart, lung, and liver (Al-Shaeli et al., 2020).

Although *N. caninum* is not considered a zoonotic parasite, serological studies indicate the possible capacity of *N. caninum* to infect humans, particularly immunocompromised individuals (Tranas et al., 1999; Lobato et al., 2006; Oshiro et al., 2015) and pregnant women. Recent reports revealed *N. caninum* in samples of umbilical cord blood and placental tissue in pregnant women. The seroprevalence in these women can vary between 8 and

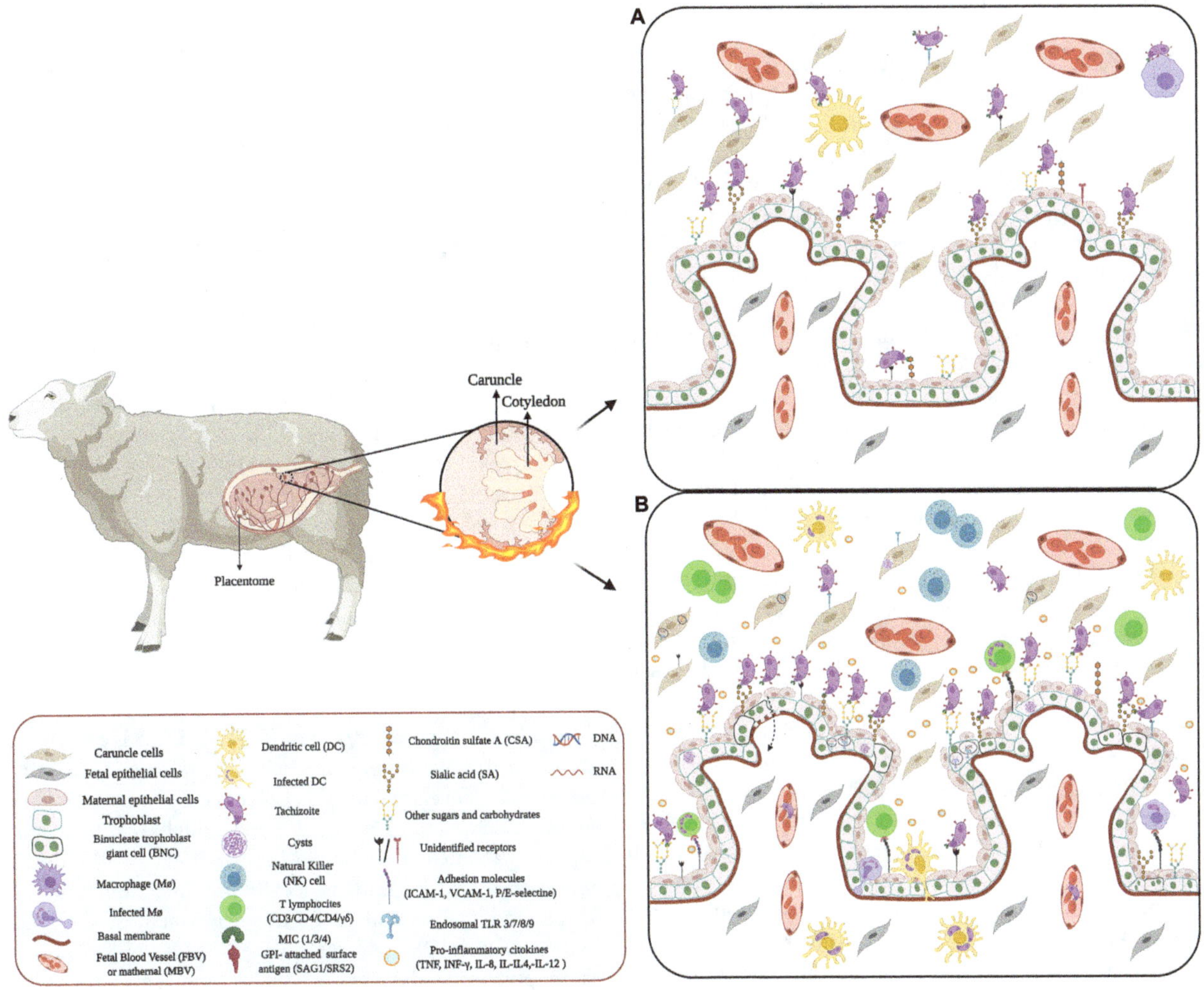

FIGURE 4 | Host–pathogen interaction between *Neospora* and placenta: **(A)** Adhesion of Neospora. Neospora adhesion to the placenta can occur through proteins belonging to the SAG, SRS, and MIC families. These proteins expressed on the surface of the parasite act as surface antigens and ligands for molecules present on the surface of placental cells. Possibly, these protein proteins could bind to proteoglycans and placental adhesion molecules. **(B)** Microenvironment and inflammatory response against *Neospora*. Inflammation in the IVS and caruncle could be attributed to chemokines and cytokines secreted by maternal Mo, T cell, as well as ST and caruncle cells. Many of these cytokines and chemokines promote cell recruitment. Additionally, infection of some cells of the maternal immune system, such DCs, and MΦ, by *Neospora* alters the migration of these cells, using them as Trojan horses.

24% (Ibrahim et al., 2009; Duarte et al., 2020) and is associated with the presence of domestic animals (Duarte et al., 2020). The biological similarities between *N. caninum* and *T. gondii* suggest the possibility of *N. caninum* transmission between humans (Petersen et al., 1999). Moreover, in studies where pregnant monkeys were inoculated with *N. caninum*, the transplacental transmission was evident; in the fetus, similar lesions as those caused by *T. gondii* can be observed (Barr et al., 1994; Ho et al., 1997). In mice, the congenital transmission of *N. caninum* occurs in 85% of the litters born from infected mothers (Cole et al., 1995).

Adhesion of *N. caninum* to the Placenta

Neospora caninum can actively invade a large variety of nucleated cells *in vitro* and *in vivo* conditions (Naguleswaran et al., 2002; Hemphill et al., 2004; Lei et al., 2005); its mechanisms are very similar to those proposed for *T. gondii*, where a first stage of low-affinity adhesion and a second stage of firm apical attachment can be observed (Hemphill et al., 2004; Carruthers and Boothroyd, 2007).

The initial adhesion is mediated by tachyzoite surface antigens belonging to the SAG-related sequence proteins (SRS) family and homologous to the *T. gondii* SAGs family (Howe et al., 1998). SAG1 and SRS2 are two main immuno-dominant antigens of *N. caninum* tachyzoites (Dong et al., 2012; Sinnott et al., 2017) that binds to host cells (Hemphill et al., 2013). In addition, SRS allows parasite adhesion through binding to GAGs expressed on the host cell's surface, especially CSA and SA (Dubey et al., 2017). The latter is crucial for self-recognition by complement factor H (Varki and Gagneux, 2012) and fetal defense against maternal complement attack (Abeln et al., 2019).

Then the apical attachment is mediated mainly by MIC (Lovett et al., 2000; Naguleswaran et al., 2002; Reid et al., 2012; Wang J. et al., 2017), MIC2 and MIC19 are unique to *N. caninum* (Reid et al., 2012). *N. caninum* MIC proteins have domains similar to those found in vertebrate ECM proteins, including thrombospondin (TPS) -like, integrin-like domain (Pereira et al., 2011) and SA- binding adhesive repeat- (MAR)-like domain (Friedrich et al., 2010). Thus, MICs can bind through GAGs to various receptors present on the surface of target cells (Dubey et al., 2017), and mediate cell adhesion (Keller et al., 2002; Wang J. et al., 2017). MIC1, MIC3, and MIC4 bind to host cells through sulfated proteoglycans (Naguleswaran et al., 2002; Keller et al., 2004; Friedrich et al., 2010). *N. caninum* proliferation varies between the different cells of the placenta (Gibney et al., 2008). Studies in bovine placenta cell lines have shown that caruncular cells appear to be more resistant to *Neospora* infection than trophoblasts due to their expression of adhesion molecules (Jiménez-Pelayo et al., 2017, 2019) and phagocytic activity (Machado et al., 2007; Jiménez-Pelayo et al., 2017). However, this resistance also depends on the virulence of the isolate (Jiménez-Pelayo et al., 2017). On the other hand, *N. caninum* shows a predilection for the fetal chorionic epithelium and placental blood vessels (Buxton et al., 1998).

There are few reports related to the adhesion molecules that participate in the placenta and *N. caninum* interaction. However, SRS2 participates in the adhesion of *N. caninum* to the trophoblast (**Figure 4A**) and the development of an effective immune response against transplacental transmission (Nishikawa et al., 2001; Haldorson et al., 2005, 2006), but the receptor for SRS2 has not yet been identified (Naguleswaran et al., 2002; **Figure 4A**). Nevertheless, the presence of SA and glycoproteins expressed on the surface of binucleate trophoblast giant cells (BNCs) in the ovine placenta (Jones et al., 1997; Klisch et al., 2006) could be involved in *N. caninum* adhesion to the placenta (**Figure 4A**).

Modulation of gene expression in the host cell is also a mechanism for *N. caninum* to invade and cross the placental barrier (Horcajo et al., 2017; Dorsch et al., 2019). Thus, infection of immortalized bovine trophoblasts with *N. caninum* induces the expression MMPs involved in ECM degradation (Cui et al., 2017; Horcajo et al., 2017). Additionally, infection by *N. caninum* alters the glycosylation pattern in the glycocalyx and apical cytoplasm of trophoblast (Dorsch et al., 2019; **Figure 4A**). The BNCs and the uterine epithelium also shows changes in sugars, including α-D-GalNAc, α-D-Man, β-D-Gal, α-D-Gluc, and NeuNac (Vonlaufen et al., 2004; Dorsch et al., 2019; **Figure 4A**). The expression of the adhesion molecules *E*-selectin, *P*-selectin, VCAM-1, and ICAM-1 is also altered, possibly through paracrine activation, through the pro-inflammatory cascade activation, which involves the release of IL-1b, IL-8, and MCP-1 leading to cell activation and subsequent expression of the adhesion molecules (Taubert et al., 2006).

Neospora caninum can also hijack immune cells to circumvent biological barriers. Thus, infection of DCs by tachyzoites enhances the translocation of parasites across cell monolayers (Collantes-Fernandez et al., 2012; **Figure 4A**). Furthermore, similar to *T. gondii* (Lambert et al., 2006; Lambert and Barragan, 2010), infection of DCs by *N. caninum* induce a migratory phenotype in these cells, enhancing its dissemination. In addition, *N. caninum* can infect MΦ and NK, cells and take advantage of their basal or inducible mobile properties (Boysen et al., 2006; Dion et al., 2011) (**Figures 4A,B**).

Immune Response Against *Neospora*

The immune response at the maternal-fetal interface against *N. caninum* is characterized by a mixture of Th1 and Th2 responses, implying the presence of pro-and anti-inflammatory cytokines (Cantón et al., 2014b; Hecker et al., 2015; Arranz-Solís et al., 2016; Gutiérrez-Expósito et al., 2020; **Figure 4B**). Although these responses play a vital role in controlling parasite multiplication, they are responsible for placental damage that might lead to abortion (Maley et al., 2006; Rosbottom et al., 2011; Cantón et al., 2014a; Gutiérrez-Expósito et al., 2020).

The role of the innate immune response in the placenta against *N. caninum* has been studied mainly in cattle. The parasite is recognized by endosomal TLRs (3, 7, 8, and 9), which are upregulated in response to Neospora infection (**Figure 4B**; Marin et al., 2017).

Similar to *T. gondii* infection, TLR 3/7 and 8 is associated with the control of *N. caninum* intracellular infection. TLR7 activation leads to the development of a protective Th1 response (Andrade et al., 2013; Castillo et al., 2018) through MyD88-dependent signaling (Mineo et al., 2009; Miranda et al., 2019) inducing the secretion of pro-inflammatory cytokines including IFN-γ, IL-12, IL-18, and TNF-α, and promotes recruitment of T lymphocyte (CD3, CD4, CD8, and γδ) subsets, MΦ, NK cells (NKp46 subpopulation) (Maley et al., 2006; Cantón et al., 2014a,b; Hecker et al., 2015; Arranz-Solís et al., 2016; Gutiérrez-Expósito et al., 2020; **Figure 4B**).

In addition, the Th2 (IL-4) and regulatory (IL-10) cytokines also show alterations during *N. caninum* infection (López-Pérez et al., 2010; Rosbottom et al., 2011). Thus, the increase of IL-4 attenuates the effects of the pro-inflammatory response and enhances susceptibility to *N. caninum* favoring congenital transmission (López-Pérez et al., 2010). On the other hand, IL-10 has a regulatory effect on IFN-γ and TNF-α mediated response (Eperon et al., 1999; Quinn et al., 2004) and might also promote the invasion and intracellular replication of *N. caninum* and consequently its transmission.

CONCLUSION

Apicomplexa are a large group of intracellular parasites that are distributed globally. Some of those parasites pose significant risks to pregnancy in humans and animals. The interaction between the parasites and hosts is the most critical factor in determining the success or failure of infection. During congenital infection, the parasites must break through the placental barrier and modulate host defenses. Apicomplexan parasites, despite having some differences during their life cycle, these parasites use very similar adhesion mechanisms to the placenta, based fundamentally on the alteration and modulation of the expression of molecules present on the surface of placental cells, including the trophoblast. Additionally, the presence of these parasites induces alterations in the immune response and a change in the Th1/Th2 balance, promoting the activation of defense mechanisms in the placenta based fundamentally on cellular immunity. This cellular immunity, mediated by different populations of T lymphocytes, secretion of chemokines, and pro-inflammatory cytokines, negatively affect the placental function and fetal growth that might ultimately cause fetal death and abortion.

Thus, better knowledge about changes in host gene expression, parasite strategies for modulating the host's immune system, among others, should clarify the mechanisms of congenital transmission of those parasites.

AUTHOR CONTRIBUTIONS

MR-P prepared the draft of the manuscript the figures. LM, MR, AL, CC, EP-P, JG-M, and SA corrected the draft and figures and participated in the different rounds of correcting the manuscript. UK corrected the manuscript into its final version for submission.

REFERENCES

Abbasi, M., Kowalewska-Grochowska, K., Bahar, M. A., Kilani, R. T., Winkler-Lowen, B., and Guilbert, L. J. (2003). Infection of placental trophoblasts by Toxoplasma gondii. *J. Infect. Dis.* 188, 608–616. doi: 10.1086/377132

Abeln, M., Albers, I., Peters-Bernard, U., Flächsig-Schulz, K., Kats, E., Kispert, A., et al. (2019). Sialic acid is a critical fetal defense against maternal complement attack. *J. Clin. Invest.* 129, 422–436. doi: 10.1172/JCI99945

Abrams, E. T., Brown, H., Chensue, S. W., Turner, G. D. H., Tadesse, E., Lema, V. M., et al. (2003). Host response to malaria during pregnancy: placental monocyte recruitment is associated with elevated beta chemokine expression. *J. Immunol.* 170, 2759–2764. doi: 10.4049/jimmunol.170.5.2759

Aderinboye, O., and Syed, S. S. (2010). Congenital babesiosis in a four-week-old female infant. *Pediatr. Infect. Dis. J.* 29:188. doi: 10.1097/INF.0b013e3181c3c971

Aikawa, M., Pongponratn, E., Tegoshi, T., Nakamura, K.-I., Nagatake, T., Cochrane, A., et al. (1992). A study on the pathogenesis of human cerebral malaria and cerebral babesiosis. *Memórias Instituto Oswaldo Cruz* 87, 297–301. doi: 10.1590/S0074-02761992000700051

Allred, D. R. (2019). Variable and Variant Protein Multigene Families in Babesia bovis Persistence. *Pathogens* 8:athogens8020076. doi: 10.3390/pathogens8020076

Allred, D. R., Carlton, J. M., Satcher, R. L., Long, J. A., Brown, W. C., Patterson, P. E., et al. (2000). The ves multigene family of B. bovis encodes components of rapid antigenic variation at the infected erythrocyte surface. *Mol. Cell* 5, 153–162. doi: 10.1016/s1097-2765(00)80411-6

Al-Shaeli, S. J. J., Ethaeb, A. M., and Gharban, H. A. J. (2020). Molecular and histopathological identification of ovine neosporosis (Neospora caninum) in aborted ewes in Iraq. *Vet. World* 13, 597–603. doi: 10.14202/vetworld.2020.597-603

Ander, S. E., Rudzki, E. N., Arora, N., Sadovsky, Y., Coyne, C. B., and Boyle, J. P. (2018). Human Placental Syncytiotrophoblasts Restrict Toxoplasma gondii Attachment and Replication and Respond to Infection by Producing Immunomodulatory Chemokines. *mBio* 9, 1678–1617. doi: 10.1128/mBio.01678-17

Andrade, W. A., Souza, M., do, C., Martinez, E. R., Nagpal, K., Dutra, M. S., et al. (2013). Combined action of Nucleic Acid-Sensing Toll-Like Receptors (TLRs) and TLR11/TLR12 heterodimers imparts resistance to Toxoplasma gondii in mice. *Cell Host Microbe* 13, 42–53. doi: 10.1016/j.chom.2012.12.003

Arranz-Solís, D., Benavides, J., Regidor-Cerrillo, J., Horcajo, P., Castaño, P., del Carmen, et al. (2016). Systemic and local immune responses in sheep after Neospora caninum experimental infection at early, mid and late gestation. *Vet. Res.* 47:0290. doi: 10.1186/s13567-015-0290-0

Arranz-Solís, D., Mukhopadhyay, D., and Saeij, J. J. P. (2021). Toxoplasma Effectors that Affect Pregnancy Outcome. *Trends Parasitol.* 37, 283–295. doi: 10.1016/j.pt.2020.10.013

Autino, B., Corbett, Y., Castelli, F., and Taramelli, D. (2012). Pathogenesis of Malaria in Tissues and Blood. *Mediterr. J. Hematol. Infect. Dis.* 4:061. doi: 10.4084/MJHID.2012.061

Azimi-Nezhad, M. (2014). Vascular endothelial growth factor from embryonic status to cardiovascular pathology. *Rep. Biochem. Mol. Biol.* 2, 59–69.

Azzouz, N., Kamena, F., Laurino, P., Kikkeri, R., Mercier, C., Cesbron-Delauw, M.-F., et al. (2013). Toxoplasma gondii secretory proteins bind to sulfated heparin structures. *Glycobiology* 23, 106–120. doi: 10.1093/glycob/cws134

Baba, M., Batanova, T., Kitoh, K., and Takashima, Y. (2017). Adhesion of Toxoplasma gondii tachyzoite-infected vehicle leukocytes to capillary endothelial cells triggers timely parasite egression. *Sci. Rep.* 7:5675. doi: 10.1038/s41598-017-05956-z

Bachmeyer, C., Mouchnino, G., Thulliez, P., and Blum, L. (2006). Congenital toxoplasmosis from an HIV-infected woman as a result of reactivation. *J. Infect.* 52, e55–e57. doi: 10.1016/j.jinf.2005.05.004

Barbosa, B. F., Paulesu, L., Ietta, F., Bechi, N., Romagnoli, R., Gomes, A. O., et al. (2014). Susceptibility to Toxoplasma gondii proliferation in BeWo human trophoblast cells is dose-dependent of macrophage migration inhibitory factor (MIF), via ERK1/2 phosphorylation and prostaglandin E2 production. *Placenta* 35, 152–162. doi: 10.1016/j.placenta.2013.12.013

Barboza, R., Lima, F. A., Reis, A. S., Murillo, O. J., Peixoto, E. P. M., Bandeira, C. L., et al. (2017). TLR4-Mediated Placental Pathology and Pregnancy Outcome in Experimental Malaria. *Sci. Rep.* 7:8623. doi: 10.1038/s41598-017-08299-x

Barboza, R., Reis, A. S., da Silva, L. G., Hasenkamp, L., Pereira, K. R. B., Câmara, N. O. S., et al. (2014). MyD88 signaling is directly involved in the development of murine placental malaria. *Infect. Immun.* 82, 830–838. doi: 10.1128/IAI.01288-13

Barfod, L., Dalgaard, M. B., Pleman, S. T., Ofori, M. F., Pleass, R. J., and Hviid, L. (2011). Evasion of immunity to Plasmodium falciparum malaria by IgM masking of protective IgG epitopes in infected erythrocyte surface-exposed PfEMP1. *PNAS* 108, 12485–12490. doi: 10.1073/pnas.1103708108

Barr, B. C., Conrad, P. A., Sverlow, K. W., Tarantal, A. F., and Hendrickx, A. G. (1994). Experimental fetal and transplacental Neospora infection in the nonhuman primate. *Lab. Invest.* 71, 236–242.

Barragan, A., Brossier, F., and Sibley, L. D. (2005). Transepithelial migration of Toxoplasma gondii involves an interaction of intercellular adhesion molecule 1 (ICAM-1) with the parasite adhesin MIC2. *Cell. Microbiol.* 7, 561–568. doi: 10.1111/j.1462-5822.2005.00486.x

Baruch, D. I., Gormely, J. A., Ma, C., Howard, R. J., and Pasloske, B. L. (1996). Plasmodium falciparum erythrocyte membrane protein 1 is a parasitized erythrocyte receptor for adherence to CD36, thrombospondin, and intercellular adhesion molecule 1. *Proc. Natl. Acad. Sci. U S A.* 93, 3497–3502. doi: 10.1073/pnas.93.8.3497

Beeson, J. G., Amin, N., Kanjala, M., and Rogerson, S. J. (2002). Selective Accumulation of Mature Asexual Stages of Plasmodium falciparum-Infected Erythrocytes in the Placenta. *Infect. Immun.* 70, 5412–5415. doi: 10.1128/IAI.70.10.5412-5415.2002

Beeson, J. G., and Brown, G. V. (2004). Plasmodium falciparum-infected erythrocytes demonstrate dual specificity for adhesion to hyaluronic acid and chondroitin sulfate A and have distinct adhesive properties. *J. Infect. Dis.* 189, 169–179. doi: 10.1086/380975

Beeson, J. G., Brown, G. V., Molyneux, M. E., Mhango, C., Dzinjalamala, F., and Rogerson, S. J. (1999). Plasmodium falciparum Isolates from Infected Pregnant Women and Children Are Associated with Distinct Adhesive and Antigenic Properties. *J. Infect. Dis.* 180, 464–472. doi: 10.1086/314899

Benavente, E. D., Oresegun, D. R., de Sessions, P. F., Walker, E. M., Roper, C., Dombrowski, J. G., et al. (2018). Global genetic diversity of var2csa in

Plasmodium falciparum with implications for malaria in pregnancy and vaccine development. *Sci. Rep.* 8:15429. doi: 10.1038/s41598-018-33767-3

Benirschke, K., Kaufmann, P., and Baergen, P. (2012). *Pathology of the Human Placenta*, 6 th Edn. New York, NY: SpringerLink.

Berger, S. S., Turner, L., Wang, C. W., Petersen, J. E. V., Kraft, M., Lusingu, J. P. A., et al. (2013). Plasmodium falciparum expressing domain cassette 5 type PfEMP1 (DC5-PfEMP1) bind PECAM1. *PLoS One* 8:e69117. doi: 10.1371/journal.pone.0069117

Bhatia, R., Rajwaniya, D., and Agrawal, P. (2016). Congenital Malaria due to Plasmodium Vivax Infection in a Neonate. *Case Rep. Pediatr.* 2016:1929046. doi: 10.1155/2016/1929046

Blader, I. J., and Saeij, J. P. (2009). Communication between Toxoplasma gondii and its host: impact on parasite growth, development, immune evasion, and virulence. *APMIS* 117, 458–476. doi: 10.1111/j.1600-0463.2009.02453.x

Blumenschein, T. M. A., Friedrich, N., Childs, R. A., Saouros, S., Carpenter, E. P., Campanero-Rhodes, M. A., et al. (2007). Atomic resolution insight into host cell recognition by Toxoplasma gondii. *EMBO J.* 26, 2808–2820. doi: 10.1038/sj.emboj.7601704

Bosman, A.-M., Oosthuizen, M. C., Venter, E. H., Steyl, J. C., Gous, T. A., and Penzhorn, B. L. (2013). Babesia lengau associated with cerebral and haemolytic babesiosis in two domestic cats. *Parasit. Vectors* 6:128. doi: 10.1186/1756-3305-6-128

Boysen, P., Klevar, S., Olsen, I., and Storset, A. K. (2006). The Protozoan Neospora caninum Directly Triggers Bovine NK Cells To Produce Gamma Interferon and To Kill Infected Fibroblasts. *Infect. Immun.* 74, 953–960. doi: 10.1128/IAI.74.2.953-960.2006

Briand, V., Le Hesran, J.-Y., Mayxay, M., Newton, P. N., Bertin, G., Houzé, S., et al. (2016). Prevalence of malaria in pregnancy in southern Laos: a cross-sectional survey. *Malaria J.* 15:436. doi: 10.1186/s12936-016-1492-2

Buxton, D., Maley, S. W., Wright, S., Thomson, K. M., Rae, A. G., and Innes, E. A. (1998). The pathogenesis of experimental neosporosis in pregnant sheep. *J. Comparat. Pathol.* 118, 267–279. doi: 10.1016/S0021-9975(07)80003-X

Cantón, G. J., Katzer, F., Maley, S. W., Bartley, P. M., Benavides-Silván, J., Palarea-Albaladejo, J., et al. (2014a). Cytokine expression in the placenta of pregnant cattle after inoculation with Neospora caninum. *Vet. Immunol. Immunopathol.* 161, 77–89. doi: 10.1016/j.vetimm.2014.07.004

Cantón, G. J., Katzer, F., Maley, S. W., Bartley, P. M., Benavides-Silván, J., Palarea-Albaladejo, J., et al. (2014b). Inflammatory infiltration into placentas of Neospora caninum challenged cattle correlates with clinical outcome of pregnancy. *Vet. Res.* 45:11. doi: 10.1186/1297-9716-45-11

Capellini, I., Nunn, C. L., and Barton, R. A. (2015). Microparasites and Placental Invasiveness in Eutherian Mammals. *PLoS One* 10:e0132563. doi: 10.1371/journal.pone.0132563

Carlier, Y., Truyens, C., Deloron, P., and Peyron, F. (2012). Congenital parasitic infections: A review. *Acta Tropica* 121, 55–70. doi: 10.1016/j.actatropica.2011.10.018

Carruthers, V., and Boothroyd, J. C. (2007). Pulling together: an integrated model of Toxoplasma cell invasion. *Curr. Opin. Microbiol.* 10, 83–89. doi: 10.1016/j.mib.2006.06.017

Castillo, C., Liempi, A., Medina, L., and Kemmerling, I. C. (2018). Antiparasitic Mechanisms of the Human Placenta. *Chagas Dis. Basic Investigat. Challenges* 2018:73569. doi: 10.5772/intechopen.73569

Castillo, C., Muñoz, L., Carrillo, I., Liempi, A., Gallardo, C., Galanti, N., et al. (2017a). Ex vivo infection of human placental chorionic villi explants with Trypanosoma cruzi and Toxoplasma gondii induces different Toll-like receptor expression and cytokine/chemokine profiles. *Am. J. Reprod. Immunol.* 78:12660. doi: 10.1111/aji.12660

Castillo, C., Muñoz, L., Carrillo, I., Liempi, A., Medina, L., Galanti, N., et al. (2017b). Toll-like receptor-2 mediates local innate immune response against Trypanosoma cruzi in ex vivo infected human placental chorionic villi explants. *Placenta* 60, 40–46. doi: 10.1016/j.placenta.2017.10.005

Chakraborty, A. (2016). Understanding the biology of the Plasmodium falciparum apicoplast; an excellent target for antimalarial drug development. *Life Sci.* 158, 104–110. doi: 10.1016/j.lfs.2016.06.030

Chakraborty, S., Roy, S., Mistry, H. U., Murthy, S., George, N., Bhandari, V., et al. (2017). Potential Sabotage of Host Cell Physiology by Apicomplexan Parasites for Their Survival Benefits. *Front. Immunol.* 8:01261. doi: 10.3389/fimmu.2017.01261

Chan, J.-A., Fowkes, F. J. I., and Beeson, J. G. (2014). Surface antigens of Plasmodium falciparum-infected erythrocytes as immune targets and malaria vaccine candidates. *Cell. Mol. Life Sci.* 71, 3633–3657. doi: 10.1007/s00018-014-1614-3

Chau, K., Hennessy, A., and Makris, A. (2017). Placental growth factor and pre-eclampsia. *J. Hum. Hypertens* 31, 782–786. doi: 10.1038/jhh.2017.61

Chen, C.-P., and Aplin, J. D. (2003). Placental extracellular matrix: gene expression, deposition by placental fibroblasts and the effect of oxygen. *Placenta* 24, 316–325. doi: 10.1053/plac.2002.0904

Chêne, A., Briand, V., Ibitokou, S., Dechavanne, S., Massougbodji, A., Deloron, P., et al. (2014). Placental cytokine and chemokine profiles reflect pregnancy outcomes in women exposed to Plasmodium falciparum infection. *Infect. Immun.* 82, 3783–3789. doi: 10.1128/IAI.01922-14

Chesnokov, O., Merritt, J., Tcherniuk, S. O., Milman, N., and Oleinikov, A. V. (2018). Plasmodium falciparum infected erythrocytes can bind to host receptors integrins αVβ3 and αVβ6 through DBLδ1_D4 domain of PFL2665c PfEMP1 protein. *Sci. Rep.* 8:17871. doi: 10.1038/s41598-018-36071-2

Chishti, A. H. (2015). Malaria selectively targets pregnancy receptors. *Blood* 125, 217–218. doi: 10.1182/blood-2014-11-610634

Chotivanich, K., Udomsangpetch, R., Suwanarusk, R., Pukrittayakamee, S., Wilairatana, P., Beeson, J. G., et al. (2012). Plasmodium vivax Adherence to Placental Glycosaminoglycans. *PLoS One* 7:0034509. doi: 10.1371/journal.pone.0034509

Clark, R. L. (2019). Genesis of placental sequestration in malaria and possible targets for drugs for placental malaria. *Birth Defects Res.* 111, 569–583. doi: 10.1002/bdr2.1496

Coban, C., Ishii, K. J., Kawai, T., Hemmi, H., Sato, S., Uematsu, S., et al. (2005). Toll-like receptor 9 mediates innate immune activation by the malaria pigment hemozoin. *J. Exp. Med.* 201, 19–25. doi: 10.1084/jem.20041836

Cole, R. A., Lindsay, D. S., Blagburn, B. L., and Dubey, J. P. (1995). Vertical Transmission of Neospora caninum in Mice. *J. Parasitol.* 81, 730–732. doi: 10.2307/3283962

Collantes-Fernandez, E., Arrighi, R. B. G., Álvarez-García, G., Weidner, J. M., Regidor-Cerrillo, J., Boothroyd, J. C., et al. (2012). Infected Dendritic Cells Facilitate Systemic Dissemination and Transplacental Passage of the Obligate Intracellular Parasite Neospora caninum in Mice. *PLoS One* 7:e32123. doi: 10.1371/journal.pone.0032123

Collins, W. E., and Jeffery, G. M. (2005). Plasmodium ovale: parasite and disease. *Clin. Microbiol. Rev.* 18, 570–581. doi: 10.1128/CMR.18.3.570-581.2005

Conroy, A. L., McDonald, C. R., Silver, K. L., Liles, W. C., and Kain, K. C. (2011). Complement activation: a critical mediator of adverse fetal outcomes in placental malaria? *Trends Parasitol.* 27, 294–299. doi: 10.1016/j.pt.2011.02.005

Cooke, B. M., Mohandas, N., Cowman, A. F., and Coppel, R. L. (2005). Cellular adhesive phenomena in apicomplexan parasites of red blood cells. *Vet. Parasitol.* 132, 273–295. doi: 10.1016/j.vetpar.2005.07.002

Cornett, J. K., Malhotra, A., and Hart, D. (2012). Vertical Transmission of Babesiosis From a Pregnant, Splenectomized Mother to Her Neonate. *Infect. Dis. Clin. Pract.* 20, 408–410. doi: 10.1097/IPC.0b013e31825b20c1

Cox, F. E. G. (1982). "Babesiosis in Rodents and Humans," in *Animal Models in Parasitology: A Symposium held at the Royal Zoological Society, Regents Park, London, in March 1981*, ed. D. G. Owen (London: Macmillan Education UK), 83–91. doi: 10.1007/978-1-349-06136-5_5

Crawford, J., Grujic, O., Bruic, E., Czjzek, M., Grigg, M. E., and Boulanger, M. J. (2009). Structural Characterization of the Bradyzoite Surface Antigen (BSR4) from Toxoplasma gondii, a Unique Addition to the Surface Antigen Glycoprotein 1-related Superfamily. *J. Biol. Chem.* 284, 9192–9198. doi: 10.1074/jbc.M808714200

Cui, N., Hu, M., and Khalil, R. A. (2017). Biochemical and Biological Attributes of Matrix Metalloproteinases. *Prog. Mol. Biol. Transl. Sci.* 147, 1–73. doi: 10.1016/bs.pmbts.2017.02.005

de Oliveira Gomes, A., de Oliveira Silva, D. A., Silva, N. M., de Freitas Barbosa, B., Franco, P. S., Angeloni, M. B., et al. (2011). Effect of Macrophage Migration Inhibitory Factor (MIF) in Human Placental Explants Infected with Toxoplasma gondii Depends on Gestational Age. *Am. J. Pathol.* 178, 2792–2801. doi: 10.1016/j.ajpath.2011.02.005

De Silva, D. H. G., Mendis, K. N., Premaratne, U. N., Jayatilleke, S. M. D., and Soyza, P. E. (1982). Congenital malaria due to Plasmodium vivax: a case report from Sri Lanka. *Transact. R. Soc. Trop. Med. Hygiene* 76, 33–35. doi: 10.1016/0035-9203(82)90011-6

Debierre-Grockiego, F., Campos, M. A., Azzouz, N., Schmidt, J., Bieker, U., Resende, M. G., et al. (2007). Activation of TLR2 and TLR4 by Glycosylphosphatidylinositols Derived from Toxoplasma gondii. *J. Immunol.* 179, 1129–1137.

del Campo, J., Heger, T. J., Rodríguez-Martínez, R., Worden, A. Z., Richards, T. A., Massana, R., et al. (2019). Assessing the Diversity and Distribution of Apicomplexans in Host and Free-Living Environments Using High-Throughput Amplicon Data and a Phylogenetically Informed Reference Framework. *Front. Microbiol.* 10:02373. doi: 10.3389/fmicb.2019.02373

Denkers, E. Y. (2010). Toll-Like Receptor Initiated Host Defense against Toxoplasma gondii. *J. Biomed. Biotechnol.* 2010:737125. doi: 10.1155/2010/737125

Diallo, M., Aldebert, D., Moreau, J.-C., Ndiaye, M., and Jambou, R. (2008). Decrease of lymphoid dendritic cells in blood from malaria-infected pregnant women. *Int. J. Parasitol.* 38, 1557–1565. doi: 10.1016/j.ijpara.2008.04.013

Dion, Ş., Germon, S., Guiton, R., Ducournau, C., and Dimier-Poisson, I. (2011). Functional activation of T cells by dendritic cells and macrophages exposed to the intracellular parasite Neospora caninum. *Int. J. Parasitol.* 41, 685–695. doi: 10.1016/j.ijpara.2011.01.008

Dobaño, C., Berthoud, T., Manaca, M. N., Nhabomba, A., Guinovart, C., Aguilar, R., et al. (2018). High production of pro-inflammatory cytokines by maternal blood mononuclear cells is associated with reduced maternal malaria but increased cord blood infection. *Malar. J.* 17:177. doi: 10.1186/s12936-018-2317-2

Dobbs, K. R., and Dent, A. E. (2016). Plasmodium malaria and antimalarial antibodies in the first year of life. *Parasitology* 143, 129–138. doi: 10.1017/S0031182015001626

Dombrowski, J. G., de Souza, R. M., Silva, N. R. M., Barateiro, A., Epiphanio, S., Gonçalves, L. A., et al. (2018). Malaria during pregnancy and newborn outcome in an unstable transmission area in Brazil: A population-based record linkage study. *PLoS One* 13:e0199415. doi: 10.1371/journal.pone.0199415

Donahoe, S. L., Lindsay, S. A., Krockenberger, M., Phalen, D., and Šlapeta, J. (2015). A review of neosporosis and pathologic findings of Neospora caninum infection in wildlife. *Int. J. Parasitol. Parasites Wildl.* 4, 216–238. doi: 10.1016/j.ijppaw.2015.04.002

Dong, J., Otsuki, T., Kato, T., and Park, E. Y. (2012). Development of a diagnostic method for neosporosis in cattle using recombinant Neospora caninum proteins. *BMC Biotechnol.* 12:19. doi: 10.1186/1472-6750-12-19

Dorsch, M. A., de Yaniz, M. G., Fiorani, F., Hecker, Y. P., Odeón, A. C., Morrell, E. L., et al. (2019). A Descriptive Study of Lectin Histochemistry of the Placenta in Cattle following Inoculation of Neospora caninum. *J. Comparat. Pathol.* 166, 45–53. doi: 10.1016/j.jcpa.2018.10.172

Dos Santos, T. R., Faria, G., da, S. M., Guerreiro, B. M., Dal Pietro, N. H. P., da, S., et al. (2016). Congenital Toxoplasmosis in Chronically Infected and Subsequently Challenged Ewes. *PLoS One* 11:e0165124. doi: 10.1371/journal.pone.0165124

Duarte, P. O., Oshiro, L. M., Zimmermann, N. P., Csordas, B. G., Dourado, D. M., Barros, J. C., et al. (2020). Serological and molecular detection of Neospora caninum and Toxoplasma gondii in human umbilical cord blood and placental tissue samples. *Sci. Rep.* 10, 65991–65991. doi: 10.1038/s41598-020-65991-1

Duaso, J., Rojo, G., Cabrera, G., Galanti, N., Bosco, C., Maya, J. D., et al. (2010). Trypanosoma cruzi induces tissue disorganization and destruction of chorionic villi in an ex vivo infection model of human placenta. *Placenta* 31, 705–711. doi: 10.1016/j.placenta.2010.05.007

Dubey, J. P. (2003). Review of Neospora caninum and neosporosis in animals. *Kor. J. Parasitol.* 41, 1–16. doi: 10.3347/kjp.2003.41.1.1

Dubey, J. P., Graham, D. H., Dahl, E., Sreekumar, C., Lehmann, T., Davis, M. F., et al. (2003). Toxoplasma gondii isolates from free-ranging chickens from the United States. *J. Parasitol.* 89, 1060–1062. doi: 10.1645/GE-124R

Dubey, J. P., Hemphill, A., Calero-Bernal, R., and Schares, G. (2017). *Neosporosis in animals*, 1st Edn. Florida, FL: CRC Press.

Dubey, J. P., Schares, G., and Ortega-Mora, L. M. (2007). Epidemiology and Control of Neosporosis and Neospora caninum. *Clin. Microbiol. Rev.* 20, 323–367. doi: 10.1128/CMR.00031-06

Dubey, J. P., Verma, S. K., Ferreira, L. R., Oliveira, S., Cassinelli, A. B., Ying, Y., et al. (2014). Detection and survival of Toxoplasma gondii in milk and cheese from experimentally infected goats. *J. Food Prot.* 77, 1747–1753. doi: 10.4315/0362-028X.JFP-14-167

Duncanson, P., Terry, R. S., Smith, J. E., and Hide, G. (2001). High levels of congenital transmission of Toxoplasma gondii in a commercial sheep flock. *Int. J. Parasitol.* 31, 1699–1703. doi: 10.1016/S0020-7519(01)00282-X

Efstratiou, A., Galon, E. M. S., Wang, G., Umeda, K., Kondoh, D., Terkawi, M. A., et al. (2020). Babesia microti Confers Macrophage-Based Cross-Protective Immunity Against Murine Malaria. *Front. Cell. Infect. Microbiol.* 10:00193. doi: 10.3389/fcimb.2020.00193

Eperon, S., Brönnimann, K., Hemphill, A., and Gottstein, B. (1999). Susceptibility of B-cell deficient C57BL/6 (microMT) mice to Neospora caninum infection. *Parasite Immunol.* 21, 225–236. doi: 10.1046/j.1365-3024.1999.00223.x

Esernio-Jenssen, D., Scimeca, P. G., Benach, J. L., and Tenenbaum, M. J. (1987). Transplacental/perinatal babesiosis. *J. Pediatr.* 110, 570–572. doi: 10.1016/s0022-3476(87)80552-8

Ferro, E. A. V., Mineo, J. R., Ietta, F., Bechi, N., Romagnoli, R., Silva, D. A. O., et al. (2008). Macrophage Migration Inhibitory Factor Is Up-Regulated in Human First-Trimester Placenta Stimulated by Soluble Antigen of Toxoplasma gondii, Resulting in Increased Monocyte Adhesion on Villous Explants. *Am. J. Pathol.* 172, 50–58. doi: 10.2353/ajpath.2008.070432

Flick, K., Scholander, C., Chen, Q., Fernandez, V., Pouvelle, B., Gysin, J., et al. (2001). Role of nonimmune IgG bound to PfEMP1 in placental malaria. *Science* 293, 2098–2100. doi: 10.1126/science.1062891

Fortier, B., Aïssi, E., Ajana, F., Dieusart, P., Denis, P., Martin, et al. (1991). Spontaneous abortion and reinfection by Toxoplasma gondii. *Lancet* 338:444. doi: 10.1016/0140-6736(91)91064-2

Fried, M., Domingo, G. J., Gowda, C. D., Mutabingwa, T. K., and Duffy, P. E. (2006). Plasmodium falciparum: chondroitin sulfate A is the major receptor for adhesion of parasitized erythrocytes in the placenta. *Exp. Parasitol.* 113, 36–42. doi: 10.1016/j.exppara.2005.12.003

Fried, M., Muga, R. O., Misore, A. O., and Duffy, P. E. (1998). Malaria elicits type 1 cytokines in the human placenta: IFN-gamma and TNF-alpha associated with pregnancy outcomes. *J. Immunol.* 160, 2523–2530.

Friedrich, N., Santos, J. M., Liu, Y., Palma, A. S., Leon, E., Saouros, S., et al. (2010). Members of a novel protein family containing microneme adhesive repeat domains act as sialic acid-binding lectins during host cell invasion by apicomplexan parasites. *J. Biol. Chem.* 285, 2064–2076. doi: 10.1074/jbc.M109.060988

Fuentes, I., Rubio, J. M., Ramírez, C., and Alvar, J. (2001). Genotypic Characterization of Toxoplasma gondii Strains Associated with Human Toxoplasmosis in Spain: Direct Analysis from Clinical Samples. *J. Clin. Microbiol.* 39, 1566–1570. doi: 10.1128/JCM.39.4.1566-1570.2001

Furtado, G. C., Cao, Y., and Joiner, K. A. (1992). Laminin on Toxoplasma gondii mediates parasite binding to the beta 1 integrin receptor alpha 6 beta 1 on human foreskin fibroblasts and Chinese hamster ovary cells. *Infect. Immun.* 60, 4925–4931. doi: 10.1128/IAI.60.11.4925-4931.1992

Gabrielli, S., Bellina, L., Milardi, G. L., Katende, B. K., Totino, V., Fullin, V., et al. (2016). Malaria in children of Tshimbulu (Western Kasai, Democratic Republic of the Congo): epidemiological data and accuracy of diagnostic assays applied in a limited resource setting. *Malar. J.* 15:81. doi: 10.1186/s12936-016-1142-8

Gallego-Lopez, G. M., Cooke, B. M., and Suarez, C. E. (2019). Interplay between Attenuation- and Virulence-Factors of Babesia bovis and Their Contribution to the Establishment of Persistent Infections in Cattle. *Pathogens* 8:athogens8030097. doi: 10.3390/pathogens8030097

Garcia-Lloret, M. I., Winkler-Lowen, B., and Guilbert, L. J. (2000). Monocytes adhering by LFA-1 to placental syncytiotrophoblasts induce local apoptosis via release of TNF-alpha. A model for hematogenous initiation of placental inflammations. *J. Leukoc. Biol.* 68, 903–908.

Gaw, S. L., Hromatka, B. S., Ngeleza, S., Buarpung, S., Ozarslan, N., Tshefu, A., et al. (2019). Differential Activation of Fetal Hofbauer Cells in Primigravidas Is Associated with Decreased Birth Weight in Symptomatic Placental Malaria. *Malar. Res. Treat.* 2019:1378174. doi: 10.1155/2019/1378174

Ge, Y. Y., Zhang, L., Zhang, G., Wu, J. P., Tan, M. J., Hu, E., et al. (2008). In pregnant mice, the infection of Toxoplasma gondii causes the decrease of CD4+CD25+-regulatory T cells - GE - 2008 - Parasite Immunology - Wiley Online Library. *Parasite Immunol.* 30, 471–481.

Geleta, G., and Ketema, T. (2016). Severe Malaria Associated with Plasmodium falciparum and P. vivax among Children in Pawe Hospital. Northwest Ethiopia. *Malar. Res. Treat.* 2016:1240962. doi: 10.1155/2016/1240962

Gibney, E. H., Kipar, A., Rosbottom, A., Guy, C. S., Smith, R. F., Hetzel, U., et al. (2008). The extent of parasite-associated necrosis in the placenta and foetal tissues of cattle following Neospora caninum infection in early and late gestation correlates with foetal death. *Int. J. Parasitol.* 38, 579–588. doi: 10.1016/j.ijpara.2007.09.015

Gilbert, R. E., Freeman, K., Lago, E. G., Bahia-Oliveira, L. M. G., Tan, H. K., Wallon, M., et al. (2008). Ocular sequelae of congenital toxoplasmosis in Brazil compared with Europe. *PLoS Negl. Trop. Dis.* 2:e277. doi: 10.1371/journal.pntd.0000277

Gillrie, M. R., Avril, M., Brazier, A. J., Davis, S. P., Stins, M. F., Smith, J. D., et al. (2015). Diverse functional outcomes of Plasmodium falciparum ligation of EPCR: potential implications for malarial pathogenesis. *Cell. Microbiol.* 17, 1883–1899. doi: 10.1111/cmi.12479

Gimenez, G., Magalhães, K. G., Belaunzarán, M. L., Poncini, C. V., Lammel, E. M., Gonzalez Cappa, S. M., et al. (2010). Lipids from attenuated and virulent Babesia bovis strains induce differential TLR2-mediated macrophage activation. *Mol. Immunol.* 47, 747–755. doi: 10.1016/j.molimm.2009.10.014

Gómez-Chávez, F., Cañedo-Solares, I., Ortiz-Alegría, L. B., Flores-García, Y., Figueroa-Damián, R., and Luna-Pastén, H. et al. (2020). A Proinflammatory immune response might determine *Toxoplasma gondii* vertical transmission and severity of clinical features in congenitally infected newborns. *Molecules* 26:390. doi: 10.3389/fimmu.2020.00390

Gómez-Chávez, F., Cañedo-Solares, I., Ortiz-Alegría, L. B., Flores-García, Y., Luna-Pastén, H., Figueroa-Damián, R., et al. (2019). Maternal Immune Response During Pregnancy and Vertical Transmission in Human Toxoplasmosis. *Front. Immunol.* 10:00285. doi: 10.3389/fimmu.2019.00285

González-Warleta, M., Castro-Hermida, J. A., Calvo, C., Pérez, V., Gutiérrez-Expósito, D., Regidor-Cerrillo, J., et al. (2018). Endogenous transplacental transmission of Neospora caninum during successive pregnancies across three generations of naturally infected sheep. *Vet. Res.* 49:106. doi: 10.1186/s13567-018-0601-3

Griffiths, S. K., and Campbell, J. P. (2015). Placental structure, function and drug transfer. *Contin. Educat. Anaesthes. Crit. Care Pain* 15, 84–89. doi: 10.1093/bjaceaccp/mku013

Gude, N. M., Roberts, C. T., Kalionis, B., and King, R. G. (2004). Growth and function of the normal human placenta. *Thromb. Res.* 114, 397–407. doi: 10.1016/j.thromres.2004.06.038

Gutiérrez-Expósito, D., González-Warleta, M., Espinosa, J., Vallejo-García, R., Castro-Hermida, J. A., Calvo, C., et al. (2020). Maternal immune response in the placenta of sheep during recrudescence of natural congenital infection of Neospora caninum. *Vet. Parasitol.* 285:109204. doi: 10.1016/j.vetpar.2020.109204

Haldorson, G. J., Mathison, B. A., Wenberg, K., Conrad, P. A., Dubey, J. P., Trees, A. J., et al. (2005). Immunization with native surface protein NcSRS2 induces a Th2 immune response and reduces congenital Neospora caninum transmission in mice. *Int. J. Parasitol.* 35, 1407–1415. doi: 10.1016/j.ijpara.2005.05.013

Haldorson, G. J., Stanton, J. B., Mathison, B. A., Suarez, C. E., and Baszler, T. V. (2006). Neospora caninum: antibodies directed against tachyzoite surface protein NcSRS2 inhibit parasite attachment and invasion of placental trophoblasts in vitro. *Exp. Parasitol.* 112, 172–178. doi: 10.1016/j.exppara.2005.11.004

Hamann, L., Bedu-Addo, G., Eggelte, T. A., Schumann, R. R., and Mockenhaupt, F. P. (2010). The toll-like receptor 1 variant S248N influences placental malaria. *Infect. Genet. Evolut.* 10, 785–789. doi: 10.1016/j.meegid.2010.05.005

Harker, K. S., Ueno, N., Wang, T., Bonhomme, C., Liu, W., and Lodoen, M. B. (2013). Toxoplasma gondii modulates the dynamics of human monocyte adhesion to vascular endothelium under fluidic shear stress. *J. Leukoc. Biol.* 93, 789–800. doi: 10.1189/jlb.1012517

He, X., Grigg, M. E., Boothroyd, J. C., and Garcia, K. C. (2002). Structure of the immunodominant surface antigen from the Toxoplasma gondii SRS superfamily. *Nat. Struct. Biol.* 9, 606–611. doi: 10.1038/nsb819

Hecker, Y. P., Cantón, G., Regidor-Cerrillo, J., Chianini, F., Morrell, E., Lischinsky, L., et al. (2015). Cell mediated immune responses in the placenta following challenge of vaccinated pregnant heifers with Neospora caninum. *Vet. Parasitol.* 214, 247–254. doi: 10.1016/j.vetpar.2015.10.015

Hemphill, A., Debache, K., Monney, T., Schorer, M., Guionaud, C., Alaeddine, F., et al. (2013). Proteins mediating the Neospora caninum-host cell interaction as targets for vaccination. *Front. Biosci.* 5:23–36. doi: 10.2741/e593

Hemphill, A., Vonlaufen, N., Naguleswaran, A., Keller, N., Riesen, M., Guetg, N., et al. (2004). Tissue culture and explant approaches to studying and visualizing Neospora caninum and its interactions with the host cell. *Microsc. Microanal.* 10, 602–620. doi: 10.1017/S1431927604040930

Hide, G. (2016). Role of vertical transmission of Toxoplasma gondii in prevalence of infection. *Expert Rev. Anti Infect. Ther.* 14, 335–344. doi: 10.1586/14787210.2016.1146131

Ho, M. S., Barr, B. C., Tarantal, A. F., Lai, L. T., Hendrickx, A. G., Marsh, A. E., et al. (1997). Detection of Neospora from tissues of experimentally infected rhesus macaques by PCR and specific DNA probe hybridization. *J. Clin. Microbiol.* 35, 1740–1745.

Horcajo, P., Jiménez-Pelayo, L., García-Sánchez, M., Regidor-Cerrillo, J., Collantes-Fernández, E., Rozas, D., et al. (2017). Transcriptome modulation of bovine trophoblast cells in vitro by Neospora caninum. *Int. J. Parasitol.* 47, 791–799. doi: 10.1016/j.ijpara.2017.08.007

Howe, D. K., Crawford, A. C., Lindsay, D., and Sibley, L. D. (1998). The p29 and p35 immunodominant antigens of Neospora caninum tachyzoites are homologous to the family of surface antigens of Toxoplasma gondii. *Infect. Immun.* 66, 5322–5328. doi: 10.1128/IAI.66.11.5322-5328.1998

Hsieh, F.-L., Turner, L., Bolla, J. R., Robinson, C. V., Lavstsen, T., and Higgins, M. K. (2016). The structural basis for CD36 binding by the malaria parasite. *Nat. Commun.* 7:12837. doi: 10.1038/ncomms12837

Hutchings, C. L., Li, A., Fernandez, K. M., Fletcher, T., Jackson, L. A., Molloy, J. B., et al. (2007). New insights into the altered adhesive and mechanical properties of red blood cells parasitized by Babesia bovis. *Mol. Microbiol.* 65, 1092–1105. doi: 10.1111/j.1365-2958.2007.05850.x

Hutson, S. L., Wheeler, K. M., McLone, D., Frim, D., Penn, R., Swisher, C. N., et al. (2015). Patterns of Hydrocephalus Caused by Congenital Toxoplasma gondii Infection Associate With Parasite Genetics. *Clin. Infect. Dis.* 61, 1831–1834. doi: 10.1093/cid/civ720

Ibrahim, H. M., Huang, P., Salem, T. A., Talaat, R. M., Nasr, M. I., Xuan, X., et al. (2009). Short report: prevalence of Neospora caninum and Toxoplasma gondii antibodies in northern Egypt. *Am. J. Trop. Med. Hyg.* 80, 263–267.

Jackson, A. P., Otto, T. D., Darby, A., Ramaprasad, A., Xia, D., Echaide, I. E., et al. (2014). The evolutionary dynamics of variant antigen genes in Babesia reveal a history of genomic innovation underlying host-parasite interaction. *Nucleic Acids Res.* 42, 7113–7131. doi: 10.1093/nar/gku322

Jacquet, A., Coulon, L., De Nève, J., Daminet, V., Haumont, M., Garcia, L., et al. (2001). The surface antigen SAG3 mediates the attachment of Toxoplasma gondii to cell-surface proteoglycans. *Mol. Biochem. Parasitol.* 116, 35–44. doi: 10.1016/s0166-6851(01)00297-3

Jeninga, M. D., Quinn, J. E., and Petter, M. (2019). ApiAP2 Transcription Factors in Apicomplexan Parasites. *Pathogens* 8:athogens8020047. doi: 10.3390/pathogens8020047

Jenkins, H. G. (1957). Congenital Malaria in England—Plasmodium Ovale. *Br. Med. J.* 1, 88–89.

Jiménez-Pelayo, L., García-Sánchez, M., Regidor-Cerrillo, J., Horcajo, P., Collantes-Fernández, E., Gómez-Bautista, M., et al. (2017). Differential susceptibility of bovine caruncular and trophoblast cell lines to infection with high and low virulence isolates of Neospora caninum. *Parasit. Vectors* 10:463. doi: 10.1186/s13071-017-2409-9

Jiménez-Pelayo, L., García-Sánchez, M., Regidor-Cerrillo, J., Horcajo, P., Collantes-Fernández, E., Gómez-Bautista, M., et al. (2019). Immune response profile of caruncular and trophoblast cell lines infected by high- (Nc-Spain7) and low-virulence (Nc-Spain1H) isolates of Neospora caninum. *Parasites Vectors* 12:218. doi: 10.1186/s13071-019-3466-z

Jones, C. J., Dantzer, V., Leiser, R., Krebs, C., and Stoddart, R. W. (1997). Localisation of glycans in the placenta: a comparative study of epitheliochorial, endotheliochorial, and haemomonochorial placentation. *Microsc. Res. Tech.* 38, 100–114. doi: 10.1002/(SICI)1097-0029(19970701/15)38:1/2<100::AID-JEMT11>3.0.CO;2-T

Joseph, J. T., Purtill, K., Wong, S. J., Munoz, J., Teal, A., Madison-Antenucci, S., et al. (2012). Vertical transmission of Babesia microti, United States. *Emerging Infect. Dis.* 18, 1318–1321. doi: 10.3201/eid1808.110988

Juliano, P. B., Blotta, M. H. S. L., and Altemani, A. M. A. (2006). ICAM-1 is overexpressed by villous trophoblasts in placentitis. *Placenta* 27, 750–757. doi: 10.1016/j.placenta.2005.07.008

Jung, C., Lee, C. Y.-F., and Grigg, M. E. (2004). The SRS superfamily of Toxoplasma surface proteins. *Int. J. Parasitol.* 34, 285–296. doi: 10.1016/j.ijpara.2003.12.004

Katz, L. M., and Dodd, R. Y. (2019). "Transfusion-Transmitted Diseases," in *Transfusion Medicine and Hemostasis*, eds B. H. Shaz and C. D. Hillyer (Amsterdam: Elsevier), 437–453. doi: 10.1016/B978-0-12-813726-0.00073-8

Keller, N., Naguleswaran, A., Cannas, A., Vonlaufen, N., Bienz, M., Björkman, C., et al. (2002). Identification of a Neospora caninum Microneme Protein (NcMIC1) Which Interacts with Sulfated Host Cell Surface Glycosaminoglycans. *Infect. Immun.* 70, 3187–3198. doi: 10.1128/IAI.70.6.3187-3198.2002

Keller, N., Riesen, M., Naguleswaran, A., Vonlaufen, N., Stettler, R., Leepin, A., et al. (2004). Identification and Characterization of a Neospora caninum Microneme-Associated Protein (NcMIC4) That Exhibits Unique Lactose-Binding Properties. *Infect. Immun.* 72, 4791–4800. doi: 10.1128/IAI.72.8.4791-4800.2004

Kelly, M. N., Kolls, J. K., Happel, K., Schwartzman, J. D., Schwarzenberger, P., Combe, C., et al. (2005). Interleukin-17/Interleukin-17 Receptor-Mediated Signaling Is Important for Generation of an Optimal Polymorphonuclear Response against Toxoplasma gondii Infection. *Infect. Immun.* 73, 617–621. doi: 10.1128/IAI.73.1.617-621.2005

Kemmerling, U., Osuna, A., Schijman, A. G., and Truyens, C. (2019). Congenital Transmission of Trypanosoma cruzi: A Review About the Interactions Between the Parasite, the Placenta, the Maternal and the Fetal/Neonatal Immune Responses. *Front. Microbiol.* 10:1854. doi: 10.3389/fmicb.2019.01854

Khan, A., Shaik, J. S., Sikorski, P., Dubey, J. P., and Grigg, M. E. (2020). Neosporosis: An Overview of Its Molecular Epidemiology and Pathogenesis. *Engineering* 6, 10–19. doi: 10.1016/j.eng.2019.02.010

Khangura, R. K., Williams, N., Cooper, S., and Prabulos, A.-M. (2019). Babesiosis in Pregnancy: An Imitator of HELLP Syndrome. *AJP Rep.* 9, e147–e152. doi: 10.1055/s-0039-1687873

Kim, K., Weiss, L. M., and Tanowitz, H. B. (2016). "Parasitic Infections," in *Murray and Nadel's Textbook of Respiratory Medicine*, eds R. J. Mason, A. Slutsky, J. F. Murray, J. A. Nadel, M. Gotway, and V. C. Broaddus (Amsterdam: Elsevier), 682.e–698.e. doi: 10.1016/B978-1-4557-3383-5.00039-7

Klisch, K., Boos, A., Friedrich, M., Herzog, K., Feldmann, M., Sousa, N., et al. (2006). The glycosylation of pregnancy-associated glycoproteins and prolactin-related protein-I in bovine binucleate trophoblast giant cells changes before parturition. *Reproduction* 132, 791–798. doi: 10.1530/REP-06-0040

Krause, P. J., Daily, J., Telford, S. R., Vannier, E., Lantos, P., and Spielman, A. (2007). Shared features in the pathobiology of babesiosis and malaria. *Trends Parasitol.* 23, 605–610. doi: 10.1016/j.pt.2007.09.005

Krishnegowda, G., Hajjar, A. M., Zhu, J., Douglass, E. J., Uematsu, S., Akira, S., et al. (2005). Induction of proinflammatory responses in macrophages by the glycosylphosphatidylinositols of Plasmodium falciparum: cell signaling receptors, glycosylphosphatidylinositol (GPI) structural requirement, and regulation of GPI activity. *J. Biol. Chem.* 280, 8606–8616. doi: 10.1074/jbc.M413541200

Lachenmaier, S. M., Deli, M. A., Meissner, M., and Liesenfeld, O. (2011). Intracellular transport of Toxoplasma gondii through the blood–brain barrier. *J. Neuroimmunol.* 232, 119–130. doi: 10.1016/j.jneuroim.2010.10.029

Lachkhem, A., Galal, L., Lahmar, I., Passebosc, K., Riahi, H., Plault, N., et al. (2021). First isolation and genotyping of Toxoplasma gondii strains from domestic animals in Tunisia. *Sci. Rep.* 11:9328. doi: 10.1038/s41598-021-88751-1

Laha, R., Das, M., and Sen, A. (2015). Morphology, epidemiology, and phylogeny of Babesia: An overview. *Trop. Parasitol.* 5, 94–100. doi: 10.4103/2229-5070.162490

Lahmar, I., Lachkhem, A., Babba, O., Slama, D., Trabelsi, A., Passebosc-Faure, K., et al. (2020). First isolation and molecular characterization of Toxoplasma gondii strains from human congenital toxoplasmosis cases in Monastir, Tunisia. *Sci. Rep.* 10:1963. doi: 10.1038/s41598-020-59060-w

Lambert, H., and Barragan, A. (2010). Modelling parasite dissemination: host cell subversion and immune evasion by Toxoplasma gondii. *Cell. Microbiol.* 12, 292–300. doi: 10.1111/j.1462-5822.2009.01417.x

Lambert, H., Hitziger, N., Dellacasa, I., Svensson, M., and Barragan, A. (2006). Induction of dendritic cell migration upon Toxoplasma gondii infection potentiates parasite dissemination. *Cell. Microbiol.* 8, 1611–1623. doi: 10.1111/j.1462-5822.2006.00735.x

Lei, Y., Davey, M., and Ellis, J. T. (2005). Attachment and invasion of Toxoplasma gondii and Neospora caninum to epithelial and fibroblast cell lines in vitro. *Parasitology* 131, 583–590. doi: 10.1017/S0031182005008310

Lekutis, C., Ferguson, D. J., Grigg, M. E., Camps, M., and Boothroyd, J. C. (2001). Surface antigens of Toxoplasma gondii: variations on a theme. *Int. J. Parasitol.* 31, 1285–1292. doi: 10.1016/s0020-7519(01)00261-2

Lennartz, F., Smith, C., Craig, A. G., and Higgins, M. K. (2019). Structural insights into diverse modes of ICAM-1 binding by Plasmodium falciparum-infected erythrocytes. *PNAS* 116, 20124–20134. doi: 10.1073/pnas.1911900116

Liempi, A., Castillo, C., Carrillo, I., Muñoz, L., Droguett, D., Galanti, N., et al. (2016). A local innate immune response against Trypanosoma cruzi in the human placenta: The epithelial turnover of the trophoblast. *Microb. Pathog.* 99, 123–129. doi: 10.1016/j.micpath.2016.08.022

Liempi, A., Castillo, C., Medina, L., Galanti, N., Maya, J. D., Parraguez, V. H., et al. (2020). Comparative ex vivo infection with Trypanosoma cruzi and Toxoplasma gondii of human, canine and ovine placenta: Analysis of tissue damage and infection efficiency. *Parasitol. Int.* 76:102065. doi: 10.1016/j.parint.2020.102065

Liempi, A., Castillo, C., Medina, L., Rojas, M., Maya, J. D., Parraguez, V. H., et al. (2019). Ex vivo infection of human placental explants with Trypanosoma cruzi and Toxoplasma gondii: Differential activation of NF kappa B signaling pathways. *Acta Trop.* 199:105153. doi: 10.1016/j.actatropica.2019.105153

Lobato, J., Silva, D. A. O., Mineo, T. W. P., Amaral, J. D. H. F., Segundo, G. R. S., Costa-Cruz, J. M., et al. (2006). Detection of Immunoglobulin G Antibodies to Neospora caninum in Humans: High Seropositivity Rates in Patients Who Are Infected by Human Immunodeficiency Virus or Have Neurological Disorders. *Clin. Vaccine Immunol.* 13, 84–89. doi: 10.1128/CVI.13.1.84-89.2006

López-Pérez, I. C., Collantes-Fernández, E., Rojo-Montejo, S., Navarro-Lozano, V., Risco-Castillo, V., Pérez-Pérez, V., et al. (2010). Effects of Neospora caninum Infection at Mid-Gestation on Placenta in a Pregnant Mouse Model. *J. Parasitol.* 96, 1017–1020.

Lovett, J. L., Howe, D. K., and Sibley, L. D. (2000). Molecular characterization of a thrombospondin-related anonymous protein homologue in Neospora caninum. *Mol. Biochem. Parasitol.* 107, 33–43. doi: 10.1016/S0166-6851(99)00228-5

Lucchi, N. W., Peterson, D. S., and Moore, J. M. (2008). Immunologic activation of human syncytiotrophoblast by Plasmodium falciparum. *Malaria J.* 7:42. doi: 10.1186/1475-2875-7-42

Lucchi, N. W., Sarr, D., Owino, S. O., Mwalimu, S. M., Peterson, D. S., and Moore, J. M. (2011). Natural hemozoin stimulates syncytiotrophoblast to secrete chemokines and recruit peripheral blood mononuclear cells. *Placenta* 32, 579–585. doi: 10.1016/j.placenta.2011.05.003

Machado, R. Z., Mineo, T. W. P., Landim, L. P., Carvalho, A. F., Gennari, S. M., and Miglino, M. A. (2007). Possible role of bovine trophoblast giant cells in transplacental transmission of Neospora caninum in cattle. *Rev. Bras. Parasitol. Vet.* 16, 21–25.

Maciel, E., Siqueira, I., Queiroz, A. C., and Melo, A. (2000). Toxoplasma gondii myelitis in a patient with adult T-cell leukemia-lymphoma. *Arquivos Neuro Psiquiatria* 58, 1107–1109. doi: 10.1590/S0004-282X2000000600019

Maldonado, Y. A., Read, J. S., and Committee on Infectious Diseases. (2017). Diagnosis, Treatment, and Prevention of Congenital Toxoplasmosis in the United States. *Pediatrics* 139:3860. doi: 10.1542/peds.2016-3860

Maley, S. W., Buxton, D., Macaldowie, C. N., Anderson, I. E., Wright, S. E., Bartley, P. M., et al. (2006). Characterization of the Immune Response in the Placenta of Cattle Experimentally Infected with Neospora caninum in Early Gestation. *J. Comparat. Pathol.* 135, 130–141. doi: 10.1016/j.jcpa.2006.07.001

Manger, I. D., Hehl, A. B., and Boothroyd, J. C. (1998). The Surface of Toxoplasma Tachyzoites Is Dominated by a Family of Glycosylphosphatidylinositol-Anchored Antigens Related to SAG1. *Infect. Immun.* 66, 2237–2244.

Marin, M. S., Hecker, Y. P., Quintana, S., Pérez, S. E., Leunda, M. R., Cantón, G. J., et al. (2017). Toll-like receptors 3, 7 and 8 are upregulated in the placental caruncle and fetal spleen of Neospora caninum experimentally infected cattle. *Vet. Parasitol.* 236, 58–61. doi: 10.1016/j.vetpar.2017.02.002

Martínez-Ocampo, F. (2018). Genomics of Apicomplexa. *Farm Anim. Dis. Recent Omic Trends New Strateg. Treat.* 2018:72633. doi: 10.5772/intechopen.72633

Marty, P., Bongain, A., Rahal, A., Thulliez, P., Wasfi, D., Lambert, J. C., et al. (1994). Prenatal diagnosis of severe fetal toxoplasmosis as a result of toxoplasmic reactivation in an HIV-1 seropositive woman. *Prenat. Diagn.* 14, 414–415. doi: 10.1002/pd.1970140514

Masocha, W., and Kristensson, K. (2012). Passage of parasites across the blood-brain barrier. *Virulence* 3, 202–212. doi: 10.4161/viru.19178

Matejevic, D., Neudeck, H., Graf, R., Müller, T., and Dietl, J. (2001). Localization of hyaluronan with a hyaluronan-specific hyaluronic acid binding protein in the placenta in pre-eclampsia. *Gynecol. Obstet. Invest.* 52, 257–259. doi: 10.1159/000052986

Maubert, B., Guilbert, L. J., and Deloron, P. (1997). Cytoadherence of Plasmodium falciparum to intercellular adhesion molecule 1 and chondroitin-4-sulfate expressed by the syncytiotrophoblast in the human placenta. *Infect. Immun.* 65, 1251–1257.

McAuley, J. B. (2014). Congenital Toxoplasmosis. *J. Pediatric. Infect. Dis. Soc.* 3, S30–S35. doi: 10.1093/jpids/piu077

McLean, A. R., Ataide, R., Simpson, J. A., Beeson, J. G., and Fowkes, F. J. (2015). Malaria and immunity during pregnancy and postpartum: a tale of two species. *Parasitology* 142, 999–1015. doi: 10.1017/S0031182015000074

Melamed, J., Eckert, G. U., Spadoni, V. S., Lago, E. G., and Uberti, F. (2010). Ocular manifestations of congenital toxoplasmosis. *Eye* 24, 528–534. doi: 10.1038/eye.2009.140

Mesquita, L. P., Costa, R. C., Nogueira, C. I., Abreu, C. C., Orlando, D. R., Ascari Junior, I., et al. (2018). Placental lesions associated with abortion and stillbirth in goats naturally infected by Neospora caninum. *Pesquisa Veterinária Brasileira* 38, 444–449. doi: 10.1590/1678-5150-pvb-4598

Metwally, N. G., Tilly, A.-K., Lubiana, P., Roth, L. K., Dörpinghaus, M., Lorenzen, S., et al. (2017). Characterisation of Plasmodium falciparum populations selected on the human endothelial receptors P-selectin, E-selectin, CD9 and CD151. *Sci. Rep.* 7:4069. doi: 10.1038/s41598-017-04241-3

Milian, I. C. B., Silva, R. J., Manzan-Martins, C., Barbosa, B. F., Guirelli, P. M., Ribeiro, M., et al. (2019). Increased Toxoplasma gondii Intracellular Proliferation in Human Extravillous Trophoblast Cells (HTR8/SVneo Line) Is Sequentially Triggered by MIF, ERK1/2, and COX-2. *Front. Microbiol.* 10:852. doi: 10.3389/fmicb.2019.00852

Mineo, T. W. P., Benevides, L., Silva, N. M., and Silva, J. S. (2009). Myeloid differentiation factor 88 is required for resistance to Neospora caninum infection. *Vet. Res.* 40:2009015. doi: 10.1051/vetres/2009015

Miranda, V. D. S., França, F. B. F., da Costa, M. S., Silva, V. R. S., Mota, C. M., Barros, P., et al. (2019). Toll-Like Receptor 3-TRIF Pathway Activation by Neospora caninum RNA Enhances Infection Control in Mice. *Infect. Immun.* 87, 739–718. doi: 10.1128/IAI.00739-18

Mondragon, R., Howe, D. K., Dubey, J. P., and Sibley, L. D. (1998). Genotypic analysis of Toxoplasma gondii isolates from pigs. *J. Parasitol.* 84, 639–641.

Moormann, A. M., Sullivan, A. D., Rochford, R. A., Chensue, S. W., Bock, P. J., Nyirenda, T., et al. (1999). Malaria and pregnancy: placental cytokine expression and its relationship to intrauterine growth retardation. *J. Infect. Dis.* 180, 1987–1993. doi: 10.1086/315135

Moraes, L. V., de, Tadokoro, C. E., Gómez-Conde, I., Olivieri, D. N., and Penha-Gonçalves, C. (2013). Intravital Placenta Imaging Reveals Microcirculatory Dynamics Impact on Sequestration and Phagocytosis of Plasmodium-Infected Erythrocytes. *PLoS Pathog.* 9:e1003154. doi: 10.1371/journal.ppat.1003154

Mosqueda, J., Olvera-Ramírez, A., Aguilar-Tipacamú, G., and Cantó, G. (2012). Current Advances in Detection and Treatment of Babesiosis. *Curr. Med. Chem.* 19, 1504–1518. doi: 10.2174/092986712799828355

Multhaup, A., Huppertz, B., Göhner, C., Böhringer, M., Mai, M., Markert, U., et al. (2018). N-cadherin knockdown leads to disruption of trophoblastic and endothelial cell interaction in a 3D cell culture model - New insights in trophoblast invasion failure. *Cell Adh. Migr.* 12, 259–270. doi: 10.1080/19336918.2017.1386822

Muñoz, L., Castillo, C., Carrillo, I., Salinas, A., Liempi, A., Droguett, D., et al. (2016). The ex vivo infection of human placental chorionic villi explants with Trypanosoma cruzi and Toxoplasma gondii is mediated by different toll-like receptors. *Placenta* 45:86. doi: 10.1016/j.placenta.2016.06.089

Muthusamy, A., Achur, R. N., Bhavanandan, V. P., Fouda, G. G., Taylor, D. W., and Gowda, D. C. (2004). Plasmodium falciparum-infected erythrocytes adhere both in the intervillous space and on the villous surface of human placenta by binding to the low-sulfated chondroitin sulfate proteoglycan receptor. *Am. J. Pathol.* 164, 2013–2025. doi: 10.1016/S0002-9440(10)63761-3

Naguleswaran, A., Cannas, A., Keller, N., Vonlaufen, N., Björkman, C., and Hemphill, A. (2002). Vero cell surface proteoglycan interaction with the microneme protein NcMIC(3) mediates adhesion of Neospora caninum tachyzoites to host cells unlike that in Toxoplasma gondii. *Int. J. Parasitol.* 32, 695–704. doi: 10.1016/s0020-7519(02)00014-0

New, D. L., Quinn, J. B., Qureshi, M. Z., and Sigler, S. J. (1997). Vertically Transmitted Babesiosis. *J. Pediatr.* 131, 163–164. doi: 10.1016/S0022-3476(97)70143-4

Ngô, H. M., Zhou, Y., Lorenzi, H., Wang, K., Kim, T.-K., Zhou, Y., et al. (2017). Toxoplasma Modulates Signature Pathways of Human Epilepsy, Neurodegeneration & Cancer. *Sci. Rep.* 7:11496. doi: 10.1038/s41598-017-10675-6

Nishikawa, Y., Xuan, X., Nagasawa, H., Igarashi, I., Fujisaki, K., Otsuka, H., et al. (2001). Prevention of vertical transmission of Neospora caninum in BALB/c mice by recombinant vaccinia virus carrying NcSRS2 gene. *Vaccine* 19, 1710–1716. doi: 10.1016/s0264-410x(00)00407-2

Nunes, M. C., and Scherf, A. (2007). Plasmodium falciparum during pregnancy: a puzzling parasite tissue adhesion tropism. *Parasitology* 134, 1863–1869. doi: 10.1017/S0031182007000133

O'Connor, R. M., and Allred, D. R. (2000). Selection of Babesia bovis-infected erythrocytes for adhesion to endothelial cells coselects for altered variant erythrocyte surface antigen isoforms. *J. Immunol.* 164, 2037–2045. doi: 10.4049/jimmunol.164.4.2037

Okamgba, O. C., Ifeanyichukwu, M. O., Ilesanmi, A. O., and Chigbu, L. N. (2018). Variations in the leukocyte and cytokine profiles between placental and maternal circulation in pregnancy-associated malaria. *Res. Rep. Trop. Med.* 9, 1–8. doi: 10.2147/RRTM.S137829

Oldenhove, G., Bouladoux, N., Wohlfert, E. A., Hall, J. A., Chou, D., Dos santos, L., et al. (2009). Decrease of Foxp3+ Treg Cell Number and Acquisition of Effector Cell Phenotype during Lethal Infection. *Immunity* 31, 772–786. doi: 10.1016/j.immuni.2009.10.001

Olupot-Olupot, P., Eregu, E. I. E., Naizuli, K., Ikiror, J., Acom, L., and Burgoine, K. (2018). Neonatal and congenital malaria: a case series in malaria endemic eastern Uganda. *Malar. J.* 17:171. doi: 10.1186/s12936-018-2327-0

Ordi, J., Ismail, M. R., Ventura, P. J., Kahigwa, E., Hirt, R., Cardesa, A., et al. (1998). Massive chronic intervillositis of the placenta associated with malaria infection. *Am. J. Surg. Pathol.* 22, 1006–1011. doi: 10.1097/00000478-199808000-00011

Ortiz-Alegría, L. B., Caballero-Ortega, H., Cañedo-Solares, I., Rico-Torres, C. P., Sahagún-Ruiz, A., Medina-Escutia, M. E., et al. (2010). Congenital toxoplasmosis: candidate host immune genes relevant for vertical transmission and pathogenesis. *Genes Immun.* 11, 363–373. doi: 10.1038/gene.2010.21

Oshiro, L. M., Motta-Castro, A. R. C., Freitas, S. Z., Cunha, R. C., Dittrich, R. L., Meirelles, A. C. F., et al. (2015). Neospora caninum and Toxoplasma gondii serodiagnosis in human immunodeficiency virus carriers. *Revista Sociedade Brasileira Med. Trop.* 48, 568–572. doi: 10.1590/0037-8682-0151-2015

Ossani, R. A., Borges, H. A. T., Souza, A. P., Sartor, A. A., Miletti, L. C., Federle, M., et al. (2017). Toxoplasma gondii in milk of naturally infected dairy ewes on west mesoregion of Santa Catarina state, Brazil. *Arq. Bras. Med. Vet. Zootec.* 69, 1294–1300. doi: 10.1590/1678-4162-9177

Ouédraogo, A., Tiono, A. B., Diarra, A., Bougouma, E. C. C., Nébié, I., Konaté, A. T., et al. (2012). Transplacental Transmission of Plasmodium falciparum in a Highly Malaria Endemic Area of Burkina Faso. *J. Trop. Med.* 2012:109705. doi: 10.1155/2012/109705

Ozarslan, N., Robinson, J. F., and Gaw, S. L. (2019). Circulating Monocytes, Tissue Macrophages, and Malaria. *J. Trop. Med.* 2019:3720838. doi: 10.1155/2019/3720838

Ozawa, S., Haynie, D. G., Bessias, S., Laing, S. K., Ngamasana, E. L., Yemeke, T. T., et al. (2019). Modeling the Economic Impact of Substandard and Falsified Antimalarials in the Democratic Republic of the Congo. *Am. J. Trop. Med. Hyg.* 100, 1149–1157. doi: 10.4269/ajtmh.18-0334

Pappas, G., Roussos, N., and Falagas, M. E. (2009). Toxoplasmosis snapshots: global status of Toxoplasma gondii seroprevalence and implications for pregnancy and congenital toxoplasmosis. *Int. J. Parasitol.* 39, 1385–1394. doi: 10.1016/j.ijpara.2009.04.003

Parekh, F. K., Davison, B. B., Gamboa, D., Hernandez, J., and Branch, O. H. (2010). Placental Histopathologic Changes Associated with Subclinical Malaria Infection and Its Impact on the Fetal Environment. *Am. J. Trop. Med. Hyg.* 83, 973–980. doi: 10.4269/ajtmh.2010.09-0445

Parroche, P., Lauw, F. N., Goutagny, N., Latz, E., Monks, B. G., Visintin, A., et al. (2007). Malaria hemozoin is immunologically inert but radically enhances innate responses by presenting malaria DNA to Toll-like receptor 9. *Proc. Natl. Acad. Sci. U S A.* 104, 1919–1924. doi: 10.1073/pnas.0608745104

Parrodi, F., Wright, I. G., Kerr, J. D., and Dobson, C. (1990). In vitro adherence of erythrocytes infected with Babesia bigemina and Babesia rodhainito thrombospondin. *Int. J. Parasitol.* 20, 899–903. doi: 10.1016/0020-7519(90) 90028-L

Passos, S. T., Silver, J. S., O'Hara, A. C., Sehy, D., Stumhofer, J. S., and Hunter, C. A. (2010). IL-6 promotes NK cell production of IL-17 during toxoplasmosis. *J. Immunol.* 184, 1776–1783. doi: 10.4049/jimmunol.0901843

Pedroni, M. J., Sondgeroth, K. S., Gallego-Lopez, G. M., Echaide, I., and Lau, A. O. (2013). Comparative transcriptome analysis of geographically distinct virulent and attenuated Babesia bovis strains reveals similar gene expression changes through attenuation. *BMC Genomics* 14:763. doi: 10.1186/1471-2164-14-763

Pehrson, C., Mathiesen, L., Heno, K. K., Salanti, A., Resende, M., Dzikowski, R., et al. (2016). Adhesion of Plasmodium falciparum infected erythrocytes in ex vivo perfused placental tissue: a novel model of placental malaria. *Malaria J.* 15:292. doi: 10.1186/s12936-016-1342-2

Penazzato, M., Rampon, O., Canale, E. D., Rossi, A. D., Mazza, A., D'Elia, R., et al. (2007). Congenital Plasmodium ovale malaria in an infant born to HIV positive mother. *J. Pediatr. Infect. Dis.* 2, 167–169.

Pereira, L. M., Candido-Silva, J. A., De Vries, E., and Yatsuda, A. P. (2011). A new thrombospondin-related anonymous protein homologue in Neospora caninum (NcMIC2-like1). *Parasitology* 138, 287–297. doi: 10.1017/S0031182010001290

Petersen, E., Lebech, M., Jensen, L., Lind, P., Rask, M., Bagger, P., et al. (1999). Neospora caninum infection and repeated abortions in humans. *Emerg. Infect. Dis.* 5, 278–280.

Pfaff, A. W., Georges, S., Abou-Bacar, A., Letscher-Bru, V., Klein, J.-P., Mousli, M., et al. (2005). Toxoplasma gondii regulates ICAM-1 mediated monocyte adhesion to trophoblasts. *Immunol. Cell Biol.* 83, 483–489. doi: 10.1111/j.1440-1711.2005.01356.x

PLoS Neglected Tropical Disease (2020). *PLoS Neglected Tropical Diseases.* Available online at: https://journals.plos.org/plosntds/s/journal-information. %20Accessed%201%20April%202020. (accessed August 21, 2020).

Pollard, A. M., Onatolu, K. N., Hiller, L., Haldar, K., and Knoll, L. J. (2008). Highly polymorphic family of glycosylphosphatidylinositol-anchored surface antigens with evidence of developmental regulation in Toxoplasma gondii. *Infect. Immun.* 76, 103–110. doi: 10.1128/IAI.01170-07

Pons, J. C., Sigrand, C., Grangeot-Keros, L., Frydman, R., and Thulliez, P. (1995). [Congenital toxoplasmosis: transmission to the fetus of a pre-pregnancy maternal infection]. *Presse. Med.* 24, 179–182.

Qiu, J., Wang, L., Zhang, R., Ge, K., Guo, H., Liu, X., et al. (2016). Identification of a TNF-α inducer MIC3 originating from the microneme of non-cystogenic, virulent Toxoplasma gondii. *Sci. Rep.* 6:39407. doi: 10.1038/srep39407

Quinn, H. E., Miller, C. M. D., and Ellis, J. T. (2004). The cell-mediated immune response to Neospora caninum during pregnancy in the mouse is associated with a bias towards production of interleukin-4. *Int. J. Parasitol.* 34, 723–732. doi: 10.1016/j.ijpara.2004.01.007

Ralph, S. A., van Dooren, G. G., Waller, R. F., Crawford, M. J., Fraunholz, M. J., Foth, B. J., et al. (2004). Tropical infectious diseases: metabolic maps and functions of the Plasmodium falciparum apicoplast. *Nat. Rev. Microbiol.* 2, 203–216. doi: 10.1038/nrmicro843

Recht, J., Siqueira, A. M., Monteiro, W. M., Herrera, S. M., Herrera, S., and Lacerda, M. V. G. (2017). Malaria in Brazil, Colombia, Peru and Venezuela: current challenges in malaria control and elimination. *Malaria J.* 16:273. doi: 10.1186/s12936-017-1925-6

Reichel, M. P., Alejandra Ayanegui-Alcérreca, M., Gondim, L. F. P., and Ellis, J. T. (2013). What is the global economic impact of Neospora caninum in cattle - the billion dollar question. *Int. J. Parasitol.* 43, 133–142. doi: 10.1016/j.ijpara.2012.10.022

Reid, A. J., Vermont, S. J., Cotton, J. A., Harris, D., Hill-Cawthorne, G. A., Könen-Waisman, S., et al. (2012). Comparative genomics of the apicomplexan parasites Toxoplasma gondii and Neospora caninum: Coccidia differing in host range and transmission strategy. *PLoS Pathog.* 8:e1002567. doi: 10.1371/journal.ppat.1002567

Reis, A. S., Barboza, R., Murillo, O., Barateiro, A., Peixoto, E. P. M., Lima, F. A., et al. (2020). Inflammasome activation and IL-1 signaling during placental malaria induce poor pregnancy outcomes. *Sci. Adv.* 6:eaax6346. doi: 10.1126/sciadv.aax6346

Rico-Torres, C. P., Vargas-Villavicencio, J. A., and Correa, D. (2016). Is Toxoplasma gondii type related to clinical outcome in human congenital infection? Systematic and critical review. *Eur. J. Clin. Microbiol. Infect. Dis.* 35, 1079–1088. doi: 10.1007/s10096-016-2656-2

Ripoll, J. G., Rizvi, M. S., King, R. L., and Daniels, C. E. (2018). Severe Babesia microti infection presenting as multiorgan failure in an immunocompetent host. *BMJ Case. Rep.* 2018:224647. doi: 10.1136/bcr-2018-224647

Robbins, J. R., Zeldovich, V. B., Poukchanski, A., Boothroyd, J. C., and Bakardjiev, A. I. (2012). Tissue barriers of the human placenta to infection with Toxoplasma gondii. *Infect. Immun.* 80, 418–428. doi: 10.1128/IAI.05899-11

Robert-Gangneux, F., and Dardé, M.-L. (2012). Epidemiology of and Diagnostic Strategies for Toxoplasmosis. *Clin. Microbiol. Rev.* 25, 264–296. doi: 10.1128/CMR.05013-11

Robert-Gangneux, F., Murat, J.-B., Fricker-Hidalgo, H., Brenier-Pinchart, M.-P., Gangneux, J.-P., and Pelloux, H. (2011). The placenta: a main role in congenital toxoplasmosis? *Trends Parasitol.* 27, 530–536. doi: 10.1016/j.pt.2011.09.005

Robinson, D. P., and Klein, S. L. (2012). Pregnancy and pregnancy-associated hormones alter immune responses and disease pathogenesis. *Horm. Behav.* 62, 263–271. doi: 10.1016/j.yhbeh.2012.02.023

Rosbottom, A., Gibney, H., Kaiser, P., Hartley, C., Smith, R. F., Robinson, R., et al. (2011). Up Regulation of the Maternal Immune Response in the Placenta of Cattle Naturally Infected with Neospora caninum. *PLoS One* 6:e15799. doi: 10.1371/journal.pone.0015799

Rowe, J. H., Ertelt, J. M., Aguilera, M. N., Farrar, M. A., and Way, S. S. (2011). Foxp3(+) regulatory T cell expansion required for sustaining pregnancy compromises host defense against prenatal bacterial pathogens. *Cell Host Microbe* 10, 54–64. doi: 10.1016/j.chom.2011.06.005

Saetre, K., Godhwani, N., Maria, M., Patel, D., Wang, G., Li, K. I., et al. (2018). Congenital Babesiosis After Maternal Infection With Borrelia burgdorferi and Babesia microti. *J. Pediat. Infect. Dis. Soc.* 7, e1–e5. doi: 10.1093/jpids/pix074

Safeukui, I., Buffet, P. A., Deplaine, G., Perrot, S., Brousse, V., Sauvanet, A., et al. (2018). Sensing of red blood cells with decreased membrane deformability by the human spleen. *Blood Adv.* 2, 2581–2587. doi: 10.1182/bloodadvances.2018024562

Salazar Gonzalez, R. M., Shehata, H., O'Connell, M. J., Yang, Y., Moreno-Fernandez, M. E., Chougnet, C. A., et al. (2014). Toxoplasma gondii-Derived Profilin Triggers Human Toll-Like Receptor 5-Dependent Cytokine Production. *J. Innate Immun.* 6, 685–694. doi: 10.1159/000362367

Salomaki, E. D., and Kolisko, M. (2019). There Is Treasure Everywhere: Reductive Plastid Evolution in Apicomplexa in Light of Their Close Relatives. *Biomolecules* 9:biom9080378. doi: 10.3390/biom9080378

Sanecka, A., and Frickel, E.-M. (2012). Use and abuse of dendritic cells by Toxoplasma gondii. *Virulence* 3, 678–689. doi: 10.4161/viru.22833

Sartelet, H., Garraud, O., Rogier, C., Milko-Sartelet, I., Kaboret, Y., Michel, G., et al. (2000). Hyperexpression of ICAM-1 and CD36 in placentas infected with Plasmodium falciparum: a possible role of these molecules in sequestration of infected red blood cells in placentas. *Histopathology* 36, 62–68. doi: 10.1046/j.1365-2559.2000.00742.x

Sasai, M., and Yamamoto, M. (2019). Innate, adaptive, and cell-autonomous immunity against Toxoplasma gondii infection. *Exp. Mol. Med.* 51, 1–10. doi: 10.1038/s12276-019-0353-9

Sasai, M., Pradipta, A., and Yamamoto, M. (2018). Host immune responses to Toxoplasma gondii. *Int. Immunol.* 30:dxy004. doi: 10.1093/intimm/dxy004

Schetters, T. (2019). Mechanisms Involved in the Persistence of Babesia canis Infection in Dogs. *Pathogens* 8:athogens8030094. doi: 10.3390/pathogens8030094

Schoeman, J. P. (2009). Canine babesiosis. *Onderstepoort J. Vet. Res.* 76, 59–66.

Sethi, S., Alcid, D., Kesarwala, H., and Tolan, R. W. (2009). Probable Congenital Babesiosis in Infant, New Jersey, USA. *Emerg. Infect. Dis.* 15, 788–791. doi: 10.3201/eid1505.070808

Sharma, L., and Shukla, G. (2017). Placental Malaria: A New Insight into the Pathophysiology. *Front. Med.* 4:00117. doi: 10.3389/fmed.2017.00117

Shoda, L. K. M., Kegerreis, K. A., Suarez, C. E., Roditi, I., Corral, R. S., Bertot, G. M., et al. (2001). DNA from Protozoan Parasites Babesia bovis, Trypanosoma cruzi, and T. brucei Is Mitogenic for B Lymphocytes and Stimulates Macrophage Expression of Interleukin-12, Tumor Necrosis Factor Alpha, and Nitric Oxide. *Infect. Immun.* 69, 2162–2171. doi: 10.1128/IAI.69.4.2162-2171.2001

Shoda, L. K., Palmer, G. H., Florin-Christensen, J., Florin-Christensen, M., Godson, D. L., and Brown, W. C. (2000). Babesia bovis-stimulated macrophages express interleukin-1beta, interleukin-12, tumor necrosis factor alpha, and nitric oxide and inhibit parasite replication in vitro. *Infect. Immun.* 68, 5139–5145. doi: 10.1128/iai.68.9.5139-5145.2000

Sinnott, F. A., Monte, L. G., Collares, T. F., Silveira, R. M., and Borsuk, S. (2017). Review on the immunological and molecular diagnosis of neosporosis (years 2011-2016). *Vet. Parasitol.* 239, 19–25. doi: 10.1016/j.vetpar.2017.04.008

Skariah, S., Arnaboldi, P., Dattwyler, R. J., Sultan, A. A., Gaylets, C., Walwyn, O., et al. (2017). Elimination of *Babesia microti* Is Dependent on Intraerythrocytic Killing and CD4 + T Cells. *J.I.* 199, 633–642. doi: 10.4049/jimmunol.1601193

Smith, J. D. (2014). The role of PfEMP1 adhesion domain classification in Plasmodium falciparum pathogenesis research. *Mol. Biochem. Parasitol.* 195, 82–87. doi: 10.1016/j.molbiopara.2014.07.006

Sommerville, C., Richardson, J. M., Williams, R. A. M., Mottram, J. C., Roberts, C. W., Alexander, J., et al. (2013). Biochemical and Immunological Characterization of Toxoplasma gondii Macrophage Migration Inhibitory Factor. *J. Biol. Chem.* 288, 12733–12741. doi: 10.1074/jbc.M112.419911

Sondgeroth, K. S., McElwain, T. F., Allen, A. J., Chen, A. V., and Lau, A. O. (2013). Loss of neurovirulence is associated with reduction of cerebral capillary sequestration during acute Babesia bovis infection. *Parasites Vect.* 6:181. doi: 10.1186/1756-3305-6-181

Soulard, V., Amadoudji Zin, M., Fitting, C., Ibitokou, S., Oesterholt, M., Luty, A. J. F., et al. (2011). Placental Malaria-Associated Suppression of Parasite-Specific Immune Response in Neonates Has No Major Impact on Systemic CD4 T Cell Homeostasis ∇. *Infect. Immun.* 79, 2801–2809. doi: 10.1128/IAI.00203-11

Stelzer, S., Basso, W., Benavides Silván, J., Ortega-Mora, L. M., Maksimov, P., Gethmann, J., et al. (2019). Toxoplasma gondii infection and toxoplasmosis in farm animals: Risk factors and economic impact. *Food Waterborne Parasitol.* 15:e00037. doi: 10.1016/j.fawpar.2019.e00037

Sugiyama, T., Cuevas, L. E., Bailey, W., Makunde, R., Kawamura, K., Kobayashi, M., et al. (2001). Expression of Intercellular Adhesion Molecule 1 (ICAM-1) in Plasmodium falciparum -infected Placenta. *Placenta* 22, 573–579. doi: 10.1053/plac.2001.0692

Suguitan, A. L., Leke, R. G. F., Fouda, G., Zhou, A., Thuita, L., Metenou, S., et al. (2003). Changes in the Levels of Chemokines and Cytokines in the Placentas of Women with Plasmodium falciparum Malaria. *J. Infect. Dis.* 188, 1074–1082. doi: 10.1086/378500

Sun, Y., Li, S.-G., Jiang, J.-F., Wang, X., Zhang, Y., Wang, H., et al. (2014). Babesia venatorum Infection in Child. China. *Emerg. Infect. Dis.* 20, 896–897. doi: 10.3201/eid2005.121034

Surra, N. D., and Jesus, J. E. (2015). The anemic and thrombocytopenic febrile neonate. *J. Emerg. Med.* 48, 675–678. doi: 10.1016/j.jemermed.2014.11.026

Taubert, A., Krüll, M., Zahner, H., and Hermosilla, C. (2006). Toxoplasma gondii and Neospora caninum infections of bovine endothelial cells induce endothelial adhesion molecule gene transcription and subsequent PMN adhesion. *Vet. Immunol. Immunopathol.* 112, 272–283. doi: 10.1016/j.vetimm.2006.03.017

Tegegne, D., Kelifa, A., Abdurahaman, M., and Yohannes, M. (2016). Seroepidemiology and associated risk factors of Toxoplasma gondii in sheep and goats in Southwestern Ethiopia. *BMC Vet. Res.* 12:280. doi: 10.1186/s12917-016-0906-2

Tegegne, Y., Asmelash, D., Ambachew, S., Eshetie, S., Addisu, A., and Jejaw Zeleke, A. (2019). The Prevalence of Malaria among Pregnant Women in Ethiopia: A Systematic Review and Meta-Analysis. *J. Parasitol. Res.* 2019:8396091. doi: 10.1155/2019/8396091

Terkawi, M. A., Cao, S., Herbas, M. S., Nishimura, M., Li, Y., Moumouni, P. F. A., et al. (2015). Macrophages Are the Determinant of Resistance to and Outcome of Nonlethal Babesia microti Infection in Mice. *Infect. Immun.* 83, 8–16. doi: 10.1128/IAI.02128-14

Tołkacz, K., Bednarska, M., Alsarraf, M., Dwużnik, D., Grzybek, M., Welc-Falęciak, R., et al. (2017). Prevalence, genetic identity and vertical transmission of Babesia microti in three naturally infected species of vole, Microtus spp. (Cricetidae). *Parasites Vect.* 10:66. doi: 10.1186/s13071-017-2007-x

Tomavo, S. (1996). "The Major Surface Proteins of Toxoplasma gondii: Structures and Functions," in *Toxoplasma gondii Current Topics in Microbiology and Immunology*, ed. U. Gross (Berlin: Springer), 45–54. doi: 10.1007/978-3-642-51014-4_4

Torgerson, P. R., and Mastroiacovo, P. (2013). The global burden of congenital toxoplasmosis: a systematic review. *Bull. World Health Organ.* 91, 501–508. doi: 10.2471/BLT.12.111732

Tranas, J., Heinzen, R. A., Weiss, L. M., and McAllister, M. M. (1999). Serological Evidence of Human Infection with the Protozoan Neospora caninum. *Clin. Diagn. Lab. Immunol.* 6, 765–767.

Tufts, D. M., and Diuk-Wasser, M. A. (2018). Transplacental transmission of tick-borne Babesia microti in its natural host Peromyscus leucopus. *Parasit. Vectors* 11:286. doi: 10.1186/s13071-018-2875-8

Tuikue Ndam, N. G., Salanti, A., Bertin, G., Dahlbäck, M., Fievet, N., Turner, L., et al. (2005). High Level of var2csa Transcription by Plasmodium falciparum Isolated from the Placenta. *J. Infect. Dis.* 192, 331–335. doi: 10.1086/430933

Turkey, S. A., Abbas, A. A.-H., Hathal, H. D., and Abdulrasul, E. A. (2019). The Role of TLR4 Gene Polymorphism and Haplotypes in the Susceptibility to Toxoplasmosis in Iraqi Aborted Women. *J. Pure Appl. Microbiol.* 13, 1151–1157.

Umbers, A. J., Boeuf, P., Clapham, C., Stanisic, D. I., Baiwog, F., Mueller, I., et al. (2011). Placental Malaria-Associated Inflammation Disturbs the Insulin-like Growth Factor Axis of Fetal Growth Regulation. *J. Infect. Dis.* 203, 561–569. doi: 10.1093/infdis/jiq080

Valdès, V., Legagneur, H., Watrin, V., Paris, L., and Hascoët, J. M. (2011). Congenital toxoplasmosis due to maternal reinfection during pregnancy. *Arch. Pediatr.* 18, 761–763.

van Duivenvoorde, L. M., Voorberg-van, der Wel, A., van der Werff, N. M., Braskamp, G., Remarque, E. J., et al. (2010). Suppression of Plasmodium cynomolgi in rhesus macaques by coinfection with Babesia microti. *Infect. Immun.* 78, 1032–1039. doi: 10.1128/IAI.00921-09

Vannier, E., and Krause, P. J. (2012). Human babesiosis. *N. Engl. J. Med.* 366, 2397–2407. doi: 10.1056/NEJMra1202018

Varki, A., and Gagneux, P. (2012). Multifarious roles of sialic acids in immunity. *Ann. N Y. Acad. Sci.* 1253, 16–36. doi: 10.1111/j.1749-6632.2012.06517.x

Vásquez, A. M., Segura, C., and Blair, S. (2013). Induction of pro-inflammatory response of the placental trophoblast by Plasmodium falciparum infected erythrocytes and TNF. *Malar. J.* 12:421. doi: 10.1186/1475-2875-12-421

Vogel, N., Kirisits, M., Michael, E., Bach, H., Hostetter, M., Boyer, K., et al. (1996). Congenital toxoplasmosis transmitted from an immunologically competent mother infected before conception. *Clin. Infect. Dis.* 23, 1055–1060.

Vonlaufen, N., Guetg, N., Naguleswaran, A., Müller, N., Björkman, C., Schares, G., et al. (2004). In Vitro Induction of Neospora caninum Bradyzoites in Vero Cells Reveals Differential Antigen Expression, Localization, and Host-Cell Recognition of Tachyzoites and Bradyzoites. *Infect. Immun.* 72, 576–583. doi: 10.1128/IAI.72.1.576-583.2004

Vottier, G., Arsac, M., Farnoux, C., Mariani-Kurkdjian, P., Baud, O., and Aujard, Y. (2008). Congenital malaria in neonates: two case reports and review of the literature. *Acta Paediatrica* 97, 505–508. doi: 10.1111/j.1651-2227.2008.00690.x

Votýpka, J., Modrý, D., Oborník, M., Šlapeta, J., and Lukeš, J. (2017). "Apicomplexa," in *Handbook of the Protists*, eds J. M. Archibald, A. G. B. Simpson, C. H. Slamovits, L. Margulis, M. Melkonian, D. J. Chapman, et al. (Cham: Springer International Publishing), 1–58. doi: 10.1007/978-3-319-32669-6_20-1

Wahlgren, M., Goel, S., and Akhouri, R. R. (2017). Variant surface antigens of Plasmodium falciparum and their roles in severe malaria. *Nat. Rev. Microbiol.* 15, 479–491. doi: 10.1038/nrmicro.2017.47

Wang, J., Tang, D., Li, W., Xu, J., Liu, Q., and Liu, J. (2017). A new microneme protein of Neospora caninum, NcMIC8 is involved in host cell invasion. *Exp. Parasitol.* 175, 21–27. doi: 10.1016/j.exppara.2017.01.004

Wang, M. F., and Lai, S. C. (2013). Fibronectin degradation by MMP-2/MMP-9 in the serum of pregnant women and umbilical cord with Toxoplasma gondii infection. *J. Obstet. Gynaecol.* 33, 370–374. doi: 10.3109/01443615.2013.769501

Wang, X., Xiao, Y.-P., Bouchut, A., Al-Khedery, B., Wang, H., and Allred, D. R. (2012). Characterization of the Unusual Bidirectional ves Promoters Driving VESA1 Expression and Associated with Antigenic Variation in Babesia bovis. *Eukaryotic Cell* 11, 260–269. doi: 10.1128/EC.05318-11

Wang, Z.-D., Liu, H.-H., Ma, Z.-X., Ma, H.-Y., Li, Z.-Y., Yang, Z.-B., et al. (2017). Toxoplasma gondii Infection in Immunocompromised Patients: A Systematic

Review and Meta-Analysis. *Front. Microbiol.* 8:00389. doi: 10.3389/fmicb.2017.00389

WHO (2019). *World malaria report 2019*. Geneva: WHO. Available online at: https://www.who.int/publications-detail-redirect/9789241565721 (accessed August 18, 2020)

Wobeser, B. K., Godson, D. L., Rejmanek, D., and Dowling, P. (2009). Equine protozoal myeloencephalitis caused by Neospora hughesi in an adult horse in Saskatchewan. *Can. Vet. J.* 50, 851–853.

Wright, I. G., Goodger, B. V., McKenna, R. V., and Mahoney, D. F. (1979). AcuteBabesia bovis infection: A study of the vascular lesions in kidney and lung. *Z. Parasitenkd.* 60, 19–27. doi: 10.1007/BF00928968

Wujcicka, W., Wilczyński, J., and Nowakowska, D. (2013). SNPs in toll-like receptor (TLR) genes as new genetic alterations associated with congenital toxoplasmosis? *Eur. J. Clin. Microbiol. Infect. Dis.* 32, 503–511. doi: 10.1007/s10096-012-1763-y

Wujcicka, W., Wilczyński, J., and Nowakowska, D. (2014). Do the placental barrier, parasite genotype and Toll-like receptor polymorphisms contribute to the course of primary infection with various Toxoplasma gondii genotypes in pregnant women? *Eur. J. Clin. Microbiol. Infect. Dis.* 33, 703–709. doi: 10.1007/s10096-013-2017-3

Wujcicka, W., Wilczyński, J., and Nowakowska, D. (2017). Genetic alterations within TLR genes in development of Toxoplasma gondii infection among Polish pregnant women. *Adv. Med. Sci.* 62, 216–222. doi: 10.1016/j.advms.2017.02.002

Xiao, J., Garcia-Lloret, M., Winkler-Lowen, B., Miller, R., Simpson, K., and Guilbert, L. J. (1997). ICAM-1-mediated adhesion of peripheral blood monocytes to the maternal surface of placental syncytiotrophoblasts: implications for placental villitis. *Am. J. Pathol.* 150, 1845–1860.

Yager, P. H., Luginbuhl, L. M., and Dekker, J. P. (2014). Case records of the Massachusetts General Hospital. Case 6-2014. A 35-day-old boy with fever, vomiting, mottled skin, and severe anemia. *N. Engl. J. Med.* 370, 753–762. doi: 10.1056/NEJMcpc1208155

Yarovinsky, F. (2014). Innate immunity to Toxoplasma gondii infection. *Nat. Rev. Immunol.* 14, 109–121. doi: 10.1038/nri3598

Yarovinsky, F., and Sher, A. (2006). Toll-like receptor recognition of Toxoplasma gondii. *Int. J. Parasitol.* 36, 255–259. doi: 10.1016/j.ijpara.2005.12.003

Yarovinsky, F., Zhang, D., Andersen, J. F., Bannenberg, G. L., Serhan, C. N., Hayden, M. S., et al. (2005). TLR11 activation of dendritic cells by a protozoan profilin-like protein. *Science* 308, 1626–1629.

Yavuz, E., Aydin, F., Seyhan, A., Topuz, S., Karagenc, Y., Tuzlali, S., et al. (2006). Granulomatous villitis formed by inflammatory cells with maternal origin: a rare manifestation type of placental toxoplasmosis. *Placenta* 27, 780–782. doi: 10.1016/j.placenta.2005.07.002

Yi, W., Bao, W., Rodriguez, M., Liu, Y., Singh, M., Ramlall, V., et al. (2018). Robust adaptive immune response against Babesia microti infection marked by low parasitemia in a murine model of sickle cell disease. *Blood Adv.* 2, 3462–3478. doi: 10.1182/bloodadvances.2018026468

Young, K. M., Corrin, T., Wilhelm, B., Uhland, C., Greig, J., Mascarenhas, M., et al. (2019). Zoonotic Babesia: A scoping review of the global evidence. *PLoS One* 14:e0226781. doi: 10.1371/journal.pone.0226781

Zeldovich, V. B., Clausen, C. H., Bradford, E., Fletcher, D. A., Maltepe, E., Robbins, J. R., et al. (2013). Placental syncytium forms a biophysical barrier against pathogen invasion. *PLoS Pathog.* 9:e1003821. doi: 10.1371/journal.ppat.1003821

Zhang, H., Hu, X., Liu, X., Zhang, R., Fu, Q., and Xu, X. (2012). The Treg/Th17 imbalance in Toxoplasma gondii-infected pregnant mice. *Am. J. Reprod. Immunol.* 67, 112–121. doi: 10.1111/j.1600-0897.2011.01065.x

Zhao, L., Jiang, R., Jia, N., Ning, N., Zheng, Y., Huo, Q., et al. (2020). Human Case Infected With Babesia venatorum: A 5-Year Follow-Up Study. *Open Forum Infect. Dis.* 7:ofaa062. doi: 10.1093/ofid/ofaa062

Zhu, J., Krishnegowda, G., Li, G., and Gowda, D. C. (2011). Proinflammatory responses by glycosylphosphatidylinositols (GPIs) of Plasmodium falciparum are mainly mediated through the recognition of TLR2/TLR1. *Exp. Parasitol.* 128, 205–211. doi: 10.1016/j.exppara.2011.03.010

11

The Impact of Infection in Pregnancy on Placental Vascular Development and Adverse Birth Outcomes

Andrea M. Weckman[1†], Michelle Ngai[2†], Julie Wright[1], Chloe R. McDonald[2] and Kevin C. Kain[1,2,3]*

[1]Department of Laboratory Medicine and Pathobiology, University of Toronto, Toronto, ON, Canada, [2]SAR Laboratories, Sandra Rotman Centre for Global Health, University Health Network-Toronto General Hospital, Toronto, ON, Canada, [3]Tropical Disease Unit, Division of Infectious Diseases, Department of Medicine, University of Toronto, Toronto, ON, Canada

Correspondence:
Kevin C. Kain
kevin.kain@uhn.ca

[†]These authors share co-first authorship

Healthy fetal development is dependent on nutrient and oxygen transfer *via* the placenta. Optimal growth and function of placental vasculature is therefore essential to support *in utero* development. Vasculogenesis, the *de novo* formation of blood vessels, and angiogenesis, the branching and remodeling of existing vasculature, mediate the development and maturation of placental villi, which form the materno-fetal interface. Several lines of evidence indicate that systemic maternal infection and consequent inflammation can disrupt placental vasculogenesis and angiogenesis. The resulting alterations in placental hemodynamics impact fetal growth and contribute to poor birth outcomes including preterm delivery, small-for-gestational age (SGA), stillbirth, and low birth weight (LBW). Furthermore, pathways involved in maternal immune activation and placental vascularization parallel those involved in normal fetal development, notably neurovascular development. Therefore, immune-mediated disruption of angiogenic pathways at the materno-fetal interface may also have long-term neurological consequences for offspring. Here, we review current literature evaluating the influence of maternal infection and immune activation at the materno-fetal interface and the subsequent impact on placental vascular function and birth outcome. Immunomodulatory pathways, including chemokines and cytokines released in response to maternal infection, interact closely with the principal pathways regulating placental vascular development, including the angiopoietin-Tie-2, vascular endothelial growth factor (VEGF), and placental growth factor (PlGF) pathways. A detailed mechanistic understanding of how maternal infections impact placental and fetal development is critical to the design of effective interventions to promote placental growth and function and thereby reduce adverse birth outcomes.

Keywords: infection, pregnancy, placenta, vascular development, adverse birth outcomes

INTRODUCTION

Each year an estimated 20 million infants are born low birth weight (LBW) (<2,500 g) and 14.9 million are born preterm (Lee et al., 2013). Preterm birth (PTB) is the leading direct cause of under 5 mortality, responsible for more than 1 million deaths per year (Liu et al., 2016). According to the Global Burden of Disease Study, the disability-adjusted life years attributable to PTB is 77 million, comparable to the estimates for HIV or malaria (Murray et al., 2012). While these adverse birth outcomes predominantly occur in low- and middle-income countries (Blencowe et al., 2012), rates are increasing globally, and have been consistently linked with increased risks of long-term health consequences for offspring including cardiovascular disease, diabetes, obesity, and neurodevelopmental disorders (Bilbo and Schwarz, 2009; Calkins and Devaskar, 2011). The burden of infectious diseases in pregnancy (e.g., malaria, HIV, sexually transmitted infections) is also highest in low- and middle-income countries, and a growing body of evidence indicates that these prevalent infections contribute to poor birth outcomes by inflammation-mediated disruption of placental development and function (Watson-Jones et al., 2002; Chico et al., 2017; Conroy et al., 2017; McDonald et al., 2018, 2019).

Fetal development is governed by tightly regulated processes at the materno-fetal interface. Placental vasculogenesis and angiogenesis mediate placental vascular development, which is critical to nutrient and oxygen delivery to the developing fetus. These processes are primarily regulated by mediators in the vascular endothelial growth factor (VEGF) and angiopoietin families (Geva et al., 2002). Dysregulation of these factors is associated with inadequate placental vascularization, leading to hemodynamic placental insufficiency, inadequate delivery of nutrients and oxygen to the fetus, and consequently adverse birth outcomes (Kaufmann et al., 2003). Inflammatory and angiogenic pathways are interdependent and co-regulatory, suggesting that the host response to maternal infection could dysregulate pathways essential for placental vascular development. Here, we review the impact of systemic maternal infections resulting in immune activation at the materno-fetal interface – and its subsequent impact on placental vascularization – adverse birth outcomes, and later-life neurocognitive deficits in offspring.

PLACENTAL DEVELOPMENT: VASCULOGENESIS AND ANGIOGENESIS

The placenta forms the primary interface between mother and fetus, and a healthy functioning placenta is essential for a successful pregnancy. The placenta is a multi-function organ, acting as the site of materno-fetal nutrient, oxygen and waste exchange; producing hormones and growth factors critical for pregnancy progression and maintenance; and acting as a barrier to protect the fetus from maternal immune attack, toxins, and infectious pathogens (Wang and Zhao, 2010). These functions all rely on proper vascularization and perfusion of the placenta, and disruptions to placental vascular development and adaptation are associated with adverse pregnancy outcomes including preeclampsia, small-for-gestational age (SGA), PTB, and stillbirth (Kingdom, 1998; Gagnon, 2003; Wang and Zhao, 2010; Romero et al., 2011; Conroy et al., 2013; Morgan, 2016; Silver, 2018).

Placental vascular development begins early in pregnancy and undergoes adaptations across gestation. On the maternal side, uteroplacental circulation is established by the end of the first trimester (Wang and Zhao, 2010). Maternal vascular adaptation involves remodeling of the uterine spiral arteries by invasive fetal-derived extravillous trophoblasts to enable low-resistance blood flow into the intervillous space of the placenta (Wang and Zhao, 2010; Pollheimer et al., 2018). On the fetal side, primary placental villi begin to develop around day 13 post-conception, and fetoplacental vascularization of villi begins around 21 days post-conception (Kingdom et al., 2000; Kaufmann et al., 2004; Demir et al., 2006). The tertiary villi around which maternal blood flows in the intervillous space act as the functional units of the materno-fetal interface. Fetal-derived syncytiotrophoblasts are the primary mediators of exchange, protein-production, and defense at the materno-fetal interface.

Vascularization of placental villi involves the sequential processes of vasculogenesis and angiogenesis. Vasculogenesis is the *de novo* formation of blood vessels *via* differentiation of mesenchymal cells to hemangiogenic stem cells and then endothelial precursors (Demir et al., 2007). The VEGF family of ligands and receptors are heavily involved in the regulation of both vasculogenesis and angiogenesis. VEGF and its receptors (VEGFR-1 and -2) are expressed very early in placental development, and the production of VEGF by cytotrophoblasts and Hofbauer cells is thought to drive early placental vasculogenesis and subsequent angiogenesis (Kaufmann et al., 2004; Demir et al., 2006, 2007).

Angiogenesis begins at approximately 32 days post-conception (Kaufmann et al., 2004). From this point until term, the placental vascular network needed to support the rapidly growing fetus is built predominantly *via* branching and non-branching angiogenesis. The molecular mediation of angiogenesis requires tight temporal and spatial coordination and interaction between VEGF and angiopoietin protein family signaling (Ahmed and Perkins, 2000; Carmeliet, 2000; Yancopoulos et al., 2000; Geva et al., 2002; Charnock-Jones et al., 2004; Kaufmann et al., 2004; Benirschke et al., 2012). VEGF, placental growth factor (PlGF), and their inhibitor soluble fms-like tyrosine kinase-1 (sFlt-1) are produced by trophoblasts, and their balance is critical to healthy placental vascular development (Ahmed and Perkins, 2000; Kingdom et al., 2000; Charnock-Jones et al., 2004; Kaufmann et al., 2004). The timing and ratio of angiopoietin-1 (Ang-1) and its antagonist angiopoietin-2 (Ang-2) signaling through their receptor Tie2 is also essential for placental vascularization. Ang-1 promotes vascular maturation and stability, whereas Ang-2 allows for the destabilization and endothelial plasticity required for VEGF to drive angiogenesis and vascular remodeling (Carmeliet, 2000; Yancopoulos et al., 2000; Geva et al., 2002). These functions are reflected in the longitudinal dynamics of Ang-1 and -2 in healthy pregnancies: Ang-1 is initially low and increases across pregnancy as placental vasculature becomes more established, while Ang-2 decreases across pregnancy (Geva et al., 2002). Several groups have hypothesized that the tightly regulated longitudinal dynamics

---

Abbreviations: Ang-1 and -2, Angiopoietin-1 and -2; cART, Combined antiretroviral therapy; CMV, Cytomegalovirus; dNK, Decidual natural killer cells; IL, Interleukin; INF, Interferon; LBW, Low birth weight; NO, Nitric oxide; PlGF, Placental growth factor; PTB, Preterm birth; sFlt-1, Soluble fms-like tyrosine kinase-1; SGA, Small-for-gestational age; TNF, Tumor necrosis factor; VEGF, Vascular endothelial growth factor.

of VEGF and PlGF, as well as Ang-1 and -2, provide a molecular basis for the temporal transition from vasculogenesis to branching and then non-branching angiogenesis that underlies placental vascular development (**Figure 1**; Ahmed and Perkins, 2000; Geva et al., 2002; Kaufmann et al., 2004).

VEGF, PlGF, and VEGFR-1 are expressed on extravillous and villous trophoblasts, as well as Hofbauer cells in human placentas (Charnock-Jones et al., 1994; Ahmed et al., 1995; Clark et al., 1996; Khaliq et al., 1996; Vuorela et al., 1997). Their signaling has a role in trophoblast function including proliferation, differentiation, and nitric oxide (NO) production (Charnock-Jones et al., 1994; Ahmed et al., 1997; Athanassiades et al., 1998; Athanassiades and Lala, 1998; Khaliq et al., 1999). Ang-1 and -2 and their receptor Tie2 are also expressed in villous and

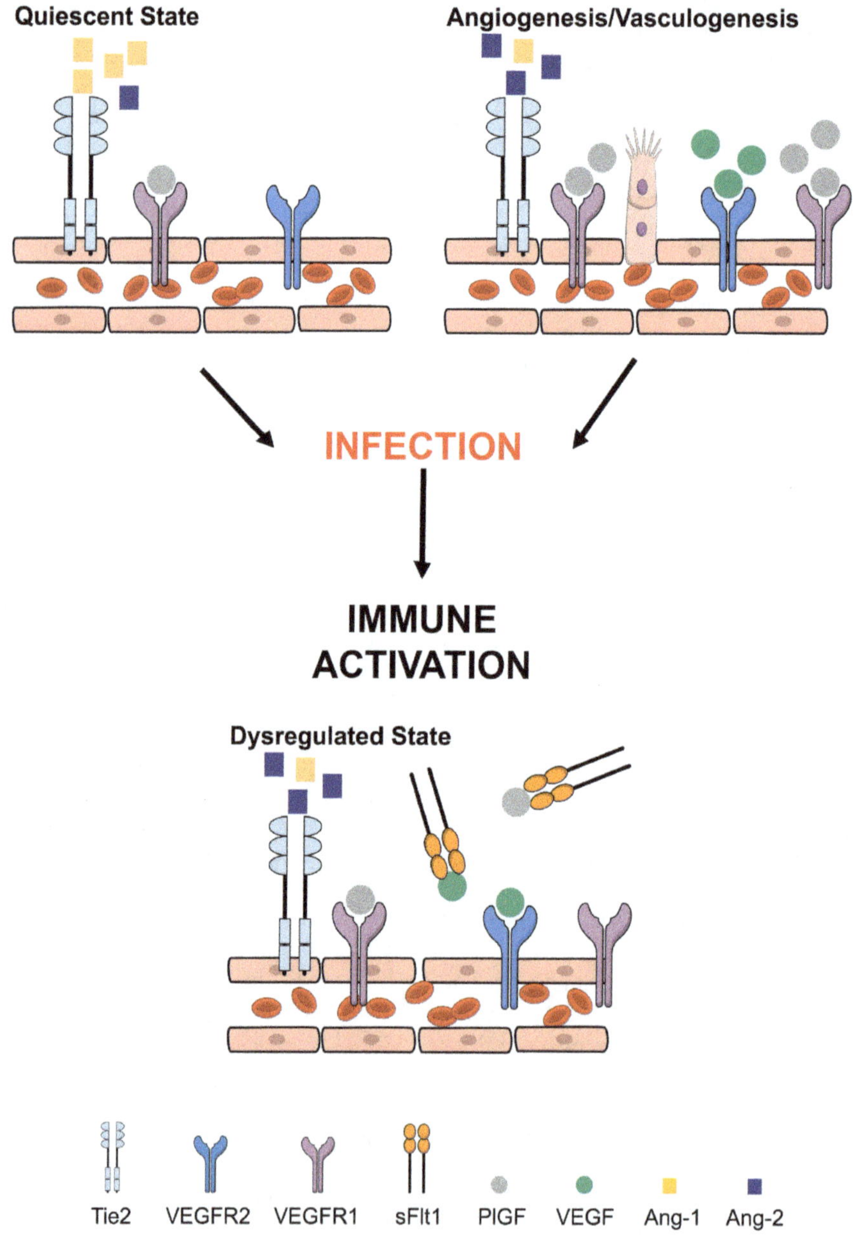

FIGURE 1 | Overview of key angiogenic and vasculogenic factors mediating placental function and how they may be disrupted in the context of maternal infection. Placental vasculogenesis and angiogenesis are processes that are vital for placental vascular development and function. These processes depend on a fine balance between pro-angiogenic and anti-angiogenic pathways. The vascular endothelial growth factor (VEGF) family of proteins (including PlGF – placental growth factor) are pro-angiogenic mediators. VEGF and PlGF bind VEGF receptor 1 [fms-like tyrosine kinase (Flt-1)] to induce vessel proliferation and sprouting. Alternative splicing of Flt-1 results in soluble Flt-1 (sFlt-1) that is anti-angiogenic. Angiopoietin-1 (Ang-1) binds its tyrosine-kinase receptor Tie2 inducing vessel maturation, whereas angiopoietin-2 (Ang-2) promotes vessel destabilization and angiogenesis. Tight control of these pathways is essential for proper vascular development, remodeling, robust placental function, and healthy birth outcomes. Maternal infection (e.g., malaria, HIV-1) can result in immune activation and inflammation which dysregulates these tightly regulated processes, contributing to poor birth outcomes.

extravillous trophoblasts in specific cell-type and temporal patterns across pregnancy, and *in vitro* studies reported a role for Ang/Tie2 signaling in trophoblast NO production and migration (Dunk et al., 2000; Goldman-Wohl et al., 2000; Seval et al., 2008).

Collectively, these data support critical roles for the VEGF and angiopoietin pathways in both fetoplacental vascularization (i.e., vasculogenesis and angiogenesis in the villi) and trophoblast function, as well as uteroplacental remodeling (i.e. trophoblast-mediated maternal spiral artery remodeling). With such diverse and interdependent roles for angiogenic factors across placental development, it is not surprising that their dysregulation has been associated with pathologic pregnancies and adverse birth outcomes.

PLACENTAL DEVELOPMENT: A ROLE FOR INFLAMMATORY MEDIATORS

In a healthy pregnancy, the maternal immune system adapts to protect the semi-allogeneic fetus and placenta. Circulating levels of both cytokines [e.g., interferon (IFN)-γ, tumor necrosis factor (TNF), etc.] and components of the complement system (e.g., C3a, C5a, etc.) are altered across normal pregnancy (Kraus et al., 2010; Regal et al., 2015). Several cell types in the placenta including maternal and fetal-derived placental cells, as well as specialized immune cells like decidual natural killer cells (dNK), produce, express and/or secrete inflammatory cytokines and complement regulatory proteins at the materno-fetal interface in a healthy pregnancy (Bowen et al., 2002; Weckman et al., 2018). These inflammatory mediators play a dual role in immunity and processes of normal placental development including extravillous trophoblast proliferation and invasion necessary for uterine spiral artery remodeling (Albieri et al., 1999; Bowen et al., 2002; Hanna et al., 2006; Bulla et al., 2008; Pollheimer et al., 2018). Furthermore, dNKs play an important role in placental vascular development *via* the production of angiogenic factors including VEGF, PlGF, Ang-1, and Ang-2 (Hanna et al., 2006; Le Bouteiller, 2013). Trophoblasts also increase VEGF production in response to cytokine stimulation, and monocytes will increase production of sFlt-1 in response to complement activation (Choi et al., 2002; Girardi et al., 2006; Conroy et al., 2009). Inflammatory and angiogenic systems are interdependent and tightly regulated across pregnancy. Together, their regulation is critical to placental vascular development. Therefore, disruption of either system could lead to a cascade of downstream events with negative impacts on placental vascular development and birth outcomes.

ABNORMAL PLACENTAL VASCULAR DEVELOPMENT UNDERLIES PREGNANCY COMPLICATIONS

There is abundant evidence for defective maternal spiral artery remodeling (Khong et al., 1986; Hustin et al., 1990; Pijnenborg et al., 1991; Kingdom et al., 2000; Romero et al., 2011; Fisher, 2015; Burton and Jauniaux, 2018; Pollheimer et al., 2018), abnormal villous development and vascularization (Jackson et al., 1995; Kingdom and Kaufmann, 1997; Kingdom et al., 2000; Vedmedovska et al., 2011; Burton and Jauniaux, 2018; Silver, 2018; Travaglino et al., 2019), and impaired umbilical blood flow (Trudinger et al., 1985; Salafia et al., 1997; Ferrazzi et al., 2000; Zhu et al., 2016) in a range of pregnancy outcomes with placental pathologies including preeclampsia, SGA, PTB, spontaneous abortion, and stillbirth.

Dysregulation of specific angiogenic mediators has also been associated with placental insufficiency and adverse pregnancy outcomes. The balance between angiogenic and anti-angiogenic factors, and the resulting alterations to placental vasculature, is modulated by multiple factors including oxygen homeostasis, external agents (e.g., drugs), infection, and inflammation (Khaliq et al., 1999; Kaufmann et al., 2004; Girardi et al., 2006; Conroy et al., 2013; McDonald et al., 2018; Mohammadi et al., 2018). Seminal preclinical studies established the importance of a precise angiogenic balance *in utero*, as both an absence and excess of VEGF and the angiopoietins were associated with abnormal embryonic development or lethality (Carmeliet et al., 1996; Suri et al., 1996; Maisonpierre et al., 1997; Miquerol et al., 2000). These findings have been extended to human studies, where multiple adverse pregnancy outcomes have been linked to dysregulation of circulating levels of angiogenic mediators critical for normal placental development including VEGF, PlGF, and sFlt-1, Ang-1 and -2, and soluble endoglin (Sharkey et al., 1996; Levine et al., 2004, 2006; Venkatesha et al., 2006; Chaiworapongsa et al., 2009; Romero et al., 2010; Conroy et al., 2013, 2017; Darling et al., 2014; McDonald et al., 2015b, 2018; Straughen et al., 2017).

As discussed above, there is a tight interrelationship between inflammatory pathways and angiogenic balance during placental development. Consequently, adverse pregnancy outcomes including spontaneous PTB and SGA have been associated with simultaneous dysregulation of both pathways (Girardi et al., 2006; Conroy et al., 2013; Darling et al., 2014; McDonald et al., 2015b). These data strongly support a role for disrupted placental development, due to inflammatory and angiogenic dysregulation at the materno-fetal interface, as a common pathway in the pathobiology of adverse birth outcomes.

MATERNAL INFECTION DISRUPTS PLACENTAL VASCULAR DEVELOPMENT

An important contributor to disruption of the inflammatory and angiogenic environment at the materno-fetal interface is maternal infection. Infections due to the TORCH pathogens [*Toxoplasma gondii*, others, rubella virus, cytomegalovirus (CMV), and herpes simplex virus] may result in adverse pregnancy outcomes *via* vertical transmission to the fetus (Coyne and Lazear, 2016). However, even in the absence of congenital infection, maternal infections such as malaria and

HIV have been linked with adverse birth outcomes including PTB, LBW, SGA, and stillbirth (Desai et al., 2007; Wedi et al., 2016; Rogerson et al., 2018). Despite increased coverage of treatment for infections in pregnancy such as malaria and HIV, rates of adverse birth outcomes remain high (Madanitsa et al., 2016; Santosa et al., 2019), and a better understanding of the pathophysiology underlying infection-induced adverse birth outcomes is needed. Increasing evidence suggests placental vascular pathology may be an important contributor to the link between maternal infection and adverse birth outcomes.

A growing body of evidence has linked maternal infection with abnormal placental pathology and altered maternal and fetal hemodynamics. Histopathological examination of human placentas have reported abnormal placental villous architecture and maternal vascular malperfusion in the context of viral, bacterial and parasitic maternal infections (Carmona-Fonseca et al., 2013; Ahmed et al., 2014; Chaikitgosiyakul et al., 2014; Kim et al., 2015; Kalk et al., 2017; Ribeiro et al., 2017; Moeller et al., 2018). Preclinical studies have also demonstrated significantly altered placental vascularization, vascular remodeling, and oxygen transport in response to maternal infection (Tabata et al., 2012; Conroy et al., 2013; Hirsch et al., 2018; McDonald et al., 2018; Phillips et al., 2018). In humans, maternal infections including influenza, *Helicobacter pylori*, malaria, and HIV have been associated with impaired maternal and fetal hemodynamics (e.g., high arterial resistance) (Dorman et al., 2002; Griffin et al., 2012; Hernandez-Andrade et al., 2014; McClure et al., 2014; Di Simone et al., 2017; Ome-Kaius et al., 2017). The available evidence implicates abnormalities in placental vascularization and function as a common driver behind infection-induced adverse birth outcomes, even in non-congenital infections.

Mechanistically, dysregulation of angiogenic mediators including sFlt-1, Ang-1, and -2, soluble endoglin, and PlGF and altered placental vascular structure and function has been reported in the context of maternal infections (e.g., malaria, HIV, CMV, and acute pyelonephritis) associated with adverse birth outcomes (Chaiworapongsa et al., 2010; Silver et al., 2010, 2011; Conroy et al., 2013, 2017; Ataíde et al., 2015; Gustafsson et al., 2015; McDonald et al., 2018). Inflammatory mediators including cytokines [e.g., interleukin (IL)-1, INF-γ, and TNF] and the complement system exhibit regulatory cross-talk with angiogenic factors critical to placental development (Naldini and Carraro, 2005; Fiedler and Augustin, 2006; Girardi et al., 2006; Conroy et al., 2009, 2013). There is evidence for systemic inflammation in bacterial, viral, and parasitic maternal infections (Horton et al., 2008; Conroy et al., 2013; Cérbulo-Vázquez et al., 2014; Romero et al., 2016; Fried et al., 2017; Wilkinson et al., 2017; Harjunmaa et al., 2018; McDonald et al., 2019), and statistical modeling suggests a hierarchical relationship between dysregulated inflammation, angiogenesis, and adverse birth outcomes (Conroy et al., 2013). Collectively, these studies suggest inflammation-mediated dysregulation of the tight angiogenic balance required for placental development as a shared mechanism underlying adverse birth outcomes in maternal infection (**Figure 2**).

FETAL DEVELOPMENT IS IMPACTED BY DYSREGULATION OF THE INFLAMMATORY-ANGIOGENIC AXIS IN MATERNAL INFECTION

Many pathways critical to placental vascular development are mirrored in fetal vascular development. Normal vasculogenesis, angiogenesis, and materno-fetal hemodynamics are critical to organ growth *in utero*. Mounting evidence supports the hypothesis that disruption of these processes *via* maternal immune activation may cause defects in development of the fetal lungs, heart, and brain, with long-term consequences for offspring (Bilbo and Schwarz, 2009; McAdams et al., 2012; Burton and Jauniaux, 2018). The nature of the disruption to fetal development may depend on timing of infection. For example, studies suggest disruption to placental development and hemodynamics, especially in the first month of pregnancy, could be reflected in fetal cardiac abnormalities and congenital heart disease (Linask, 2013; Linask et al., 2014; Burton and Jauniaux, 2018). Dysregulation of inflammatory and angiogenic factors (i.e., *via* maternal infection) during a critical period of lung development is associated with bronchopulmonary dysplasia and increased neonatal mortality in the first 28 days of life (Thébaud and Abman, 2007; McAdams et al., 2012; Procianoy et al., 2015). Furthermore, a large and rapidly growing body of evidence has linked maternal immune activation and dysregulation of angiogenesis with impaired fetal neurodevelopment and long-lasting neurocognitive and neuropsychiatric sequelae for offspring (Knuesel et al., 2014; Estes and McAllister, 2016; Brown and Meyer, 2018).

Neurodevelopment is an intricate and strictly orchestrated process. Proper molecular signaling during critical gestational and postnatal periods is required for the establishment of effective neural networks (Stiles and Jernigan, 2010). Immune cells and cytokines such as microglia, complement, and IL-6 play an integral role in mediating these signals, and are tightly regulated at the materno-fetal interface (Billiards et al., 2006; Smith et al., 2007; Bilbo and Schwarz, 2009; Gallagher et al., 2013; McDonald et al., 2013; Graham et al., 2018; Prins et al., 2018; Rudolph et al., 2018; Spann et al., 2018; Rasmussen et al., 2019). In response to bacterial, viral, and parasitic infections, the maternal immune system is activated, exposing the fetus to cytokines and immune cells that are capable of passing through the immature fetal blood brain barrier and potentially impacting fetal neurodevelopment (Dammann and Leviton, 1997; Prins et al., 2018).

Evidence of the association between maternal immune activation and neuropsychiatric disorders, including schizophrenia (SZ), autism spectrum disorder (ASD) and bipolar disorder (BD), has accumulated in both epidemiological studies and preclinical models (Knuesel et al., 2014; Estes

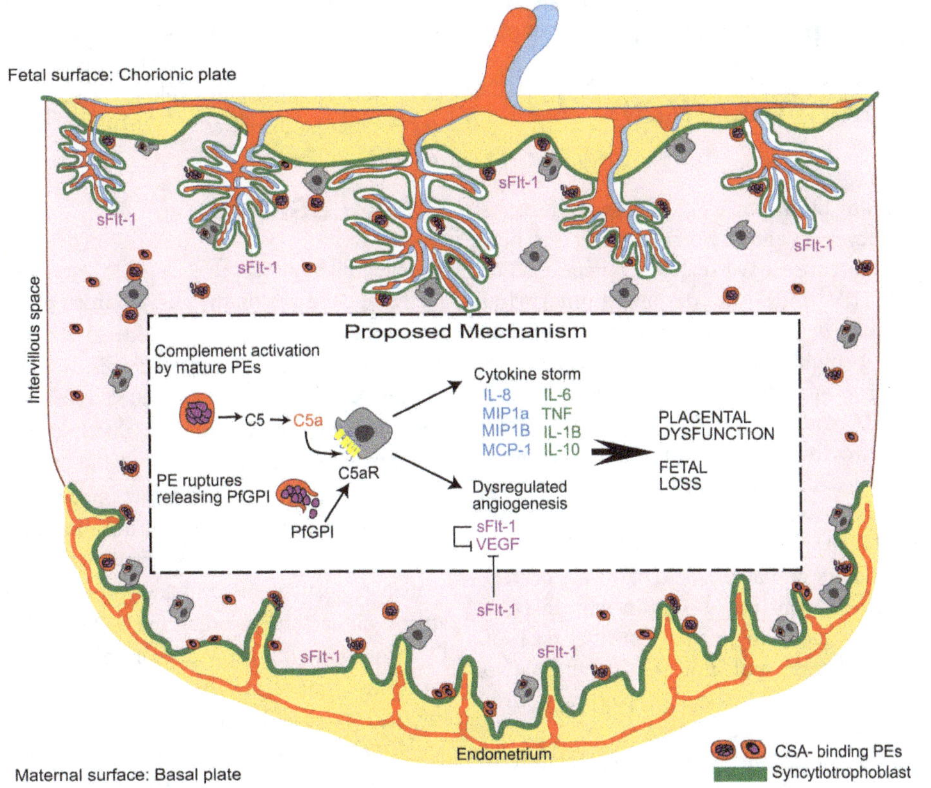

FIGURE 2 | Malaria in pregnancy as a model for infection-driven dysregulation of placental vascular development as a common mechanism underlying adverse birth outcomes. During malaria in pregnancy, parasitized erythrocytes (PE) activate the maternal complement cascade. Complement component C5a acts synergistically with circulating parasite-associated bioactive molecules (i.e., *Plasmodium falciparum* glycosylphosphatidylinositol anchor molecules; *Pf*GPI) to trigger an inflammatory response at the materno-fetal interface. This inflammatory host response dysregulates the tight balance of angiogenic factors required for placental vascular development leading to aberrant placental vascularization, placental dysfunction, and adverse birth outcomes. Existing evidence for other infections during pregnancy supports this model as a common mechanism underlying adverse birth outcomes in maternal infection [reproduced from Conroy et al., 2009].

and McAllister, 2016; Brown and Meyer, 2018). Maternal immune activation *via* individual cytokines (e.g., IL-6 and IL-2), viral/bacterial mimics [e.g., polyinosinic:polycytidylic acid, poly(I:C); lipopolysaccharides, LPS], and actual infections (e.g., malaria, influenza, urinary tract infections) have been associated with long-term behavioral consequences for exposed offspring (Cai et al., 2000; Ponzio et al., 2007; Smith et al., 2007; Giovanoli et al., 2013; Knuesel et al., 2014; McDonald et al., 2015a; Choi et al., 2016; Brown and Meyer, 2018). Altered expression of proinflammatory mediators with dual roles in inflammation and neurodevelopment have been implicated in this link. Proinflammatory cytokine IL-6, which induced psychiatric behavioral outcomes in a seminal preclinical study of maternal immune activation (Smith et al., 2007), also has roles in neurogenesis, synapse formation, white matter development, and dendritic spine architecture (Wei et al., 2012; Gallagher et al., 2013; Rasmussen et al., 2019). Complement components including C5a, C3, and C1q also have well-characterized dual roles in maternal response to infection and neurodevelopment (i.e., synaptic pruning), and dysregulation of complement has been implicated in maternal infection-associated neurocognitive deficits in offspring (Stevens et al., 2007; Schafer et al., 2012; McDonald et al., 2015a; Weckman et al., 2018).

Furthermore, evidence points toward a direct connection and cross-talk between pathways critical to angiogenesis and neurodevelopment; proteins including VEGF family members have important roles in both processes (Carmeliet, 2003). Interestingly, VEGF participates in signaling required for the intricate growth and patterning of nerves and blood vessels alongside one another in the developing brain (Carmeliet, 2003). This indicates that disruption of the angiogenic environment (possibly downstream of maternal infection and inflammation) at the materno-fetal interface could also impact neurocognitive development with potential long-term neurological consequences for the offspring. In support of this contention, micro-CT images of malaria-exposed murine offspring showed alterations to fetal neurovasculature that was C5a-C5aR signaling-dependent (McDonald et al., 2015a). Since C5a activation seems to be upstream of angiogenic dysregulation in malaria in pregnancy (**Figure 2**; Conroy et al., 2009, 2013), these preclinical data support a model whereby maternal host response to infection in pregnancy could induce disruptions to fetal neurodevelopment *via* both angiogenic and inflammatory mechanisms.

ABNORMAL PLACENTAL DEVELOPMENT AS A DRIVER OF INFECTION-INDUCED ADVERSE BIRTH OUTCOMES HAS IMPLICATIONS FOR TREATMENT STRATEGIES

An increased understanding of the impact of maternal infections on placental vascular development has implications for new intervention strategies to reduce adverse birth outcomes. For example in maternal HIV infection, despite antiretroviral treatment women exhibited dysregulation of angiogenic factors (i.e., increased circulating soluble endoglin and decreased PlGF concentrations, resulting in an anti-angiogenic state) that were associated with PTB, SGA and stillbirth (Conroy et al., 2017). Women receiving antiretrovirals and cotrimoxazole that were co-infected with HIV and malaria exhibited systemic inflammation (i.e. increased soluble TNF receptor-2) that was also associated with PTB (McDonald et al., 2019). Persistent dysregulation of inflammatory and angiogenic pathways critical to placental vascular development could explain why rates of adverse birth outcomes remain high even in the face of appropriate antimicrobial therapy and indicate that alternative strategies, including modifying host response pathways, may be necessary to reduce poor birth outcomes.

Considering the early stage at which placental vasculature is established, the timing of infection during pregnancy has important implications for prevention/treatment strategies. Increasing evidence suggests that early infection with malaria in pregnancy increases the risk of adverse birth outcomes including SGA *via* disruption to placental development (Griffin et al., 2012; Moeller et al., 2018). Since current malaria drug-based prevention strategies are not implemented until the second trimester, this could represent an important gap in the prevention of infection-induced dysregulation of placental development and resulting adverse birth outcomes (Huynh et al., 2015). The use of combined antiretroviral therapy (cART) in pregnancy has also been associated with dysregulated angiogenesis, compromised placental vascular development, and adverse birth outcomes, especially when initiated early in pregnancy (Mohammadi et al., 2018). In pre-clinical studies, supplementing cART-treated mice with progesterone prevented placental abnormalities, indicating that this addition to current treatment strategies might improve pregnancy outcomes by targeting dysregulated placental vascular development. In support of this contention, a study in a large cohort of women in Papua New Guinea demonstrated the ability of sulphadoxine-pyrimethamine and azithromycin to improve adverse birth outcomes by regulating inflammatory (e.g., C-reactive protein) and angiogenic factors (e.g., soluble endoglin, sFlt-1) critical to placental vascular development (Unger et al., 2019).

CONCLUSIONS

Despite Millennium and Sustainable Development Goals to improve maternal-child health, the global burden of adverse birth outcomes remains high. This is in part due to a critical knowledge gap in our understanding of the mechanisms underlying adverse birth outcomes, and consequently limited or ineffective strategies. Several lines of evidence suggest that infection-driven dysregulation of inflammation and angiogenesis at the materno-fetal interface is a common mechanism underlying inadequate placental and fetal development, and adverse birth outcomes. Placental vascular development and vascular adaptation requires tight temporal and spatial regulation of cytokines, the complement system, and angiogenic factors including the VEGF and angiopoietin families. Dysregulation of those systems in the context of maternal infection leads to aberrations in spiral artery remodeling, placental vascularization and villous architecture, and deleterious materno-fetal hemodynamics that are associated with adverse birth outcomes. Current interventions for infections in pregnancy including malaria and HIV target only the pathogen and not the host response that may drive poor birth outcomes. This may explain, at least in part, why rates of adverse birth outcomes remain high. Further, dysregulation of inflammatory and angiogenic factors at the materno-fetal interface can lead to impairments in fetal neurodevelopment including neurogenesis and neurovascular development, with long term cognitive and behavioral sequelae for offspring. Considering the importance of the relationship between infection-induced dysregulation and adverse birth outcomes, future research should focus on therapeutics that target early placental development as a strategy to reduce the global burden of adverse birth outcomes.

AUTHOR CONTRIBUTIONS

CM and KK managed project conception and oversight. AW, MN, JW, and CM contributed to research, analysis, and writing of the manuscript. All authors contributed to manuscript revisions and approved the final manuscript.

REFERENCES

Ahmed, A., Dunk, C., Kniss, D., and Wilkes, M. (1997). Role of VEGF receptor-1 (Flt-1) in mediating calcium-dependent nitric oxide release and limiting DNA synthesis in human trophoblast cells. *Lab. Investig.* 76, 779–791.

Ahmed, A., Li, X. F., Dunk, C., Whittle, M. J., Rushton, D. I., and Rollason, T. (1995). Colocalisation of vascular endothelial growth factor and its Flt-1 receptor in human placenta. *Growth Factors* 12, 235–243.

Ahmed, A., and Perkins, J. (2000). Angiogenesis and intrauterine growth restriction. *Best Pract. Res. Clin. Obstet. Gynaecol.* 14, 981–998. doi: 10.1053/beog.2000.0139

Ahmed, R., Singh, N., ter Kuile, F. O., Bharti, P. K., Singh, P. P., Desai, M., et al. (2014). Placental infections with histologically confirmed *Plasmodium falciparum* are associated with adverse birth outcomes in India: a cross-sectional study. *Malar. J.* 13:232. doi: 10.1186/1475-2875-13-232

Albieri, A., Kipnis, T., and Bevilacqua, E. (1999). A possible role for activated complement component 3 in phagocytic activity exhibited by the mouse trophoblast. *Am. J. Reprod. Immunol.* 41, 343–352. doi: 10.1111/j.1600-0897.1999.tb00448.x

Ataíde, R., Murillo, O., Dombrowski, J. G., Souza, R. M., Lima, F. A., Lima, G. F. M. C., et al. (2015). Malaria in pregnancy interacts with and alters the angiogenic profiles of the placenta. *PLoS Negl. Trop. Dis.* 9:e0003824. doi: 10.1371/journal.pntd.0003824

Athanassiades, A., Hamilton, G. S., and Lala, P. K. (1998). Vascular endothelial growth factor stimulates proliferation but not migration or invasiveness in human extravillous trophoblast1. *Biol. Reprod.* 59, 643–654. doi: 10.1095/biolreprod59.3.643

Athanassiades, A., and Lala, P. K. (1998). Role of placenta growth factor (PIGF) in human extravillous trophoblast proliferation, migration and invasiveness. *Placenta* 19, 465–473. doi: 10.1016/S0143-4004(98)91039-6

Benirschke, K., Burton, G. J., and Baergen, R. N. (eds.) (2012). "Architecture of normal villous trees" in *Pathology of the human placenta* (Berlin, Heidelberg: Springer), 101–144.

Bilbo, S. D., and Schwarz, J. M. (2009). Early-life programming of later-life brain and behavior: a critical role for the immune system. *Front. Behav. Neurosci.* 3:14. doi: 10.3389/neuro.08.014.2009

Billiards, S. S., Haynes, R. L., Folkerth, R. D., Trachtenberg, F. L., Liu, L. G., Volpe, J. J., et al. (2006). Development of microglia in the cerebral white matter of the human fetus and infant. *J. Comp. Neurol.* 497, 199–208. doi: 10.1002/cne.20991

Blencowe, H., Cousens, S., Oestergaard, M. Z., Chou, D., Moller, A., Narwal, R., et al. (2012). National, regional, and worldwide estimates of preterm birth rates in the year 2010 with time trends since 1990 for selected countries: a systematic analysis and implications. *Lancet* 379, 2162–2172. doi: 10.1016/S0140-6736(12)60820-4

Bowen, J. M., Chamley, L., Mitchell, M. D., and Keelan, J. A. (2002). Cytokines of the placenta and extra-placental membranes: biosynthesis, secretion and roles in establishment of pregnancy in women. *Placenta* 23, 239–256. doi: 10.1053/plac.2001.0781

Brown, A. S., and Meyer, U. (2018). Maternal immune activation and neuropsychiatric illness: a translational research perspective. *Am. J. Psychiatry* 175, 1073–1083. doi: 10.1176/appi.ajp.2018.17121311

Bulla, R., Agostinis, C., Bossi, F., Rizzi, L., Debeus, A., Tripodo, C., et al. (2008). Decidual endothelial cells express surface-bound C1q as a molecular bridge between endovascular trophoblast and decidual endothelium. *Mol. Immunol.* 45, 2629–2640. doi: 10.1016/j.molimm.2007.12.025

Burton, G. J., and Jauniaux, E. (2018). Development of the human placenta and fetal heart: synergic or independent? *Front. Physiol.* 9:373. doi: 10.3389/fphys.2018.00373

Cai, Z., Pan, Z. L., Pang, Y., Evans, O. B., and Rhodes, P. G. (2000). Cytokine induction in fetal rat brains and brain injury in neonatal rats after maternal lipopolysaccharide administration. *Pediatr. Res.* 47, 64–72. doi: 10.1203/00006450-200001000-00013

Calkins, K., and Devaskar, S. U. (2011). Fetal origins of adult disease. *Curr. Probl. Pediatr. Adolesc. Health Care* 41, 158–176. doi: 10.1016/j.cppeds.2011.01.001

Carmeliet, P. (2000). Mechanisms of angiogenesis and arteriogenesis. *Nat. Med.* 6, 389–395. doi: 10.1038/74651

Carmeliet, P. (2003). Blood vessels and nerves: common signals, pathways and diseases. *Nat. Rev. Genet.* 4, 710–720. doi: 10.1038/nrg1158

Carmeliet, P., Ferreira, V., Breier, G., Pollefeyt, S., Kieckens, L., Gertsenstein, M., et al. (1996). Abnormal blood vessel development and lethality in embryos lacking a single VEGF allele. *Nature* 380, 435–439. doi: 10.1038/380435a0

Carmona-Fonseca, J., Arango, E., and Maestre, A. (2013). Placental malaria in Colombia: histopathologic findings in *Plasmodium vivax* and *P. falciparum* infections. *Am. J. Trop. Med. Hyg.* 88, 1093–1101. doi: 10.4269/ajtmh.12-0363

Cérbulo-Vázquez, A., Figueroa-Damián, R., Arriaga-Pizano, L. A., Hernández-Andrade, E., Mancilla-Herrera, I., Flores-Mejía, L. A., et al. (2014). Pregnant women infected with pandemic H1N1pdm2009 influenza virus displayed overproduction of peripheral blood CD69+ lymphocytes and increased levels of serum cytokines. *PLoS One* 9:e107900. doi: 10.1371/journal.pone.0107900

Chaikitgosiyakul, S., Rijken, M. J., Muehlenbachs, A., Lee, S. J., Chaisri, U., Viriyavejakul, P., et al. (2014). A morphometric and histological study of placental malaria shows significant changes to villous architecture in both *Plasmodium falciparum* and *Plasmodium vivax* infection. *Malar. J.* 13:4. doi: 10.1186/1475-2875-13-4

Chaiworapongsa, T., Romero, R., Gotsch, F., Kusanovic, J. P., Mittal, P., Kim, S. K., et al. (2010). Acute pyelonephritis during pregnancy changes the balance of angiogenic and anti-angiogenic factors in maternal plasma. *J. Matern. Fetal Neonatal Med.* 23, 167–178. doi: 10.3109/14767050903067378

Chaiworapongsa, T., Romero, R., Tarca, A., Kusanovic, J. P., Mittal, P., Kim, S. K., et al. (2009). A subset of patients destined to develop spontaneous preterm labor has an abnormal angiogenic/anti-angiogenic profile in maternal plasma: evidence in support of pathophysiologic heterogeneity of preterm labor derived from a longitudinal study. *J. Matern. Fetal Neonatal Med.* 22, 1122–1139. doi: 10.3109/14767050902994838

Charnock-Jones, D. S., Kaufmann, P., and Mayhew, T. M. (2004). Aspects of human fetoplacental vasculogenesis and angiogenesis. I. Molecular regulation. *Placenta* 25, 103–113. doi: 10.1016/j.placenta.2003.10.004

Charnock-Jones, D. S., Sharkey, A. M., Boocock, C. A., Ahmed, A., Plevin, R., Ferrara, N., et al. (1994). Vascular endothelial growth factor receptor localization and activation in human trophoblast and choriocarcinoma cells. *Biol. Reprod.* 51, 524–530. doi: 10.1095/biolreprod51.3.524

Chico, R. M., Chaponda, E. B., Ariti, C., and Chandramohan, D. (2017). Sulfadoxine-pyrimethamine exhibits dose-response protection against adverse birth outcomes related to malaria and sexually transmitted and reproductive tract infections. *Clin. Infect. Dis.* 64, 1043–1051. doi: 10.1093/cid/cix026

Choi, S. J., Park, J. Y., Lee, Y. K., Choi, H. I., Lee, Y. S., Koh, C.-M., et al. (2002). Effects of cytokines on VEGF expression and secretion by human first trimester trophoblast cell line. *Am. J. Reprod. Immunol.* 48, 70–76. doi: 10.1034/j.1600-0897.2002.01071.x

Choi, G. B., Yim, Y. S., Wong, H., Kim, S., Kim, H., Kim, S. V., et al. (2016). The maternal interleukin-17a pathway in mice promotes autism-like phenotypes in offspring. *Science* 351, 933–939. doi: 10.1126/science.aad0314

Clark, D. E., Smith, S. K., Sharkey, A. M., and Charnock-Jones, D. S. (1996). Localization of VEGF and expression of its receptors flit and KDR in human placenta throughout pregnancy. *Hum. Reprod.* 11, 1090–1098. doi: 10.1093/oxfordjournals.humrep.a019303

Conroy, A. L., McDonald, C. R., Gamble, J. L., Olwoch, P., Natureeba, P., Cohan, D., et al. (2017). Altered angiogenesis as a common mechanism underlying preterm birth, small for gestational age, and stillbirth in women living with HIV. *Am. J. Obstet. Gynecol.* 217, 684.e1–684.e17. doi: 10.1016/j.ajog.2017.10.003

Conroy, A., Serghides, L., Finney, C., Owino, S. O., Kumar, S., Gowda, D. C., et al. (2009). C5a enhances dysregulated inflammatory and angiogenic responses to malaria in vitro: potential implications for placental malaria. *PLoS One* 4, 1–10. doi: 10.1371/journal.pone.0004953

Conroy, A. L., Silver, K. L., Zhong, K., Rennie, M., Ward, P., Sarma, J. V., et al. (2013). Complement activation and the resulting placental vascular insufficiency drives fetal growth restriction associated with placental malaria. *Cell Host Microbe* 13, 215–226. doi: 10.1016/j.chom.2013.01.010

Coyne, C. B., and Lazear, H. M. (2016). Zika virus – reigniting the TORCH. *Nat. Rev. Microbiol.* 14, 707–715. doi: 10.1038/nrmicro.2016.125

Dammann, O., and Leviton, A. (1997). Maternal intrauterine infection, cytokines, and brain damage in the preterm newborn. *Pediatr. Res.* 42, 1–8. doi: 10.1203/00006450-199707000-00001

Darling, A. M., McDonald, C. R., Conroy, A. L., Hayford, K. T., Liles, W. C., Wang, M., et al. (2014). Angiogenic and inflammatory biomarkers in midpregnancy and small-for-gestational-age outcomes in Tanzania. *Am. J. Obstet. Gynecol.* 211, 509.e1–509.e8. doi: 10.1016/j.ajog.2014.05.032

Demir, R., Kayisli, U. A., Cayli, S., and Huppertz, B. (2006). Sequential steps during vasculogenesis and angiogenesis in the very early human placenta. *Placenta* 27, 535–539. doi: 10.1016/j.placenta.2005.05.011

Demir, R., Seval, Y., and Huppertz, B. (2007). Vasculogenesis and angiogenesis in the early human placenta. *Acta Histochem.* 109, 257–265. doi: 10.1016/j.acthis.2007.02.008

Desai, M., ter Kuile, F. O., Nosten, F., McGready, R., Asamoa, K., Brabin, B., et al. (2007). Epidemiology and burden of malaria in pregnancy. *Lancet Infect. Dis.* 7, 93–104. doi: 10.1016/S1473-3099(07)70021-X

Di Simone, N., Tersigni, C., Cardaropoli, S., Franceschi, F., Di Nicuolo, F., Castellani, R., et al. (2017). *Helicobacter pylori* infection contributes to placental impairment in preeclampsia: basic and clinical evidences. *Helicobacter* 22:e12347. doi: 10.1111/hel.12347

Dorman, E. K., Shulman, C. E., Kingdom, J., Bulmer, J. N., Mwendwa, J., Peshu, N., et al. (2002). Impaired uteroplacental blood flow in pregnancies complicated by falciparum malaria. *Ultrasound Obstet. Gynecol.* 19, 165–170. doi: 10.1046/j.0960-7692.2001.00545.x

Dunk, C., Shams, M., Nijjar, S., Rhaman, M., Qiu, Y., Bussolati, B., et al. (2000). Angiopoietin-1 and Angiopoietin-2 activate trophoblast Tie-2 to promote growth and migration during placental development. *Am. J. Pathol.* 156, 2185–2199. doi: 10.1016/S0002-9440(10)65089-4

Estes, M. L., and McAllister, A. K. (2016). Maternal immune activation: implications for neuropsychiatric disorders. *Science* 353, 772–777. doi: 10.1126/science.aag3194

Ferrazzi, E., Rigano, S., Bozzo, M., Bellotti, M., Giovannini, N., Galan, H., et al. (2000). Umbilical vein blood flow in growth-restricted fetuses. *Ultrasound Obstet. Gynecol.* 16, 432–438. doi: 10.1046/j.1469-0705.2000.00208.x

Fiedler, U., and Augustin, H. G. (2006). Angiopoietins: a link between angiogenesis and inflammation. *Trends Immunol.* 27, 552–558. doi: 10.1016/j.it.2006.10.004

Fisher, S. J. (2015). Why is placentation abnormal in preeclampsia? *Am. J. Obstet. Gynecol.* 213, S115–S122. doi: 10.1016/j.ajog.2015.08.042

Fried, M., Kurtis, J. D., Swihart, B., Pond-Tor, S., Barry, A., Sidibe, Y., et al. (2017). Systemic inflammatory response to malaria during pregnancy is associated with pregnancy loss and preterm delivery. *Clin. Infect. Dis.* 65, 1729–1735. doi: 10.1093/cid/cix623

Gagnon, R. (2003). Placental insufficiency and its consequences. *Eur. J. Obstet. Gynecol. Reprod. Biol.* 110, S99–S107. doi: 10.1016/S0301-2115(03)00179-9

Gallagher, D., Norman, A. A., Woodard, C. L., Yang, G., Fujitani, M., Vessey, J. P., et al. (2013). Transient maternal IL-6 mediates long-lasting changes in neural stem cell pools by deregulating an endogenous self-renewal pathway. *Cell Stem Cell* 13, 564–576. doi: 10.1016/j.stem.2013.10.002

Geva, E., Ginzinger, D. G., Zaloudek, C. J., Moore, D. H., Byrne, A., and Jaffe, R. B. (2002). Human placental vascular development: vasculogenic and angiogenic (branching and nonbranching) transformation is regulated by vascular endothelial growth factor-A, angiopoietin-1, and angiopoietin-2. *J. Clin. Endocrinol. Metab.* 87, 4213–4224. doi: 10.1210/jc.2002-020195

Giovanoli, S., Engler, H., Engler, A., Richetto, J., Voget, M., Willi, R., et al. (2013). Stress in puberty unmasks latent neuropathological consequences of prenatal immune activation in mice. *Science* 339, 1095–1099. doi: 10.1126/science.1228261

Girardi, G., Yarilin, D., Thurman, J. M., Holers, V. M., and Salmon, J. E. (2006). Complement activation induces dysregulation of angiogenic factors and causes fetal rejection and growth restriction. *J. Exp. Med.* 203, 2165–2175. doi: 10.1084/jem.20061022

Goldman-Wohl, D. S., Ariel, I., Greenfield, C., Lavy, Y., and Yagel, S. (2000). Tie-2 and angiopoietin-2 expression at the fetal-maternal interface: a receptor ligand model for vascular remodelling. *Mol. Hum. Reprod.* 6, 81–87. doi: 10.1093/molehr/6.1.81

Graham, A. M., Rasmussen, J. M., Rudolph, M. D., Heim, C. M., Gilmore, J. H., Styner, M., et al. (2018). Maternal systemic interleukin-6 during pregnancy is associated with newborn amygdala phenotypes and subsequent behavior at 2 years of age. *Biol. Psychiatry* 83, 109–119. doi: 10.1016/j.biopsych.2017.05.027

Griffin, J. B., Lokomba, V., Landis, S. H., Thorp, J. M., Herring, A. H., Tshefu, A. K., et al. (2012). *Plasmodium falciparum* parasitaemia in the first half of pregnancy, uterine and umbilical artery blood flow, and foetal growth: a longitudinal Doppler ultrasound study. *Malar. J.* 11:319. doi: 10.1186/1475-2875-11-319

Gustafsson, R. K. L., Jeffery, H. C., Yaiw, K.-C., Wilhelmi, V., Kostopoulou, O. N., Davoudi, B., et al. (2015). Direct infection of primary endothelial cells with human cytomegalovirus prevents angiogenesis and migration. *J. Gen. Virol.* 96, 3598–3612. doi: 10.1099/jgv.0.000301

Hanna, J., Goldman-Wohl, D., Hamani, Y., Avraham, I., Greenfield, C., Natanson-Yaron, S., et al. (2006). Decidual NK cells regulate key developmental processes at the human fetal-maternal interface. *Nat. Med.* 12, 1065–1074. doi: 10.1038/nm1452

Harjunmaa, U., Doyle, R., Järnstedt, J., Kamiza, S., Jorgensen, J., Stewart, C., et al. (2018). Periapical infection may affect birth outcomes via systemic inflammation. *Oral Dis.* 24, 847–855. doi: 10.1111/odi.12817

Hernandez-Andrade, E., Figueroa, R., Cerbulo-Vazquez, A., Benavides-Serralde, J. A., Borbón, G. P., and Ramírez, J. M. (2014). Fetal hemodynamic changes in pregnant women with influenza AH1N1 infection and reduced arterial partial pressure of oxygen. *Ultrasound Obstet. Gynecol.* 44, 492–494. doi: 10.1002/uog.13417

Hirsch, A. J., Roberts, V. H. J., Grigsby, P. L., Haese, N., Schabel, M. C., Wang, X., et al. (2018). Zika virus infection in pregnant rhesus macaques causes placental dysfunction and immunopathology. *Nat. Commun.* 9:263. doi: 10.1038/s41467-017-02499-9

Horton, A. L., Boggess, K. A., Moss, K. L., Jared, H. L., Beck, J., and Offenbacher, S. (2008). Periodontal disease early in pregnancy is associated with maternal systemic inflammation among African American women. *J. Periodontol.* 79, 1127–1132. doi: 10.1902/jop.2008.070655

Hustin, J., Jauniaux, E., and Schaaps, J. P. (1990). Histological study of the materno-embryonic interface in spontaneous abortion. *Placenta* 11, 477–486. doi: 10.1016/S0143-4004(05)80193-6

Huynh, B.-T., Cottrell, G., Cot, M., and Briand, V. (2015). Burden of malaria in early pregnancy: a neglected problem? *Clin. Infect. Dis.* 60, 598–604. doi: 10.1093/cid/ciu848

Jackson, M. R., Walsh, A. J., Morrow, R. J., Mullen, J. B., Lye, S. J., and Ritchie, J. W. (1995). Reduced placental villous tree elaboration in small-for-gestational-age pregnancies: relationship with umbilical artery Doppler waveforms. *Am. J. Obstet. Gynecol.* 172, 518–525. doi: 10.1016/0002-9378(95)90566-9

Kalk, E., Schubert, P., Bettinger, J. A., Cotton, M. F., Esser, M., Slogrove, A., et al. (2017). Placental pathology in HIV infection at term: a comparison with HIV-uninfected women. *Tropical Med. Int. Health* 22, 604–613. doi: 10.1111/tmi.12858

Kaufmann, P., Black, S., and Huppertz, B. (2003). Endovascular trophoblast invasion: implications for the pathogenesis of intrauterine growth retardation and preeclampsia. *Biol. Reprod.* 69, 1–7. doi: 10.1095/biolreprod.102.014977

Kaufmann, P., Mayhew, T. M., and Charnock-Jones, D. S. (2004). Aspects of human fetoplacental vasculogenesis and angiogenesis. II. Changes during normal pregnancy. *Placenta* 25, 114–126. doi: 10.1016/j.placenta.2003.10.009

Khaliq, A., Dunk, C., Jiang, J., Shams, M., Li, X. F., Acevedo, C., et al. (1999). Hypoxia down-regulates placenta growth factor, whereas fetal growth restriction up-regulates placenta growth factor expression: molecular evidence for "placental hyperoxia" in intrauterine growth restriction. *Lab. Investig.* 79, 151–170.

Khaliq, A., Li, X. F., Shams, M., Sisi, P., Acevedo, C. A., Whittle, M. J., et al. (1996). Localisation of placenta growth factor (PIGF) in human term placenta. *Growth Factors* 13, 243–250.

Khong, T. Y., De Wolf, F., Robertson, W. B., and Brosens, I. (1986). Inadequate maternal vascular response to placentation in pregnancies complicated by pre-eclampsia and by small-for-gestational age infants. *Br. J. Obstet. Gynaecol.* 93, 1049–1059.

Kim, C. J., Romero, R., Chaemsaithong, P., and Kim, J.-S. (2015). Chronic inflammation of the placenta: definition, classification, pathogenesis, and clinical significance. *Am. J. Obstet. Gynecol.* 213, S53–S69. doi: 10.1016/j.ajog.2015.08.041

Kingdom, J. (1998). Adriana and Luisa Castellucci Award Lecture 1997. Placental pathology in obstetrics: adaptation or failure of the villous tree? *Placenta* 19, 347–351. doi: 10.1016/S0143-4004(98)90073-X

Kingdom, J., Huppertz, B., Seaward, G., and Kaufmann, P. (2000). Development of the placental villous tree and its consequences for fetal growth. *Eur. J. Obstet. Gynecol. Reprod. Biol.* 92, 35–43. doi: 10.1016/S0301-2115(00)00423-1

Kingdom, J. C., and Kaufmann, P. (1997). Oxygen and placental villous development: origins of fetal hypoxia. *Placenta* 18, 613–621; discussion 623–626. doi: 10.1016/S0143-4004(97)90000-X

Knuesel, I., Chicha, L., Britschgi, M., Schobel, S. A., Bodmer, M., Hellings, J. A., et al. (2014). Maternal immune activation and abnormal brain development across CNS disorders. *Nat. Rev. Neurol.* 10, 643–660. doi: 10.1038/nrneurol.2014.187

Kraus, T. A., Sperling, R. S., Engel, S. M., Lo, Y., Kellerman, L., Singh, T., et al. (2010). Peripheral blood cytokine profiling during pregnancy and post-partum periods. *Am. J. Reprod. Immunol.* 64, 411–426. doi: 10.1111/j.1600-0897.2010.00889.x

Le Bouteiller, P. (2013). Human decidual NK cells: unique and tightly regulated effector functions in healthy and pathogen-infected pregnancies. *Front. Immunol.* 4:404. doi: 10.3389/fimmu.2013.00404

Lee, A. C., Katz, J., Blencowe, H., Cousens, S., Kozuki, N., Vogel, J. P., et al. (2013). National and regional estimates of term and preterm babies born small for gestational age in 138 low-income and middle-income countries in 2010. *Lancet Glob. Health* 1, e26–e36. doi: 10.1016/S2214-109X(13)70006-8

Levine, R. J., Lam, C., Qian, C., Yu, K. F., Maynard, S. E., Sachs, B. P., et al. (2006). Soluble endoglin and other circulating antiangiogenic factors in preeclampsia. *N. Engl. J. Med.* 355, 992–1005. doi: 10.1056/NEJMoa055352

Levine, R. J., Maynard, S. E., Qian, C., Lim, K.-H., England, L. J., Yu, K. F., et al. (2004). Circulating angiogenic factors and the risk of preeclampsia. *N. Engl. J. Med.* 350, 672–683. doi: 10.1056/NEJMoa031884

Linask, K. K. (2013). The heart-placenta axis in the first month of pregnancy: induction and prevention of cardiovascular birth defects. *J. Pregnancy* 2013:320413. doi: 10.1155/2013/320413

Linask, K. K., Han, M., and Bravo-Valenzuela, N. J. M. (2014). Changes in vitelline and utero-placental hemodynamics: implications for cardiovascular development. *Front. Physiol.* 5. doi: 10.3389/fphys.2014.00390

Liu, L., Oza, S., Hogan, D., Chu, Y., Perin, J., Zhu, J., et al. (2016). Global, regional, and national causes of under-5 mortality in 2000-15: an updated systematic analysis with implications for the sustainable development goals. *Lancet* 388, 3027–3035. doi: 10.1016/S0140-6736(16)31593-8

Madanitsa, M., Kalilani, L., Mwapasa, V., van Eijk, A. M., Khairallah, C., Ali, D., et al. (2016). Scheduled intermittent screening with rapid diagnostic tests and treatment with dihydroartemisinin-piperaquine versus intermittent preventive therapy with sulfadoxine-pyrimethamine for malaria in pregnancy in Malawi: an open-label randomized controlled trial. *PLoS Med.* 13:e1002124. doi: 10.1371/journal.pmed.1002124

Maisonpierre, P. C., Suri, C., Jones, P. F., Bartunkova, S., Wiegand, S. J., Radziejewski, C., et al. (1997). Angiopoietin-2, a natural antagonist for Tie2 that disrupts in vivo angiogenesis. *Science* 277, 55–60. doi: 10.1126/science.277.5322.55

McAdams, R. M., Vanderhoeven, J., Beyer, R. P., Bammler, T. K., Farin, F. M., Liggitt, H. D., et al. (2012). Choriodecidual infection downregulates angiogenesis and morphogenesis pathways in fetal lungs from *Macaca nemestrina*. *PLoS One* 7:e46863. doi: 10.1371/journal.pone.0046863

McClure, E. M., Meshnick, S. R., Lazebnik, N., Mungai, P., King, C. L., Hudgens, M., et al. (2014). A cohort study of *Plasmodium falciparum* malaria in pregnancy and associations with uteroplacental blood flow and fetal anthropometrics in Kenya. *Int. J. Gynecol. Obstet.* 126, 78–82. doi: 10.1016/j.ijgo.2014.01.016

McDonald, C. R., Cahill, L. S., Gamble, J. L., Elphinstone, R., Gazdzinski, L. M., Zhong, K. J. Y., et al. (2018). Malaria in pregnancy alters l-arginine bioavailability and placental vascular development. *Sci. Transl. Med.* 10:eaan6007. doi: 10.1126/scitranslmed.aan6007

McDonald, C. R., Cahill, L. S., Ho, K. T., Yang, J., Kim, H., Silver, K. L., et al. (2015a). Experimental malaria in pregnancy induces neurocognitive injury in uninfected offspring via a C5a-C5a receptor dependent pathway. *PLoS Pathog.* 11:e1005140. doi: 10.1371/journal.ppat.1005140

McDonald, C. R., Darling, A. M., Conroy, A. L., Tran, V., Cabrera, A., Liles, W. C., et al. (2015b). Inflammatory and angiogenic factors at mid-pregnancy are associated with spontaneous preterm birth in a cohort of Tanzanian women. *PLoS One* 10:e0134619. doi: 10.1371/journal.pone.0134619

McDonald, C. R., Elphinstone, R. E., and Kain, K. C. (2013). The impact of placental malaria on neurodevelopment of exposed infants: a role for the complement system? *Trends Parasitol.* 29, 213–219. doi: 10.1016/j.pt.2013.03.005

McDonald, C. R., Weckman, A. M., Conroy, A. L., Olwoch, P., Natureeba, P., Kamya, M. R., et al. (2019). Systemic inflammation is associated with malaria and preterm birth in women living with HIV on antiretrovirals and co-trimoxazole. *Sci. Rep.* 9:6758. doi: 10.1038/s41598-019-43191-w

Miquerol, L., Langille, B. L., and Nagy, A. (2000). Embryonic development is disrupted by modest increases in vascular endothelial growth factor gene expression. *Development* 127, 3941–3946.

Moeller, S. L., Nyengaard, J. R., Larsen, L. G., Nielsen, K., Bygbjerg, I. C., Msemo, O. A., et al. (2018). Malaria in early pregnancy and the development of the placental vasculature. *J. Infect. Dis.* jiy735. doi: 10.1093/infdis/jiy735

Mohammadi, H., Papp, E., Cahill, L., Rennie, M., Banko, N., Pinnaduwage, L., et al. (2018). HIV antiretroviral exposure in pregnancy induces detrimental placenta vascular changes that are rescued by progesterone supplementation. *Sci. Rep.* 8:6552. doi: 10.1038/s41598-018-24680-w

Morgan, T. K. (2016). Role of the placenta in preterm birth: a review. *Am. J. Perinatol.* 33, 258–266. doi: 10.1055/s-0035-1570379

Murray, C. J. L., Vos, T., Lozano, R., Naghavi, M., Flaxman, A. D., Michaud, C., et al. (2012). Disability-adjusted life years (DALYs) for 291 diseases and injuries in 21 regions, 1990-2010: a systematic analysis for the global burden of disease study 2010. *Lancet* 380, 2197–2223. doi: 10.1016/S0140-6736(12)61689-4

Naldini, A., and Carraro, F. (2005). Role of inflammatory mediators in angiogenesis. *Curr. Drug Targets Inflamm. Allergy* 4, 3–8. doi: 10.2174/1568010053622830

Ome-Kaius, M., Karl, S., Wangnapi, R. A., Bolnga, J. W., Mola, G., Walker, J., et al. (2017). Effects of *Plasmodium falciparum* infection on umbilical artery resistance and intrafetal blood flow distribution: a Doppler ultrasound study from Papua New Guinea. *Malar. J.* 16:35. doi: 10.1186/s12936-017-1689-z

Phillips, P., Brown, M. B., Progulske-Fox, A., Wu, X.-J., and Reyes, L. (2018). *Porphyromonas gingivalis* strain-dependent inhibition of uterine spiral artery remodeling in the pregnant rat. *Biol. Reprod.* 99, 1045–1056. doi: 10.1093/biolre/ioy119

Pijnenborg, R., Anthony, J., Davey, D. A., Rees, A., Tiltman, A., Vercruysse, L., et al. (1991). Placental bed spiral arteries in the hypertensive disorders of pregnancy. *Br. J. Obstet. Gynaecol.* 98, 648–655.

Pollheimer, J., Vondra, S., Baltayeva, J., Beristain, A. G., and Knöfler, M. (2018). Regulation of placental extravillous trophoblasts by the maternal uterine environment. *Front. Immunol.* 9:2597. doi: 10.3389/fimmu.2018.02597

Ponzio, N. M., Servatius, R., Beck, K., Marzouk, A., and Kreider, T. (2007). Cytokine levels during pregnancy influence immunological profiles and neurobehavioral patterns of the offspring. *Ann. N. Y. Acad. Sci.* 1107, 118–128. doi: 10.1196/annals.1381.013

Prins, J. R., Eskandar, S., Eggen, B. J. L., and Scherjon, S. A. (2018). Microglia, the missing link in maternal immune activation and fetal neurodevelopment; and a possible link in preeclampsia and disturbed neurodevelopment? *J. Reprod. Immunol.* 126, 18–22. doi: 10.1016/j.jri.2018.01.004

Procianoy, R., Hentges, C., and Silveira, R. (2015). Vascular endothelial growth factor/placental growth factor heterodimer levels in preterm infants with bronchopulmonary dysplasia. *Am. J. Perinatol.* 33, 480–485. doi: 10.1055/s-0035-1566294

Rasmussen, J. M., Graham, A. M., Entringer, S., Gilmore, J. H., Styner, M., Fair, D. A., et al. (2019). Maternal interleukin-6 concentration during pregnancy is associated with variation in frontolimbic white matter and cognitive development in early life. *NeuroImage* 185, 825–835. doi: 10.1016/j.neuroimage.2018.04.020

Regal, J. F., Gilbert, J. S., and Burwick, R. M. (2015). The complement system and adverse pregnancy outcomes. *Mol. Immunol.* 67, 56–70. doi: 10.1016/j.molimm.2015.02.030

Ribeiro, C. F., Lopes, V. G. S., Brasil, P., Pires, A. R. C., Rohloff, R., and Nogueira, R. M. R. (2017). Dengue infection in pregnancy and its impact on the placenta. *Int. J. Infect. Dis.* 55, 109–112. doi: 10.1016/j.ijid.2017.01.002

Rogerson, S. J., Desai, M., Mayor, A., Sicuri, E., Taylor, S. M., and van Eijk, A. M. (2018). Burden, pathology, and costs of malaria in pregnancy: new developments for an old problem. *Lancet Infect. Dis.* 18, e107–e118. doi: 10.1016/S1473-3099(18)30066-5

Romero, R., Chaemsaithong, P., Docheva, N., Korzeniewski, S. J., Tarca, A. L., Bhatti, G., et al. (2016). Clinical chorioamnionitis at term IV: the maternal plasma cytokine profile. *J. Perinat. Med.* 44, 77–98. doi: 10.1515/jpm-2015-0103

Romero, R., Chaiworapongsa, T., Erez, O., Tarca, A. L., Gervasi, M. T., Kusanovic, J. P., et al. (2010). An imbalance between angiogenic and anti-angiogenic factors precedes fetal death in a subset of patients: results of a longitudinal study. *J. Matern. Fetal Neonatal Med.* 23, 1384–1399. doi: 10.3109/14767051003681121

Romero, R., Kusanovic, J. P., Chaiworapongsa, T., and Hassan, S. S. (2011). Placental bed disorders in preterm labor, preterm PROM, spontaneous abortion and abruptio placentae. *Best Pract. Res. Clin. Obstet. Gynaecol.* 25, 313–327. doi: 10.1016/j.bpobgyn.2011.02.006

Rudolph, M. D., Graham, A. M., Feczko, E., Miranda-Dominguez, O., Rasmussen, J. M., Nardos, R., et al. (2018). Maternal IL-6 during pregnancy can be estimated from newborn brain connectivity and predicts future working memory in offspring. *Nat. Neurosci.* 21, 765–772. doi: 10.1038/s41593-018-0128-y

Salafia, C., Pezzullo, J., Minior, V., and Divon, M. (1997). Placental pathology of absent and reversed end-diastolic flow in growth-restricted fetuses. *Obstet. Gynecol.* 90, 830–836. doi: 10.1016/S0029-7844(97)00473-0

Santosa, W. B., Staines-Urias, E., Tshivuila-Matala, C. O. O., Norris, S. A., and Hemelaar, J. (2019). Perinatal outcomes associated with maternal HIV and antiretroviral therapy in pregnancies with accurate gestational age in South Africa. *AIDS* 33, 1623–1633. doi: 10.1097/QAD.0000000000002222

Schafer, D. P., Lehrman, E. K., Kautzman, A. G., Koyama, R., Mardinly, A. R., Yamasaki, R., et al. (2012). Microglia sculpt postnatal neural circuits in an activity and complement-dependent manner. *Neuron* 74, 691–705. doi: 10.1016/j.neuron.2012.03.026

Seval, Y., Sati, L., Celik-Ozenci, C., Taskin, O., and Demir, R. (2008). The distribution of angiopoietin-1, angiopoietin-2 and their receptors tie-1 and tie-2 in the very early human placenta. *Placenta* 29, 809–815. doi: 10.1016/j.placenta.2008.06.009

Sharkey, A. M., Cooper, J. C., Balmforth, J. R., McLaren, J., Clark, D. E., Charnock-Jones, D. S., et al. (1996). Maternal plasma levels of vascular endothelial growth factor in normotensive pregnancies and in pregnancies complicated by pre-eclampsia. *Eur. J. Clin. Investig.* 26, 1182–1185. doi: 10.1046/j.1365-2362.1996.830605.x

Silver, R. M. (2018). Examining the link between placental pathology, growth restriction, and stillbirth. *Best Pract. Res. Clin. Obstet. Gynaecol.* 49, 89–102. doi: 10.1016/j.bpobgyn.2018.03.004

Silver, K. L., Conroy, A. L., Leke, R. G. F., Leke, R. J. I., Gwanmesia, P., Molyneux, M. E., et al. (2011). Circulating soluble endoglin levels in pregnant women in Cameroon and Malawi – associations with placental malaria and fetal growth restriction. *PLoS One* 6:e24985. doi: 10.1371/annotation/e9946f72-821d-45ea-bcd4-3fa3ff89a5fe

Silver, K. L., Zhong, K., Leke, R. G. F., Taylor, D. W., and Kain, K. C. (2010). Dysregulation of angiopoietins is associated with placental malaria and low birth weight. *PLoS One* 5:e9481. doi: 10.1371/journal.pone.0009481

Smith, S. E. P., Li, J., Garbett, K., Mirnics, K., and Patterson, P. H. (2007). Maternal immune activation alters fetal brain development through interleukin-6. *J. Neurosci.* 27, 10695–10702. doi: 10.1523/JNEUROSCI.2178-07.2007

Spann, M. N., Monk, C., Scheinost, D., and Peterson, B. S. (2018). Maternal immune activation during the third trimester is associated with neonatal functional connectivity of the salience network and fetal to toddler behavior. *J. Neurosci.* 38, 2877–2886. doi: 10.1523/JNEUROSCI.2272-17.2018

Stevens, B., Allen, N. J., Vazquez, L. E., Howell, G. R., Christopherson, K. S., Nouri, N., et al. (2007). The classical complement cascade mediates CNS synapse elimination. *Cell* 131, 1164–1178. doi: 10.1016/j.cell.2007.10.036

Stiles, J., and Jernigan, T. L. (2010). The basics of brain development. *Neuropsychol. Rev.* 20, 327–348. doi: 10.1007/s11065-010-9148-4

Straughen, J. K., Misra, D. P., Helmkamp, L., and Misra, V. K. (2017). Preterm delivery as a unique pathophysiologic state characterized by maternal soluble FMS-like tyrosine kinase 1 and uterine artery resistance during pregnancy: a longitudinal cohort study. *Reprod. Sci.* 24, 1583–1589. doi: 10.1177/1933719117698574

Suri, C., Jones, P. F., Patan, S., Bartunkova, S., Maisonpierre, P. C., Davis, S., et al. (1996). Requisite role of angiopoietin-1, a ligand for the TIE2 receptor, during embryonic angiogenesis. *Cell* 87, 1171–1180. doi: 10.1016/S0092-8674(00)81813-9

Tabata, T., Petitt, M., Fang-Hoover, J., Rivera, J., Nozawa, N., Shiboski, S., et al. (2012). Cytomegalovirus impairs cytotrophoblast-induced lymphangiogenesis and vascular remodeling in an in vivo human placentation model. *Am. J. Pathol.* 181, 1540–1559. doi: 10.1016/j.ajpath.2012.08.003

Thébaud, B., and Abman, S. H. (2007). Bronchopulmonary dysplasia: where have all the vessels gone? Roles of angiogenic growth factors in chronic lung disease. *Am. J. Respir. Crit. Care Med.* 175, 978–985. doi: 10.1164/rccm.200611-1660PP

Travaglino, A., Raffone, A., Saccone, G., Migliorini, S., Maruotti, G. M., Esposito, G., et al. (2019). Placental morphology, apoptosis, angiogenesis and epithelial mechanisms in early-onset preeclampsia. *Eur. J. Obstet. Gynecol. Reprod. Biol.* 234, 200–206. doi: 10.1016/j.ejogrb.2018.12.039

Trudinger, B. J., Giles, W. B., Cook, C. M., Bombardieri, J., and Collins, L. (1985). Fetal umbilical artery flow velocity waveforms and placental resistance: clinical significance. *Br. J. Obstet. Gynaecol.* 92, 23–30.

Unger, H. W., Hansa, A. P., Buffet, C., Hasang, W., Teo, A., Randall, L., et al. (2019). Sulphadoxine-pyrimethamine plus azithromycin may improve birth outcomes through impacts on inflammation and placental angiogenesis independent of malarial infection. *Sci. Rep.* 9:2260. doi: 10.1038/s41598-019-38821-2

Vedmedovska, N., Rezeberga, D., Teibe, U., Melderis, I., and Donders, G. G. G. (2011). Placental pathology in fetal growth restriction. *Eur. J. Obstet. Gynecol. Reprod. Biol.* 155, 36–40. doi: 10.1016/j.ejogrb.2010.11.017

Venkatesha, S., Toporsian, M., Lam, C., Hanai, J., Mammoto, T., Kim, Y. M., et al. (2006). Soluble endoglin contributes to the pathogenesis of preeclampsia. *Nat. Med.* 12, 642–649. doi: 10.1038/nm1429

Vuorela, P., Hatva, E., Lymboussaki, A., Kaipainen, A., Joukov, V., Persico, M. G., et al. (1997). Expression of vascular endothelial growth factor and placenta growth factor in human placental. *Biol. Reprod.* 56, 489–494. doi: 10.1095/biolreprod56.2.489

Wang, Y., and Zhao, S. (2010). *Vascular biology of the placenta*. Morgan & Claypool Life Sciences. Available at: http://www.ncbi.nlm.nih.gov/pubmed/21452443 (Accessed January 16, 2019).

Watson-Jones, D., Changalucha, J., Gumodoka, B., Weiss, H., Rusizoka, M., Ndeki, L., et al. (2002). Syphilis in pregnancy in Tanzania. I. Impact of maternal syphilis on outcome of pregnancy. *J. Infect. Dis.* 186, 940–947. doi: 10.1086/342952

Weckman, A., Tran, V., and Kain, K. C. (2018). "Complement and malaria in pregnancy" in *Complement activation in malaria immunity and pathogenesis*. ed. J. A. Stoute (Springer, Cham).

Wedi, C. O. O., Kirtley, S., Hopewell, S., Corrigan, R., Kennedy, S. H., and Hemelaar, J. (2016). Perinatal outcomes associated with maternal HIV infection: a systematic review and meta-analysis. *Lancet HIV* 3, e33–e48. doi: 10.1016/S2352-3018(15)00207-6

Wei, H., Chadman, K. K., McCloskey, D. P., Sheikh, A. M., Malik, M., Brown, W. T., et al. (2012). Brain IL-6 elevation causes neuronal circuitry imbalances and mediates autism-like behaviors. *Biochim. Biophys. Acta* 1822, 831–842. doi: 10.1016/j.bbadis.2012.01.011

Wilkinson, A. L., Pedersen, S. H., Urassa, M., Michael, D., Andreasen, A., Todd, J., et al. (2017). Maternal systemic or cord blood inflammation is associated with birth anthropometry in a Tanzanian prospective cohort. *Tropical Med. Int. Health* 22, 52–62. doi: 10.1111/tmi.12799

Yancopoulos, G. D., Davis, S., Gale, N. W., Rudge, J. S., Wiegand, S. J., and Holash, J. (2000). Vascular-specific growth factors and blood vessel formation. *Nature* 407, 242–248. doi: 10.1038/35025215

Zhu, M. Y., Milligan, N., Keating, S., Windrim, R., Keunen, J., Thakur, V., et al. (2016). The hemodynamics of late-onset intrauterine growth restriction by MRI. *Am. J. Obstet. Gynecol.* 214, 367.e1–367.e17. doi: 10.1016/j.ajog.2015.10.004

12

Transfusion-Transmitted Zika Virus Infection in Pregnant Mice Leads to Broad Tissue Tropism with Severe Placental Damage and Fetal Demise

Wanbo Tai[1†], Denis Voronin[1†], Jiawei Chen[1], Weili Bao[1], Debra A. Kessler[1], Beth Shaz[1], Shibo Jiang[1,2], Karina Yazdanbakhsh[1] and Lanying Du[1]*

[1] Lindsley F. Kimball Research Institute, New York Blood Center, New York, NY, United States, [2] Key Laboratory of Medical Molecular Virology of MOE/MOH, Fudan University, Shanghai, China

***Correspondence:**
Lanying Du
ldu@nybc.org

[†]These authors have contributed equally to this work

Zika virus (ZIKV) infection during pregnancy can cause significant problems, particularly congenital Zika syndrome. Nevertheless, the potential deleterious consequences and associated mechanisms of transfusion-transmitted ZIKV infection on pregnant individuals and their fetuses and babies have not been investigated. Here we examined transmissibility of ZIKV through blood transfusion in ZIKV-susceptible pregnant A129 mice. Our data showed that transfused-transmitted ZIKV at the early infection stage led to significant viremia and broad tissue tropism in the pregnant recipient mice, which were not seen in those transfused with ZIKV-positive (ZIKV$^+$) plasma at later infection stages. Importantly, pregnant mice transfused with early-stage, but not later stages, ZIKV$^+$ plasma also exhibited severe placental infection with vascular damage and apoptosis, fetal infection and fetal damage, accompanied by fetal and pup death. Overall, this study suggests that transfusion-related transmission of ZIKV during initial stage of infection, which harbors high plasma viral titers, can cause serious adverse complications in the pregnant recipients and their fetuses and babies.

Keywords: Zika virus, blood transmissibility, broad tissue tropism, placental infection, fetal demise

INTRODUCTION

Zika virus (ZIKV), a flavivirus in the *Flaviviridae* family, was first identified in rhesus monkeys in 1947 (Dick et al., 1952; Wikan and Smith, 2016). Similar to other flaviviruses, including dengue virus, yellow fever virus, West Nile virus, and Japanese encephalitis virus, ZIKV is a positive-stranded RNA virus, whose genome encodes structural proteins, including capsid, pre-membrane (prM)/membrane (M), and envelope (E), as well as seven non-structural proteins (Dai et al., 2016; Sirohi et al., 2016; Zhao et al., 2016). ZIKV E protein is a major protein in receptor binding and fusion, and it consists of ectodomain, e.g., domain I (EDI), II (EDII), and III (EDIII), stem region, and transmembrane region (Dai et al., 2016; Kostyuchenko et al., 2016).

Most people infected with ZIKV have no clinical symptoms or only exhibit mild symptoms, without requiring hospitalization. However, ZIKV infection during pregnancy can cause significant problems, particularly congenital Zika syndrome, which involves congenital brain abnormalities, microcephaly at birth, and motor anomalies and epilepsy in infants, as well as other malformations

(Melo et al., 2016; Mlakar et al., 2016; Cui et al., 2017; Krauer et al., 2017; Zorrilla et al., 2017; Chimelli et al., 2018; Pessoa et al., 2018). In addition, ZIKV infection is linked to Guillain-Barre syndrome (GBS), a severe neurological disease (Cao-Lormeau et al., 2016; Roze et al., 2017; Salinas et al., 2017; Simon et al., 2018). The association of ZIKV infection with these unexpected diseases has thus brought worldwide attention to study this virus and its pathogenic mechanisms.

Several mouse models are developed to study ZIKV infection and associated pathology, and to evaluate the efficacy of ZIKV vaccines and therapeutics. We and others have shown the susceptibility of type I interferon receptor (IFNAR)-deficient A129 mice, as well as type I and II interferon receptor (IFNAR/IFNGR)-deficient AG129 and AG6 mice, to ZIKV, and identified candidate vaccines and therapeutic agents that protect against ZIKV infection in these mouse models (Aliota et al., 2016; Cui et al., 2017; Du et al., 2017; Wu et al., 2017; Sumathy et al., 2017; Yu et al., 2017; Espinosa et al., 2018; Tai et al., 2018; Jiang and Du, 2019).

As seen with other mosquito-borne flaviviruses (Harrington et al., 2003; Iwamoto et al., 2003; Wilder-Smith et al., 2009; Aubry et al., 2015), ZIKV has acquired the ability to infect humans via blood or blood components (Barjas-Castro et al., 2016; Motta et al., 2016; Musso et al., 2016; Benjamin, 2017; Bloch et al., 2018). ZIKV RNA was identified in blood donations, and the risk of ZIKV transmission by blood donations does exist, even in the regions with low disease circulation (Galel et al., 2017; Williamson et al., 2017; Magnus et al., 2018). Nevertheless, the transmissibility of ZIKV through blood transfusion and associated pathogenic mechanisms, particularly in pregnant women and their fetuses or babies, are poorly understood. The present study aimed to answer these questions in ZIKV-susceptible pregnant A129 mice. Our data have demonstrated that transfusion with plasma from high-dose, early-stage ZIKV infection led to significant viremia and broad tissue tropism, particularly brain, in pregnant mice. In addition, such transfusion-transmitted ZIKV infection also resulted in severe placental vascular damage, apoptosis, and inflammation, as well as fetal damage and fetal and pup demise. In contrast, transfusion with ZIKV-positive (ZIKV$^+$) plasma at later stages of ZIKV infection, which contained low-titer or no ZIKV, did not enable significant ZIKV replication and/or congenital Zika infection.

MATERIALS AND METHODS

Ethics Statement

Adult (6–8-week-old) and pregnant [8–12-week-old, embryonic day (E7–9 and E10–12)] A129 mice were used in the study. The animal studies were carried out in strict accordance with the recommendations in the Guide for the Care and Use of Laboratory Animals of the National Institutes of Health. The protocols were approved by the Committee on the Ethics of Animal Experiments of the New York Blood Center (Permit Numbers: 344.00 and 345.01).

Virus and Plasma at Different Stages After ZIKV Infection

To understand transmissibility of ZIKV through blood transfusion and determine which stage(s) of ZIKV infection after ZIKV$^+$ plasma transfusion that will not cause severe consequences to the pregnant recipients, plasma from early, middle, and late stages of ZIKV infection was prepared (**Figure 1**). A contemporary ZIKV strain, R103451, which has demonstrated effective infectivity in A129 mice (Tai et al., 2018), was used in the study. To set up ZIKV$^+$ plasma transfusion and eliminate potential effects of other factors, such as preexisting antibodies, in the plasma to be transfused, plasma from naive A129 mice was manually added with a non-lethal, low-dose ZIKV (~90 plaque forming unit: PFU), and transfused into adult A129 mice (200 μl/mouse, 18 mice/group) via retro-orbital injection. Here a non-lethal ZIKV dose was used to maintain mouse survival during the long-term observation period. Plasma was collected from the mice at defined time points after transfusion, and pooled at early, middle, and late stages of infection for subsequent transfusion experiments. To prepare plasma at early-stage ZIKV infection containing a high ZIKV titer (early stage: high dose), adult A129 mice was transfused with plasma (200 μl/mouse, 18 mice/group) with manually added ZIKV (~10^4 PFU), and plasma was collected on days 3 and 5 after transfusion. Plasma from A129 mice transfused with normal plasma (200 μl/mouse, 12 mice/group) was collected for control experiments.

Plasma Transfusion, Sample Collection and Evaluation

Three experiments were designed for evaluating potential consequences of transfusion with plasma containing ZIKV at different infection stages to pregnant mice. First, the aforementioned plasma collected from mice at early, middle, and late stages of ZIKV infection with calculated ZIKV titers was transfused into pregnant (E10–12) A129 mice (200 μl/mouse, 6 mice/group) via retro-orbital injection. Six days later, plasma, tissues, placentas, fetuses, and amniotic fluid were collected for detecting viral replication and for subsequent experiments described below. Second, pregnant (E7–9 and E10–12) A129 mice were transfused with early-stage (high dose) ZIKV$^+$ plasma (200 μl/mouse, 6 mice/group), and uteri and placentas were collected 6 days post-transfusion to compare for placental morphology and fetal changes. Third, pregnant (E10–12) A129 mice transfused with early-stage (high dose) ZIKV$^+$ plasma (200 μl/mouse, 6 mice/group) were counted for newborn pups with or without survival. A129 mice transfused with normal plasma (200 μl/mouse, 6 mice/group) were used as controls.

Quantitative Reverse Transcriptase PCR (qRT-PCR)

ZIKV RNA copies in the collected samples were detected by qRT-PCR (Tai et al., 2018). Briefly, RNA was extracted using QIAamp MinElute Virus Spin Kit (for plasma and amniotic fluid) (Qiagen)

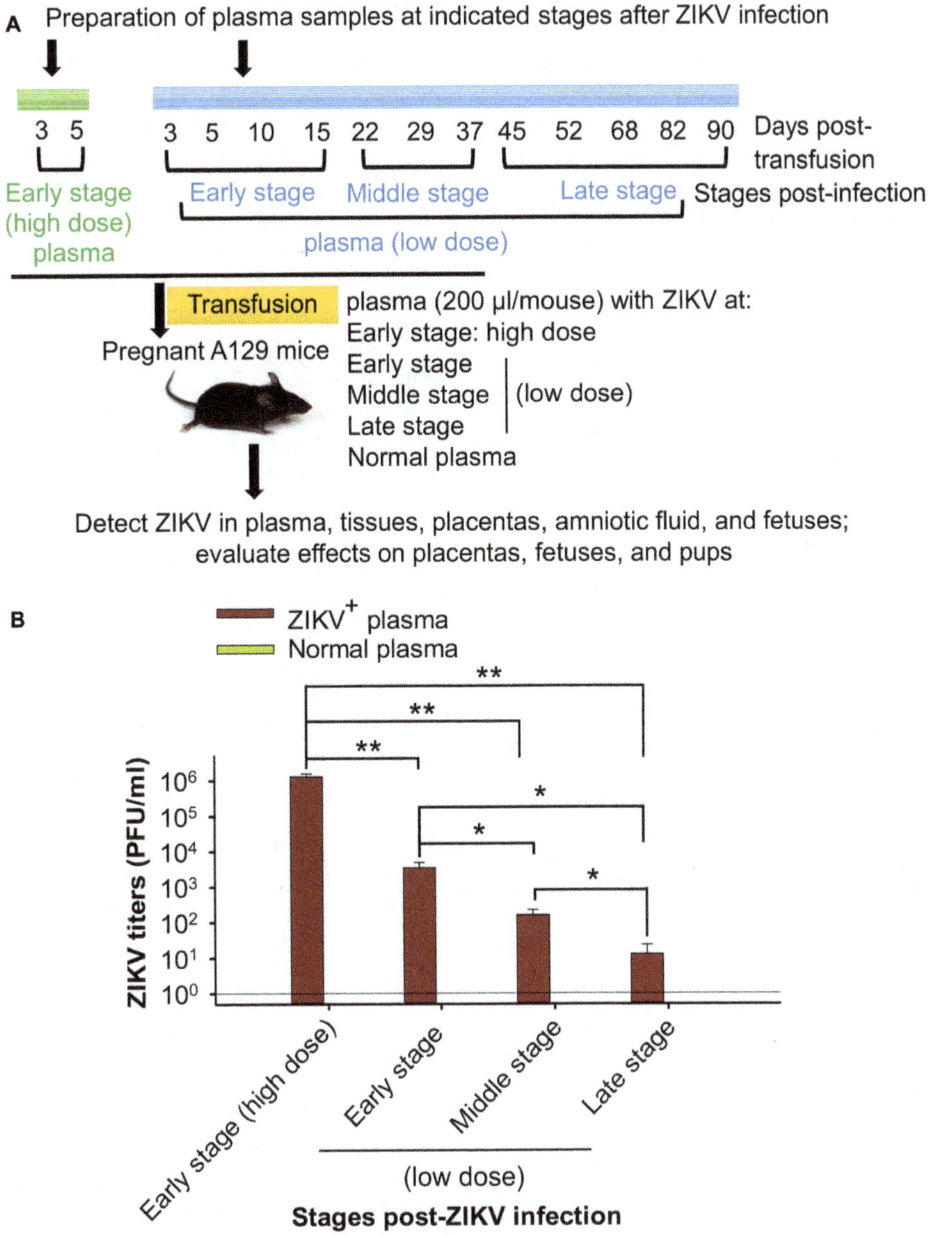

FIGURE 1 | Sample preparation and experimental design. **(A)** Schematic diagram of plasma preparation and experimental procedure. Adult A129 mice were transfused with naive mouse plasma inoculated with or without a non-lethal, low-dose of ZIKV (~90 PFU). Blood was then collected at the indicated time points to prepare for the pooled plasma at early, middle, and late stages post-ZIKV infection (low dose, shown in blue). In addition, adult A129 mice were transfused with naive mouse plasma with or without ZIKV (~10^4 PFU), and blood was collected on days 3 and 5 post-transfusion for preparation of pooled plasma containing high-titer ZIKV at early infection stage (early stage: high dose, shown in green). The above pooled plasma at different stages post-ZIKV infection was transfused to pregnant A129 mice (200 µl/mouse, 6 mice/group) for subsequent experiments. **(B)** Detection of ZIKV titers of above pooled plasma from different infection stages by plaque assay. The ZIKV titers are expressed as PFU/ml, based on which each mouse receiving plasma containing specific ZIKV titer at early stage (high dose), early-, middle-, and late-stages (low dose) was calculated. * and ** indicate significant differences between early stage (high dose) and other stages, between low dose of early stage and middle or late stage, or between low dose of middle and late stages, of ZIKV infection. The data are presented as means ± s.e.m of duplicate wells. The experiments were repeated twice, and similar results were obtained. Normal plasma: control plasma from A129 mice transfused with normal plasma without ZIKV (0 PFU).

and RNeasy Mini Kit (for tissues) (Qiagen), and quantified using one-step qRT-PCR in the presence of Power SYBR Green PCR Master Mix, MultiScribe Reverse Transcriptase, and Ambion^{TM} RNase Inhibitor (Thermo Fisher Scientific) in ViiA 7 Master Cycler PCR System (Thermo Fisher Scientific). The forward (5′-TTGGTCATGATACTGCTGATTGC-3′) and reverse (5′-CCTTCCACAAAGTCCCTATTGC-3′) primers were used for the amplification. To establish a standard curve of qRT-PCR, the M-E genes of ZIKV (strain R103451, 141–1800 bp) were amplified and cloned into pCR2.1-TOPO vector (Thermo Fisher Scientific) to construct a recombinant plasmid. This plasmid was serially diluted at 10-fold, and a linear standard curve at 10^2 to 10^{10} RNA copies (correlation coefficient R^2 value > 0.99; detection limit: $\sim10^2$ RNA copies) was selected to calculate ZIKV RNA in the plasma-transfused mouse samples. ZIKV RNA was purified from about 40 μl (for plasma or amniotic fluid) or 40 mg (for tissues) of transfused samples, so the detection limit per milliliter (ml) or gram (g) was about 2.5 × 10^3 RNA copies.

Measurement of ZIKV Titers

Plaque-forming assay was carried out to measure ZIKV titers in collected samples (Wu et al., 2017; Tai et al., 2018). Briefly, diluted plasma, amniotic fluid, and tissue lysates were transferred onto Vero E6 cells (ATCC) and incubated at 37°C for 1 h. The cells were further overlaid with DMEM (Thermo Fisher Scientific) containing 1% carboxymethyl cellulose (MilliporeSigma) and 2% FBS (Atlanta Biologicals), cultured at 37°C for four to five days, and stained with 0.5% crystal violet (MilliporeSigma). Viral titers are presented as PFU/ml or PFU/g of test samples.

Immunofluorescence Staining

Harvested maternal brain and placentas were fixed in 4% paraformaldehyde (MilliporeSigma), embedded in paraffin, and sectioned (Sapparapu et al., 2016; Yuan et al., 2017). The tissue slides were deparaffinized, blocked with 2% BSA (MilliporeSigma) for 30 min, and then incubated with human anti-ZIKV (EDIII-specific monoclonal antibody (mAb) ZV-64, 1:200, Absolute Antibody) and rabbit anti-vimentin antibody (1:300, Abcam), respectively, at 4°C overnight. For caspase-3 staining, the deparaffinized tissue slides were fixed and permed with FIX and PERM Cell Permeabilization Kit (Thermo Fisher Scientific), then blocked and incubated with rabbit anti-active caspase-3 antibody (1:200, Abcam) as described above. After washing with PBS, the slides were incubated with anti-human FITC (for ZIKV) or anti-rabbit Alexa Fluor® 647 (1:300, Abcam; for vimentin and caspase-3)-conjugated antibodies for 1 h. The slides were counter-stained with DAPI (4′,6-diamidino-2-phenylindole, 300 nM, Thermo Fisher Scientific) for nuclei for 5 min, and mounted in a VectaMount Permanent Mounting Medium (Vector Laboratories). All slides were imaged on confocal microscope (Zeiss LSM 880). Images were prepared using Adobe Photoshop and ZEN software, and the fluorescent signals were quantified by ImageJ software for the relative intensity (particle analysis) using a standard protocol (Wu et al., 2003). Specifically, the pictures were set up image type at 8-bit, and those from the experiment and control groups were adjusted to the same thresholds. The fluorescence intensity of the particles was then analyzed to get positive counts of each picture.

Transmission Electron Microscope (TEM)

Tissues were dissected in PBS, and 3 mm^3 fragments were fixed with 2.5% glutaraldehyde (MilliporeSigma) and 2% paraformaldehyde in sodium cacodylate buffer (0.1 M, MilliporeSigma) for at least 2 h. After fixation, samples were washed three times in sodium cacodylate buffer (0.1 M) and post-fixed by 2% OsO4 (MilliporeSigma) for 1 h. Samples were then washed and dehydrated using a series of ethanol concentrations (50–100%) with a final wash of propylene oxide (MilliporeSigma). Samples were embedded in plastic (Epon 812, EMS) and prepared for sectioning. Ultrathin sections were contrasted with UranyLess (EMS) and lead citrate (MilliporeSigma), and analyzed under the Tecnai G2 Spirit TEM.

Detection of Inflammatory Cytokines and Chemokines

Inflammatory cytokines and chemokines were measured in collected placentas and amniotic fluid using Mouse Inflammatory Cytokines Multi-Analyte ELISArray Kit and Mouse Common Chemokines Multi-Analyte ELISArray Kit according to the manufacturer's instructions (Qiagen). Briefly, mouse placental lysates and amniotic fluid were incubated with respective cytokine and chemokine capture antibodies pre-coated in the ELISA plates for 2 h at room temperature. After three washes, the plates were sequentially incubated with detection antibody for 1 h, and Avidin-HRP conjugate for 30 min at room temperature. The plates were then, respectively, incubated with development solution and stop solution to stop the reaction. Absorbance at 450 nm was measured by ELISA plate reader (Tecan).

Statistical Analysis

The values are presented as means with standard error (s.e.m). Statistical significance among different groups was calculated using GraphPad Prism Statistical Software. For data comparing viral RNA copies, viral titers, and fluorescence staining (shown on a log-based scale), Welch's t-test was used, and for other data, two-tailed Student's t-test was applied. *, ** and *** represent $P < 0.05$, $P < 0.01$, and $P < 0.001$, respectively.

RESULTS

Preparation of Plasma Samples at Different Stages of ZIKV Infection

To prepare plasma at early, middle, and late infection stages with low-dose ZIKV, plasma containing ZIKV at a non-lethal dose ($\sim$90 PFU), which was previously identified via intraperitoneal (i.p.) route (Tai et al., 2018), was transfused into A129 mice, and blood was collected and pooled for plasma from defined time points after transfusion (**Figure 1A**) to detect for ZIKV viral titers. To prepare plasma at early stage (high dose) of ZIKV infection, mice were inoculated with a high, lethal-dose of ZIKV [$\sim10^4$ PFU: previously identified through i.p. route (Tai et al., 2018)] and plasma collected at early stage post-ZIKV infection (day 3 and 5 after transfusion) (**Figure 1A**). This plasma contains significantly higher ZIKV titers than the plasma collected from mice receiving non-lethal, low-dose ZIKV at early, middle, and late stages of infection. In addition, ZIKV titers in the plasma of mice from early and middle infection stages (low dose) were also significantly higher than those from later infection stages (low dose) (**Figure 1B**).

Transfusion of High-Dose Early-Stage ZIKV+ Plasma to Pregnant A129 Mice Caused Significant Viremia and Broad Tissue Tropism, Including Brain

To investigate tissue distribution of ZIKV in pregnant A129 mice following transfusion with ZIKV+ plasma, we performed the following analyses.

First, we measured viral load on day 6 post-transfusion, an optimal time point for detecting viral RNA levels and viral titers in tissues and blood (Dowall et al., 2016). We found that pregnant mice (E10–12) receiving plasma at the early-stage ZIKV infection containing a high titer ($\sim 2.6 \times 10^5 \pm 5 \times 10^4$ PFU) of ZIKV (early stage: high dose) exhibited severe ZIKV viremia, with significantly higher levels of ZIKV RNA (**Figure 2A**) and ZIKV titers (**Figure 2B**) than those receiving plasma containing a lower titer, early-stage (low dose) ZIKV+ ($\sim 690 \pm 285$ PFU). In contrast, pregnant mice receiving middle- ($\sim 32 \pm 13$ PFU) and late-stage ($\sim 3 \pm 2$ PFU) (low dose) ZIKV+ plasma had undetectable levels of viremia similar to normal plasma-transfused mice (**Figures 2A,B**). These data reveal that establishment of transfusion-transmitted ZIKV infection in pregnant mice might occur only with early-stage infected plasma containing high-dose ZIKV.

Second, analysis of tissues, including brain, on day 6 post-transfusion demonstrated that pregnant (E10–12) mice transfused with early-stage high-dose ZIKV+ plasma had significantly higher ZIKV RNA (**Figure 2C**) and ZIKV titers (**Figure 2D**) in lung, spleen, kidney, heart, liver, muscle, and brain than mice receiving plasma from early stage (low dose) of ZIKV infection. In contrast, ZIKV RNA and ZIKV titers were undetectable in the above tissues of mice transfused with middle- and late-stage (low dose) ZIKV+ plasma, or normal plasma (**Figures 2C,D**). The presence of ZIKV in brain tissues of pregnant mice transfused with early-stage high-dose ZIKV+ plasma was confirmed by immunofluorescence staining of ZIKV E protein using a ZIKV EDIII-specific mAb (**Figure 3A**), which

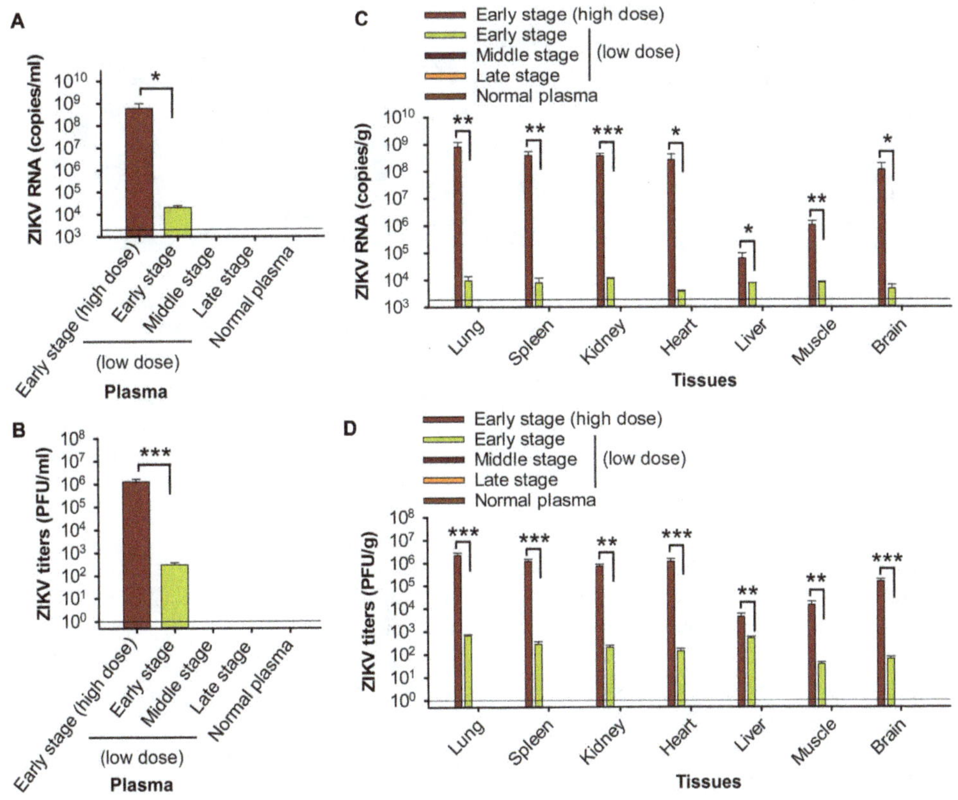

FIGURE 2 | Transfusion of pregnant A129 mice with early-stage (high dose) ZIKV+ plasma resulted in significant viremia and broad tissue tropism. Pregnant (E10–12) A129 mice were transfused with ZIKV+ plasma from early, middle, and late stages, respectively, and plasma and tissues were collected 6 days post-transfusion for below tests. Plasma ZIKV RNA **(A)** and ZIKV titers **(B)** were detected by qRT-PCR and plaque assay, respectively. Tissue ZIKV RNA **(C)** and viral titers **(D)** were detected by qRT-PCR and plaque assay, respectively. *, **, and *** indicate significant differences between early stage (high dose) and early stage (low dose) post-transfusion with ZIKV+ plasma. The data are presented as means ± s.e.m ($n = 6$ mice/group). In **(A)** and **(C)**, the limit of detection, shown as the horizontal lines, was about 2.5×10^3 copies/ml (for **A**) or 2.5×10^3 copies/g (for **C**) of ZIKV RNA. This was determined based on a detection limit of 10^2 copies in a linear standard curve (at serial dilutions of 10^2 to 10^{10} copies) of ZIKV RNA, as described in Materials and Methods. In **(B)** and **(D)**, the detection limit was about 1 PFU/ml (for **B**) or 1 PFU/g (for **D**). The experiments were repeated twice, and similar results were obtained. Normal plasma: control plasma from A129 mice transfused with normal plasma without ZIKV.

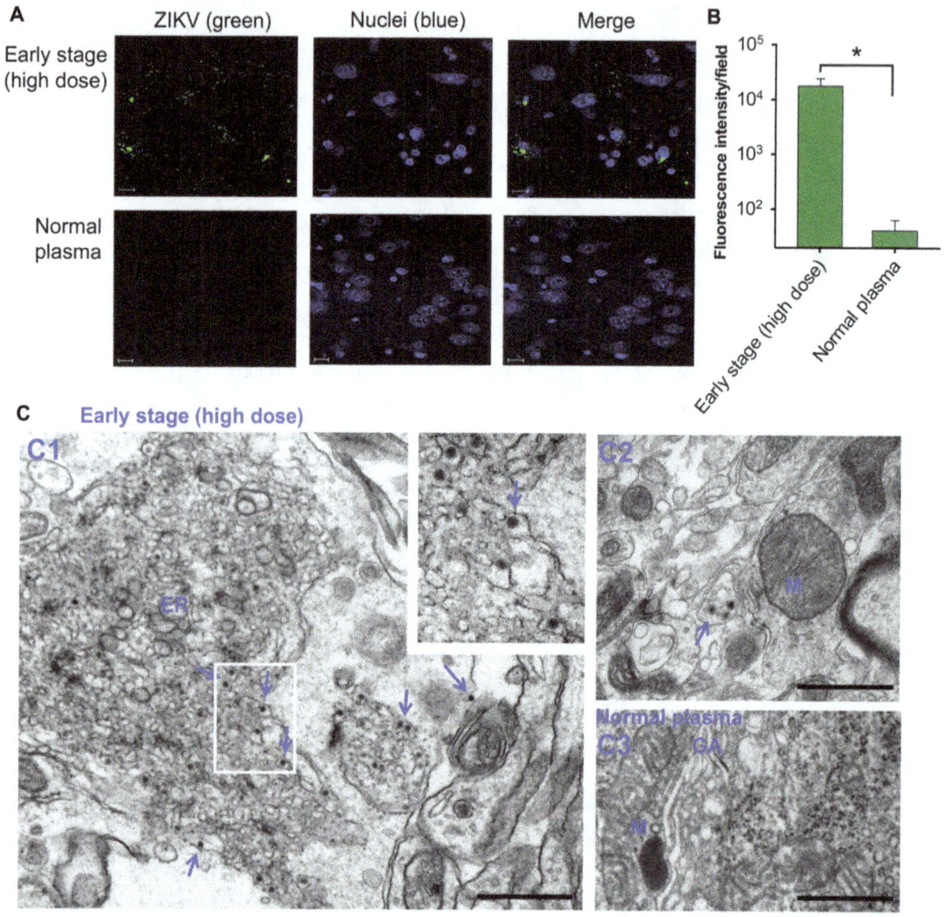

FIGURE 3 | Identification of ZIKV particles in brain tissues of pregnant A129 (E10–12) mice transfused with early-stage (high dose) ZIKV$^+$ plasma. **(A)** Immunofluorescence staining of brain tissues collected 6 days post-transfusion. Brain sections were stained for ZIKV (green) using ZIKV EDIII-specific mAb ZV-64, and representative images are listed. Nuclei were stained with DAPI, and are shown in blue. Magnification: 63X; Scale bar: 10 μm. **(B)** Quantification of ZIKV staining in **(A)** was calculated by ImageJ software for the relative intensity (particle analysis) of ZIKV staining with fluorescent signals. The data are presented as mean fluorescence intensity (e.g., ZIKV$^+$ staining) in each field ± s.e.m (n = 6, "n" indicates numbers of image from different brain tissues), and * indicates significant differences between early stage (high dose) and normal plasma groups. **(C)** TEM analysis of above brain tissues. Microphotographs of ZIKV particles formed in brain tissues of mice transfused with early-stage (high dose) ZIKV$^+$ plasma (C1–C2) or normal plasma (C3). Short arrows indicate ZIKV particles. ER, endoplasmic reticulum; M, mitochondria; GA, golgi apparatus. Scale bar: 500 nm. Normal plasma groups (A–C) indicate control mice transfused with normal plasma without ZIKV.

showed significantly more ZIKV staining than in those of mice transfused with normal plasma (**Figure 3B**), as well as by TEM analysis, which revealed multiple particles (~50–80 nm) in highly vacuolated cells, indicative of ZIKV infection (**Figure 3C**).

The above data indicate that transfusion of ZIKV$^+$ plasma from high-dose early-stage, but not later stages, of ZIKV infection leads to severe complications in pregnant A129 recipient mice, causing high viremia and broad tissue tropism, particularly brain.

Transfusion of High-Dose Early-Stage ZIKV$^+$ Plasma to Pregnant A129 Mice Resulted in Severe Placental Infection, as Well as Vascular Damage and Apoptosis in Placentas

To further investigate whether transfusion-transmitted ZIKV causes placental infection and damage, pregnant (E10–12) A129 mice were transfused with ZIKV$^+$ plasma from different infection stages, and placentas were analyzed on day 6 post-transfusion.

Significantly higher levels of ZIKV RNA (**Figure 4A**, top) and viral titers (**Figure 4A**, bottom) were detected in the placentas of mice transfused with early-stage (high dose) ZIKV$^+$ plasma than those receiving ZIKV$^+$ plasma at early and middle stages (low dose) of ZIKV infection, whereas both ZIKV RNA and viral titers were undetectable in the placentas of mice transfused with late-stage (low dose) ZIKV$^+$ plasma or normal plasma. Immunofluorescence staining also demonstrated strong signals with ZIKV-specific mAb in the placentas of early-stage (high dose) ZIKV$^+$ plasma-transfused mice (**Figure 4B**), and greater numbers of ZIKV$^+$ signals than those of control mice (**Figure 4C**). TEM analysis of infected placental tissues revealed high numbers of particles (~50–80 nm) in the early-stage (high dose) ZIKV$^+$ plasma-transfused placental tissues. In addition,

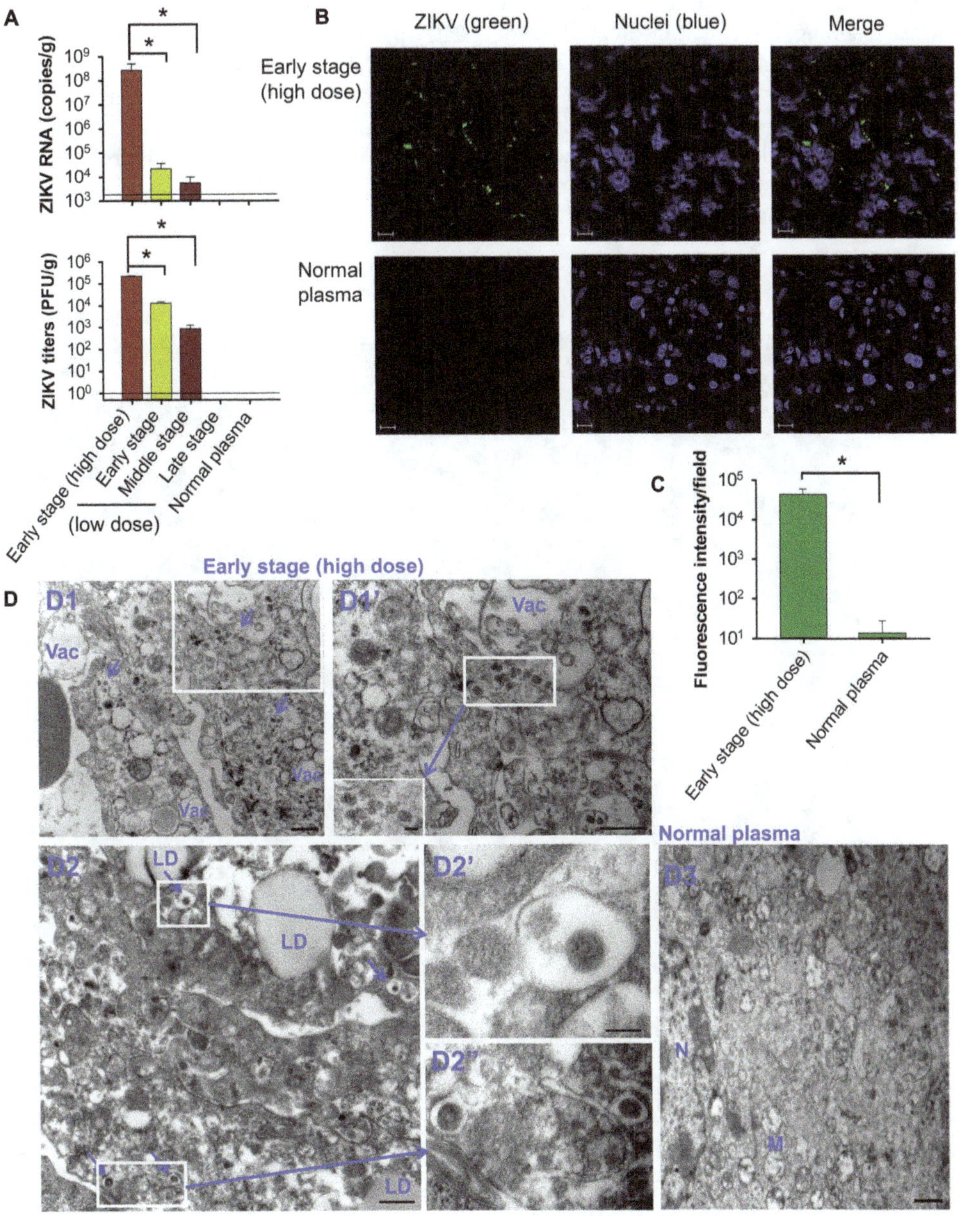

FIGURE 4 | Transfusion of pregnant A129 mice with early-stage (high dose) ZIKV$^+$ plasma led to significant placental infection. Pregnant (E10–12) A129 mice were transfused with ZIKV$^+$ plasma from early, middle, and late stages, respectively, and placentas were collected 6 days after transfusion for below tests. Detection of ZIKV RNA by qRT-PCR (**A**, top) and ZIKV titers by plaque assay (**A**, bottom). The data are presented as means ± s.e.m (n = 6 mice/group). * indicates significant differences between early stage (high dose) and early or middle stages (low dose). The detection limit, shown as the horizontal lines, for qRT-PCR and plaque assay was about 2.5×10^3 RNA copies/g and 1 PFU/g, respectively. **(B)** Immunofluorescence staining of placental tissues of pregnant mice transfused with early-stage (high dose) ZIKV$^+$ plasma. ZIKV (green) was stained using ZIKV EDIII-specific mAb ZV-64. Nuclei were stained with DAPI, and are shown in blue. Representative images are listed. Magnification: 63X; Scale bar: 10 μm. **(C)** Quantification of ZIKV staining in (B) was calculated by ImageJ software for the relative intensity (particle analysis) of ZIKV staining with fluorescent signals. The data are presented as mean fluorescence intensity (e.g., ZIKV$^+$ staining) in each field ± s.e.m (n = 6, "n" indicates numbers of image from different placentas). * indicates significant differences between early stage (high dose) and normal plasma groups. **(D)** TEM analysis of placental tissues collected from the mice transfused with early-stage (high dose) ZIKV$^+$ plasma. D1–D2, microphotographs show ZIKV particles in the placentas of ZIKV$^+$ plasma-transfused mice. Infected cells were highly vacuolated and abundant with lipid droplets. Short arrows indicate ZIKV particles. D3, placental tissues collected from normal plasma-transfused mice. Vac, vacuole; LD, lipid droplet; M, mitochondria; N, nuclei. Scale bar: 500 nm for D1, D1", D2, and D3, and 100 nm for D1' insertion, D2', and D2". Normal plasma: control plasma from A129 mice transfused with normal plasma without ZIKV.

the cytoplasm of placental cells of mice transfused with ZIKV$^+$ plasma, but not normal plasma control, had an abundance of vacuoles and large lipid droplets (**Figure 4D**).

To identify potential mechanisms of placental damage, placentas from pregnant mice transfused with high-dose early-stage ZIKV$^+$ plasma were also investigated for vascular damage and apoptosis. By immunofluorescence microscopy, diminished staining for vimentin, a marker for fetal capillary endothelium and fetal blood vessels in mouse placentas (Sapparapu et al., 2016; Miner et al., 2016), was detected in placentas from mice transfused with ZIKV$^+$ plasma, with significantly reduced numbers of vimentin$^+$ signals than those of the mice transfused with normal plasma (**Figures 5A,C**), suggesting damaged vasculature associated with early-stage ZIKV$^+$ plasma transfusion. The placentas of mice transfused with high-dose early-stage ZIKV$^+$ plasma also stained positive for activated form of caspase-3, an apoptotic marker (Yuan et al., 2017), with significantly higher numbers than those from normal plasma-transfused mice (**Figures 5B,C**), demonstrating considerable cell death, consistent with reduced vimentin expression.

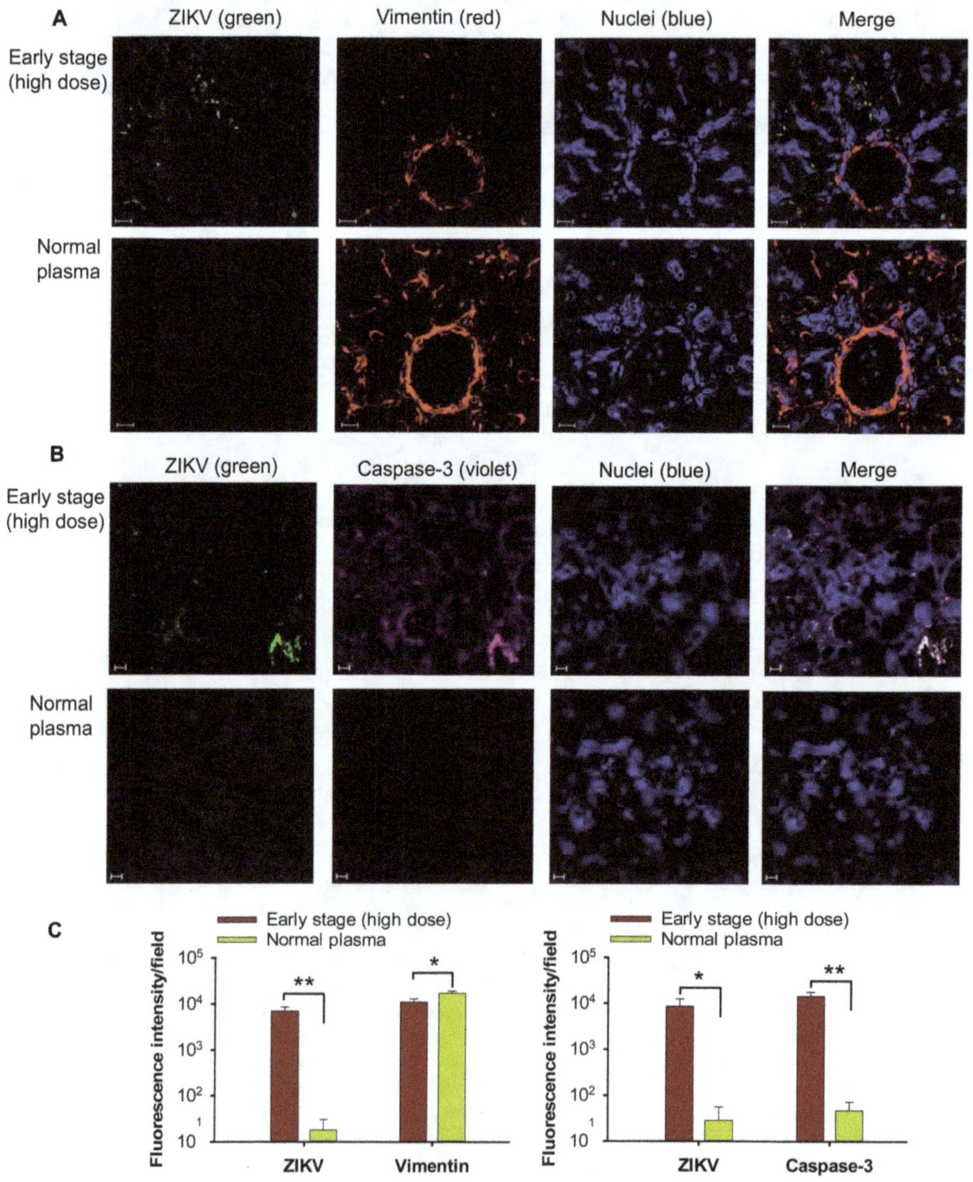

FIGURE 5 | Transfusion of pregnant A129 mice with early-stage (high dose) ZIKV$^+$ plasma caused vascular damage and apoptosis in placentas. Placentas were collected from pregnant (E10–12) A129 mice transfused with early-stage (high dose) ZIKV$^+$ plasma 6 days after transfusion, and used for below tests. Representative images of immunofluorescence staining of vimentin **(A)** and activated form of caspase-3 **(B)** in placentas are shown. ZIKV (green), vimentin (red), and activated caspase-3 (violet) were stained with anti-ZIKV, anti-vimentin, and anti-active caspase-3 antibodies, respectively. Nuclei were stained with DAPI, and are shown in blue. Magnification: 63X. Scale bar: 10 μm. **(C)** Quantification of vimentin and caspase-3 staining in **(A)** and **(B)** by ImageJ software as described above. The data are presented as mean fluorescence intensity for ZIKV$^+$, vimentin$^+$, or caspase-3$^+$ staining in each field ± s.e.m (n = 6, "n" indicates numbers of image from different placentas). * and ** indicate significant differences between early stage (high dose) and normal plasma groups. Normal plasma: control plasma from A129 mice transfused with normal plasma without ZIKV.

Altogether, these data indicate severe placental infection, vascular damage, and apoptosis following transfusion of pregnant A129 mice with early-stage ZIKV$^+$ plasma containing high titer ($\sim 2.6 \times 10^5 \pm 5 \times 10^4$ PFU) of infectious particles.

Transfusion of High-Dose Early-Stage ZIKV$^+$ Plasma to Pregnant A129 Mice Resulted in Severe Fetal Infection and Damage, Leading to Fetal and Pup Death

To test the impact of transfusion-transmitted ZIKV infection during pregnancy on fetuses and newborn pups, we first measured ZIKV in fetal amniotic fluid and embryonic brain tissue from pregnant (E10–12) A129 mice 6 days after transfusion with ZIKV$^+$ plasma. We found significantly higher ZIKV RNA (**Figure 6A**) and viral titers (**Figure 6B**), in amniotic fluid and embryonic brain of the pregnant mice transfused with early-stage (high dose) ZIKV$^+$ plasma than with plasma of early and/or middle stages (low dose) of ZIKV infection. There were also significantly higher ZIKV RNA and viral titers in amniotic fluid of the mice transfused with early-stage (low dose) than middle-stage (low dose) ZIKV$^+$ plasma. In contrast, ZIKV RNA and viral titers were undetectable in aforementioned samples of the mice transfused with other stages (low dose) of ZIKV$^+$ plasma, or normal plasma (**Figures 6A,B**).

To investigate effects of transfusion-transmitted ZIKV infection during gestation, pregnant A129 mice at E7–9 and E10–12 were transfused with early-stage (high dose) ZIKV$^+$ plasma, and then evaluated for uterus and placental morphology and fetus conditions 6 days after transfusion. All fetuses from ZIKV$^+$ plasma-transfused pregnant (E7–9) mice died in uteri and had experienced severe resorption (**Figure 6Ca**). In addition, these fetuses displayed significant growth restriction compared to those from the pregnant mice transfused with normal plasma (**Figure 6Cb**). Also, placentas from pregnant (E10–12) mice transfused with ZIKV$^+$ plasma presented obvious congestion, with significantly smaller diameter than those of the mice transfused with normal plasma (**Figure 6Cc**). Particularly, the size of the fetuses from ZIKV$^+$ plasma-transfused pregnant (E10–12) mice was significantly smaller than that of the fetuses from normal plasma-transfused mice (**Figure 6Cd**), suggesting significant fetal growth restriction during pregnancy in the ZIKV$^+$ plasma-transfused mice.

We further monitored the survival of newborn pups from pregnant (E10–12) A129 mice transfused with early-stage (high dose) ZIKV$^+$ plasma. Fewer pups were born to ZIKV$^+$ plasma-transfused pregnant mice than to normal plasma-transfused mice, and all pups from the former group died by 24 h after birth (**Figure 6D**).

The above data demonstrate that while transfusion of pregnant A129 mice with low-dose ZIKV$^+$ plasma at early ($\sim 690 \pm 285$ PFU), middle ($\sim 32 \pm 13$ PFU), and late ($\sim 3 \pm 2$ PFU) stages of infection led to low to no ZIKV replication in fetuses, transfusion with early-stage (high dose) ZIKV$^+$ ($\sim 2.6 \times 10^5 \pm 5 \times 10^4$ PFU) plasma caused severe congenital fetal infection, fetal damage, and reduced fetal growth, leading to fetal and pup death.

Transfusion of High-Dose Early-Stage ZIKV$^+$ Plasma to Pregnant A129 Mice Resulted in Inflammation With Increased Cytokines and Chemokines

To evaluate whether transfusion-transmitted ZIKV causes inflammation to pregnant mice and their fetuses, placentas and fetal amniotic fluid from pregnant (E10–12) A129 mice 6 days after transfusion were tested for inflammatory cytokines and chemokines using Multi-Analyte ELISArray Kits. Significantly higher expression of IL-1α, G-CSF, MCP-1 (CCL-2), SDF-1 (CXCL-12), and KC (CXCL-1) was identified in the ZIKV$^+$ plasma (early-stage, high dose)-transfused mouse placentas than those of the mice transfused with normal plasma (**Figures 7A,B**). In addition to the cytokines and chemokines described above, fetal amniotic fluid of the mice transfused with ZIKV$^+$ plasma also demonstrated significantly increased production of inflammatory cytokine IL-6 and chemokines MIG (CXCL-9) and Eotaxin (CCL-11), as compared with that of the normal plasma-transfused mice (**Figures 7C,D**). These data suggest that early-stage (high dose) ZIKV$^+$ plasma transfusion may lead to significant inflammation in the pregnant mice, and that fetuses might experience a more severe inflammatory response than maternal placentas.

DISCUSSION

ZIKV may be transmitted through blood transfusion. ZIKV RNA was detected in asymptomatic blood donors during the ZIKV outbreak, posing a serious threat to blood safety (Musso et al., 2016; Bierlaire et al., 2017; Slavov et al., 2017; Willyard, 2017). Here, we used ZIKV-susceptible pregnant A129 mice to study transmissibility of ZIKV through transfusion and evaluate viremia, tissue tropism, placental infection and damage, and associated pathogenic mechanisms, as well as fetal damage and fetal and pup death. Overall, the data suggest that transfusion-transmitted ZIKV from early-stage infection can cause significant viremia, broad tissue tropism, and inflammation, with devastating effects during pregnancy, particularly on the fetuses.

To establish transfusion process with ZIKV$^+$ plasma, minimize potential impact of preexisting antibodies or other factors in the transfused plasma, and maintain the recipient mice to survive during the observation period, we manually inoculated normal plasma with a contemporary ZIKV strain (R103451) at non-lethal, low-dose (e.g., ~90 PFU) (Tai et al., 2018), transfused it to A129 mice, and collected plasma at early, middle, and late ZIKV infection stages after transfusion to test ZIKV titers. Surprisingly, viremia was detectable in the transfused mouse plasma after 45 days, with early-stage infection having the highest ZIKV titer. It has been shown that viral load in human maternal sera can be detectable for 14 weeks, and that ZIKV RNAs are detected in maternal sera 8 weeks after the onset of clinical symptoms, which potentially result from viral replication in the fetuses or placentas where the latter might serve as a reservoir (Driggers et al., 2016; Suy et al., 2016). Here

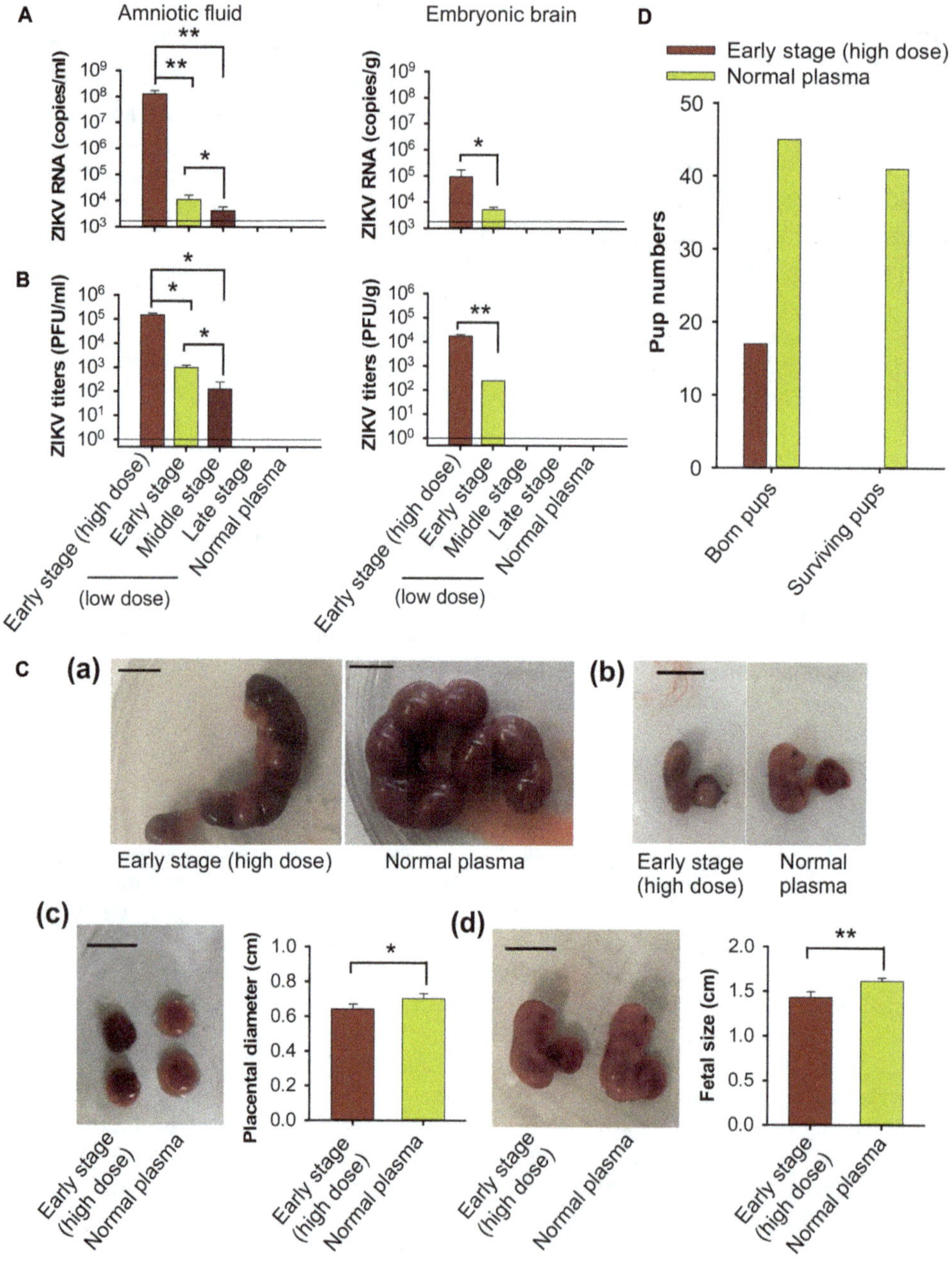

FIGURE 6 | Transfusion of pregnant A129 mice with early-stage (high dose) ZIKV$^+$ plasma led to significant fetal infection and fetal and pup death. Pregnant (E10–12) A129 mice were transfused with ZIKV$^+$ plasma from early, middle, and late stages, respectively. ZIKV RNA and ZIKV titers were detected by qRT-PCR **(A)** and plaque assay **(B)** in amniotic fluid and embryonic brain collected 6 days post-transfusion. The detection limit, shown as the horizontal lines, was about 2.5×10^3 RNA copies/ml and 1 PFU/ml (for amniotic fluid), or 2.5×10^3 RNA copies/g and 1 PFU/g (for embryonic brain), respectively, for qRT-PCR and plaque assay. * and ** indicate significant differences between early stage (high dose) and early or middle stages (low dose), or between early and middle stages (low dose). The data are presented as means ± s.e.m (n = 6 mice/group). **(C)** Morphology of mouse uteri and placentas and conditions of fetuses 6 days after transfusion of early-stage (high dose) ZIKV$^+$ plasma. **(a)** E13–15 uteri from pregnant mice transfused at E7–9. **(b)** Representative images of fetuses in **(a)**. **(c)** E16–18 placentas from pregnant mice transfused at E10–12. **(d)** Representative images of E16–18 fetuses in **(c)**. Scale bar: 1 cm. Placental diameter in **(c)** and fetal size in **(d)** are shown. * and ** indicate significant differences between early stage (high dose) and normal plasma groups. The data are presented as means ± s.e.m (n = 6 mice/group). **(D)** Total born and surviving pups 24 h after birth from pregnant (E10–12) mice transfused with early-stage (high dose) ZIKV$^+$ plasma. Normal plasma: control plasma from A129 mice transfused with normal plasma without ZIKV.

we speculate that persistent ZIKV viremia post non-lethal, low-dose ZIKV$^+$ plasma transfusion might be partially due to viral replication in organs that could act as potential reservoirs.

To determine which stages of ZIKV infection with the identified viral titers that will not cause problems to the transfused pregnant recipients, plasma collected above at early,

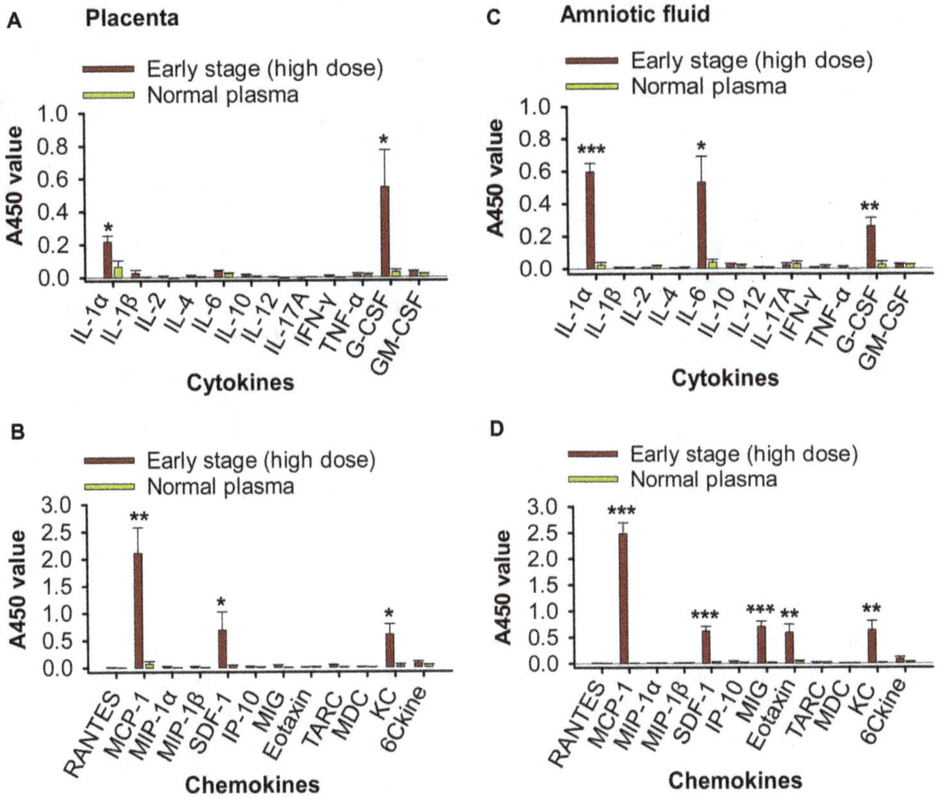

FIGURE 7 | Transfusion of pregnant A129 mice with early-stage (high dose) ZIKV+ plasma led to significant inflammation. Placentas **(A,B)** and amniotic fluid **(C,D)** collected from pregnant (E10–12) A129 mice 6 days post-transfusion of early-stage (high dose) ZIKV+ plasma were detected by Multi-Analyte ELISArray Kits for inflammatory cytokines **(A,C)** and chemokines **(B,D)**. *, **, and *** indicate significant differences between early stage (high dose) and normal plasma groups, and the data are presented as means ± s.e.m (*n* = 6 mice/group). Normal plasma: control plasma from A129 mice transfused with normal plasma without ZIKV.

middle, and late stages of ZIKV infection was transfused into pregnant A129 mice. We found that significantly higher viremia was identified in the pregnant mice receiving early-stage (high-dose) ZIKV$^+$ plasma than other stages of ZIKV$^+$ plasma, suggesting that transfusion-transmitted ZIKV infection at early stage containing high-titer ZIKV will lead to rapid ZIKV replication. Although ZIKV titers were significantly lower in the pregnant mice transfused with plasma at early-stage (low dose) ZIKV infection, it remains possible that such transfusion might have long-term effects.

ZIKV infection may trigger GBS (severe neuropathies) (Savino et al., 2017; Zhou et al., 2017; Hygino da Cruz et al., 2018; Wu et al., 2018) and it is closely associated with congenital Zika diseases (microcephaly and brain abnormalities) in humans (Franca et al., 2016; Shapiro-Mendoza et al., 2017; Zorrilla et al., 2017). ZIKV RNA replication has been identified in human brain and placental tissues (Bhatnagar et al., 2017). Our data show that while pregnant mice had low to no brain and congenital ZIKV infection upon transfusion with early-, middle-, and late-stage plasma containing the low-titer ZIKV, they had significant brain infection with identified ZIKV particles in the infected brain tissue after receiving the high-titer ZIKV$^+$ plasma. Notably, such transfusion also caused severe ZIKV replication in the placentas, amniotic fluid, and fetal brain, as well as inflammation in the placentas and fetal amniotic fluid, and had detrimental effects on the placentas, fetuses and newborn babies, causing fetal damage, and fetal and pup death. Overall, since elevated viral titers were associated with increased cell death and damaged vasculature in the placentas, loss of placental integrity in pregnant mice may have been a contributor of increased fetal and newborn mortality.

Clearly, identification of transfusion-transmitted ZIKV infection in brain and placental tissues of pregnant mice, as well as associated fetal damage and pup death by vertical transmission during pregnancy, further reinforce the need for surveillance measures to detect ZIKV in blood products. Our data from mouse studies also suggest that low ZIKV plasma titers might not be associated with establishment of transfusion-transmitted ZIKV infection in brain, placentas, and fetuses. It is thus reassuring that only high-titer ZIKV infection drives complications in pregnant mice and/or their fetuses and pups, suggesting that high risk of transfusion-transmitted ZIKV infection may be restricted to high viral titers at the early stage. Since murine and human placentas present different developmental anatomy and distinct co-expression patterns of certain genes (Georgiades et al., 2002; Soncin et al., 2018), infectious doses required for efficient ZIKV transfusion transmission in mouse and human placentas may differ. Thus, the transfusion studies performed in mice might not be completely consistent in human settings. It is possible that humans receiving ZIKV-containing plasma or blood at different doses, particularly low dose, might have distinct consequences from mice. Nevertheless, considering that murine placentas have paralleling development to the first half of human placental development (through gestational week 16), and that there are still some similarities between human and mouse placentas in terms of structures and cell types (Georgiades et al., 2002; Soncin et al., 2018), the current data provide important information to infection window period and evaluate risk of transfusion-associated transmission by ZIKV through blood products in humans.

Our study has identified potential differences in transfusion-induced ZIKV tissue tropism and/or associated pathology compared to transmission by other routes. For example, ZIKV subcutaneous (S.C.) inoculation leads to detectable virus in peripheral nervous tissues, lymphoid tissues, joints, and uterus at day 7 post-infection (Hirsch et al., 2017). Other studies have shown that ZIKV infection via mosquito bite (e.g., route for human ZIKV infection) alters ZIKV tissue tropism, but the distribution is limited to hemolymphatic tissues, reproductive tract tissues, kidney, and liver (Dudley et al., 2017). More recently, ZIKV infection and congenital Zika syndrome were found to be also associated with critical human congenital heart disease (Angelidou et al., 2018). It is noted that pregnant mice infected with ZIKV through different routes also present variant symptoms, viral replication, and pathology in placentas, fetuses, and pups, and the doses required for efficient viral infection may vary. For instance, pregnant immunocompetent mice, such as BALB/c and C57BL/6, do not generally show significant clinical symptoms, viral replication, and tissue tropism via S.C., I.P., or intravenous (I.V.) routes after high-dose ZIKV infection ($\geq 10^5$ PFU), except for some fetal infection or fetal abnormalities (fetal resorption or growth restriction) (Yu et al., 2017; Caine et al., 2018; Szaba et al., 2018). However, pregnant C57BL/6 or BALB/c mice injected with anti-IFNAR antibodies may have significant viral replication in placentas and fetal heads after I.V. or S.C. infection of ZIKV (10^5–10^6 PFU) (Turner et al., 2017; Caine et al., 2018; Li et al., 2018). Particularly, A129 and AG129 mice infected with ZIKV through S.C. or I.P. routes demonstrate severe placental injury, fetal brain injury, shorter skull length, reduced size in fetuses and pups, or fetal and pup demise, with viral doses ranging from 10^2–10^4 PFU, focus forming unit (FFU), 50% tissue culture infectious doses ($TCID_{50}$), or 50% cell culture infectious doses ($CCID_{50}$) (Miner et al., 2016; Caine et al., 2018; Julander et al., 2018; Tai et al., 2018). Here we found that transfusion of A129 mice with early-stage $ZIKV^+$ (2.6×10^5 PFU) plasma induced broad tissue tropism 6 days post-transfusion, resulting in high viral titers in lung, spleen, kidney, heart, liver, muscle, brain, and placentas, as well as severe fetal infection and damage, accompanying with fetal and pup death. This consequence could be partially contributed to the high-dose ZIKV contained in the transfused plasma. Although other infection stages of plasma with the low-dose ZIKV did not cause significant tissue tropism at short-term (6 days) post-transfusion, ZIKV might replicate slowly but continuously, leading to long-term effects. It should be clarified that the ZIKV tissue tropisms and associated pathology resulting from various infection routes, as described above, did not count for different virus strains used for infection, hosts, age of animals, or time points post-infection. Therefore, comparative studies of viral titers by various routes of ZIKV transmission are needed to determine whether more severe outcome is linked to transfusion-transmitted ZIKV infection, and to develop a more comprehensive profile of ZIKV tropism in all tissues and related outcome to help better understand ZIKV pathogenesis.

To summarize, we report on the transmissibility and pathogenesis of transfusion-transmitted ZIKV infection in ZIKV-susceptible pregnant A129 mice. The data indicate that transfusion of plasma containing ZIKV at early-stage infection harboring high-titer ZIKV has serious consequences for pregnant mice, their fetuses and newborn pups. In contrast, transfusion-associated transmission with plasma from later stages of ZIKV infection, which contained low-titer ZIKV, might not be associated with ZIKV replication and have no serious outcome during pregnancy. Overall, the consequences from transfusion-transmitted ZIKV infection in the pregnant mice are positively correlated with ZIKV titers in the transfused plasma. Taken together, our data may help future design of studies to perform risk assessment of ZIKV transmissibility by blood transfusion in humans.

AUTHOR CONTRIBUTIONS

WT, SJ, KY, and LD designed the experiments. WT, DV, JC, and WB performed the experiments. WT, DV, JC, WB, DK, and BS analyzed the data. WT, DV, BS, SJ, KY, and LD wrote and revised the manuscript.

REFERENCES

Aliota, M. T., Caine, E. A., Walker, E. C., Larkin, K. E., Camacho, E., and Osorio, J. E. (2016). Characterization of lethal Zika virus infection in AG129 mice. *PLoS. Negl. Trop. Dis.* 10:e0004682. doi: 10.1371/journal.pntd.0004682

Angelidou, A., Michael, Z., Hotz, A., Friedman, K., Emani, S., LaRovere, K., et al. (2018). Is there more to Zika? Complex cardiac disease in a case of congenital Zika syndrome. *Neonatology* 113, 177–182. doi: 10.1159/000484656

Aubry, M., Finke, J., Teissier, A., Roche, C., Broult, J., Paulous, S., et al. (2015). Seroprevalence of arboviruses among blood donors in French Polynesia, 2011-2013. *Int. J. Infect. Dis.* 41, 11–12. doi: 10.1016/j.ijid.2015.10.005

Barjas-Castro, M. L., Angerami, R. N., Cunha, M. S., Suzuki, A., Nogueira, J. S., Rocco, I. M., et al. (2016). Probable transfusion-transmitted Zika virus in Brazil. *Transfusion* 56, 1684–1688. doi: 10.1111/trf.13681

Benjamin, R. J. (2017). Zika virus in the blood supply. *Blood* 129, 144–145. doi: 10.1182/blood-2016-12-751925

Bhatnagar, J., Rabeneck, D. B., Martines, R. B., Reagan-Steiner, S., Ermias, Y., Estetter, L. B., et al. (2017). Zika virus RNA replication and persistence in brain and placental tissue. *Emerg. Infect. Dis.* 23, 405–414. doi: 10.3201/eid2303.161499

Bierlaire, D., Mauguin, S., Broult, J., and Musso, D. (2017). Zika virus and blood transfusion: the experience of French Polynesia. *Transfusion* 57, 729–733. doi: 10.1111/trf.14028

Bloch, E. M., Ness, P. M., Tobian, A. A. R., and Sugarman, J. (2018). Revisiting blood safety practices given emerging data about Zika virus. *N. Engl. J. Med.* 378, 1837–1841. doi: 10.1056/NEJMsb1704752

Caine, E. A., Jagger, B. W., and Diamond, M. S. (2018). Animal models of Zika virus infection during pregnancy. *Viruses* 10:E598. doi: 10.3390/v10110598

Cao-Lormeau, V. M., Blake, A., Mons, S., Lastere, S., Roche, C., Vanhomwegen, J., et al. (2016). Guillain-barre syndrome outbreak associated with Zika virus infection in French Polynesia: a case-control study. *Lancet* 387, 1531–1539. doi: 10.1016/S0140-6736(16)00562-6

Chimelli, L., Moura, P. S., Avvad-Portari, E., Farias, M. V., Araujo, Z. A., Prado, C. D., et al. (2018). Persistence of Zika virus after birth: clinical, virological, neuroimaging, and neuropathological documentation in a 5-month infant with congenital Zika syndrome. *J. Neuropathol. Exp. Neurol.* 77, 193–198. doi: 10.1093/jnen/nlx116

Cui, L., Zou, P., Chen, E., Yao, H., Zheng, H., Qiang, Q., et al. (2017). Visual and motor deficits in grown-up mice with congenital Zika virus infection. *eBioMedicine* 20, 193–201. doi: 10.1016/j.ebiom.2017.04.029

Dai, L., Song, J., Lu, X., Deng, Y. Q., Musyoki, A. M., Cheng, H., et al. (2016). Structures of the Zika virus envelope protein and its complex with a flavivirus broadly protective antibody. *Cell Host Microbe* 19, 696–704. doi: 10.1016/j.chom.2016.04.013

Dick, G. W., Kitchen, S. F., and Haddor, A. J. (1952). Zika virus. I. Isolations and serological specificity. *Trans. R. Soc. Trop. Med. Hyg.* 46, 509–520. doi: 10.1016/0035-9203(52)90042-4

Dowall, S. D., Graham, V. A., Rayner, E., Atkinson, B., Hall, G., Watson, R., et al. (2016). A susceptible mouse model for Zika virus infection. *PLoS Negl. Trop. Dis.* 10:e0004658. doi: 10.1371/journal.pntd.0004658

Driggers, R. W., Ho, C. Y., Korhonen, E. M., Kuivanen, S., Jaaskelainen, A. J., Smura, T., et al. (2016). Zika virus infection with prolonged maternal viremia and fetal brain abnormalities. *N. Engl. J. Med.* 374, 2142–2151. doi: 10.1056/NEJMoa1601824

Du, L., Zhou, Y., and Jiang, S. (2017). The latest advancements in Zika virus vaccine development. *Expert Rev. Vaccines* 16, 951–954. doi: 10.1080/14760584.2017.1363648

Dudley, D. M., Newman, C. M., Lalli, J., Stewart, L. M., Koenig, M. R., Weiler, A. M., et al. (2017). Infection via mosquito bite alters Zika virus tissue tropism and replication kinetics in rhesus macaques. *Nat. Commun.* 8:2096. doi: 10.1038/s41467-017-02222-8

Espinosa, D., Mendy, J., Manayani, D., Vang, L., Wang, C., Richard, T., et al. (2018). Passive transfer of immune sera induced by a Zika virus-like particle vaccine protects AG129 mice against lethal Zika virus challenge. *eBioMedicine* 27, 61–70. doi: 10.1016/j.ebiom.2017.12.010

Franca, G. V., Schuler-Faccini, L., Oliveira, W. K., Henriques, C. M., Carmo, E. H., Pedi, V. D., et al. (2016). Congenital Zika virus syndrome in Brazil: a case series of the first 1501 livebirths with complete investigation. *Lancet* 388, 891–897. doi: 10.1016/S0140-6736(16)30902-3

Galel, S. A., Williamson, P. C., Busch, M. P., Stanek, D., Bakkour, S., Stone, M., et al. (2017). First Zika-positive donations in the continental United States. *Transfusion* 57, 762–769. doi: 10.1111/trf.14029

Georgiades, P., Ferguson-Smith, A. C., and Burton, G. J. (2002). Comparative developmental anatomy of the murine and human definitive placentae. *Placenta* 23, 3–19. doi: 10.1053/plac.2001.0738

Harrington, T., Kuehnert, M. J., Kamel, H., Lanciotti, R. S., Hand, S., Currier, M., et al. (2003). West nile virus infection transmitted by blood transfusion. *Transfusion* 43, 1018–1022. doi: 10.1046/j.1537-2995.2003.00481.x

Hirsch, A. J., Smith, J. L., Haese, N. N., Broeckel, R. M., Parkins, C. J., Kreklywich, C., et al. (2017). Zika virus infection of rhesus macaques leads to viral persistence in multiple tissues. *PLoS Pathog.* 13:e1006219. doi: 10.1371/journal.ppat.1006219

Hygino da Cruz, L. C. Jr., Nascimento, O. J. M., Lopes, F. P. P. L., and da Silva, I. R. F. (2018). Neuroimaging findings of Zika virus-associated neurologic complications in adults. *AJNR Am. J. Neuroradiol.* 39, 1967–1974. doi: 10.3174/ajnr.A5649

Iwamoto, M., Jernigan, D. B., Guasch, A., Trepka, M. J., Blackmore, C. G., Hellinger, W. C., et al. (2003). Transmission of west nile virus from an organ donor to four transplant recipients. *N. Engl. J. Med.* 348, 2196–2203. doi: 10.1056/NEJMoa022987

Jiang, S., and Du, L. (2019). Advances in the research and development of therapeutic antibodies against the Zika virus. *Cell. Mol. Immunol.* 16, 107–108. doi: 10.1038/s41423-018-0043-x

Julander, J. G., Siddharthan, V., Park, A. H., Preston, E., Mathur, P., Bertolio, M., et al. (2018). Consequences of in utero exposure to Zika virus in offspring of AG129 mice. *Sci. Rep.* 8:9384. doi: 10.1038/s41598-018-27611-x

Kostyuchenko, V. A., Lim, E. X., Zhang, S., Fibriansah, G., Ng, T. S., Ooi, J. S., et al. (2016). Structure of the thermally stable Zika virus. *Nature* 533, 425–428. doi: 10.1038/nature17994

Krauer, F., Riesen, M., Reveiz, L., Oladapo, O. T., Martinez-Vega, R., Porgo, T. V., et al. (2017). Zika virus infection as a cause of congenital brain abnormalities and guillain-barre syndrome: systematic review. *PLoS Med.* 14:e1002203. doi: 10.1371/journal.pmed.1002203

Li, X. F., Dong, H. L., Wang, H. J., Huang, X. Y., Qiu, Y. F., Ji, X., et al. (2018). Development of a chimeric Zika vaccine using a licensed live-attenuated flavivirus vaccine as backbone. *Nat. Commun.* 9:673. doi: 10.1038/s41467-018-02975-w

Magnus, M. M., Esposito, D. L. A., Costa, V. A. D., Melo, P. S., Costa-Lima, C., Fonseca, B. A. L. D., et al. (2018). Risk of Zika virus transmission by blood donations in Brazil. *Hematol. Transfus. Cell Ther.* 40, 250–254. doi: 10.1016/j.htct.2018.01.011

Melo, A. S., Aguiar, R. S., Amorim, M. M., Arruda, M. B., Melo, F. O., Ribeiro, S. T., et al. (2016). Congenital Zika virus infection: beyond neonatal microcephaly. *JAMA Neurol.* 73, 1407–1416. doi: 10.1001/jamaneurol.2016.3720

Miner, J. J., Cao, B., Govero, J., Smith, A. M., Fernandez, E., Cabrera, O. H., et al. (2016). Zika virus infection during pregnancy in mice causes placental damage and fetal demise. *Cell* 165, 1081–1091. doi: 10.1016/j.cell.2016.05.008

Mlakar, J., Korva, M., Tul, N., Popovic, M., Poljsak-Prijatelj, M., Mraz, J., et al. (2016). Zika virus associated with microcephaly. *N. Engl. J. Med.* 374, 951–958. doi: 10.1056/NEJMoa1600651

Motta, I. J., Spencer, B. R., Cordeiro da Silva, S. G., Arruda, M. B., Dobbin, J. A., Gonzaga, Y. B., et al. (2016). Evidence for transmission of Zika virus by platelet transfusion. *N. Engl. J. Med.* 375, 1101–1103. doi: 10.1056/NEJMc1607262

Musso, D., Stramer, S. L., and Busch, M. P. (2016). Zika virus: a new challenge for blood transfusion. *Lancet* 387, 1993–1994. doi: 10.1016/S0140-6736(16)30428-7

Pessoa, A., van der Linden, V., Yeargin-Allsopp, M., Carvalho, M. D. C. G., Ribeiro, E. M., Van Naarden, B. K., et al. (2018). Motor abnormalities and epilepsy in infants and children with evidence of congenital Zika virus infection. *Pediatrics* 141, S167–S179. doi: 10.1542/peds.2017-2038F

Roze, B., Najioullah, F., Ferge, J. L., Dorleans, F., Apetse, K., Barnay, J. L., et al. (2017). Guillain-Barre syndrome associated with Zika virus infection in martinique in 2016: a prospective study. *Clin. Infect. Dis.* 65, 1462–1468. doi: 10.1093/cid/cix588

Salinas, J. L., Walteros, D. M., Styczynski, A., Garzon, F., Quijada, H., Bravo, E., et al. (2017). Zika virus disease-associated guillain-barre syndrome-barranquilla, Colombia 2015-2016. *J. Neurol. Sci.* 381, 272–277. doi: 10.1016/j.jns.2017.09.001

Sapparapu, G., Fernandez, E., Kose, N., Bin, C., Fox, J. M., Bombardi, R. G., et al. (2016). Neutralizing human antibodies prevent Zika virus replication and fetal disease in mice. *Nature* 540, 443–447. doi: 10.1038/nature20564

Savino, W., Messias, C. V., Mendes-da-Cruz, D. A., Passos, P., Ferreira, A. C., and Nascimento, O. J. (2017). Zika virus infection in the elderly: possible relationship with guillain-barre syndrome. *Gerontology* 63, 210–215. doi: 10.1159/000453579

Shapiro-Mendoza, C. K., Rice, M. E., Galang, R. R., Fulton, A. C., VanMaldeghem, K., Prado, M. V., et al. (2017). Pregnancy outcomes after maternal Zika virus infection during pregnancy - U.S. territories, January 1, 2016-April 25, 2017. *MMWR Morb. Mortal. Wkly. Rep.* 66, 615–621. doi: 10.15585/mmwr.mm6623e1

Simon, O., Acket, B., Forfait, C., Girault, D., Gourinat, A. C., Millon, P., et al. (2018). Zika virus outbreak in new caledonia and guillain-barre syndrome: a case-control study. *J. Neurovirol.* 24, 362–368. doi: 10.1007/s13365-018-0621-9

Sirohi, D., Chen, Z., Sun, L., Klose, T., Pierson, T. C., Rossmann, M. G., et al. (2016). The 3.8 Å resolution cryo-EM structure of Zika virus. *Science* 352, 467–470. doi: 10.1126/science.aaf5316

Slavov, S. N., Hespanhol, M. R., Rodrigues, E. S., Levi, J. E., Ubiali, E. M. A., Covas, D. T., et al. (2017). Zika virus RNA detection in asymptomatic blood donors during an outbreak in the northeast region of Sao Paulo State, Brazil, 2016. *Transfusion* 57, 2897–2901. doi: 10.1111/trf.14322

Soncin, F., Khater, M., To, C., Pizzo, D., Farah, O., Wakeland, A., et al. (2018). Comparative analysis of mouse and human placentae across gestation reveals species-specific regulators of placental development. *Development* 145:dev156273. doi: 10.1242/dev.156273

Sumathy, K., Kulkarni, B., Gondu, R. K., Ponnuru, S. K., Bonguram, N., Eligeti, R., et al. (2017). Protective efficacy of Zika vaccine in AG129 mouse model. *Sci. Rep.* 7:46375. doi: 10.1038/srep46375

Suy, A., Sulleiro, E., Rodo, C., Vazquez, E., Bocanegra, C., Molina, I., et al. (2016). Prolonged Zika virus viremia during pregnancy. *N. Engl. J. Med.* 375, 2611–2613. doi: 10.1056/NEJMc1607580

Szaba, F. M., Tighe, M., Kummer, L. W., Lanzer, K. G., Ward, J. M., Lanthier, P., et al. (2018). Zika virus infection in immunocompetent pregnant mice causes fetal damage and placental pathology in the absence of fetal infection. *PLoS Pathog.* 14:e1006994. doi: 10.1371/journal.ppat.1006994

Tai, W., He, L., Wang, Y., Sun, S., Zhao, G., Luo, C., et al. (2018). Critical neutralizing fragment of Zika virus EDIII elicits cross-neutralization and protection against divergent Zika viruses. *Emerg. Microbes Infect.* 7:7. doi: 10.1038/s41426-017-0007-8

Turner, L. H., Kinder, J. M., Wilburn, A., D'Mello, R. J., Braunlin, M. R., Jiang, T. T., et al. (2017). Preconceptual Zika virus asymptomatic infection protects against secondary prenatal infection. *PLoS Pathog.* 13:e1006684. doi: 10.1371/journal.ppat.1006684

Wikan, N., and Smith, D. R. (2016). Zika virus: history of a newly emerging arbovirus. *Lancet Infect. Dis.* 16:e119–e126. doi: 10.1016/S1473-3099(16)30010-X

Wilder-Smith, A., Chen, L. H., Massad, E., and Wilson, M. E. (2009). Threat of dengue to blood safety in dengue-endemic countries. *Emerg. Infect. Dis.* 15, 8–11. doi: 10.3201/eid1501.071097

Williamson, P. C., Linnen, J. M., Kessler, D. A., Shaz, B. H., Kamel, H., Vassallo, R. R., et al. (2017). First cases of Zika virus-infected US blood donors outside states with areas of active transmission. *Transfusion* 57, 770–778. doi: 10.1111/trf.14041

Willyard, C. (2017). Screening: in the blood. *Nature* 549, S19–S21. doi: 10.1038/549S19a

Wu, K. H., Madigan, M. C., Billson, F. A., and Penfold, P. L. (2003). Differential expression of GFAP in early v late AMD: a quantitative analysis. *Br. J. Ophthalmol.* 87, 1159–1166. doi: 10.1136/bjo.87.9.1159

Wu, S., Zeng, Y., Lerner, A., Gao, B., and Law, M. (2018). Nervous system injury and neuroimaging of Zika virus infection. *Front. Neurol.* 9:227. doi: 10.3389/fneur.2018.00227

Wu, Y., Li, S., Du, L., Wang, C., Zou, P., Hong, B., et al. (2017). Neutralization of Zika virus by germline-like human monoclonal antibodies targeting cryptic epitopes on envelope domain III. *Emerg. Microbes Infect.* 6:e89. doi: 10.1038/emi.2017.79

Yu, Y., Deng, Y. Q., Zou, P., Wang, Q., Dai, Y., Yu, F., et al. (2017). A peptide-based viral inactivator inhibits Zika virus infection in pregnant mice and fetuses. *Nat. Commun.* 8:15672. doi: 10.1038/ncomms15672

Yuan, L., Huang, X. Y., Liu, Z. Y., Zhang, F., Zhu, X. L., Yu, J. Y., et al. (2017). A single mutation in the prM protein of Zika virus contributes to fetal microcephaly. *Science* 358, 933–936. doi: 10.1126/science.aam7120

Zhao, H., Fernandez, E., Dowd, K. A., Speer, S. D., Platt, D. J., Gorman, M. J., et al. (2016). Structural basis of Zika virus-specific antibody protection. *Cell* 166, 1016–1027. doi: 10.1016/j.cell.2016.07.020

Zhou, K., Wang, L., Yu, D., Huang, H., Ji, H., and Mo, X. (2017). Molecular and cellular insights into Zika virus-related neuropathies. *J. Neurovirol.* 23, 341–346. doi: 10.1007/s13365-017-0514-3

Zorrilla, C. D., Garcia, G. I., Garcia, F. L., and De La Vega, A. (2017). Zika virus infection in pregnancy: maternal, fetal, and neonatal considerations. *J. Infect. Dis.* 216, S891–S896. doi: 10.1093/infdis/jix448

13

Placental Macrophage (Hofbauer Cell) Responses to Infection during Pregnancy

Georgia Fakonti, Paschalia Pantazi, Vladimir Bokun and Beth Holder*

Institute of Reproductive and Developmental Biology, Department of Metabolism, Digestion and Reproduction, Imperial College London, London, United Kingdom

***Correspondence:**
Beth Holder
b.holder@imperial.ac.uk

Background: Congenital infection of the fetus *via* trans-placental passage of pathogens can result in severe morbidity and mortality. Even without transmission to the fetus, infection of the placenta itself is associated with pregnancy complications including pregnancy loss and preterm birth. Placental macrophages, also termed Hofbauer cells (HBCs), are fetal-origin macrophages residing in the placenta that are likely involved in responding to placental infection and protection of the developing fetus. As HBCs are the only immune cell present in the villous placenta, they represent one of the final opportunities for control of infection and prevention of passage to the developing fetus.

Objective and Rationale: The objective of this review was to provide a systematic overview of the literature regarding HBC responses during infection in pregnancy, including responses to viral, bacterial, and parasitic pathogens.

Methods: PubMed and Scopus were searched on May 20th, 2021, with no limit on publication date, to identify all papers that have studied placental macrophages/Hofbauer cells in the context of infection. The following search strategy was utilized: (hofbauer* OR "hofbauer cells" OR "hofbauer cell" OR "placental macrophage" OR "placental macrophages") AND [infect* OR virus OR viral OR bacteri* OR parasite* OR pathogen* OR LPS OR "poly(i:c)" OR toxoplasm* OR microb* OR HIV)].

Outcomes: 86 studies were identified for review. This included those that investigated HBCs in placentas from pregnancies complicated by maternal infection and *in vitro* studies investigating HBC responses to pathogens or Pathogen-Associated Molecular Patterns (PAMPs). HBCs can be infected by a variety of pathogens, and HBC hyperplasia was a common observation. HBCs respond to pathogen infection and PAMPs by altering their transcriptional, translational and secretion profiles. Co-culture investigations demonstrate that they can replicate and transmit pathogens to other cells. In other cases, they may eliminate the pathogen through a variety of mechanisms including phagocytosis, cytokine-mediated pathogen elimination, release of macrophage extracellular traps and HBC-antibody-mediated neutralization. HBC responses differ across gestation and may be influenced by pre-existing immunity. Clinical information, including gestational age at infection, gestational age of the samples, mode of sample collection and pregnancy outcome were missing for the majority of studies.

Keywords: Hofbauer cells, placental macrophages, placenta, congenital infection, virus

INTRODUCTION

The maternal-fetal interface is the site of *in utero* pathogen transmission from mother to the fetus during pregnancy. The maternal decidua, which is in close contact with the placenta, contains several immune cell types including macrophages, natural killer cells, innate lymphoid cells and T cells. In contrast, the only immune cells present in placental tissue are macrophages termed Hofbauer cells (HBCs). These macrophages are of fetal origin and have been detected from the sixth week of pregnancy to the end of gestation (1). HBCs help maintain homeostatic conditions in the placenta by regulating processes such as angiogenesis, vasculogenesis (2, 3), tissue remodeling and (4) development (5) and immune regulation (6), as well as orchestrating responses to infection and directly responding to pathogens that access the placenta. The functional variability of HBCs reflects the phenotypic diversity and plasticity of macrophages and allows adaptation to different microenvironments (7–10).

Pathogens can be transmitted from mother to fetus either *via* infection of the placenta or fetal membranes (often viral), ascension of the reproductive tract (often bacterial) or by transmission during childbirth (viral, bacterial, fungal). Infection that occurs whilst the baby is *in utero* is termed congenital infection. Each year congenital anomalies lead to approximately 300,000 neonatal deaths during the first month of their lives (11). Globally, approximately 190,000 cases of congenital toxoplasmosis (12) and 1,000,000 incidences of congenital syphilis (13) are reported each year. Pathogens capable of causing congenital infection have historically been classified as members of the 'TORCH complex': **T**oxoplasma gondii, **O**thers (syphilis, Hepatitis B), **R**ubella, **C**ytomegalovirus (CMV) and **H**erpes simplex virus (HSV) (14). Other pathogens such as Zika virus (ZIKV), Human Immunodeficiency Virus (HIV), Varicella-zoster virus (VZV), *Listeria monocytogenes* and *Treponema pallidum* have subsequently been added to this group (15). Congenital infection can be associated with considerable morbidity and mortality, depending on the developmental stage of the fetus at the time of infection and the causative pathogen (16, 17). Consequences include neurodevelopmental delays, hearing loss (18), microencephaly and other major neurological abnormalities (19).

Placental infection with or without concomitant pathogen transmission to the fetal compartment can cause distinct histopathological findings in the placental tissue. Specifically, infectious processes in the placenta can be accompanied by villitis, a destructive inflammation of the chorionic villi associated with lower birth weight (20), or chorioamnionitis (CA), inflammation of the fetal membranes often associated with spontaneous preterm birth (21). Evidence accumulated since the start of the COVID-19 pandemic indicates that SARS-CoV-2 could be an example of a pathogen capable of infecting the placenta but not readily transferred transplacentally to the fetus in most cases (22, 23). SARS-CoV-2 protein and RNA have been detected in the syncytiotrophoblast cells and less so in other cell types in the placenta, while marked inflammation and lymphohistiocytic infiltration were noted as a consequence of placental infection (24–26). Whilst the presence of pronounced inflammation in this case can be damaging to the placental tissue, it could be essential for preventing further SARS-CoV-2 spread and subsequent *in utero* infection, a scenario with a worse potential outcome. Several published studies of placental SARS-CoV-2 infection are lacking in their methodology and terminology; the importance of proper sampling and techniques for accurate definition of placental SARS-CoV-2 infection was recently published (27).

Given the significant medical, societal and economic impacts of placental and fetal infection in pregnancy (28, 29), and the easy accessibility to these tissue macrophages at the end of pregnancy, it is surprising that we do not better understand the roles that Hofbauer cells play in infective processes. This information can help in the establishment of new preventive strategies and therapeutic interventions to protect individuals at a very vulnerable stage of the life course. There are several excellent previous reviews of HBC biology and their role in normal and pathological pregnancy (10, 28, 29). This scoping review follows systematic review methodology to synthesize the literature specifically regarding the role of HBCs in infection during pregnancy.

METHODS

Search Strategy

Studies without any publication year limit were retrieved from PubMed and Scopus on 20th May 2021 using a combination of key words designed to capture all articles that have investigated HBCs and infection. The keywords were selected to be in the title/abstract for PubMed and title/abstract/keywords for Scopus search to identify results focused on the main research question. The search was as follows: (hofbauer* OR "hofbauer cells" OR "hofbauer cell" OR "placental macrophage" OR "placental macrophages") AND [infect* OR virus OR viral OR bacteri* OR parasite* OR pathogen* OR lps OR "poly (i:c)" OR toxoplasm* OR microb* OR HIV)]. Additional keywords were tested without identifying any additional studies, and therefore were excluded from the final search (**Supplementary Material - Table 1**).

Inclusion and Exclusion Criteria

Only studies that used human material from infected patients and investigated HBCs responses were included. Studies that investigated HBCs (isolated from human placenta) in combination with pathogens or pathogen-associated molecular patterns (PAMPs) were also included. Excluded criteria included (a) usage of animal models or cell lines without the use of any primary human placental macrophages (b) reviews and book chapters (c) studies not written in English. Duplicates found during title/abstract screening or/and full-text screening and studies without full text available were also excluded (**Supplementary Material - Table 2**).

Study Screening

For article screening and Preferred Reporting Items for Systematic Reviews and Meta-Analyses (PRISMA) flow diagram creation (**Figure 1**), the Covidence systematic review platform was used. The articles were screened independently by two reviewers (G. F. and P. P.) for eligibility. A third reviewer (B. H.) resolved any conflicts that arose during the screening. For the purposes of this review the risk of bias for each study was not evaluated since no cohort studies nor randomized control trials were present.

Data Extraction and Analysis

To facilitate the interpretation of the final list of results, the following data were extracted from the articles: article identification (title, authors, journal and publication year), study design (case-control, *in vitro*), health status of the samples (normal pregnancy, villitis, CA and preeclampsia), mode of sample collection (birth, termination, miscarriage and stillbirth), gestational age (first, second or third trimester), sample type (placental tissue, explants and isolated HBCs), method of HBC isolation (digestion and centrifugation, positive selection with anti-CD14 immunobeads, negative selection using anti-CD10 and anti-epidermal growth factor receptor (EGFR) immunobeads or other), sample treatment (co-culture, *in vitro* exposure to pathogen or PAMPs), methods to identify infection, placental infection prevalence, fetal infection, HBC infection, HBC hyperplasia, gene transcription and protein expression or secretion and the main findings are summarized in tables across results section.

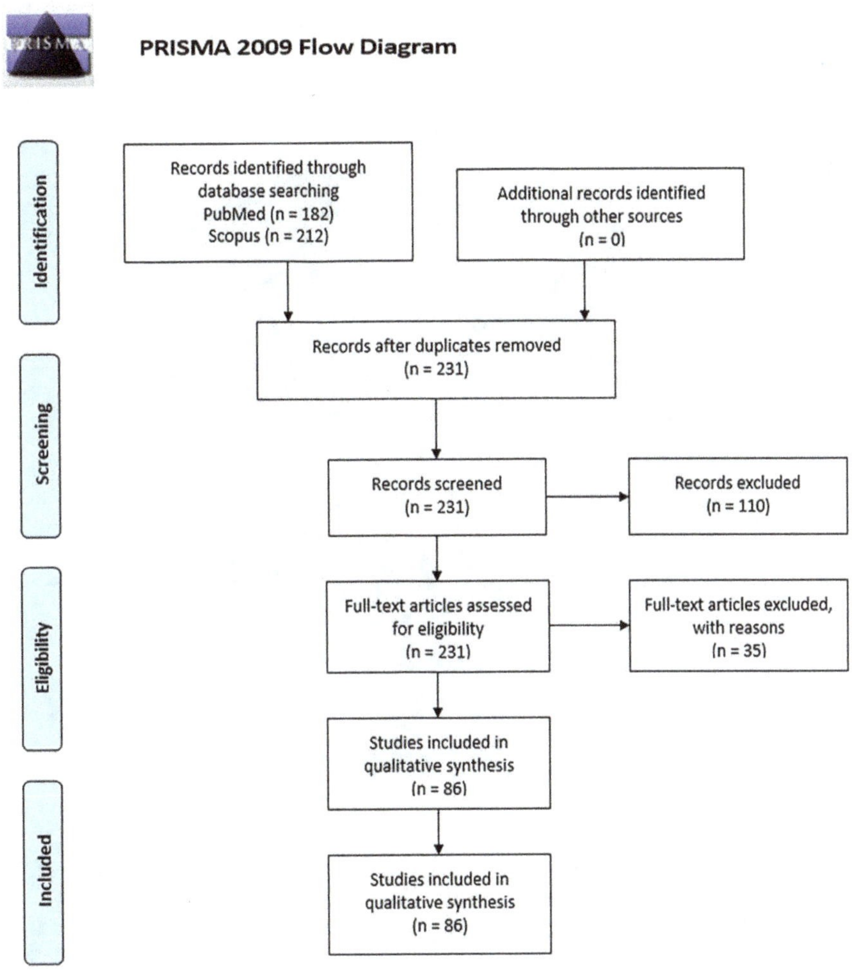

FIGURE 1 | PRISMA 2009 flow diagram of literature search and records selection.

RESULTS

Studies Identified

From a total of 231 studies initially screened, 86 were included (**Figure 1**). Of these, 37 were *in vitro* studies using isolated HBCs or explants, 47 were observational studies using placental tissue, which included case-control studies and case reports and 2 studied both. The results were divided into 4 main groups based on the type of infection; HBCs in: 1) viral infection (n=67) including infections by HIV (n=26), ZIKV (n=17), CMV (n=8) and others; 2) bacterial infection (n=7); 3) parasitic infection, which were all studies of *Plasmodium falciparum* (n=4); or 4) response to Pathogen-Associated Molecular Patterns (PAMPs) (n=13). An overview of the study of HBCs and infection is shown in **Figure 2**.

HBCs in Viral Infection

HIV-1 Observational Studies

HIV-1 was the most investigated pathogen in observational studies (n=6/9) (30–35). Placentas were obtained from mothers after pregnancy termination, pregnancy loss or delivery (**Table 1**). HIV-1 infection of the placenta was detected in 27% to 100% of samples. Infection of HBCs was assessed through observation of viral protein (n=5), reporting 30% - 100% of samples with infected HBCs and through detection of viral nucleic acid (n=4), reporting infected HBCs in 16% to 100% patients (**Table 1**). The proportion of infected HBCs in each placenta was missing from most studies; however, Lewis et al. (30) reported that one in five HBCs were positive for HIV-1 and Backé et al. (33) reported the presence of a few positive HBCs.

Four studies examined HBC infection and transplacental transmission (30, 33, 34, 37). HIV-1 was detected in embryonic precursor blood cells in three first trimester fetuses with infected HBCs, underlying a possible role of HBCs in fetal infection during early gestation (30). Backé et al. (33) reported 12 asymptomatic offspring from 13 HIV-1 antigen-positive placentas and one infected offspring from four HIV-1-positive placentas. Sheikh et al. (34) reported three cases of HIV-1 *in utero* transmission in women with syphilis, one of them also having chorioamnionitis, and observed that HBC infection indicated a possible involvement of HBCs in offspring infection during late pregnancy. Cases of chorioamnionitis were reported in three studies (34, 35, 37); however, only the study of Bhoopat et al. (35) investigated the contribution of

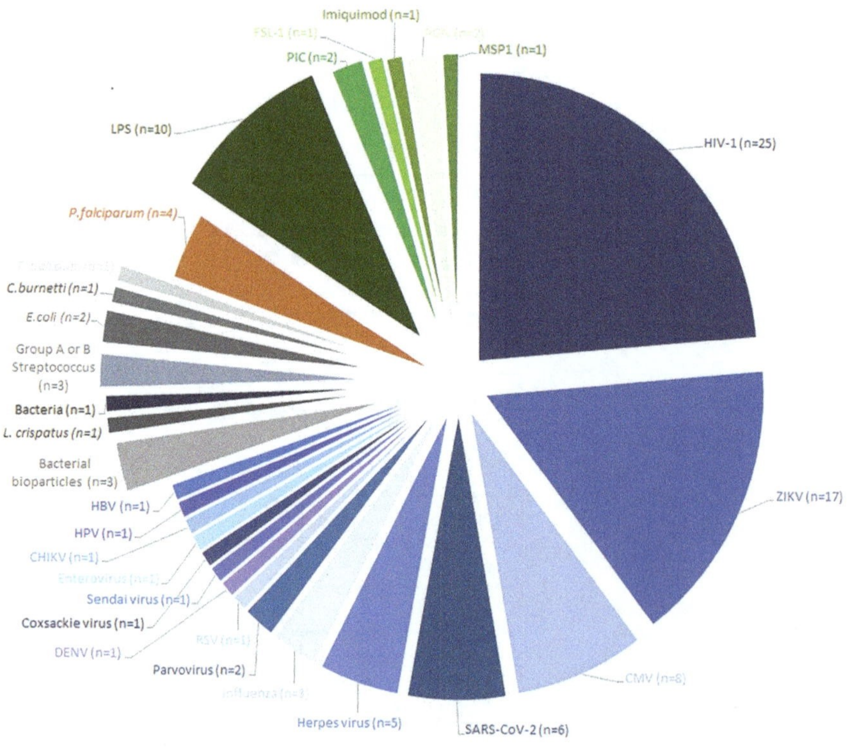

FIGURE 2 | Overview of all studies that have investigated pathogen infection or pathogen responses in Hofbauer cells. All identified studies published before 20th May 2021 were categorized by pathogen, or Pathogen-Associated Molecular Pattern (PAMP) studied. Viral infections are represented in blue, bacterial infections in grey, parasitic infections in orange and PAMP treatments in green. The number of articles that investigated each pathogen or PAMP is indicated in parentheses. HIV Human Immunodeficiency Virus, ZIKV Zika virus, CMV Cytomegalovirus, RSV Respiratory syncytial virus, DENV Dengue virus, CHIKV Chikungunya virus, HPV Human papillomavirus, HBV Hepatitis B virus, L. crispatus Lactobacillus crispatus, E.coli Escherichia coli, T.pallidum Treponema pallidum, C.burnetti Coxiella burnetii, P.falciparum Plasmodium falciparum, LPS lipopolysaccharide, PIC Polyinosinic:polycytidylic acid, FSL-1 Pam2CGDPKHPKSF-synthetic lipopeptide, PGN Peptidoglycan, MSP1 Merozoite surface protein.

TABLE 1 | Hofbauer cells in observational studies of viral infection.

Virus	Samples studied by trimester (outcome)				HBC infection diagnosis method	Key outcome(s) in HBCs		Reference
	1st	2nd	3rd <37w	3rd ≥37w		HBC infection detected (no.)	HBC hyperplasia (%)	
HIV-1	3 (TOP)	–	–	–	Protein & RNA	+ (3/3 protein) & + (2/3 nucleic acid)	NR	Lewis et al. (30)
	23 (TOP) gestational age between 6-39w & 11 term (LB)				Protein	+ (10/23 & 5/11)	NR	Backé et al. (31)
	9 gestational age NR (NR)				Protein	+ (4/9)	NR	Martin et al. (32)
	48 gestational age NR (LB)				Protein & RNA	+ (NR)	NR	Backé et al. (33)
	–	–	–	23 (LB)	NR	NR	NR	Behbahani et al. (36)
	–	–	2 (LB)	1 (LB)	RNA	+ (3/3)	NR	Sheikh et al. (34)
	24; 8-20w (TOP)		–	–	Protein & RNA	+ (8/24 protein) & + (4/24 nucleic acid)	NR	Bhoopat et al. (35)
	–	–	–	40 (LB)	NR	NR	NR	Pillay et al. (37)
	–	–	–	99 (LB)	NR	NR	NR	Martinez et al. (38)
ZIKV	1 (PL)	–	–	2 (LB)	Protein	+ (1/1)	+ (100%)	de Noronha et al. (39)
	–	1 (TOP)	–	–	RNA	+ (1/1)	+ (100%)	Rosenberg et al. (40)
	–	1 (TOP)	1 (PL)	–	RNA	+ (1/1)	+ (100%)	Schwartz, (41)
	1 (PL)	–	3 (LB)	19 (LB) & 1 (PL)	Protein	+ (NR)	+ (35%)	de Noronha et al. (42)
		1 (PL)	–	–	Protein	+ (1/1)	+ (100%)	Rabelo et al. (43)
	–	3 (TOP)	–	–	NR	NR	+ (100%)	Beaufrère et al. (44)
	–	–	–	3 (LB)	Protein	+ (3/3)	- (0%)	Lum et al. (45)
	–	–	–	1 (LB)	NR	NR	+ (100%)	Santos et al. (46)
	–	–	4 (LB)	–	NR	NR	+ (100%)	Miranda et al. (47)
CMV	–	1 (PL)	1 (PL) & 3 (LB)	1 (PL)	Protein	–	NR	Mühlemann et al. (48)
	–	3 (PL)	1 (LB & neonatal death)	–	Protein	–	+ (100%)	Schwartz et al. (49)
	–	1 (PL)	4 (3 LB & 1 PL)	1 (PL)	Protein	–	NR	Mühlemann et al. (50)
	3 gestational age NR (NR)				DNA	+ (NR)	+ (100%)	Euscher et al. (51)
	–	–	4 between 28-41w (PL or/and LB & neonatal death)		DNA	+ (NR)	NR	Satosar et al. (52)
Coxsackie virus	–	6 cases gestational age 25-43w (LB)			Protein + RNA	+ (NR) & + (NR)	+ (NR)	Euscher et al. (51)
HSV	1 case of infection gestational age NR (NR)				DNA	+ (1/1)	- (0%)	Euscher et al. (51)
	–	–	2 cases between 28-41w (PL or/ and LB)		DNA	+ (NR)	NR	Satosar et al. (52)
Enterovirus	–	–	23 cases between 28-41w (PL or/and LB & neonatal death)		Protein & RNA	+ (12/23) & + (NR)	NR	Satosar et al. (52)
Parvovirus	–	–	2 cases between 28-41w (PL or/ and LB & neonatal death)		DNA	- (NR)	NR	Satosar et al. (52)
	1 gestational age NR (PL)				DNA	- (1/1)	+ (100%)	Euscher et al. (51)
H5N1	–	1 (PL)	–	–	NR	NR	NR	Yao et al. (53)
	–	1 (PL)	–	–	Protein & RNA	+ (1/1)	NR	Gu et al. (54)
HBV	–	–	–	28 (LB)	NR	NR	NR	Liu et al. (55)
HPV	100 (54 TOP + 46 PL)		68 (LB)	103 (LB)	DNA	+ (1/1)	NR	Ambühl et al. (56)
DENV	–	–	1 (PL)	–	Protein	+ (1/1)	+ (100%)	Nunes et al. (57)

(Continued)

TABLE 1 | Continued

Virus	Samples studied by trimester (outcome)				HBC infection diagnosis method	Key outcome(s) in HBCs		Reference
	1st	2nd	3rd <37w	3rd ≥37w		HBC infection detected (no.)	HBC hyperplasia (%)	
Chikungunya virus	4 (PL)		–	–	Protein	+ (3/4)	NR	Salomão et al. (58)
SARS-CoV-2	–	–	–	1 (LB)	Protein & RNA	+ (1/1)	+ (100%)	Facchetti et al. (26)
	–	1 (PL)	8 (LB)	10 (LB)	NR	NR	+ (5.5%)	Hecht et al. (25)
	–	–	–	1 (LB)	Protein & RNA	- (1/1)	+ (100%)	Morotti et al. (59)
	–	1 (LB)	–	4 (LB)	Protein & RNA	+ (5/5)	NR	Verma et al. (60)
	–	–	1 (LB)	7(LB)	Protein & RNA	- (8/8)	- (100%)	Gao et al. (61)

TOP, Termination of pregnancy; LB, Live birth; NR, Not reported; PL, Pregnancy loss (stillbirth/miscarriage); HIV-1, Human immunodeficiency virus 1; ZIKV, Zika virus; CMV, Cytomegalovirus; HSV, Herpes simplex virus; H5N1, Influenza virus A; subtype H5N1; HBV, Hepatitis B virus; HPV, human papilloma virus; DENV, Dengue virus; SARS-CoV-2, Severe acute respiratory syndrome coronavirus 2.

chorioamnionitis in vertical transmission of HIV-1. In this study, 24 first and second trimester therapeutic abortions from HIV-1 seropositive women were examined and placental histological analysis revealed five cases of chorioamnionitis (35). Of these five cases, four were associated with fetal viral transmission, suggesting a link between HBC infection, placental inflammation and HIV-1 in vertical transmission during early pregnancy.

The three remaining observational studies of HIV in HBCs were focused on proteins associated with the immune response or viral entry. One study investigated the placental expression of HIV-1 co-receptors, C-C chemokine receptor type 5 (CCR5) and C-X-C chemokine receptor type 4 (CXCR4) in 16 non-transmitting and 7 transmitting HIV-1 women (36). They reported expression of both co-receptors in HBCs but not in trophoblast cells and identified that placental CCR5:CXCR4 ratio was significantly higher in transmitting women; however, they did not further investigate whether the alteration was due to upregulation or downregulation of co-receptors in HBCs. Also, higher expression levels of DC-SIGN and DC-SIGNR, lectins that recognize viral PAMPs, were reported in placentas from 25 women with HIV-1 and 15 women with HIV-1 and CA compared to HIV-negative women, and HBCs were reported to express both proteins (37). No difference in the expression of the natural killer inhibitory receptor ligand, HLA-E, was documented in placental tissue from 99 HIV-infected mothers compared to uninfected group in another study (38). Though HLA-E was expressed in HBCs, differences between HIV-positive and negative women were not examined.

HIV-1 *In Vitro* Studies

Fifteen studies examined the permissiveness of HBCs to HIV-1 using *in vitro* challenge (**Table 2**). Of these, infection was reported through detection of HIV-1 nucleic acid (34, 62, 63, 67, 68, 73, 75, 77) or protein (62, 65, 66, 70, 73, 76). Productive infection was also measured by extracellular protein (62–66, 68, 69, 71, 75, 77), extracellular reverse transcriptase activity (62), infectious virions in supernatant (62, 65) or/and microscopy (75, 76). Of the 17 studies, eight investigated susceptibility to HIV-1 infection in HBCs compared to monocytes or monocyte-derived macrophages (MDMs) through p24 detection in supernatants (n=8) or/and viral nucleic acid (n=5) (62, 63, 69, 73, 75). These studies reported HIV-1 replication in HBCs but reduced ability to replicate the virus compared to fetal MDMs, adult blood and cord MDMs. Even upon GM-CSF treatment, HBCs produced fewer virions compared to fetal MDMs (62) and adult MDMs (64). The distinct difference in viral replication was not due to increased cell death, cytopathic effects (62, 64, 68, 75) or inefficient particle assembly/release (75), but due to restriction at the transcriptional level (73).

Permissiveness of HBCs depends on the HIV-1 strain utilized (63, 65, 68, 94). For example, Fear et al. (68) highlighted differences in viral replication among seven clinical and two laboratory-adapted strains, such as the macrophage-tropic HIV-Bal, and showed that only the laboratory-adapted strains and not the clinical isolates were able to replicate in HBCs.

Co-culture experiments of HBCs with different cell types *in vitro* have shown the importance of cell-cell interactions and cytokines in viral replication and hence a potential role of HBCs in viral dissemination. Viral replication in HIV-1-infected HBCs was enhanced after co-culture with CEM, a highly permissive T-cell line (62). Co-culture of infected syncytiotrophoblasts with non-infected HBCs increased HIV-1 gene expression in the former cells and secretion of IL6 and TNF-a by HBCs (70, 75).

Furthermore, intrinsic HBC factors could increase the risk of vertical HIV-1 transmission. The potential role of DC-SIGN in intrauterine transmission was discussed in the study of Boily-Larouche et al. (74), who detected the expression of DC-SIGN on HBCs derived from placentas of HIV-1-positive and -negative mothers and found that specific promoter variants enhanced the risk of vertical transmission. Reduced DC-SIGN expression was observed after promoter variant induction in HBCs from placentas of HIV-1-negative mothers and not those from HIV-1-exposed mothers (74). Decreased HIV-1 replication was observed when isolated HBCs from term placentas were infected with HIV-1 following small interfering ribonucleic acid (siRNA) knockdown of the proteinase inhibitor Cystatin B (CSTB). The levels of CSTB were lower in HBCs compared to MDMs isolated from seronegative donors, while viral protein was more abundant in MDMs (71). CSTB interacts with signal transducer and activator of transcription (STAT)-1 in

TABLE 2 | Hofbauer cells in *in vitro* studies of viral infection.

Virus	Samples studied by trimester (outcome)				Model(s) of infection	Immuno-purification of HBCs	Diagnosis of HBC infection/ viral production (no.)	Key outcome(s) in HBCs	Reference
	1st	2nd	3rd <37w	3rd ≥37w					
HIV-1	3 (NR)		3 (NR)		Cells & co-culture	No	RT activity, antigen release, virion release, PCR-Southern & IF	Productive HIV-1 infection	Mano and Chermann (62)
	–	–	–	NR (LB)	Cells	No	ISH & antigen release	Productive HIV-1 infection. HIV-1 clinical isolates exhibit different tropism	Kesson et al. (63)
		NR			Cells	No	Antigen release	Infection peak at 3-7 days with no subsequent rise up to 60 days. HIV-1 replication in HBCs not affected by PHA-PBMCs nor treatment with GM-CSF or TNF-α	Kesson et al. (64)
	–	–	–	5 (LB)	Cells	No	Antigen release, infectious virions in supernatant & IF	Different HIV-1 replication rates between HIV-1 strains and HBC donors	McGann et al. (65)
	–	–	–	NR (LB)	Cells	No	IF & antigen release	HBC displayed a similar increase in p24 as adult and cord blood monocytes in response to HIV-1$_{baL}$ monocyte-tropic strain	Meléndez-Guerrero et al. (66)
	–	–	–	NR (LB)	Cells	No	PCR	Zidovudine and progesterone suppress HIV-1 replication in HBCs	Lee et al. (67)
	–	–	–	NR (LB)	Cells	No	PCR & antigen release	Varying susceptibility to different HIV-1 strains and isolates	Fear et al. (68)
	–	–	–	NR (LB)	Cells	No	Antigen release	Altered cytokine secretion	Plaud-Valentin et al. (69)
	–	–	–	6 (LB)	Explants	No	IS-PCR	Infection of HBCs in placental explants	Sheikh et al. (34)
	–	–	–	5 (LB)	Cells & co-culture	No	IF	Infected syncytiotrophoblast transmits the virus to HBCs which release cytokines that induce HIV-1 replication	Bácsi et al. (70)
	–	–	–	4 (LB)	Cells	No	Antigen release	Different HIV-1 replication and viral protein abundance in HBCs and MDMs	Luciano-Montalvo et al. (71)
	–	–	–	4 (LB)	Cells	No	NR	The levels of STAT-1-tyr phosphorylation are lower in HIV-1 infected HBCs	Luciano-Montalvo and Meléndez (72)
	–	–	–	3 (LB)	Cells	No	PCR & Western blot	Lower HIV-1 replication in HBCs compared to MDMs due to restricted transcription	García-Crespo et al. (73)
	–	–	–	9 (LB)	Cells	No	NR	DC-SIGN promoter variants in HBCs influence HIV-1 transmission from mother to child	Boily-Larouche et al. (74)
	–	–	–	40 (LB)	Cells & co-culture	CD14^{pos}	Antigen release, PCR & electron microscopy	HBCs display reduced replication and ability to transmit HIV-1$_{baL}$ to PBMCs compared to MDMs; stimulation of HBCs with IL-10, TGF-β, IFN-γ reduces infection in HBCs	Johnson and Chakraborty (75)
	–	–	–	20 (LB)	Cells	CD14^{pos}	IF & electron microscopy	HIV-1 assembles in VCCs accessible to neutralizing antibodies which reduce viral replication *via* FcγRI	Johnson et al. (76)
	–	–	–	10 (LB)	Cells	CD14^{pos}	Antigen release & PCR	CMV infected HBCs enhance HIV-1 replication in HBCs	Johnson et al. (77)
ZIKV	26 (TOP)	–	–	–	Cells & explants	CD14^{pos}	RNA (6) & antigen (4)	ZIKV infects HBCs and damages the placenta architecture	El Costa et al. (78)
	–	–	–	3 (LB)	Cells & explants	CD10^{neg}/ EGFR^{neg}	RNA (3) & antigen (3)	ZIKV infects HBCs *in vitro*	Jurado et al. (79)
	4 (TOP)	–	–	–	Explants	N/A	Antigen (4)	ZIKV infects HBCs *in vitro* and expresses important viral entry cofactors	Tabata et al. (80)
	–	–	–	5 (LB)	Cells	CD14^{pos}	RNA, antigen & plaque assay (5)	ZIKV can replicate in HBCs with infection rate and antiviral response varying among donors	Quicke et al. (81)

(Continued)

TABLE 2 | Continued

Virus	Samples studied by trimester (outcome)				Model(s) of infection	Immuno-purification of HBCs	Diagnosis of HBC infection/ viral production (no.)	Key outcome(s) in HBCs	Reference
	1st	2nd	3rd <37w	3rd ≥37w					
	7 (TOP)	–	–	–	Explants	N/A	Antigen (6)	HBC infection rate varies among strains and donors	Tabata et al. (82)
	–	–	–	12 (LB)	Cells	CD14^{pos}	RNA & antigen	JAK-STAT signalling influences the ability of HBCs to produce mature virions	Gavegnano et al. (83)
	–	4 (TOP)	–	–	Cells & explants	CD14^{pos}	RNA, antigen & plaque assay (3)	Pre-existing DENV antibodies enhance the HBC infection with ZIKV	Zimmerman et al. (84)
	3 (NR)	–	–	–	Explants	N/A	Antigen	ZIKV NS1 induced shedding of HA and HS, altered expression of CD44 and LYVE-1, and increased placental explant permeability	Puerta-Guardo et al. (85)
CMV	–	–	–	5 (LB)	Cells & co-culture	No	Antigen	IL-8 and TGF-1β released upon HBC-syncytiotrophoblast contact stimulates CMV replication in the STB	Bácsi et al. (86)
	–	–	–	NR (LB)	Cells	CD14^{pos}	Antigen	Poxvirus-based vaccine-induced neutralizing antibodies prevent CMV infection of HBCs	Wussow et al. (87)
	–	–	–	10 (LB)	Cells & co-culture	CD14^{pos}	GFP positive cells	CMV induces TNF-α and IL-6 secretion and supresses STAT2 phosphorylation to supress type I interferon response	Johnson et al. (77)
HSV-2	6 (LB)				Cells	No	IF & viral titre measurement	HBCs are not very permissive to HSV and do not support productive replication	Plaeger-Marshall et al. (88)
HSV-2	Number and gestational age NR (LB)				Cells	No	IF, viral titration & microscopy (NR)	HBCs prevent HSV-2 and echovirus-type 19 infection	Oliveira et al. (89)
Echovirus-type 19									
Sendai virus	–	–	36 – 42w (LB)		Cells	No	Quantify viral concentration in culture media	Sendai virus induces HBC IFN-β secretion	Toth et al. (90)
RSV	–	–	–	5 (LB)	Cells	CD10^{neg}/ EGFR^{neg}	IF, PCR & Western blot (5)	HBCs are permissive to RSV infection and can transfer the virus to neighbouring cells	Bokun et al. (91)
γ-herpesvirus-(MHV-68)	–	–	–	7 (LB)	Cells & co-culture	CD10^{neg}/ EGFR^{neg}	PCR	Infected HBCs secrete IL-1β which activates HUVECs to generate a pro-neutrophilic response	Hendrix et al. (92)
SARS-CoV-2	–	–	–	10 (LB)	Cells	CD10^{neg}/ EGFR^{neg}	IF	No HBC infection with SARS-CoV-2	Lu-Culligan et al. (93)

HIV-1, Human immunodeficiency virus 1; NR, Not reported; RT, Reverse transcriptase; LB, Live birth; PCR, Polymerase chain reaction; IF, Immunofluorescence; ISH, In situ hybridization; PHA-PBMCs, Phytohemagglutinin stimulated peripheral blood cells; GM-CSF, Granulocyte-macrophage colony-stimulating factor; TNF, Tumor necrosis factor; IS-PCR, In situ PCR; MDMs, Monocyte-derived macrophages; DC-SIGN, Dendritic Cell-Specific Intercellular adhesion molecule-3-Grabbing Non-integrin; IL, Interleukin; TGF, Transforming growth factor; IFN, Interferon; VCCs, Virus containing compartments; FcγRI, Fc-gamma receptor 1; CMV, Cytomegalovirus; ZIKV, Zika virus; TOP, Termination of pregnancy; STB, Syncytiotrophoblast; GFP, Green fluorescent protein; HSV(-2), Herpes simplex virus (2); RSV, Respiratory syncytial virus; HUVECs, Human umbilical vein endothelial cells; SARS-CoV-2, sever acute respiratory syndrome coronavirus 2.

both HBCs and MDMs, with the levels of STAT-1 tyrosine phosphorylation being higher in HBCs compared to MDMs and in uninfected HBCs compared to infected. Protein analysis of HBCs indicated an altered pattern of activation and signal transduction upon HIV-1 infection. Notably, the levels of STAT-1 serine phosphorylation didn't alter upon infection and the different levels of phosphorylation suggest distinct regulation pathways (72). In addition, using primary HBCs from 10 term pregnancies, an increased susceptibility for HIV-1 and increased HIV-1 replication within HBCs was reported following CMV infection *in vitro* (77).

Finally, despite the ability of HBCs to replicate HIV-1, several factors can interrupt viral dissemination. Exogenous administration of IL-10 and TGF-β limited viral replication within HBCs while TNF-α pre-treatment significantly increased it (75). However, HBC co-culture with TNF-α or phytohemagglutinin (PHA)-stimulated peripheral blood mononuclear cells (PBMCs), which promotes the activation of T-cells, did not affect viral replication in HBCs (64). Of particular note, suppression of viral replication in HBCs was observed when treated with progesterone and zidovudine (67). HBCs were permissive to HIV-1 and formed virus-containing compartments (VCCs) enriched in tetraspanins, endosomal and lysosomal markers, and VCCs were accessible to neutralizing antibodies that could limit viral replication in HBCs through FcγRI (76).

ZIKV Observational Studies

In 2015-16, there was a Zika virus (ZIKV) epidemic, mainly affecting countries in South and Central America, as well as South East Asia, the Pacific Islands and parts of North America (95).

During this epidemic, it was discovered that ZIKV can be transmitted vertically to the fetus, causing severe developmental complications including microcephaly (96, 97). This led to a number of studies that sought to study ZIKV infection in the placenta. Of these, nine studies investigated HBC infection and/or hyperplasia (increased HBC numbers) (**Table 1**) (39–47).

In situ analyses of placental tissue from ZIKV-infected pregnant women revealed ZIKV placental infection in 35% - 100% of samples (39–47) and HBC hyperplasia in all, except for one case-control study (45). In HBCs, ZIKV infection was assessed through detection of ZIKV protein (39, 42, 43, 45) or ZIKV ribonucleic acid (RNA) (40, 41) and both ZIKV RNA and protein were found in HBCs. No study investigated the presence of both ZIKV RNA and protein in HBCs nor reported the proportion of infected HBCs.

A range of gestational ages was studied, demonstrating the infection of HBCs in the first, second and third trimester. Most studies were small ($n \leq 3$) (39–41, 43–46), but one larger study of 20 term placenta samples (42) suggested that ZIKV probably infects HBCs by term in all cases of maternal infection. A few studies reported the potential infection timepoint at which maternal infection occurred: first (39, 40, 42, 44–46), second (40, 42, 45) and third (39, 42, 45) pregnancy trimester.

Some studies reported fetal outcomes such as fetal infection or congenital malformations and HBC infection or/and hyperplasia (41, 43–47). Santos et al. (46) reported a case of placental inflammation, HBC hyperplasia and fetal infection. HBC hyperplasia in ZIKV-infected pregnancies has been observed in the presence (41) and absence (44) of placental inflammation and was correlated with fetal infection in both cases. Fetal defects were reported in cases with HBC hyperplasia (44), whereas no congenital anomalies were observed in the absence of HBC hyperplasia (45); a link between HBC hyperplasia and fetal defects could be suggested but needs further investigation. Increased numbers of HBCs expressing vascular permeability markers (vascular endothelial growth factor (VEGF)-2 and (C-C motif) ligands (CCL5) and pro-inflammatory cytokines (TNF-α and IFN-γ) were observed in immunohistochemistry experiments of a fetus with documented HBC infection and hyperplasia (43), suggesting a role of HBCs in the placental pro-inflammatory response, vascular permeability and a possible role of HBCs in transplacental transmission. Notably, fetal samples were not available for some studies and information on HBC infection/hyperplasia or fetal infection was often lacking.

ZIKV *In Vitro* Studies

Several groups have investigated ZIKV infection of HBCs *in vitro*, either by infecting isolated HBCs or placental explants (78–85) (**Table 2**). When isolated HBCs were infected *in vitro* with ZIKV, infection was identified through detection of viral protein (78–85) or/and viral RNA in HBCs (78, 79, 81, 83, 84), across all trimesters of pregnancy (78, 81, 84) (**Table 2**). However, different viral replication rates were observed among HBCs from different donors (81). An average percentage of 5% of isolated HBCs were infected (78, 81) and an average range of 10-37% in placental explants was documented (79, 82, 84). In addition, distinct infection rates were reported among different ZIKV strains in placental explants (82).

Some studies investigated the ability of ZIKV-infected HBCs and explants to produce mature virions capable of infecting other cells and thus contribute to vertical transmission. Production of virions by infected explants was observed in plaque assay experiments (82). HBCs were reported to replicate ZIKV that could infect epithelial Vero cells *in vitro* (79), and Janus kinase (JAK)-STAT signaling was important for the production of mature virions (83). Exposure of placental explants to ZIKV or/and flavivirus non-structural protein 1 (NS1) increased placental permeability, measured by dextran fluorescence permeability assay (85), suggesting a mechanism by which HBC-produced virions could potentially cross the placenta and transmit to the fetus.

HBCs express surface receptors that are important for ZIKV dissemination (80). The study of Tabata et al. (80) reported the expression of important surface viral entry cofactors T-cell immunoglobulin and mucin domain 1 (TIM1) and AXL tyrosine kinase receptors on HBCs. Co-cultivation of placental explants with duramycin, which prevents TIM1 receptor binding, reduced the viral load. However, changes in the expression of TIM1 or AXL in HBCs between infected and uninfected explants were not investigated (80).

Interestingly, a link between previously obtained immunity and ZIKV infection was recently described (84). The study of Zimmerman et al. (84) showed that pre-existing Dengue virus (DENV) antibodies enhanced ZIKV infection of HBCs *in vitro*, and the ZIKV-DENV complexes suppressed the production of antiviral effector proteins and retinoic acid-inducible gene-I-(RIG-I) like receptors, while treatment with IFN-β or blocking of FcRn binding reduced the viral replication rate (84). Regarding the presence of DENV cross-reactive antibodies *in vivo*, a few observational studies evaluated the presence of serum cross-reactive DENV antibodies with ZIKV antibodies but not with ZIKV (42, 43), while other studies reported previous DENV infection but did not check for the existence of cross-reactive antibodies (39).

ZIKV infection of HBCs and explants has been shown to alter HBC transcriptional and protein profiles (81, 83, 85). Infection of HBCs *in vitro* increased the transcription rate of several antiviral genes (IFNA, IFNB, IFIH1, DDX58, DHX58, IFIT1.2.3, OAS1, RSAD2), modestly upregulated surface proteins important for T-cell interactions (CD80, CD86 and MHC II) and elevated the secretion of cytokines/chemokines (IFN-α, IL-6, CCL2) and C-X-C motif chemokine ligand-10 (CXCL-10) (81). Of particular note, HBC activation was enhanced upon increased viral replication and, despite increased IFN-β mRNA, no IFN-β secretion was observed (81). Also, an increase in numbers of HBCs expressing DC-SIGN and HLA-DR proteins was reported (83). Downregulation of LYVE-1 - which regulates hyaluronic acid (HA) metabolism and induces HA-dependent leukocyte rolling - was observed (85). That decrease may imply an insufficient role of HBCs in maintaining vascular integrity of chorionic villi during infection and may therefore contribute to the alteration of placental permeability, as observed *in vitro* (85) and *in vivo* (43).

CMV Observational Studies

One of the most common transplacental infections in pregnancy, CMV, was examined in five observational studies (48–52) (**Table 1**). Absence of HBC infection was reported following immunohistochemistry analysis of placental tissue from CMV-infected women in two studies (48–50), while presence of viral DNA was observed (51, 52), highlighting differences in outcomes depending on the method used. Similarly to ZIKV infection studies, no study investigated the presence of both viral DNA and protein nor the percentage of infected HBCs. In addition, the trimester at which maternal infection or re-activation of infection occurred was not reported in any of the studies.

HBC hyperplasia was examined in two studies (49, 51), which found HBC hyperplasia in 100% of cases (n=7; **Table 1**) in the presence or absence of HBC infection. Euscher et al. (51) reported infection and hyperplasia of HBCs in three out of ten cases of unknown gestational ages. In contrast, Schwartz et al. (49) observed HBC hyperplasia in all four placentas from different gestational ages in absence of HBC infection.

Severe fetal or new-born outcomes were reported in the presence and absence of HBC infection (48–52). All examined cases of chorionic villitis with confirmed placental CMV infection (3 cases) exhibited fetal infection in the absence of HBC infection (48, 50). Also, three cases of lymphocytic villitis were examined and placental CMV inclusions were observed in two mothers and one reported fetal infection without identified viral positive HBCs (49). Euscher et al. (51) examined 10 cases of newborns with respiratory and neurological abnormalities and identified viral DNA in HBCs of 3 newborns, while Satosar et al. (52) examined 77 cases of Newborn mortality and morbidity and found four cases of CMV placental infection with CMV-positive HBCs.

CMV *In Vitro* Studies

Studies that have investigated HBC CMV infection and viral dissemination *in vitro* are shown in **Table 2**. Co-culture of isolated HBCs with CMV-infected syncytiotrophoblasts resulted in viral transmission to HBCs and induction of IL-8 and TGF-1β, whilst absence of the virus in co-culture experiments was reported after antibody-mediated blocking of cytokines, suggesting a role of those cytokines in viral gene expression that influences viral transmission (86). Wussow et al. (87) focused on the development of a vaccine based on modified vaccinia Ankara with CMV proteins and demonstrated that serum neutralizing antibodies against gH/gL were capable of preventing infection of HBCs, suggesting that pre-existing CMV antibodies could be captured by Fc receptors on HBCs and prevent viral spread by HBC-mediated neutralization.

Finally, changes in HBC immunophenotype during CMV infection were identified *in vitro* (77). Infection of HBCs with CMV led to upregulation of co-stimulatory (CD80) and immunoregulatory [programmed death-ligand 1 (PDL-1)] proteins and CCR5 co-receptor expression, increased the release of proinflammatory cytokines (TNF-α, IL-6), type I IFNs (IFN-α, IFN-β) and decreased the secretion of the IL-10 immunoregulatory protein (77). In addition, several antiviral gene transcripts were increased in HBCs, including type I IFNs and proteins contributing to type I IFN signaling (STAT-1, melanoma differentiation-associated protein-5 (MDA-5), RIG-I), while under-expression of STAT-2 and phosphorylated STAT-2 suggested involvement of CMV in transcription-translation interruption in HBCs (77).

Other Viruses

Apart from the effort to understand HBC response to HIV-1, ZIKV and CMV infection, the response of HBCs to other viral infections has been less extensively studied. Other viral infections examined included different types of herpes viruses (51, 52, 88, 89, 92), influenza (53, 54), parvovirus (51, 52), coxsackievirus (51), enterovirus (51), echovirus (89), Dengue virus (57), human papillomavirus (HPV) (56), hepatitis B (HBV) (55), respiratory syncytial virus (RSV) (91), Sendai virus (90), Chikungunya virus (58) and SARS-CoV-2 (25, 26, 59–61, 93).

Observational Studies of Other Viruses

Ten of thirteen observational studies investigated HBC infection by *in situ* detection of viral protein or/and viral DNA or RNA (**Table 1**). Both viral protein and RNA were detected in HBCs during coxsackievirus (51), enterovirus (52), H5N1 (54), and SARS-CoV-2 (26, 60) infection. Viral protein was also detected in HBCs following Dengue virus infection (57), viral RNA during Chikungunya virus infection (58), and viral DNA during herpes simplex virus types 1 and 2 (HSV) (51, 52) and HPV infection (56), while absence of parvovirus DNA (51, 52) and SARS-CoV-2 RNA and protein in HBCs (59, 61) was reported. Information regarding the timing of maternal infection during pregnancy was missing from all studies except the studies that investigated H5N1 infection, which occurred during the second pregnancy trimester and resulted in death (53, 54). The proportion of infected HBCs was only stated for coxsackievirus; reporting 10% positive cells for viral protein and 50% for viral RNA (51).

HBC hyperplasia was examined in eight observational studies. Coxsackievirus (51), parvovirus (51) and DENV infection (57) all induced HBC hyperplasia, whilst HBC hyperplasia was not seen during HSV infection (51). After maternal SARS-CoV-2 infection, no evidence of HBC hyperplasia was detected in one study (61), whilst three other studies identified HBC hyperplasia (25, 26, 59). For the other viral infections such as influenza, HBV, HPV and enterovirus, HBC hyperplasia was not examined.

Five of the observational studies looked at the presence of surface proteins including immunoglobulins on HBCs (25, 26, 53, 55, 60). HBCs express the human influenza receptor but not the avian receptor, with similar distribution between the infected and the control group, implying that distinct receptors or co-receptors are responsible for H5N1 entry in HBCs (53). Hepatitis B immunoglobulin (HBIG) was found on HBCs in placentas from HBV-positive mothers given intravenous HBIG (55). The proportion of HBIG was associated with fetal protection, potentially through viral neutralization by HBIG-HBCs (55). Expression of the checkpoint inhibitor PDL-1 was observed in HBCs following SARS-CoV-2 infection (26). Whether HBCs express the major SARS-CoV-2 entry receptor Angiotensin-converting enzyme 2 (ACE2) is still under debate, with one study reporting its absence in HBCs from 19 SARS-CoV-2-

exposed placentas (25) and another reporting that ACE2 is expressed in the placenta, including HBCs, but downregulated upon SARS-CoV-2 infection (60).

Infection of HBCs has also been explored as a risk factor for transplacental infection or adverse pregnancy outcome. A large observational study involving 271 HPV-positive women identified placental infection in 31 placentas, with viral DNA present in HBCs, although HPV infection was not associated with pregnancy complications such as preterm birth or miscarriage (56). Fetal infection with DENV (57) and H5N1 (54) was documented and HBCs were infected in both cases. Placental analysis during DENV infection revealed increased deposition of proinflammatory cytokines (IFN-γ, TNF-α) and chemokines (CCL2, CCL5) in HBCs and vascular permeability factors such as VEGF2, VEGF receptor in the endothelium (57), proposing a barrier interruption and possible viral transmission through infected HBCs.

In Vitro Studies of Other Viruses

In vitro studies have shown that HBCs are permissive to MHV-68 (92), Sendai virus (90) and RSV (91) but not to HSV-2 (88, 89), echovirus 19 (89) or SARS-CoV-2 infection (93) (**Table 2**). The methods utilized include protein detection by immunofluorescence (88, 89, 91, 93), viral titer quantification (88–90), electron microscopy (89), polymerase chain reaction (PCR) (91, 92) and western blot (91). For *in vitro* studies of viral infection, HBCs were mostly isolated from term placentas, with only five out of thirty studies utilizing samples from the first or second trimester - the time period where congenital infection is most damaging.

The proportion of infected HBCs has only been reported for HSV (88) infection and RSV (91). Exposure to HSV resulted in infection of 17% of HBCs, measured by viral protein, whilst only 4.4% of cells produced infectious HSV, measured by viral titer assays (88). The proportion of RSV-infected HBCs varied between 5% to 17% among donors as measured by RFP fluorescence (91). This study also proposes a contribution of HBCs to RSV dissemination. Although no detectable RSV was observed in HBC supernatant 30 days after *in vitro* infection, co-culture of infected HBCs with human bronchial epithelial cells spread the virus, suggesting a vital role of cell-to-cell interaction for viral dissemination.

Interestingly, HBCs were competent to eliminate HSV-2 and echovirus 19 infection (89). During those infections, pseudopods were emitted from HBCs, and there were increases in lipid accumulation, cellular volume, and numbers of vacuoles in cytoplasm, suggesting viral phagocytosis and degradation within HBCs (89).

An altered secretion profile has been observed upon viral infection of HBCs *in vitro*. Proinflammatory cytokines were released from HBCs during MHV-68 (IL-1β) (92), Sendai virus (IFN-β) (90) and RSV (TNF-α, IFN-γ, IL-6, IL-12) (91) infection. Interestingly, the IL-1β secretion during MHV-68 infection induced IL-8 secretion and increased pro-neutrophil response marker expression (IL-8, vascular cell adhesion molecule-1, intercellular cell adhesion molecule-1 (ICAM-1), E-selectin) in human umbilical vein endothelial cells (HUVECs) (92). This indicates a possible role of HBCs in creation or maintenance of a proinflammatory environment and activation of other cells in the placenta to counter pathogen invasion.

HBCs in Bacterial Infection

Observational Studies of Bacterial Infection

Some bacterial infections are associated with pregnancy complications followed by adverse pregnancy outcomes (98) (**Table 3**). The used search strategy obtained two observational studies which examined HBC bacterial infection or hyperplasia (52, 103). An increase in the number of HBCs was reported in *Treponema pallidum*-infected placentas from mothers with placental villitis (103). From a total of 15 cases of offspring death or illness in which placental bacterial infection was identified (using a consensus probe), mainly trophoblast rather than HBC infection was reported, in contrast to viral infection (52). The gestational age of maternal infection in pregnancy was not reported for any of these 21 cases of bacterial infection (52, 103).

In Vitro Studies of Bacterial Infection

Several groups have investigated HBC responses to bacterial infection *in vitro*, including 5 studies of GBS (104–108), *Coxiella burnetii* (109), *E. coli* (104, 105) and *Lactobacillus crispatus* and *E.coli* infections (110). Most of the studies used third trimester placentas. The sample size and gestational age were often not reported (**Table 4**).

Alterations in HBC numbers and phenotype have been reported in cases of chorioamnionitis (104). Amara et al. (104) examined nine patients with chorioamnionitis (4 grade I, 3 grade II and 2 grade III), of whom two had vaginal GBS and one had vaginal *E.coli*, three had bacteriuria and two had *E.coli* in their placentas. The numbers of HBCs were remarkably reduced in chorioamnionitis cases compared to HBCs from normal pregnancies and the expression of CD163, monocyte/macrophage scavenger receptor shed by inflammatory stimuli, was significantly increased in severe compared to moderate cases. CD163 expression was also increased in HBCs from chorioamnionitis-affected placentas with documented infections compared to those without an identified infection, suggesting this is a response to infection rather than sterile inflammation. The expression of M2 and M1 macrophage phenotype markers was similar between chorioamnionitis-positive and -negative pregnancies, and only three M1 genes (EDN1, IL-15 and IL-15RA) were reported as upregulated in HBCs from chorioamnionitis-positive cases (104).

HBCs alter their inflammatory profile to cope with *in vitro* bacterial infection. GBS infection of HBCs shifts their immunophenotype by increasing the secretion of proinflammatory cytokines (IL-6, IL-1β and TNF-α), activation of the nuclear factor kappa B (NFκβ), inflammasome assembly and upregulation of E-Selectin and the chemokine CCL4 in a protein kinase D-dependent manner (106). HBCs infected with *Coxiella burnetii* upregulate eight M1 macrophage-associated genes, whilst increased release of IFN-γ was associated with bacterial elimination (109).

In addition to the ability of HBCs to eliminate pathogen infection by cytokine induction, Doster et al. (105) proposed a

TABLE 3 | Hofbauer cells in observational studies of parasitic and bacterial infection.

Pathogen	Gestation of samples (outcome)		Trimester of infection	Diagnosis of HBC infection	HBC infection (no.)	HBC hyperplasia (no.)	Key outcome(s) in HBCs	Reference
	Preterm	Term						
Plasmodium falciparum	9 (NR)	14 (NR)	NR	NR	NR	NR	Similar CCR5 expression in HBCs from infected and uninfected women	Tkachuk et al. (99)
	–	9 (LB)	NR	NR	NR	NR	No significant difference in HBCs MIF expression between PM+ and PM- placentas	Chaisavaneeyakorn et al. (100)
	3 (LB)	14 (LB)	NR	Hemozoin detection	+ (NR)	NR	Hyperplasia of HBCs and decrease in M2 percentage associated with low-birth weight in first pregnancies	Gaw et al. (101)
	33 (CA)	8 (LB) & 26 (CA)	NR	NR	NR	NR	Identification of IgE positive HBCs	Rindsjö et al. (102)
Treponema pallidum	2 (1 LB & 1 PL)	4 (3 LB & 1 PL)	NR	NR	NR	+ (100%)	Hyperplasia of HBCs was observed in *Treponema pallidum* infected placentas	Walter et al. (103)
Various bacteria, including *E. coli, Klebsiella, Streptococcus agalactiae*	15, gestational age NR (PL and LB; numbers NR)		NR	rRNA sequence	- (NR)	NR	Mainly trophoblast rather than HBC infection was identified	Satosar et al. (52)
***E.coli, Haemophilus influenza*, GBS (CA patients)**	11 (LB) & 9 (CA)	–	NR	NR	NR	NR	Differences in HBC biology among healthy individuals and CA patients	Amara et al. (104)

NR, Not reported; CCR5, C-C chemokine receptor type 5; LB, Live birth; MIF, Migration inhibitory factor; PM, Placental malaria; PL, Pregnancy loss (stillbirth/miscarriage); E. coli, Escherichia coli; GBS, Group B Streptococcus; CA, Chorioamnionitis.

novel mechanism of bacterial elimination by the release of macrophage extracellular traps (METs). Upon GBS infection, HBCs were observed to release METs containing matrix metalloproteases capable of killing infected cells. The release of METs is not GBS-specific, with other bacteria such as *E. coli* and heat-killed GBS bacteria leading to similar MET release levels, suggesting a broad defense mechanism. Interestingly, MET release may contribute to fetal membrane weakening since METs which contained matrix metalloproteases and CD163-positive cells were found on fetal membranes (105).

TABLE 4 | Hofbauer cells in *in vitro* studies of bacterial infection.

Bacteria	Samples studied by trimester (outcome)				Model(s) of infection	Immuno-purification of HBCs	Diagnosis of HBC infection/ viral replication (no.)	Key outcome(s) in HBCs	Reference
	1st	2nd	3rd <37w	3rd ≥37w					
Unopsonized GAS bioparticles	–	–	–	3-5 (LB)	Cells	$CD14^{pos}$	Fluorometric phagocytosis assay	PGE2 regulates HBC phagocytic ability	Mason et al. (107)
Unopsonized GBS & *E.coli* bioparticles	–	–	–	3 (LB)	Cells	$CD14^{pos}$	Fluorometric phagocytosis assay	PGE2 regulates HBC phagocytic ability	Rogers et al. (108)
GBS & *E.coli*	–	9 CA (LB)	11 (LB)	–	Cells	$CD14^{pos}$	NR	HBCs from CA patients are altered compared to HBC from normal pregnancies	Amara et al. (104)
GBS, *E.coli* & killed bacteria	–	–	–	3 (LB)	*Ex-vivo* & cells	$CD14^{pos}$	Microscopy (NR)	HBCs release METs with digestion enzymes upon GBS and *E.coli* infection	Doster et al. (105)
GBS	NR				Cells	$CD14^{pos}$	Colony forming units (NR)	HBC immune response to GBS is dependent on protein kinase D	Sutton et al. (106)
Coxiella burnetii	–	–	46 (LB)		Cells	$CD14^{pos}$	PCR & microscopy (NR)	HBCs eliminate *Coxiella burnetii* through IFN-γ	Mezouar et al. (109)
Lactobacillus crispatus, E.coli* and labeled *E.coli	20 (TOP)	–	–	–	Cells	Multiparameter flow cytometry	Colony forming units (NR)	HBCs eliminate *Lactobacillus crispatus* and *E.coli*, and have phagocytic capacity	Thomas et al. (110)

GAS, Group A Streptococcus; LB, Live birth; PGE2, Prostaglandin E2; GBS, Group B Streptococcus; E. coli, Escherichia coli; NR, Not reported; CA, Chorioamnionitis; METs, Macrophage extracellular traps; PCR, Polymerase chain reaction; IFN, Interferon; TOP, Termination of pregnancy.

Finally, three studies reported the phagocytic capacity of HBCs using labelled bacteria (110) and unopsonized bacterial bioparticles (107, 108). Using unopsonized bioparticles, it has been shown that prostaglandin E2 (PGE2) regulates the phagocytic ability of HBCs to take up Group A *Streptococcus* (107), GBS and *E. coli* (108).

HBCs in Parasitic Infection

Only four observational studies of HBC responses to parasitic infections were identified, and all of them focused on *Plasmodium falciparum* (99–102) (**Table 3**). One of these investigated HBC infection indirectly, by identifying parasite disposal products in HBCs (101), one investigated the presence of IgE in association with HBCs (102), and the other two investigated HBC protein expression. Similar expression of the macrophage migration inhibitory factor (MIF) (100) and HIV-1 co-receptor CCR5 (99) was reported in HBCs between infected and uninfected women. A possible association between the HBC inflammatory response and fetal growth restriction in malaria-infected women was reported (101). Specifically, an increase in HBC numbers was observed and analysis of the CD163:CD68 balance in HBCs revealed a decrease in the M2 phenotype, which was associated with lower birth weight (101).

HBC Responses to Pathogen Associated Molecular Patterns (PAMPs)

As an alternative to studying responses to whole pathogens, several groups have investigated HBC responses to individual pathogen-associated molecular patterns (PAMPs) including lipopolysaccharide (LPS) (6, 69, 104, 109–115), merozoite surface protein 1 (MSP1) (116), polyinosinic:polycytidylic acid (PIC) and peptidoglycan (PGN) (110, 114), and Imiquimod and FSL-1 stimulation (110) (**Table 5**). HBCs were isolated mainly from third trimester placentas (n=9 studies) (6, 69, 109, 111–116), with only three studies using HBCs from the first or second trimester (6, 110, 112).

Lipopolysaccharide (LPS) was the most commonly used bacterial PAMP in HBC studies, LPS is a membrane component of gram-negative bacteria that signals mainly through toll-like receptor 4 (TLR4). One recent study performed an analysis of HBC response to LPS across gestation (6), and found a significant amount of activated HBCs expressing

TABLE 5 | Studies that investigated HBC response to PAMP(s) treatment *in vitro.*.

Treatment	Samples studied by trimester (outcome)				Model(s) of infection	Immuno purification of HBCs	Key outcome(s) in HBCs	Reference
	1st	2nd	3rd <37w	3rd ≥37w				
LPS	–	–	–	NR (LB)	Cells	No	HBCs secrete lower levels of cytokines compared to MDMs and LPS-treated HBCs	Plaud-Valentin et al. (69)
	–	–	–	12 (LB)	Cells	No	LPS treatment increased the percentage of cytokine producing HBCs	Pavlov et al. (111)
	–	9 CA (LB)	11 (LB)	–	Cells	CD14^{pos}	Differences in inflammatory response of HBCs, MGCs and HBCs from CA patients	Amara et al. (104)
	13-24 (TOP)	–	–	13-24 (LB)	Cells	No	LPS treatment increased cytokine release by HBCs	Pavlov et al. (112)
	–	–	46 (LB)		Cells	CD14^{pos}	LPS did not induce M1-like transcriptional profile in HBCs	Mezouar et al. (109)
LPS & IFN-γ	8 (TOP)		–	5 (LB)	Cells	CD14^{pos}	Difference in HBC response to LPS/IFN-γ treatment from early/midgestational and term pregnancies	Swieboda et al. (6)
	–	–	–	5 (LB)	Cells	CD10^{neg}/ EGFR^{neg}	HBCs maintain their M2 phenotype despite treatment with LPS/IFN-γ and alter their cytokine profile	Schliefsteiner et al. (113)
LPS, PIC & PGN		–	–	16 (LB)	Cells	CD10^{neg}/ EGFR^{neg}	HBC inflammatory responses can be induced despite their M2 phenotype	Young et al. (114)
MSP1	–	–	–	6 (LB)	Perfusion model	No	No immune complexes identified in HBCs	May et al. (116)
LPS & ATP	–	–	–	6 (LB)	Cells	CD10^{neg}/ EGFR^{neg}	Inflammasome activation in HBCs, release of IL-1β and pyroptotic cell death	Abrahams et al. (115)
LPS, LPS & IFN-γ, PIC, Imiquimod, PGN, FSL-1	20 (TOP)	–	–	–	–	Multiparameter flow cytometry	HBCs respond to toll-like receptor agonist stimulation Among the stimulants, FSL-1 and LPS & IFN-γ have the greatest impact FSL-1 enhanced the production of CCL-3, IL-8, IL-6, and GM-CSF LPS & IFN-γ enhanced the secretion of TNF-α, IL-1β and reduced the production of TIMP-1 and MMP-9	Thomas et al. (110)

LPS, Lipopolysaccharides; NR, Not reported; LB, Live birth; MDMs, Monocyte-derived macrophages; CA, Chorioamnionitis; MGCs Multinucleated giant cells; TOP, Termination of pregnancy; IFN, Interferon; PIC, Polyinosinic,polycytidylic acid; PGN, Peptidoglycan; MSP1, Merozoite surface protein 1; ATP, Adenosine triphosphate; IL, Interleukin; FSL-1, Pam2CGDPKHPKSF-synthetic lipopeptide; CCL, C-C motif chemokine ligand; GM-CSF, Granulocyte-macrophage colony-stimulating factor; TNF, Tumor necrosis factor; TIMP-1, TIMP metallopeptidase inhibitor 1; MMP-9, Matrix metallopeptidase 9.

tolerogenic markers in early pregnancy stages, with the number of activated cells dropping at term. Treatment with IFN-γ and LPS led to the expression of inducible nitric oxide synthase (iNOS) and STAT-1 by early/midgestational HBCs, while the M1 to M2 phenotype ratio was not affected in term HBCs. More specifically, several subtypes of M2 phenotypes were detected at term, suggesting that HBCs are a heterogenous population of macrophages with regulatory and anti-inflammatory properties orchestrated in time through pregnancy (6). Thomas et al. (110) also showed that LPS and IFN-γ treatment enhanced the secretion of inflammatory cytokines (TNF-α and IL-1β) and reduced the production of tissue remodeling factors (TIMP-1 and MMP-9), while FSL-1 (TLR2/TLR6 agonist) treatment enhanced the production of chemoattractants and cytokines (CCL-3, IL-8, IL-6, and GM-CSF) in 3rd trimester.

Mezouar et al. (109) proposed that HBCs from term placentas maintain an M2 anti-inflammatory phenotype in the presence of LPS, despite the induction of M1-like proteins and cytokines, unlike *in vitro* bacterial infections. Schliefsteiner et al. (113) examined the HBC response in the presence of LPS and IFN-γ, which did not induce M1 polarization but a decrease in the percentage of HBCs expressing M2 type associated proteins (CD206 and DC-SIGN). In addition, they observed an elevated release of proinflammatory cytokines (TNF-α and IL-12) but also release of M2-immunoregulatory (IL10), highlighting the heterogenicity of HBCs and the oversimplified classification of macrophage phenotypes (113). Plaud-Valentin et al. (69) also observed the release of TNF-α and IL-1 from IFN-γ and LPS-stimulated HBCs; however, the cytokine secretion was higher in monocyte-derived macrophages. Similarly, an increase in the percentage of HBCs with intracellular expression of proinflammatory cytokines IL-1α, IL-1β, TNF-α and IL-6 was reported upon LPS stimulation by Pavlov et al. (111). Inflammasome activation, increased release of IL-1β and pyroptosis were induced upon HBC treatment with LPS and ATP (115). Robust secretion and transcription of the IL-6 pro-inflammatory cytokine and to a smaller degree of IL-8 chemokine was documented upon HBC treatment with LPS and to a lesser extent with PIC treatment, while PGN did not affect IL-6 and IL-8 secretion (114).

LPS responses by HBCs from normal pregnancy and those with chorioamnionitis were compared by Amara et al. (104). HBCs were shown to release IL-6, IL-10 and TNF-α in response to LPS. This study also observed, for the first time, the spontaneous *in vitro* formation of multinuclear giant cells (MGCs) from HBCs in healthy pregnancies. These MGCs exhibited similar phagocytic capacity to HBCs and released smaller amounts of TNF-α in response to LPS (though similar levels of IL-6 and IL-10). Interestingly, in cases of chorioamnionitits, they saw reduced HBC numbers, potentially *via* increased apoptosis or recruitment of HBCs into inflamed fetal tissues, as well as a failure by the cells to form MGCs. LPS treatment of HBCs from chorioamnionitis patients demonstrated reduced IL-10 responses and defective activation of the signal transducer and activator of transcription 1 (STAT-1), which is important for LPS-stimulated gene expression.

DISCUSSION

Here we present a systematic scoping review of the role of Hofbauer cells in infection during pregnancy. A variety of pathogens productively infect, invade, or modulate HBCs as revealed using *in situ*, *ex vivo* and *in vitro* approaches (Summarized in **Figures 3** and **4**). HBCs can exert responses that are highly infection-restrictive and protective to the fetus (87, 92, 105, 110, 115), but can also be exploited to the advantage of the pathogen for dissemination or hiding (76, 91, 113). Therefore, HBCs appear to be a "double-edged sword" in the context of placental and congenital infection. Several studies described the presence of HBC hyperplasia during infection in the placenta, supporting their role in fetal defense against invading pathogens (25, 26, 39–44, 46, 47, 49, 51, 57, 59, 103). It is not known whether this is a result of replication of existing HBCs in the villi or through migration of additional cells from the fetus. Only one study demonstrated an increase in HBC proliferation upon infection- a study of ZIKV infection (82), hence further studies are needed to determine the potential role of HBC proliferation during infection by other pathogens.

Different pathogens and PAMPs uniquely influence HBC responses inducing alterations in their transcriptional, translational and secretion profiles. Although HBCs have been defined as M2-like macrophages that maintain an anti-inflammatory phenotype, characterized by contributions to tissue maintenance and developmental regulation (4, 5), pathogens or PAMPs have been reported to induce potent M1-like responses in these cells (109), with HBCs mounting robust pro-inflammatory cytokine responses (92, 114, 115). Conversely, HBCs have also been reported to maintain an M2-like phenotype during pathogen encounter (109, 113). A number of pro-inflammatory cytokines are released following exposure to viral and bacterial infections and upon PAMP exposure (**Figure 4**). These reported alterations in HBC profile during infection suggest that HBCs have evolved mechanisms to enable their activation and stimulation of adaptive immune responses through antigen presentation, however secretion of some cytokines could also aid in virus dissemination (70).

Of the clinically relevant viruses that are known to infect the fetus *in utero*, HIV, ZIKV and CMV have been proven as capable of establishing infection in the placenta (34, 78, 86) but specific interactions with HBCs are still far from fully characterized. Infection by HIV, for example, has been shown to occur *in vitro*, though clinical strains were inferior at infecting HBCs compared to laboratory-adapted strains (65, 66, 68), and HBCs were more resistant to production of new viral progeny than monocytes or monocyte-derived macrophages (MDMs) (71, 73), suggesting that more studies are needed to establish how efficiently HIV can replicate within HBCs. Even though the field is more recent, ZIKV infection of HBCs has been more extensively studied following the establishment of its link to congenital abnormalities such as microcephaly, and HBCs could therefore be important for ZIKV cross-placental transmission. However, it is not completely understood whether it is through productive replication or migration and cell-to-cell spread that HBCs contribute to dissemination towards the fetal

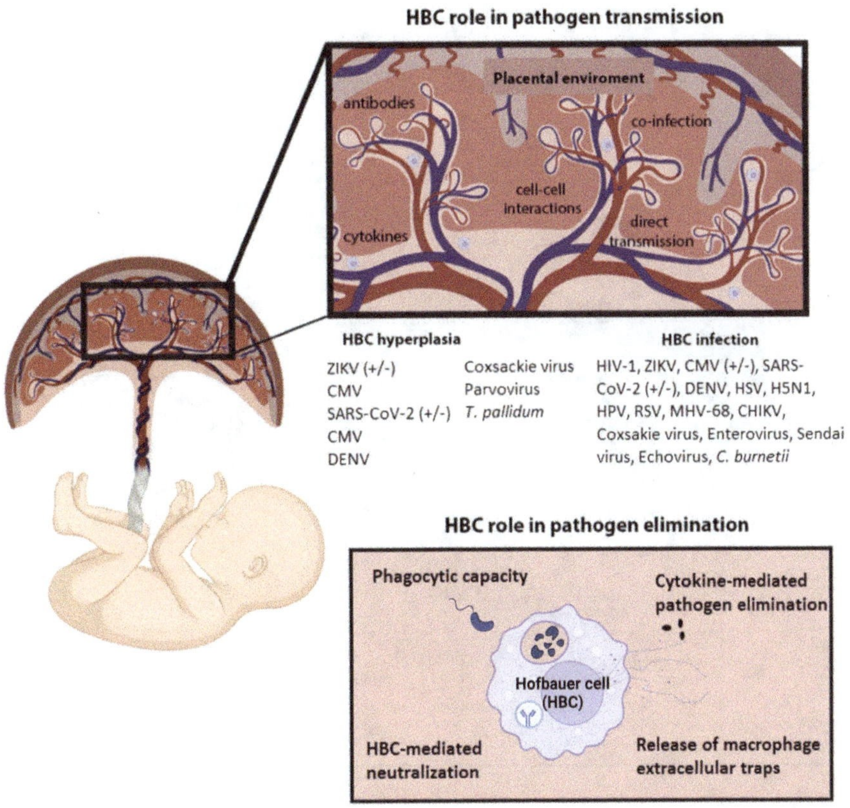

FIGURE 3 | Overview of the role of HBCs in pathogen infection and pathogen elimination. HBCs can be infected by a range of pathogens, which in some cases can replicate and transmit to other cells. Some pathogens induce HBC hyperplasia which may contribute to pathogen spread by increasing pathogen reservoirs. Release of cytokines during infection may contribute to pathogen elimination or enhance pathogen replication in HBCs. Other factors, such as antibodies and cytokines also influence HBC susceptibility to infection. However, HBCs also have the capacity to eliminate pathogen invasion by phagocytosis or the release of METs and pathogen neutralization. Created with BioRender.com.

compartment. Hyperplasia during placental ZIKV infection has been observed in a number of studies (39, 40, 42–44, 46, 47).

Despite being the most common congenital virus, CMV is not well characterized in terms of its ability to infect HBCs. *In situ* studies involve only a few samples (48–52) and the number of *in vitro* studies is small (77, 86, 87). Thus, it is not clear whether HBCs are routinely infected during placental infection by CMV. Furthermore, additional *in vitro* investigations are necessary to understand how HBCs interact with and respond to CMV and what implications that may have for preventing congenital infection. It would be of interest to explore what other viruses may escape "under the radar" during pregnancy, particularly where overt disease is not seen in the neonate. Multiple studies indicate other viruses such as HSV and coxsackie virus may also be clinically relevant and should be investigated further in the context of placental and HBC infection (51, 52). Additional studies describe capability of other viruses to infect and replicate within HBCs (26, 51, 52, 54, 56–58, 60, 90–92), though it is not known whether these also possess the ability to be systemically spread to reach the placenta and the fetal compartment due to their specific tropism profiles.

An inflammatory microenvironment induced by PAMPs, pathogens and a broader alteration of placental microenvironment may influence the profile of HBCs without direct infection (104). Most of the studies that documented placental and HBC infection identified pathogen genome or antigens within HBCs; however, identifying pathogen components does not reflect live infection. Extracellular vesicles could transfer pathogen components from infected cells to other cell types (117); however, this communication mechanism has not been investigated in HBCs. In this case, plaque assays or culture experiments could reveal the presence of live virus or bacteria, respectively, and thus reflect the capacity of HBCs to replicate pathogens. Infection-like microenvironments induced by PAMPs compared to damage-associated molecular patterns induce different HBC proliferation rates (118) and potentially different HBC expression patterns. Furthermore, supraphysiological doses of individual PAMPs used in *in vitro* experiments do not recapitulate real infection, and there are documented differences in HBC profiles between pathogen infection and PAMP treatment (109) (Summarized in **Figure 4**).

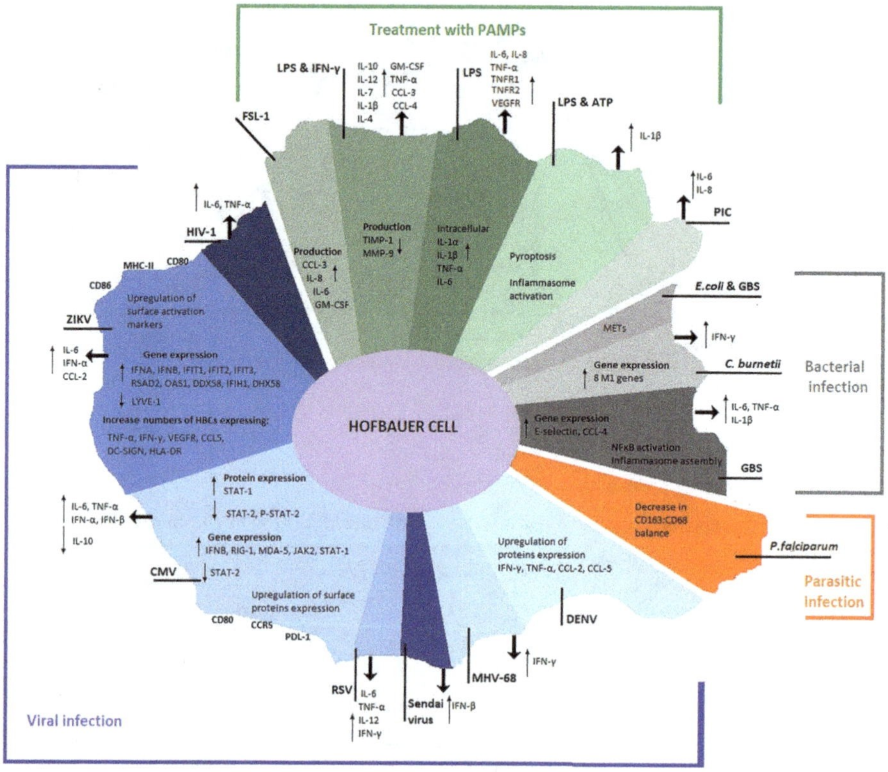

FIGURE 4 | Overview of HBC profile during pathogen infection and PAMP(s) stimulation. Alterations in HBC transcriptional, translational and secretional levels documented after pathogen infection or PAMP(s) treatment in the studies retrieved from the search strategy. Viral infections are represented in blue shades, parasitic infections in orange, bacterial infections in grey and PAMP(s) treatments in green.

TABLE 6 | Considerations for future microbial studies in placental macrophages.

Minimal reporting for clinical samples	Considerations when studying isolated HBCs
Pregnancy outcome (e.g. termination, pregnancy loss or live birth, gestation at delivery)	Isolation procedure: using initial trypsin digests of placenta will result in contamination with maternal macrophages
Presence/absence of fetal/newborn infection Presence/absence of chorioamnionitis	Isolation procedure: depletion of non-macrophage cells by immunomagnetic isolation should be performed
Fetal sex The gestation of pregnancy at maternal infection	Isolation procedure: positive immunoselection of CD14+ macrophages will cause cell activation
Method used for infection diagnosis The number of patients studied	*In vitro* direct exposure to high-dose pathogens does not recapitulate how HBCs encounter pathogens *in vivo*
Sampling methodology for placental biopsies Gestation of placental samples	HBC permissiveness to pathogens could be affected by monoculture versus co-culture with other placental cells
The proportion of HBCs with evidence of infection	
Considerations for *in vitro* pathogen challenge	**Unanswered/less explored research questions**
The strain of virus or bacteria is important – macrophage tropism and clinical strains should be considered	To what extent HBCs alter their response, susceptibility, and permissiveness to infection throughout gestation
Ability for viruses to enter cells should be clearly distinguished from ability to replicate	Whether past infection history influences infection susceptibility/ transmission during pregnancy
Techniques that measure viral infection using protein and nucleic acid should be complemented with techniques that measure live infectious virus	To what extent HBC localisation (both within villi and across the placenta) alter their phenotype and function
	The role of fetal sex in HBC responses to infection
Possibility of replication followed by entrapment inside cells should be considered and experimentally tested.	Few studies have investigated first/second trimester HBC responses to pathogens *in vitro*
Rate of infection – the use of high multiplicity of infections (MOI) may affect outcomes	In what way inflammation in response to infection may be beneficial in preventing spread to the fetus

Finally, HBCs reside in several micro-locations within the chorionic villus (119), but how these spatial differences affect permissiveness to pathogens and immune functions remains to be investigated. Specifically, HBCs within the anchoring villi are closer to the decidua than those within the floating villi. Since some pathogens are thought to infect the placenta by invading extravillous trophoblasts in the anchoring villi (14), the phenotype and the proportion of infected HBCs within anchoring villi may be different compared to HBCs in floating villi. Also, the influence of decidual cells, including immune cells, on HBC behavior could be higher in anchoring villi, which would have higher exposure to secreted factors. Current investigations of *in vitro* HBC responses have not examined the effect of HBC location on their response to pathogens and likelihood of infection; this could be beneficial to understanding their role in protecting the fetus from congenital infections.

In completing this review, we identified some themes, including strengths and weaknesses of existing studies, the significance of HBC isolation technique in interpreting findings, the importance of considering pathogen characteristics when designing these studies, which we have summarized in **Table 6**. Collectively, elucidating the nature of interactions between HBCs and placental pathogens is of vital importance and relevance to understanding the infection-induced mechanisms leading to adverse pregnancy outcomes.

AUTHOR CONTRIBUTIONS

BH conceived the review. GF led the screening of the papers, with assistance from PP and BH. GF drafted the review with BH, PP, and VB contributing to the writing and editing. All authors contributed to the article and approved the submitted version.

REFERENCES

Castellucci M, Zaccheo D, Pescetto G. A Three-Dimensional Study of the Normal Human Placental Villous Core - I. *Hofbauer Cells Cell Tissue Res* (1980) 210(2):235–47. doi: 10.1007/BF00237612

Loegl J, Hiden U, Nussbaumer E, Schliefsteiner C, Cvitic S, Lang I, et al. Hofbauer Cells of M2a, M2b and M2c Polarisation May Regulate Feto- Placental Angiogenesis. *Reproduction* (2016) 152(5):447–55. doi: 10.1530/ REP-16-0159

Seval Y, Korgun ET, Demir R. Hofbauer Cells in Early Human Placenta: Possible Implications in Vasculogenesis and Angiogenesis. *Placenta* (2007) 28(8–9):841–5. doi: 10.1016/j.placenta.2007.01.010

Khan S, Katabuchi H, Araki M, Nishimura R, Okamura H. Human Villous Macrophage-Conditioned Media Enhance Human Trophoblast Growth and Differentiation *In Vitro*. *Biol Reprod* (2000) 62(4):1075–83. doi: 10.1095/ biolreprod62.4.1075

Anteby EY, Natanson-Yaron S, Greenfield C, Goldman-Wohl D, Haimov- Kochman R, Holzer H, et al. Human Placental Hofbauer Cells Express Sprouty Proteins: A Possible Modulating Mechanism of Villous Branching. *Placenta* (2005) 26(6):476–83. doi: 10.1016/j.placenta.2004.08.008

Swieboda D, Johnson EL, Beaver J, Haddad L, Enninga EAL, Hathcock M, et al. Baby's First Macrophage: Temporal Regulation of Hofbauer Cell Phenotype Influences Ligand-Mediated Innate Immune Responses Across Gestation. *J Immunol* (2020) 204(9):2380–91. doi: 10.4049/jimmunol. 1901185

Goldstein J, Braverman M, Salafia C, Buckley P. The Phenotype of Human Placental Macrophages and Its Variation With Gestational Age. *Am J Pathol* (1988) 133(3):648–59.

Mues B, Langer D, Zwadlo G, Sorg C. Phenotypic Characterization of Macrophages in Human Term Placenta. *Immunology* (1989) 67(3):303–7.

Mosser DM, Edwards JP. Nihms84393. *Nat Rev Immunol* (2009) 8(12):958– 69. doi: 10.1038/nri2448

Zulu MZ, Martinez FO, Gordon S, Gray CM. The Elusive Role of Placental Macrophages: The Hofbauer Cell. *J Innate Immun* (2019) 11:447–56. doi: 10.1159/000497416

WHO. *Congenital Anomalies [Internet]* (2020). Available at: https://www. who. int/news-room/fact-sheets/detail/congenital-anomalies.

Torgerson PR, Mastroiacovo P. The Global Burden of Congenital Toxoplasmosis: A Systematic Review. *Bull World Health Organ* (2013) 91 (7):501–8. doi: 10.2471/ BLT.12.111732

WHO. *The Global Elimination of Congenital Syphilis: Rationale and Strategy for Action [Internet]*. Geneva: WHO Press (2007). Available at: https://apps. who.int/iris/bitstream/handle/10665/43782/9789241595858_eng.pdf? sequence=1&isAllowed=y.

Neu N, Duchon J, Zachariah P. TORCH Infections. *Clin Perinatol* (2015) 42 (1):77–103. doi: 10.1016/j.clp.2014.11.001

Arora N, Sadovsky Y, Dermody TS, Coyne CB. Microbial Vertical Transmission During Human Pregnancy. *Cell Host Microbe* (2017) 21 (5):561–7. doi: 10.1016/j.chom.2017.04.007

Boyle AK, Rinaldi SF, Norman JE, Stock SJ. Preterm Birth: Inflammation, Fetal Injury and Treatment Strategies. *J Reprod Immunol* (2017) 119:62–6. doi: 10.1016/j.jri.2016.11.008

Frenkel DL. Infectious Diseases as a Cause of Global Childhood Mortality and Morbidity: Progress in Recognition, Prevention, and Treatment. *Adv Pediatr Res* (2018) 5(14):1–11. doi: 10.24105/apr.2018.5.14

Shmueli E, Hadar E, Pardo J, Attias J, Amir J, Bilavsky E. Congenital Cytomegalovirus Infection After a Multiple Birth Pregnancy. *Pediatr Infect Dis J* (2017) 36(12):e298–302. doi: 10.1097/INF.0000000000001725

Melo AS, Aguiar RS, Amorim MMR, Arruda MB, De Oliveira Melo F, Ribeiro STC, et al. Congenital Zika Virus Infection: Beyond Neonatal Microcephaly. *JAMA Neurol* (2016) 73(12):1407–16. doi: 10.1001/ jamaneurol.2016.3720

Kovo M, Ganer Herman H, Gold E, Bar J, Schreiber L. Villitis of Unknown Etiology – Prevalence and Clinical Associations. *J Matern Neonatal Med* (2016) 29(19):3110–4. doi: 10.3109/14767058.2015.1114090

Tita ATN, Andrews WW. Diagnosis and Management of Clinical Chorioamnionitis. *Clin Perinatol* (2010) 37(2):339–54. doi: 10.1016/ j.clp.2010.02.003

Menter T, Mertz KD, Jiang S, Chen H, Monod C, Tzankov A, et al. Placental Pathology Findings During and After SARS-CoV-2 Infection: Features of Villitis and Malperfusion. *Pathobiology* (2021) 88(1):69–77. doi: 10.1159/ 000511324

Cribiù FM, Erra R, Pugni L, Rubio-Perez C, Alonso L, Simonetti S, et al.

Severe SARS-CoV-2 Placenta Infection can Impact Neonatal Outcome in the Absence of Vertical Transmission. *J Clin Invest* (2021) 131(6):1–6. doi: 10.1172/ JCI145427

Hosier H, Farhadian S, Morotti RA, Deshmukh U, Lu-Culligan A, Campbell KH, et al. SARS-CoV-2 Infection of the Placenta. *JCI* (2020) 130(9):4947–53. doi: 10.1172/JCI139569

Hecht JL, Quade B, Deshpande V, Mino-Kenudson M, Ting DT, Desai N, et al. SARS-CoV-2 can Infect the Placenta and Is Not Associated With Specific Placental Histopathology: A Series of 19 Placentas From COVID-19-Positive Mothers. *Mod Pathol* (2020) 33(11):2092–103. doi: 10.1038/ s41379-020-0639-4

Facchetti F, Bugatti M, Drera E, Tripodo C, Sartori E, Cancila V, et al. SARS-CoV2 Vertical Transmission With Adverse Effects on the Newborn Revealed Through Integrated Immunohistochemical, Electron Microscopy and Molecular Analyses of Placenta. *EBioMedicine* (2020) 59:1–8. doi: 10.1016/ j.ebiom.2020.102951

Roberts DJ, Edlow AG, Romero RJ, Coyne CB, Ting DT, Hornick JL, et al. SPECIAL REPORT: A Standardized Definition of Placental Infection by Severe Acute Respiratory Syndrome Coronavirus 2 (SARS-CoV-2), a Consensus Statement From the National Institutes of Health/ Eunice Kennedy Shriver National Institute of Child Health and Hu. *Am J Obstet Gynecol [Internet]* (2021) 2:P593. E1–9. doi: 10.1016/j.ajog.2021. 07.029

Tang Z, Abrahams VM, Mor G, Guller S. Placental Hofbauer Cells and Complications of Pregnancy. *Ann N Y Acad Sci* (2011) 1221:103–8. doi: 10.1111/j.1749-6632.2010.05932.x

Reyes L, Golos TG. Hofbauer Cells: Their Role in Healthy and Complicated Pregnancy. *Front Immunol* (2018) 9(NOV):1–8. doi: 10.3389/fimmu.2018.02628

Lewis SH, Fox HE, Lewis SH, Lewis SH, Reynolds-Kohler C, Nelson JA. HIV-1 in Trophoblastic and Villous Hofbauer Cells, and Haematological Precursors in Eight-Week Fetuses. *Lancet* (1990) 335(8689):565–8. doi: 10.1016/0140-6736(90)90349-A

Backé E, Jimenez E, Unger M, Schafer A, Jauniaux E, Vogel M. Demonstration of HIV-1 Infected Cells in Human Placenta by *In Situ* Hybridisation and Immunostaining. *J Clin Pathol* (1992) 45(10):871–4. doi: 10.1136/jcp.45.10.871

Martin AW, Brady K, Smith SI, DeCoste D, Page DV, Malpica A, et al. Immunohistochemical Localization of Human Immunodeficiency Virus P24 Antigen in Placental Tissue. *Hum Pathol* (1992) 23(4 PG-411–4):411–4. doi: 10.1016/0046-8177(92)90088-K

Backé E, Jimenez E, Unger M, Schäfer A, Vocks-Hauck M, Grosch-Wörner I, et al. Vertical Human Immunodeficiency Virus Transmission: A Study of Placental Pathology in Relation to Maternal Risk Factors. *Am J Perinatol* (1994) 11(5):326–30. doi: 10.1055/s-2007-994545

Sheikh AU, Polliotti BM, Miller RK. Human Immunedeficiency Virus Infection: *In Situ* Polymerase Chain Reaction Localization in Human Placentas After *In Utero* and *In Vitro* Infection. *Am J Obstet Gynecol* (2000) 182(1 I PG-207–213):207–13. doi: 10.1016/S0002-9378(00)70514-X

Bhoopat L, Khunamornpong S, Sirivatanapa P, Rithaporn T, Lerdsrimongkol P, Thorner PS, et al. Chorioamnionitis Is Associated With Placental Transmission of Human Immunodeficiency Virus-1 Subtype E in the Early Gestational Period. *Mod Pathol* (2005) 18(10 PG- 1357–64):1357–64. doi: 10.1038/modpathol.3800418

Behbahani H, Popek E, Garcia P, Andersson J, Spetz A-L, Landay A, et al. Up-Regulation of CCR5 Expression in the Placenta Is Associated With Human Immunodeficiency Virus-1 Vertical Transmission. *Am J Pathol* (2000) 157(6):1811–8. doi: 10.1016/S0002-9440(10)64819-5

Pillay K, Cloete M, McLeod H. Expression of DC-SIGN and DC-SIGNRs in Placentas of HIV-Positive Patients. *South Afr J HIV Med* (2014) 15(3 PG- 97–101):97–101. doi: 10.4102/sajhivmed.v15i3.8

Martinez J, Santiago MR, Martelli-Palomino G, de Souza DA, Silva TGA, Silva GEB, et al. Expression of HLA-E Molecules in the Placental Tissue of Women Infected With HIV-1 and Uninfected Women. *Placenta* (2017) 49:33–6. doi: 10.1016/j.placenta.2016.08.082

de Noronha L, Zanluca C, Azevedo MLV, Luz KG, dos Santos CND. Zika Virus Damages the Human Placental Barrier and Presents Marked Fetal Neurotropism. *Mem Inst Oswaldo Cruz* (2016) 111(5):287–93. doi: 10.1590/ 0074-02760160085

Rosenberg A, Yu W, Hill D, Reyes C, Schwartz D. Placental Pathology of Zika Virus: Viral Infection of the Placenta Induces Villous Stromal Macrophage (Hofbauer Cell) Proliferation and Hyperplasia. *Arch Pathol Lab Med* (2017) 141(1):43–8. doi: 10.5858/arpa.2016-0401-OA

Schwartz DA. Viral Infection, Proliferation, and Hyperplasia of Hofbauer Cells and Absence of Inflammation Characterize the Placental Pathology of Fetuses With Congenital Zika Virus Infection. *Arch Gynecol Obstet* (2017) 295(6):1361–8. doi: 10.1007/s00404-017-4361-5

de Noronha L, Zanluca C, Burger M, Suzukawa AA, Azevedo M, Rebutini PZ, et al. Zika Virus Infection at Different Pregnancy Stages: Anatomopathological Findings, Target Cells and Viral Persistence in Placental Tissues. *Front Microbiol* (2018) 9(SEP):1–11. doi: 10.3389/ fmicb.2018.02266

Rabelo K, Souza LJ, Salomão NG, Oliveira ERA, Sentinelli L de P, Lacerda MS, et al. Placental Inflammation and Fetal Injury in a Rare Zika Case Associated With Guillain-Barré Syndrome and Abortion. *Front Microbiol* (2018) 9:1018. doi: 10.3389/fmicb.2018.01018

Beaufrère A, Bessières B, Bonnière M, Driessen M, Alfano C, Couderc T, et al. A Clinical and Histopathological Study of Malformations Observed in Fetuses Infected by the Zika Virus. *Brain Pathol* (2019) 29(1):114–25. doi: 10.1111/bpa.12644

Lum FM, Narang V, Hue S, Chen J, McGovern N, Rajarethinam R, et al. Immunological Observations and Transcriptomic Analysis of Trimester-Specific Full-Term Placentas From Three Zika Virus-Infected Women. *Clin Transl Immunol* (2019) 8(11):e01082. doi: 10.1002/cti2.1082

Santos GR, Pinto CAL, Prudente RCS, Bevilacqua EMAF, Witkin SS, Passos SD. Histopathologic Changes in Placental Tissue Associated With Vertical Transmission of Zika Virus. *Int J Gynecol Pathol* (2020) 39(2):157–62. doi: 10.1097/PGP.0000000000000586

Miranda J, Martın-Tapia D, Valdespino-Va̋zquez Y, Alarcőn L, Espejel- Nuñez A, Guzma̋n-Huerta M, et al. Syncytiotrophoblast of Placentae From Women With Zika Virus Infection Has Altered Tight Junction Protein Expression and Increased Paracellular Permeability. *Cells* (2019) 8(10): P1174. doi: 10.3390/cells8101174

Mühlemann K, Miller RK, Metlay L, Menegus MA. Cytomegalovirus Infection of the Human Placenta: An Immunocytochemical Study. *Hum Pathol* (1992) 23(11):1234–7. doi: 10.1016/0046-8177(92)90290-J

Schwartz DA, Khan R, Stoll B. Characterization of the Fetal Inflammatory Response to Cytomegalovirus Placentitis. An Immunohistochemical Study. *Arch Pathol Lab Med* (1992) 116(1):21–7.

Mühlemann K, Miller RK, Metlay L, Menegus MA. Characterization of Placental Cytomegalovirus Infection by Immunocytochemistry. *Placenta* (1994) 15(1):215–22. doi: 10.1016/S0143-4004(05)80345-5

Euscher E, Davis J, Holzman I, Nuovo GJ. Coxsackie Virus Infection of the Placenta Associated With Neurodevelopmental Delays in the Newborn. *Obstet Gynecol* (2001) 98(6):1019–26. doi: 10.1097/00006250-200112000- 00006

Satosar A, Ramirez NC, Bartholomew D, Davis J, Nuovo GJ. Histologic Correlates of Viral and Bacterial Infection of the Placenta Associated With Severe Morbidity and Mortality in the Newborn. *Hum Pathol* (2004) 35 (5):536–45. doi: 10.1016/j.humpath.2004.01.015

Yao L, Korteweg C, Hsueh W, Gu J. Avian Influenza Receptor Expression in H5N1-Infected and Noninfected Human Tissues. *FASEB [Internet]* (2008) 22(3):733–40. doi: 10.1096/fj.06-7880com

Gu J, Xie Z, Gao Z, Liu J, Korteweg C, Ye J, et al. H5N1 Infection of the Respiratory Tract and Beyond: A Molecular Pathology Study. *Lancet* (2007) 370(9593):1137–45. doi: 10.1016/S0140-6736(07)61515-3

Liu J, Feng Y, Wang J, Li X, Lei C, Jin D, et al. An "Immune Barrier" Is Formed in the Placenta by Hepatitis B Immunoglobulin to Protect the Fetus From Hepatitis B Virus Infection From the Mother. *Hum Vaccin Immunother* (2015) 11(8):2068–76. doi: 10.1080/21645515.2015.1010890

Ambühl L, Leonhard A, Widen Zakhary C, Jørgensen A, Blaakaer J, Dybkaer K, et al. Human Papillomavirus Infects Placental Trophoblast and Hofbauer Cells, But Appears Not to Play a Causal Role in Miscarriage and Preterm Labor. *Acta Obs Gynecol Scand* (2017) 96(10):1188–96. doi: 10.1111/ aogs.13190

Nunes P, Nogueira R, Coelho J, Rodrigues F, Salomão N, José C, et al. A Stillborn Multiple Organs' Investigation From a Maternal Denv-4 Infection: Histopathological and Inflammatory Mediators Characterization. *Viruses* (2019) 11(4):P319. doi: 10.3390/v11040319

Salomão N, Brendolin M, Rabelo K, Wakimoto M, de Filippis AM, Dos Santos F, et al. Spontaneous Abortion and Chikungunya Infection: Pathological Findings. *Viruses* (2021) 13(4):1–11. doi: 10.3390/v13040554

Morotti D, Cadamuro M, Rigoli E, Sonzogni A, Gianatti A, Parolin C, et al. Molecular Pathology Analysis of SARS-CoV-2 in Syncytiotrophoblast and Hofbauer Cells in Placenta From a Pregnant Woman and Fetus With COVID-19. *Pathogens* (2021) 10(4):1–13. doi: 10.3390/pathogens10040479

Verma S, Joshi CS, Silverstein RB, He M, Carter EB, Mysorekar IU. SARS CoV-2 Colonization of Maternal and Fetal Cells of the Human Placenta Promotes Alteration of Local Renin-Angiotensin System. *Med [Internet]* (2021) 2(5):575–590.e5. doi: 10.1016/j.medj.2021.04.009

Gao L, Ren J, Xu L, Ke X, Xiong L, Tian X, et al. Placental Pathology of the Third Trimester Pregnant Women From COVID-19. *Diagn Pathol* (2021) 16(1):1–11. doi: 10.1186/s13000-021-01067-6

Mano H, Chermann JC. Replication of Human Immunodeficiency Virus Type 1 in Primary Cultured Placental Cells. *Res Virol [Internet]* (1991) 142 (2–3):95–104. doi: 10.1016/0923-2516(91)90044-4

Kesson AM, Fear WR, Kazazi F, Mathijs JM, Chang J, King NJ, et al. Human Immunodeficiency Virus Type 1 Infection of Human Placental Macrophages *In Vitro*. *J Infect Dis [Internet]* (1993) 168(3):571–9. doi: 10.1093/infdis/168.3.571

Kesson AM, Fear WR, Williams L, Chang J, King NJC, Cunningham AL. HIV Infection of Placental Macrophages: Their Potential Role in Vertical Transmission. *J Leukoc Biol* (1994) 56(3):241–6. doi: 10.1002/jlb.56.3.241

McGann KA, Collman R, Kolson DL, Gonzalez-Scarano F, Coukos G, Coutifaris C, et al. Human Immunodeficiency Virus Type 1 Causes Productive Infection of Macrophages in Primary Placental Cell Cultures. *J Infect Dis [Internet]* (1994) 169(4):746–53. doi: 10.1093/infdis/169.4.746

Meléndez-Guerrero L, Holmes R, Backé E, Polliotti B, Ibegbu C, Lee F, et al. *In Vitro* Infection of Hofbauer Cells With a Monocyte-Tropic Strain of HIV- 1. *Placenta* (1994) 15(1):33–45. doi: 10.1016/S0143-4004(05)80334-0

Lee AW, Mitra D, Laurence J. Interaction of Pregnancy Steroid Hormones and Zidovudine in Inhibition of HIV Type 1 Replication in Monocytoid and Placental Hofbauer Cells: Implications for the Prevention of Maternal-Fetal Transmission of HIV. *AIDS Res Hum Retroviruses* (1997) 13(14):1235–42. doi: 10.1089/aid.1997.13.1235

Fear WR, Kesson AM, Naif H, Lynch GW, Cunningham AL. Differential Tropism and Chemokine Receptor Expression of Human Immunodeficiency Virus Type 1 in Neonatal Monocytes, Monocyte-Derived Macrophages, and Placental Macrophages. *J Virol* (1998) 72(2):1334–44. doi: 10.1128/ JVI.72.2.1334-1344.1998

Plaud-Valentin M, Delgado R, Garcia V, Zorrilla C, Gandia J, Meléndez- Guerrero L. HIV Infection of Placental Macrophages: Effect on the Secretion of HIV Stimulatory Cytokines. *Cell Mol Biol* (1999) 45(4):423–31.

Bácsi A, Csoma E, Beck Z, Andirkó I, Kónya J, Gergely L, et al. Induction of HIV-1 Replication in Latently Infected Syncytiotrophoblast Cells by Contact With Placental Macrophages: Role of Interleukin-6 and Tumor Necrosis Factor-Alpha. *J Interferon Cytokine Res* (2001) 21(12 PG-1079–88):1079–88. doi: 10.1089/107999001317205213

Luciano-Montalvo C, Ciborowski P, Duan F, Gendelman HE, Meléndez LM. Proteomic Analyses Associate Cystatin B With Restricted HIV-1 Replication in Placental Macrophages. *Placenta* (2008) 29(12):1016–23. doi: 10.1016/ j.placenta.2008.09.005

Luciano-Montalvo C, Meléndez LM. Cystatin B Associates With Signal Transducer and Activator of Transcription 1 in Monocyte-Derived and Placental Macrophages. *Placenta* (2009) 30(5):464–7. doi: 10.1016/ j.placenta.2009.03.003

Garcıa-Crespo K, Cadilla C, Skolasky R, Meléndez LM. Restricted HIV-1 Replication in Placental Macrophages Is Caused by Inefficient Viral Transcription. *J Leukoc Biol* (2010) 87(4):633–6. doi: 10.1189/jlb.0809556

Boily-Larouche G, Milev MP, Zijenah LS, Labbé AC, Zannou DM, Humphrey JH, et al. Naturally-Occurring Genetic Variants in Human DC-SIGN Increase HIV-1 Capture, Cell-Transfer and Risk of Mother-to- Child Transmission. *PloS One* (2012) 7(7):e40706. doi: 10.1371/ journal.pone.0040706

Johnson EL, Chakraborty R. Placental Hofbauer Cells Limit HIV-1 Replication and Potentially Offset Mother to Child Transmission (MTCT) by Induction of Immunoregulatory Cytokines. *Retrovirology* (2012) 9 (101):1–11. doi: 10.1186/1742-4690-9-101

Johnson EL, Chu H, Byrareddy SN, Spearman P, Chakraborty R. Placental Hofbauer Cells Assemble and Sequester HIV-1 in Tetraspanin-Positive Compartments That Are Accessible to Broadly Neutralizing Antibodies. *J Int AIDS Soc* (2015) 18(1):1–8. doi: 10.7448/IAS.18.1.19385

Johnson EL, Boggavarapu S, Johnson ES, Lal AA, Agrawal P, Bhaumik SK, et al. Human Cytomegalovirus Enhances Placental Susceptibility and Replication of Human Immunodeficiency Virus Type 1 (HIV-1), Which May Facilitate *In Utero* HIV-1 Transmission. *J Infect Dis* (2018) 218 (9):1464–73. doi: 10.1093/infdis/jiy327

El Costa H, Gouilly J, Mansuy JM, Chen Q, Levy C, Cartron G, et al. ZIKA Virus Reveals Broad Tissue and Cell Tropism During the First Trimester of Pregnancy. *Sci Rep* (2016) 6(PG-35296):35296. doi: 10.1038/srep35296

Jurado K, Simoni MK, Tang Z, Uraki R, Hwang J, Householder S, et al. Zika Virus Productively Infects Primary Human Placenta-Specific Macrophages. *JCI Insight* (2016) 1(13):1–6. doi: 10.1172/jci.insight.88461

Tabata T, Petitt M, Puerta-Guardo H, Michlmayr D, Wang C, Fang-Hoover J, et al. Zika Virus Targets Different Primary Human Placental Cells, Suggesting Two Routes for Vertical Transmission. *Cell Host Microbe* (2016) 20(2):155–66. doi: 10.1016/j.chom.2016.07.002

Quicke KM, Bowen JR, Johnson EL, McDonald CE, Ma H, O'Neal JT, et al. Zika Virus Infects Human Placental Macrophages. *Cell Host Microbe* (2016) 20(1 PG-83–90):83–90. doi: 10.1016/j.chom.2016.05.015

Tabata T, Petitt M, Puerta-Guardo H, Michlmayr D, Harris E, Pereira L. Zika Virus Replicates in Proliferating Cells in Explants From First-Trimester Human Placentas, Potential Sites for Dissemination of Infection. *J Infect Dis* (2018) 217(8):1202–13. doi: 10.1093/infdis/jix552

Gavegnano C, Bassit LC, Cox BD, Hsiao H-M, Johnson EL, Suthar M, et al. Jak Inhibitors Modulate Production of Replication-Competent Zika Virus in Human Hofbauer, Trophoblasts, and Neuroblastoma Cells. *Pathog Immun* (2017) 2(2):199–218. doi: 10.20411/pai.v2i2.190

Zimmerman MG, Quicke KM, O'Neal JT, Arora N, Machiah D, Priyamvada L, et al. Cross-Reactive Dengue Virus Antibodies Augment Zika Virus Infection of Human Placental Macrophages. *Cell Host Microbe* (2018) 24 (5):731–42. doi: 10.1016/j.chom.2018.10.008

Puerta-Guardo H, Tabata T, Petitt M, Dimitrova M, Glasner DR, Pereira L, et al. Zika Virus Nonstructural Protein 1 Disrupts Glycosaminoglycans and Causes Permeability in Developing Human Placentas. *J Infect Dis* (2020) 221 (2):313–24. doi: 10.1093/infdis/jiz331

Bácsi A, Aranyosi J, Beck Z, Ebbesen P, Andirkó I, Szabó J, et al. Placental Macrophage Contact Potentiates the Complete Replicative Cycle of Human Cytomegalovirus in Syncytiotrophoblast Cells: Role of Interleukin-8 and Transforming Growth Factor-*b1*. *J Interf Cytokine Res* (1999) 19(10 PG- 1153–1160):1153–60. doi: 10.1089/107999099313091

Wussow F, Chiuppesi F, Martinez J, Campo J, Johnson E, Flechsig C, et al. Human Cytomegalovirus Vaccine Based on the Envelope Gh/gL Pentamer Complex. *PloS Pathog* (2014) 10(11):e1004524. doi: 10.1371/journal.ppat. 1004524

Plaeger-Marshall S, Ank BJ, Altenburger KM, Pizer LI, Johnston RB, Stiehm ER. Replication of Herpes Simplex Virus in Blood Monocytes and Placental Macrophages From Human Neonates. *Pediatr Res* (1989) 26(2):135–9. doi: 10.1203/00006450-198908000-00014

Oliveira LHS, Fonseca MEF, De Bonis M. Placental Phagocytic Cells Infected With Herpes Simplex Type 2 and Echovirus Type 19: Virological and Ultrastructural Aspects. *Placenta* (1992) 13(5):405–16. doi: 10.1016/0143- 4004(92)90048-X

Toth FD, Norskov-Lauritsen N, Juhl CB, Aboagye-Mathiesen G, Ebbesen P. Interferon Production by Cultured Human Trophoblasts and Choriocarcinoma Cell Lines Induced by Sendai Virus. *J Gen Virol* (1990) 71(12):3067–9. doi: 10.1099/0022-1317-71-12-3067

Bokun V, Moore JJ, Moore R, Smallcombe CC, Harford TJ, Rezaee F, et al. Respiratory Syncytial Virus Exhibits Differential Tropism for Distinct Human Placental Cell Types With Hofbauer Cells Acting as a Permissive Reservoir for Infection. *PloS One* (2019) 14(12 PG-e0225767):1–16. doi: 10.1371/journal.pone.0225767

Hendrix P, Tang Z, Silasi M, Racicot KE, Mor G, Abrahams VM, et al. Herpesvirus-Infected Hofbauer Cells Activate Endothelial Cells Through an IL-1*b*-Dependent Mechanism. *Placenta* (2020) 91:59–65. doi: 10.1016/ j.placenta.2020.01.010

Lu-Culligan A, Chavan AR, Vijayakumar P, Irshaid L, Courchaine EM, Milano KM, et al. SARS-CoV-2 Infection in Pregnancy is Associated With Robust Inflammatory Response at The Maternal-Fetal Interface. Medrxiv : The Preprint Server for Health Sciences. (2021). doi: 10.1101/2021.01.25. 21250452

Atwood WJ, Berger JR, Kaderman R, Tornatore CS, Major EO. Human Immunodeficiency Virus Type 1 Infection of the Brain. *Clin Microbiol Rev* (1993) 6(4):339–66. doi: 10.1128/CMR.6.4.339

Hennessey M, Fischer M, Staples JE. Zika Virus Spreads to New Areas - Region of the Americas, May 2015-January 2016. *MMWR Morb Mortal Wkly Rep* (2016) 65(3):55–8. doi: 10.15585/mmwr.mm6503e1

Soares F, Abranches AD, Villela L, Lara S, Araújo D, Nehab S, et al. Zika Virus Infection in Pregnancy and Infant Growth, Body Composition in the First Three Months of Life: A Cohort Study. *Sci Rep* (2019) 9(1):6–11. doi: 10.1038/s41598-019-55598-6

Krauer F, Riesen M, Reveiz L, Oladapo OT, Martınez-Vega R, Porgo TV, et al. Zika Virus Infection as a Cause of Congenital Brain Abnormalities and Guillain–Barré Syndrome: Systematic Review. *PloS Med* (2017) 14(1):1–27. doi: 10.1371/journal.pmed.1002203

Doyle RM, Harris K, Kamiza S, Harjunmaa U, Ashorn U, Nkhoma M, et al. Bacterial Communities Found in Placental Tissues Are Associated With Severe Chorioamnionitis and Adverse Birth Outcomes. *PloS One* (2017) 12 (7):1–23. doi: 10.1371/journal.pone.0180167

Tkachuk AN, Moormann AM, Poore JA, Rochford RA, Chensue SW, Mwapasa V, et al. Malaria Enhances Expression of CC Chemokine Receptor 5 on Placental Macrophages. *J Infect Dis* (2001) 183(6):967–72. doi: 10.1086/319248

Chaisavaneeyakorn S, Lucchi N, Abramowsky C, Othoro C, Chaiyaroj SC, Shi YP, et al. Immunohistological Characterization of Macrophage Migration Inhibitory Factor Expression in Plasmodium Falciparum- Infected Placentas. *Infect Immun* (2005) 73(6):3287–93. doi: 10.1128/ IAI.73.6.3287-3293.2005

Gaw SL, Hromatka BS, Ngeleza S, Buarpung S, Ozarslan N, Tshefu A, et al. Differential Activation of Fetal Hofbauer Cells in Primigravidas Is Associated With Decreased Birth Weight in Symptomatic Placental Malaria. Malar Res Treat (2019) 2019:1–10. doi: 10.1155/2019/1378174

Rindsjö E, Varli IH, Ofori MF, Lundquist M, Holmlund U, Papadogiannakis N, et al. Presence of IgE+ Cells in Human Placenta Is Independent of Malaria Infection or Chorioamnionitis. *Clin Exp Immunol* (2006) 144(2):204–11. doi: 10.1111/j.1365-2249.2006.03055.x

Walter P, Blot P, Ivanoff B. The Placental Lesions in Congenital Syphilis - A Study of Six Cases. *Virchows Arch A Pathol Anat Histol* (1982) 397(3):313– 26. doi: 10.1007/BF00496572

Amara AB, Gorvel L, Baulan K, Derain-Court J, Buffat C, Vérollet C, et al. Placental Macrophages Are Impaired in Chorioamnionitis, an Infectious Pathology of the Placenta. *J Immunol* (2013) 191(11):5501–14. doi: 10.4049/ jimmunol.1300988

Doster RS, Sutton JA, Rogers LM, Aronoff DM, Gaddy JA. Streptococcus Agalactiae Induces Placental Macrophages To Release Extracellular Traps Loaded With Tissue Remodeling Enzymes *via* an Oxidative Burst-Dependent Mechanism. *MBio* (2018) 9(6):1–16. doi: 10.1128/mBio. 02084-18

Sutton JA, Rogers LM, Dixon B, Kirk L, Doster R, Holly AM, et al. Protein Kinase D Mediates Inflammatory Responses of Human Placental Macrophages to Group B Streptococcus. *Am J Reprod Immunol* (2019) 81 (3 PG-e13075):1–22. doi: 10.1111/aji.13075

Mason KL, Rogers LM, Soares EM, Bani-Hashemi T, Erb Downward J, Agnew D, et al. Intrauterine Group A Streptococcal Infections Are Exacerbated by Prostaglandin E 2. *J Immunol* (2013) 191(5):2457–65. doi: 10.4049/jimmunol.1300786

Rogers LM, Anders AP, Doster RS, Gill EA, Gnecco JS, Holley JM, et al. Decidual Stromal Cell-Derived PGE2 Regulates Macrophage Responses to Microbial Threat. *Am J Reprod Immunol* (2018) 80(4):e13032. doi: 10.1111/ aji.13032

Mezouar S, Benammar I, Boumaza A, Diallo AB, Chartier C, Buffat C, et al. Full-Term Human Placental Macrophages Eliminate Coxiella Burnetii Through an IFN-*g* Autocrine Loop. *Front Microbiol* (2019) 10:1–12. doi: 10.3389/fmicb.2019.02434

Thomas J, Appios A, Zhao X, Dutkiewicz R, Donde M, Lee C, et al. Phenotypic and Functional Characterisation of First Trimester Human Placental Macrophages, Hofbauer Cells. *J Exp Med* (2020) 218(1):1–17. doi: 10.1084/jem.20200891

Pavlov O, Pavlova O, Ailamazyan E, Selkov S. Characterization of Cytokine Production by Human Term Placenta Macrophages *In Vitro*. *Am J Reprod Immunol* (2008) 60(6):556–67. doi: 10.1111/j.1600-0897.2008.00657.x

Pavlov OV, Niauri DA, Selutin AV, Selkov SA. Coordinated Expression of Tnf*a*- and VEGF-Mediated Signaling Components by Placental Macrophages in Early and Late Pregnancy. *Placenta* (2016) 42:28–36. doi: 10.1016/j.placenta.2016.04.008

Schliefsteiner C, Ibesich S, Wadsack C. Placental Hofbauer Cell Polarization Resists Inflammatory Cues *In Vitro*. *Int J Mol Sci* (2020) 21(3):1–14. doi: 10.3390/ijms21030736

Young O, Tang Z, Niven-Fairchild T, Tadesse S, Krikun G, Norwitz E, et al. Toll-Like Receptor-Mediated Responses by Placental Hofbauer Cells (HBCs): A Potential Pro-Inflammatory Role for Fetal M2 Macrophages. *Am J Reprod Immunol* (2015) 73(1):22–35. doi: 10.1111/aji.12336

Abrahams VM, Tang Z, Mor G, Guller S. NLRP3 Inflammasome Function and Pyroptotic Cell Death in Human Placental Hofbauer Cells. *J Reprod Immunol* (2020) 142(July):103214. doi: 10.1016/j.jri.2020.103214

May K, Grube M, Malhotra I, Long CA, Singh S, Mandaliya K, et al. Antibody-Dependent Transplacental Transfer of Malaria Blood-Stage Antigen Using a Human *Ex Vivo* Placental Perfusion Model. *PloS One* (2009) 4(11):e7986. doi: 10.1371/journal.pone.0007986

Urbanelli L, Buratta S, Tancini B, Sagini K, Delo F, Porcellati S, et al. The Role of Extracellular Vesicles in Viral Infection and Transmission. *Vaccines* (2019) 7(3):1–20. doi: 10.3390/vaccines7030102

Duval C, Brien ME, Gaudreault V, Boufaied I, Baker B, Jones RL, et al. Differential Effect of LPS and IL-1*b* in Term Placental Explants. *Placenta* (2019) 75(October 2018):9–15. doi: 10.1016/j.placenta.2018.11.006

Castellucci M, Kaufmann P. A Three-Dimensional Study of the Normal Human Placental Villous Core - I. The Hofbauer Cells. *Placenta* (1982) 210 (3):269–85. doi: 10.1016/S0143-4004(82)80004-0

14

Full-Term Human Placental Macrophages Eliminate *Coxiella burnetii* through an IFN-γ Autocrine Loop

Soraya Mezouar[1,2], Imene Benammar[1,2], Asma Boumaza[1,2], Aïssatou Bailo Diallo[1,2], Céline Chartier[1,2], Christophe Buffat[3], John Boudjarane[4], Philippe Halfon[5], Maria Katsogiannou[6] and Jean-Louis Mege[1,2,7]**

[1]Aix-Marseille Université, MEPHI, IRD, APHM, Marseille, France, [2]IHU-Méditerranée Infection, Marseille, France, [3]APHM, Biochemistry and Molecular Biology, Hôpital de la Conception, Marseille, France, [4]INSERM U1251, Centre de Génétique Médicale MMG, APHM, Hôpital de la Timone, Aix-Marseille Université, Marseille, France, [5]Laboratoire Alphabio, Hôpital Européen, Marseille, France, [6]Department of Obstetrics and Gynecology, Hôpital Saint Joseph, Marseille, France, [7]APHM, UF Immunologie, Marseille, France

***Correspondence:**
Soraya Mezouar
soraya.mezouar@univ-amu.fr;
soraya.mezouar@hotmail.fr
Jean-Louis Mege
jean-louis.mege@univ-amu.fr

The intracellular bacterium *Coxiella burnetii* is responsible for Q fever, an infectious disease that increases the risk of abortion, preterm labor, and stillbirth in pregnant women. It has been shown that *C. burnetii* replicates in BeWo trophoblast cell line and inhibits the activation and maturation of decidual dendritic cells. Although tissue macrophages are known to be targeted by *C. burnetii*, no studies have investigated the interplay between placental macrophages and *C. burnetii*. Here, CD14$^+$ macrophages from 46 full-term placentas were isolated by positive selection. They consisted of a mixed population of maternal and fetal origin as shown by genotype analysis. We showed that *C. burnetii* organisms infected placental macrophages after 4 h. When these infected macrophages were incubated for an additional 9-day culture, they completely eliminated organisms as shown by quantitative PCR. The ability of placental macrophages to form multinucleated giant cells was not affected by *C. burnetii* infection. The transcriptional immune response of placental macrophages to *C. burnetii* was investigated using quantitative real-time RT-PCR *on* 8 inflammatory and 10 immunoregulatory genes. *C. burnetii* clearly induced an inflammatory profile. Interestingly, the production by placental macrophages of interferon-γ, a cytokine known to be involved in efficient immune responses, was dramatically increased in response to *C. burnetii*. In addition, a clear correlation between interferon-γ production and *C. burnetii* elimination was found, suggesting that macrophages from full-term placentas eliminate *C. burnetii* under the control of an autocrine production of interferon-γ.

Keywords: *Coxiella burnetii*, inflammation, interferon-γ, macrophages, multinuclear giant cells, placenta

INTRODUCTION

The placenta is a unique chimeric organ made of fetal (chorion) and maternal (decidua) tissues at the materno-fetal interface. It is essential for nutritional exchanges and the immune tolerance of the fetus (Houser, 2012; Pinhal-Enfield et al., 2012). The latter is maintained by placental immune cells that prevent fetus rejection and protect it from infections. These immune cells mainly consist of natural killer (NK) cells and macrophages whereas T and B lymphocytes, dendritic cell,s and mast cells are less represented (Bulmer et al., 2010; Ben Amara et al., 2013; Gorvel et al., 2014; Mezouar et al., 2018, 2019c).

Placental macrophages represent 20–30% of the leukocytes found in all compartments of the placenta and their proportion increased throughout pregnancy (Bulmer et al., 2010). The phenotypic characterization of placental macrophages relies on the expression of CD68, a myeloid marker and CD14, a marker of circulating monocytes that is lacking in tissue macrophages other than placental macrophages (Ben Amara et al., 2013; Mezouar et al., 2019a). Placental macrophages include two populations of different origin. While Hofbauer cells are of fetal origin, decidual macrophages are of maternal origin (Pinhal-Enfield et al., 2012). These two populations are usually distinguished by their location within the placenta: Hofbauer cells are found in the fetal chorionic villi and decidual macrophages are found in decidua basalis (Pinhal-Enfield et al., 2012). Unfortunately, no specific phenotypic marker allows the distinction of these two populations. The role of placental macrophages in pregnancy is plural: they are involved in tissue remodeling, angiogenesis (Pongcharoen et al., 2007; Fong, 2008; Loegl et al., 2016), antigen presentation (Heikkinen et al., 2003, 2004), and maternal-fetal tolerance (Wang et al., 2018). They spontaneously form *in vitro* multinuclear giant cells (MGCs) even if the precise role of these MGCs remains to be elucidated (Ben Amara et al., 2013). It is well known that the activation status, also called polarization, of macrophages govern their biological activities: M1 macrophages are inflammatory and microbicidal whereas M2 macrophages are immunoregulatory and non-microbicidal. The M1/M2 status of macrophages is dependent on their microenvironment, especially on cytokines. Indeed, inflammatory cytokines such as tumor necrosis factor (TNF) and interferon (IFN)-γ induce a M1 polarization whereas immunoregulatory cytokines such as interleukin (IL)-10 induce a M2 polarization of macrophages (Benoit et al., 2008b; Mantovani et al., 2013). As reported for other macrophages, placental macrophages have been classified in either the M1 or M2 group. The M2 profile of placental macrophages is found at the beginning of pregnancy whereas the M1 profile is found at the end of pregnancy (Zhang et al., 2017). An inappropriate polarization of placental macrophages is associated with pregnancy complications such as abortion or miscarriage (Mezouar and Mege, 2018). Chorioamnionitis, a placental infection, interferes with placental macrophage polarization (Brown et al., 2014; Mezouar and Mege, 2018), and consists in an altered inflammatory response including decreased production of IL-10 (Ben Amara et al., 2013). For others, maintenance of the M2 polarization profile was observed (Joerink et al., 2011).

Coxiella burnetii, an intracellular gram-negative bacterium, is the causative agent of Q fever, a widespread zoonosis. *C. burnetii* infection leads to two major clinical forms. The primary infection is most often (60% of cases) asymptomatic and is usually spontaneously resolved. *C. burnetii* infection may by persist in the host for a minority of infected patients (less than 5%) leading to endocarditis or vascular infection (Raoult et al., 2005). *C. burnetii* infection of pregnant women is associated with specific problems (Carcopino et al., 2007) mainly due to the absence of clinical signs characteristic of the acute Q fever. The risk of pregnancy complications such as abortions and prematurity is high when the infection occurs during the first trimester. Malformations, stunting, or death *in utero* have also been reported (Eldin et al., 2017). Animal models of *C. burnetii* infection show that approximately 10^9 bacteria are present in 1 g of placental tissue (Sobotta et al., 2017). An imbalance of cytokine production is also observed in pregnant goats infected by *C. burnetii* (Roest et al., 2012). In *C. burnetii*-infected women, it has been suggested that abortions are related to infected and inflammatory placentas (Shinar et al., 2012).

The cellular reservoirs of *C. burnetii* in placenta are likely diverse. When human BeWo trophoblast cell line is infected with *C. burnetii*, the bacteria replicate within acid phagosomes (Ben Amara et al., 2013). The analysis of the transcriptional signature of these trophoblasts reveals the up-modulation of genes associated with inflammation pathways (Ben Amara et al., 2010). We also showed that *C. burnetii* infects placental dendritic cells and prevents their maturation and likely their ability to present antigens to the adaptive immune system (Gorvel et al., 2014). To our knowledge, the effect of *C. burnetii* infection on the functional activity of placental macrophages is unknown. In this study, we showed that isolated $CD14^+$ placental macrophages were able to eliminate *C. burnetii* within 9 days. The ability of these macrophages to spontaneously differentiate within MGCs was not affected by *C. burnetii* infection. In contrast, placental macrophages exhibited an inflammatory profile with an unexpected upregulated production of IFN-γ correlated with *C. burnetii* elimination.

MATERIALS AND METHODS

Placenta Collection

The study was approved by the "Comité d'Ethique d'Aix-Marseille Université" (number 08-012). Forty-six full-term placentas were collected at the Gynecology-Obstetrics Department of the "Hôpital de la Conception" (Marseille, France) after informed consent of the mothers. Women were devoid of pathologies, with a mean age of 34 years (21–42 years), a gestational age of 39 weeks (36–42 weeks) with main vaginal delivery (44 vaginal deliveries *versus* 2 caesarean deliveries). The placentas did not show any lesions or inflammation by macroscopically observation.

Bacteria

Coxiella burnetii Nine Mile strain (RSA496) was cultured as previously described (Ka et al., 2016). Briefly, L929 cells were infected for 8 days, sonicated, and centrifuged 10 min at 300 ×*g*.

Bacteria were collected after centrifugation at 10,000 ×*g* for 10 min, then washed and stored at −80°C. The concentration and the bacterial viability were assessed using the LIVE/DEAD BacLight bacterial viability kit (Life Technologies). In some experiments, organisms were labeled with the membrane fluorescent marker 4-(4-(dihexadecylamino)styryl)-N-methylpyridinium *iodide* (DID, Thermo Fisher Scientific) for 20 min at 37°C in phosphate buffered saline (PBS).

Isolation of Placental Macrophages

Placental macrophages were isolated as previously described (Mezouar et al., 2019a). Briefly, entire placenta tissue was digested in Hank's Balanced Salt Solution (HBSS), DNase I 2.5 mM, and 2.5% trypsin (Life Technologies). Cell suspension was filtered through 100-µm pores and deposited on a Ficoll cushion and centrifuged at 700 ×*g* for 20 min to collect mononuclear cells. Placental macrophages were isolated using magnetic beads coated with anti-CD14 antibodies (Miltenyi Biotec). The purity of isolated $CD14^+$ placental macrophages was assessed by flow cytometry and was higher than 98%.

Flow Cytometry Phenotyping of Isolated $CD14^+$ Placental Cells

The phenotype of isolated $CD14^+$ placental macrophages was assessed as follows. Cells (1×10^6 cells per assay) were stained using mice IgG1 anti-human CD14-APC (Allophycocyanin) and anti-human CD68-FITC (Fluorescein isothiocyanate) antibodies or isotype controls in PBS containing 5% Fetal Bovine Serum (FBS) for 30 min at 4°C. Cells were washed, fixed with 4% paraformaldehyde, centrifuged at 600 ×*g* for 5 min, and then diluted in PBS. Stained cells were then analyzed by flow cytometry (10,000 events/acquisition) using a BD FACS Canto II flow cytometer (BD biosciences). The results of flow cytometry were analyzed with FlowJo software.

Placental Macrophage Genotyping

To evaluate the maternal or fetal origin of isolated macrophages, the placentas of male fetuses were genotyped using a commercial kit containing probes for detection of specific centromeric regions of X and Y chromosomes, and chromosome 18 was used as control, according to the manufacturer's instructions (Fast Fish prenatal enumeration probe kit, Cytocell), as previously described (Huang et al., 2017). Briefly, after fixation using methanol and glacial acetic acid mix (3:1), placental macrophages were deposited onto a slide for fluorescence *in situ* hybridization including denaturation and hybridization of probes, and addition of Hoechst 33342 to DNA labeling. Slides were analyzed with a fluorescence microscope and the proportion of cells with maternal and fetal origin was determined.

Formation of Multinuclear Giant Cells

Placental macrophages (2×10^5 cells per assay) were incubated in 24 well plates containing glass coverslips in Dulbecco's Modified Eagle Medium (DMEM)-F12 supplemented with 10% FBS, 100 U/ml penicillin, and 50 µg/ml streptomycin (Life Technologies) for 9 days, as previously described (Ben Amara et al., 2013). Every 3 days, the presence of MGCs was determined by DNA staining and labeling of filamentous actin (F-actin) with Hoechst 3342 and phalloidin-488 (Life Technologies), respectively. The formation of MGCs was then analyzed by confocal microscopy using an LSM 800 Airyscan confocal microscope (Zeiss). The number of MGCs was determined and the results expressed in percentage of cells presenting at least two nuclei.

Lactate Dehydrogenase Assay

Isolated macrophages were incubated or not with *C. burnetii* (bacterium-to-cell ratio of 50:1) for 4 h and extensively washed to remove free bacteria (time designed as day 0). Cells were additionally cultured for 9 days, and the culture supernatants were collected at various time points. Lactate dehydrogenase release was quantified photometrically using Roche/Hitachi cobas c501 systems.

Microbicidal Activity of Placental Macrophages

Isolated macrophages (2×10^6 cells per assay) were cultured in DMEM-F12 supplemented with FBS and antibiotics. They were then incubated with *C. burnetii* (bacterium-to-cell ratio of 50:1) for 4 h and extensively washed to remove free bacteria (time designed as day 0). Placental macrophages were additionally cultured for 9 days and the uptake of bacteria was studied according two different approaches. First, macrophages were incubated with DID-labeled bacteria, stained with Hoechst 3342 and phalloidin-488, and the intracellular localization of bacteria was studied by confocal microscopy. Second, the uptake of bacteria was studied by qPCR. Briefly, DNA was extracted using a DNA Mini Kit (Qiagen), and infection was quantified using quantitative real time PCR (qPCR), as previously described (Ka et al., 2016). qPCR was performed with SYBR Green Fast Master mix (Roche Diagnostics) and the CXF Touch Real-Time PCR Detection System (Bio-Rad) using F (5′-GCACTAT TTTTAGCCG-GAACCTT-3′) and R (5′-TTGAGGAGAAAA-ACTGGATTGAGA-3′) primers that amplified a 225-bp fragment of the *C. burnetii com1* gene. A standard curve was generated using serial dilutions from a known concentration of *C. burnetii* DNA.

Inflammatory Response of Placental Macrophages

Two different approaches were used to study the inflammatory response of placental macrophages. First, the transcriptional response of 8 M1 genes and 10 M2 genes was studied by real-time quantitative PCR (qRT-PCR). For that purpose, placental macrophages (3×10^5 cells per assay) were incubated with *C. burnetii* (bacterium-to-cell ratio of 50:1), or 1 µg/ml lipopolysaccharide (LPS, Sigma-Aldrich) as control, for 6 h. Total RNA was extracted using RNeasy Mini Kit (Qiagen) and DNAse I treatment to eliminate DNA contaminants, as previously described (Mezouar et al., 2019b). The quantity and the quality of RNA were evaluated using a Nanodrop spectrophotometer (Nanodrop Technologies). Reverse transcription of isolated RNA was performed using a Moloney murine leukemia virus-reverse transcriptase kit and oligo(dT) primers (Life Technologies). qRT-PCR was performed using SYBR Green Fast Master mix (Roche Diagnostics) and a CFX Touch real-time PCR Detection System (Bio-Rad) using specific primers (Ben Amara et al., 2013) listed in **Table 1**. The results were normalized using the housekeeping *actb* gene encoding β-actin endogenous control and were expressed as relative quantity (RQ) using the following formula: $RQ = 2^{-\Delta Ct}$, where $\Delta Ct = (Ct_{Target} - Ct_{Actin})$. The threshold cycle (Ct) was defined as the number of cycles required to detect the fluorescent signal. Data were analyzed using Clustvis software.

Second, the release of IFN-γ by placental macrophages was studied using specific immunoassay kits (R & D Systems). Briefly, placental macrophages (3×10^5 cells) were stimulated or not with *C. burnetii* (bacterium-to-cell ratio of 50:1) for 6 h. The supernatants were centrifuged at 1,000 × g for 10 min and frozen at −80°C. In some experiments, placental macrophages (1×10^6 cells) were incubated or not with *C. burnetii* for 4 h and, after washing to remove free bacteria (time designed as day 0), they were cultured for 9 days. Every 3 days, supernatants were collected and the release of IFN-γ was quantified. The sensitivity of the assays was 1.0 pg/ml.

Statistical Analysis

Statistical analysis was performed using GraphPad Prism software version 7.0a (GraphPad Software, La Jolla California USA, www.graphpad.com). *In vitro* data were analyzed using the Mann-Whitney *t* test, one-way ANOVA, or ANOVA Kruskal-Wallis test. Correlations were evaluated using the non-parametric Spearman test. The results are presented as the mean score of at least three independent experiments, and $p < 0.05$ was considered statistically significant.

RESULTS

Characterization of Placental Macrophages

To ensure that placental CD14⁺ cells from healthy donors were macrophages distinct from maternal circulating monocytes, we used flow cytometry to assess the expression of CD68, a canonical macrophage marker, by $CD14^+$ cells. $CD14^+$ cells also expressed CD68 (**Figure 1A**), demonstrating that they are placental macrophages. Then, we evaluated the fetal or maternal origin of isolated $CD14^+$ placental macrophages using fluorescence *in situ* hybridization technique and fluorescent probes targeting the X and Y chromosomes (**Figure 1B**). The study of five different placentas of male fetuses showed that approximately 30% of macrophages expressed XX (maternal) chromosomes and 70% expressed XY (fetal) chromosomes. These findings showed that placental $CD14^+$ macrophages from healthy donors were a mixed population of Hofbauer cells and decidual macrophages.

TABLE 1 | List of genes associated with macrophage polarization.

Gene symbol	Forward primer (5′-3′)	Reverse primer (5′-3′)
β-actin	GGAAATCGTGCGTGACATTA	AGGAGGAAGGCTGGAAGAG
M1 genes		
CCL2	GCTGGAGAGCTACAAGAGGATCA	TCTCTCTTGAGCTTGGTGACAAAA
NOS2	TTGCAAGCTGATGGTCAAGATC	CAACCCGAGCTCCTGGAA
EDN1	CCTCCATCCCCCATACTAAATC	GTCTCCAAAAATCAAGGACAGG
HESX1	GCTCGGGGAAAACAAACC	TTCTTCTGGCATTGGGTGA
IDO1	TCATCTCACAGACCACAAGTCA	CAAAATAGGAGGCAGTTCCAGT
TNFSF10	GAAAATAATCCCCACACGCTAC	GTCACTCTCTCCACCCTCACA
IL15RA	ATCTTCCGTCCCTCATCCTAAC	CTCAGCATCTCTCCCACCTTT
CXCL9	ACACTTGCGGATATTCTGGACT	GGGAGATGGTGTGTAATTGAT
IL2RA	GTTGAAGAGGAAGGGCAAAAC	ACTGGGAAGTTGGAATGAGATG
TNF	CATCTATCTGGGAGGGGTCTTC	AGGAGGGGGTAATAAAGGGATT
M2 genes		
ALOX15	AACTTCCACCAGGCTTCTCTC	GGGGGCTGAAATAACCAAAG
CCL13	GAGCAGAGAGGCAAAGAAACA	ATGTGAAGCAGCAAGTAGATGG
CCL23	CATCTCCTACACCCCACGAA	CATTCTCACGCAAACCTGAACT
CLEC4F	GGCATTTCTGGTAGAGTTCACA	ATACTTTCTGAGTGGGCAGGA
CHN2	AGAACTGTGGCTGGAAAATGAG	GTGGTTGTCGTTGTGTGTGAG
CTSC	GAGGTTGTGTCTTGTAGCCAGT	CCCCTTTTTGTAGTGGAGGAAG
FN1	ACACCTGGAGCAAGAAGGATAA	CCACAGAGTAGACCACACCACT
HRH1	ACTTGGAGGTGGTATGTGCTG	CTCAGGGCTTGCTTCTTGTAGT
SLC4A7	CCCTCAAAACAGTCCTCCTTCT	TTTCCTCATTCTTCTGCTCCTC
CD209	GGATACAAGAGCTTAGCAGGGTG	GCGTGAAGGAGAGGAGTTGC

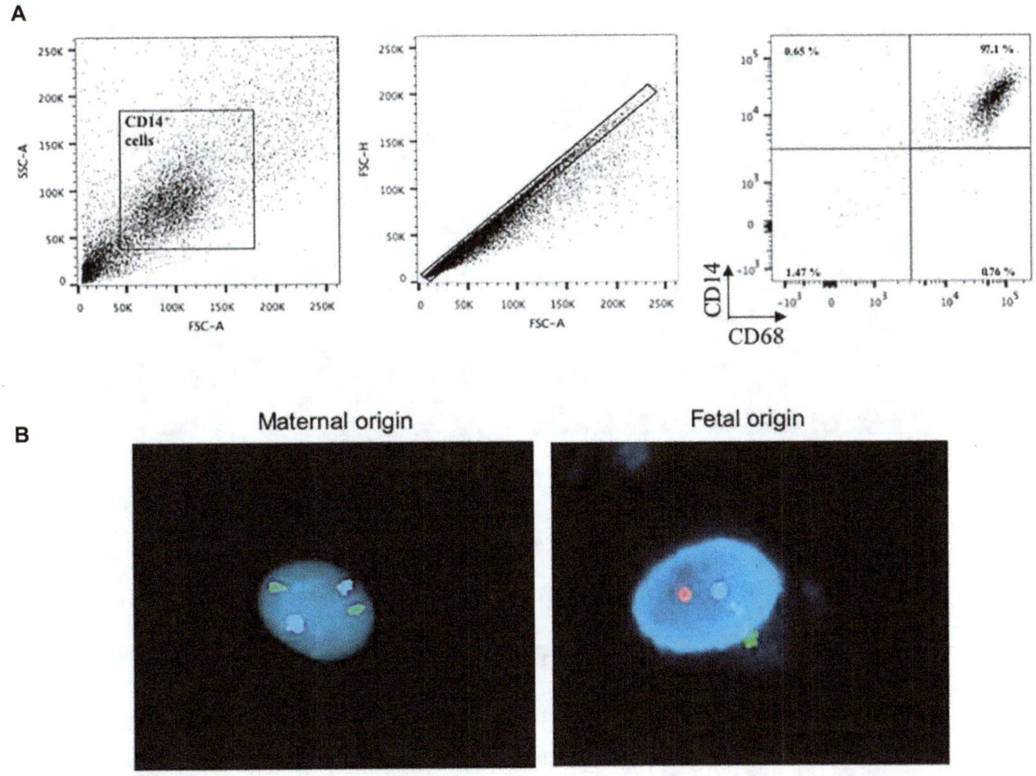

FIGURE 1 | Characterization of placental macrophages. **(A)** Placental CD14+ cells from 20 different placentas were analyzed for the expression of CD14 and CD68 by flow cytometry. Representative dot-blots are shown. **(B)** Placental macrophages from the placentas of male fetuses were analyzed for the expression of X, Y, and 18 chromosomes. Representative pictures show the X chromosome (in green), the Y chromosome (in red), and the chromosome 18 (nucleus in blue, used as control).

C. burnetii Infection of Placental Macrophages

Isolated CD14+ placental macrophages were infected or not with *C. burnetii* (bacterium-to-cell ratio of 50:1) for 4 h (**Figure 2A**) and cells were washed to remove unbound bacteria (this time was defined as day 0). Then, every 3 days of infection, the lactate dehydrogenase (LDH) release was quantified. No significant differences were observed between infected and resting placental macrophages (**Figure 2B**). The uptake, replication, or elimination of organisms by macrophages was observed (**Figure 2C**), and quantified by evaluation of the number of bacterial DNA copies using qPCR targeting the *com1* gene (**Figure 2D**). As a single *com1* gene is found per bacterium, it was easy to deduce that about 30 bacteria infected placental macrophages at day 0. A significant and steady decrease in the number of bacterial DNA copies was observed. At day 3, the number of bacterial DNA copies ($1.6 \pm 0.9 \times 10^7$) significantly ($p = 0.0049$) decreased (75%) to reach 8.11% of initial value at day 6. At day 9, the number of bacterial copies represented only 1.22% of the number found at day 0 (**Figure 2D**) with as many live bacteria as dead (**Figure 2E**). Taken together, these results provide evidence that placental macrophages were able to internalize *C. burnetii* organisms and that they had a microbicidal effect on these bacteria.

C. burnetii Infection and Multinuclear Giant Cell Formation

Because placental macrophages spontaneously form MGCs after culture, we wondered if *C. burnetii* interfered with MGC formation. Placental macrophages were infected with *C. burnetii* (bacterium-to-cell ratio of 50:1) for 4 h (day 0), washed to discard unbound bacteria and the formation of MGCs was quantified from day 0 to day 9. MGC formation was similar in uninfected and *C. burnetii*-infected macrophages (**Figure 3A**), demonstrating that *C. burnetii* did not prevent MGC formation. We then assessed the ability of these MGCs to ingest *C. burnetii*. MGCs formed after 3 days of culture were able to ingest bacteria as demonstrated by confocal imaging (**Figure 3B**). Interestingly, the formation of MGCs and *C. burnetii* DNA copies were significantly correlated ($R^2 = -0.88$, $p = 0.043$) (**Figure 3C**), suggesting that MGCs derived from placental macrophages were involved in *C. burnetii* elimination.

Molecular Mechanism of *C. burnetii* Elimination

To understand how bacteria were eliminated by placental macrophages, we investigated their transcriptional response to *C. burnetii*, and LPS as control, after 6 h of incubation. First, the expression of 8 M1-related genes including *IL-15RA*, *CXCL9*,

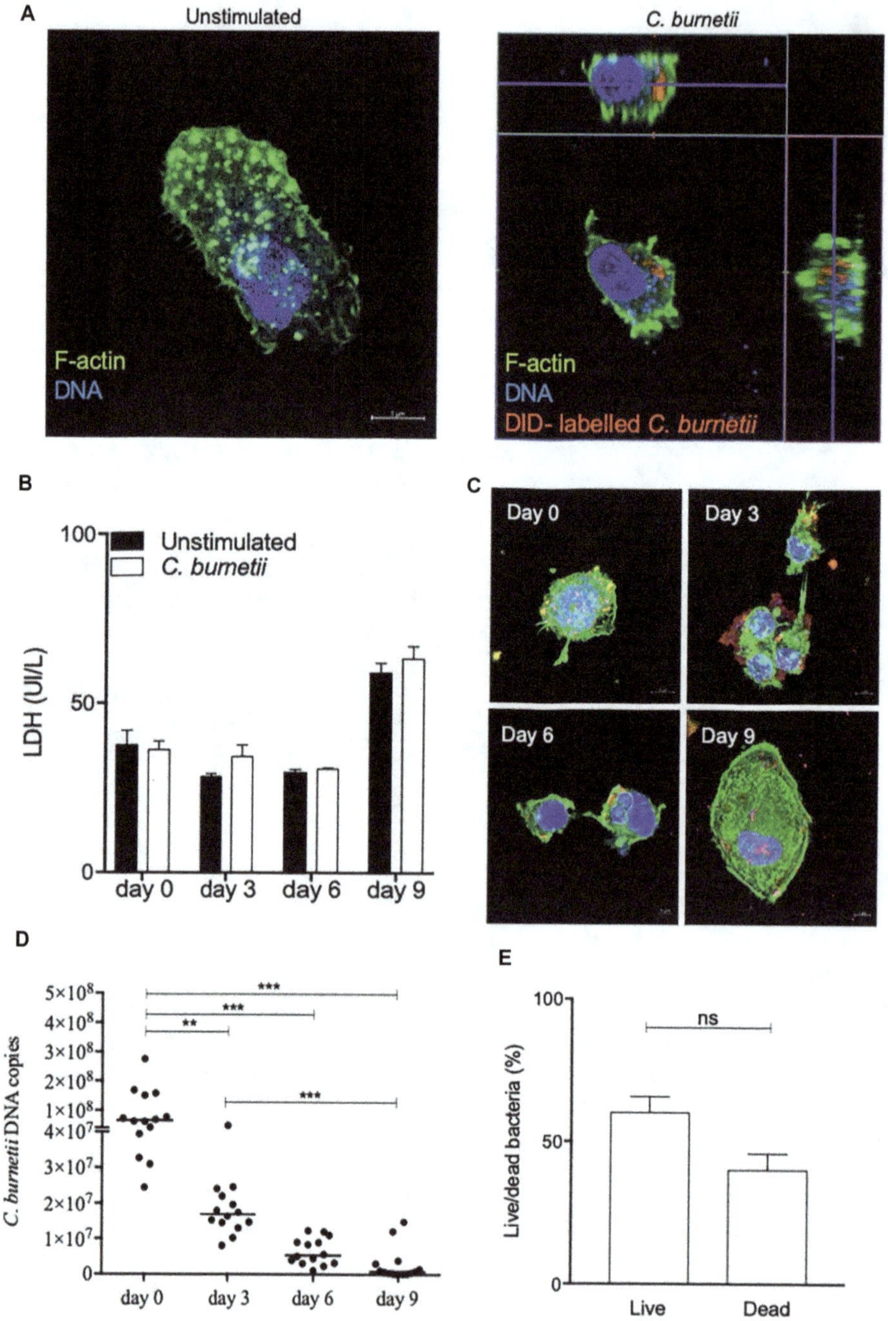

FIGURE 2 | Microbicidal activity of placental macrophages. Placental CD14⁺ macrophages (2×10^6 cells per assay) were infected or not by *C. burnetii* (bacterium-to-cell ratio of 50:1) for 4 h. **(A)** Confocal pictures show placental macrophage infected of not by DID-labeled bacteria. Infected macrophages were illustrated by the sections at the top and the right of the image was bacteria indicated in red, F-actin labeled with phalloidin-488 in green, and nucleus stained with Hoechst 3342 in blue. **(B)** Placental macrophages were incubated with *C. burnetii* for 4 h (day 0), then washed to eliminate free bacteria and incubated for 9 days. Lactate dehydrogenase (LDH) quantification was performed at each time of kinetic time of infection ($n = 4$ placentas). **(C)** Pictures of placental macrophages infected by *C. burnetii* at 0-, 3-, 6- and 9-day post-infection. Bacteria are indicated in red, F-actin labeled with phalloidin-488 in green and nucleus stained with Hoechst 3342 in blue. **(D)** Every 3 days, the number of bacterial DNA copies was evaluated by qPCR ($n = 14$ placentas). $^{**}p \leq 0.01$ and $^{***}p \leq 0.001$. **(E)** Percentage of live/dead bacteria number was evaluated per macrophages at each time (ns = not significant).

EDN1, *IDO1*, *TNF*, *TNFSF10*, *IL-2RA*, and *HESXI* and 10 M2-associated genes including *CLEC4F*, *CCL13*, *SCL4A7*, *CTSC*, *HRH1*, *CHN2*, *CD209*, *ALOX15*, *FN1*, and *CCL23* was evaluated by qRT-PCR. Using a principal component analysis approach of M1 genes, we found that unstimulated and LPS-stimulated macrophages were associated whereas *C. burnetii*-stimulated

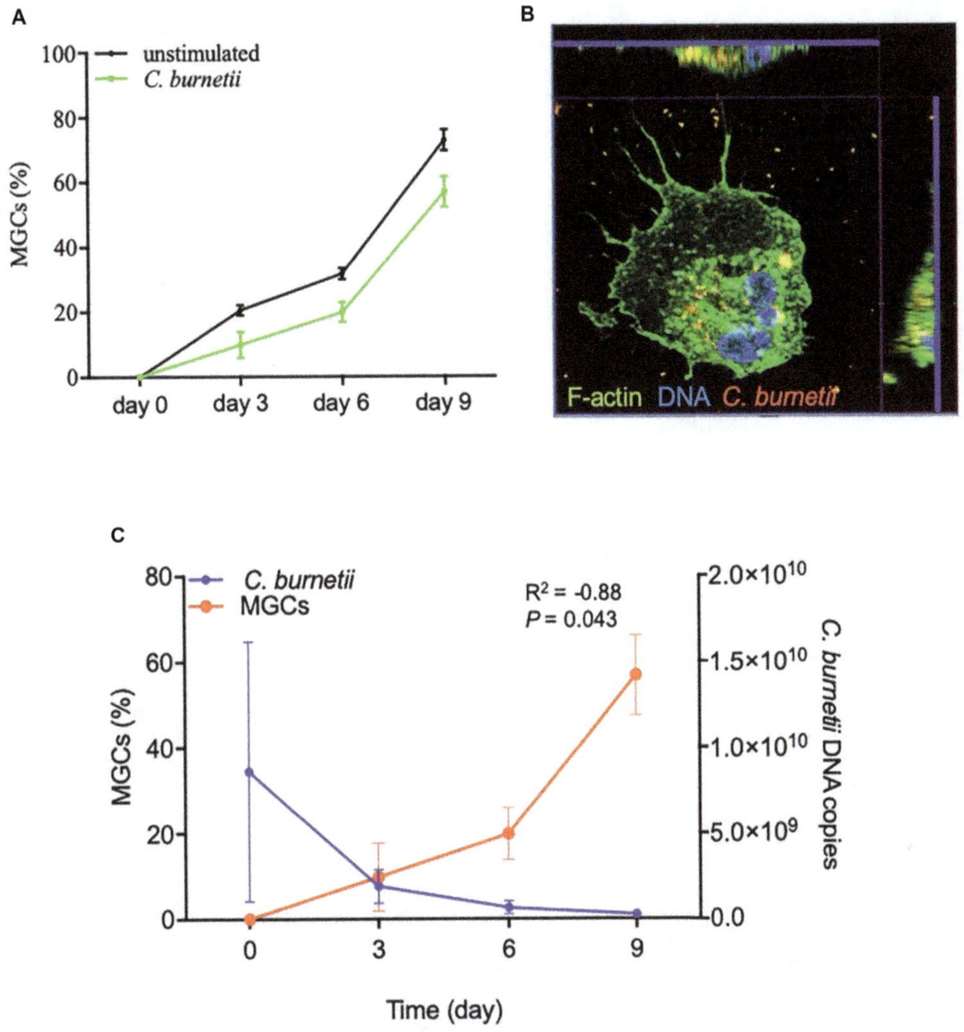

FIGURE 3 | MGC formation and *C. burnetii* infection. Isolated placental macrophages (2×10^5 cells per assay) from eight different placentas were stimulated by *C. burnetii* (bacterium-to-cell ratio of 50:1) for 4 h, then washed to eliminate unbound bacteria and cultivated for 9 days. **(A)** The time course of the number of MGCs was determined by optical determination and the results expressed in percentage of cells presenting at least two nuclei. **(B)** A representative confocal picture is shown after 3 days with F-actin labeled with phalloidin-488 in green, nucleus stained with Hoechst 3342 in blue, and bacteria in red. Intracellular bacteria were observed in the sections found at the top and the right of the image. **(C)** The analyses of MGC formation and *C. burnetii* survival performed using four placentas are correlated ($R^2 = -0.88$, $p = 0.043$).

macrophages were in an eccentric position. In contrast, the expression of M2 genes was strongly interrelated in unstimulated, LPS- and *C. burnetii*-stimulated cells (**Figure 4A**). A hierarchical clustering approach showed that modulated genes of placental macrophages stimulated by *C. burnetii* formed a cluster distinct from those of unstimulated and LPS-stimulated macrophages (**Figure 4B**). M1 genes are found in a different cluster than that of M2 genes, even if they included the *CLEC4F*, *CCL13*, and *SCLC4A7* M2-related genes. Interestingly, *C. burnetii* induced the up-modulation of all M1 genes compared to unstimulated and LPS-stimulated cells. Contrary to *C. burnetii*, LPS stimulation of placental macrophages led to the up-modulation of M2 genes. Taken together, these results demonstrated that *C. burnetii*, and not LPS, induced a M1-type transcriptional profile.

Second, we investigated IFN-γ release by placental macrophages stimulated by *C. burnetii*. Placental macrophages stimulated by *C. burnetii* induced a significant increase of IFN-γ release compared to unstimulated cells ($p = 0.038$, One-way ANOVA) (**Figure 5A**). Then, every 3 days of infection we showed a gradual increase of IFN-γ release over time ($p = 0.0041$, ANOVA Kruskal-Wallis test) (**Figure 5B**), suggesting a key role for this cytokine in cell response to bacterial infection. Finally, while investigating a relationship between IFN-γ release and *C. burnetii* survival, we showed a significant correlation between these two data ($R^2 = -1$, $p = 0.0417$, non-parametric Spearman test) (**Figure 5C**). Collectively, these results suggest that IFN-γ production was correlated with *C. burnetii* elimination.

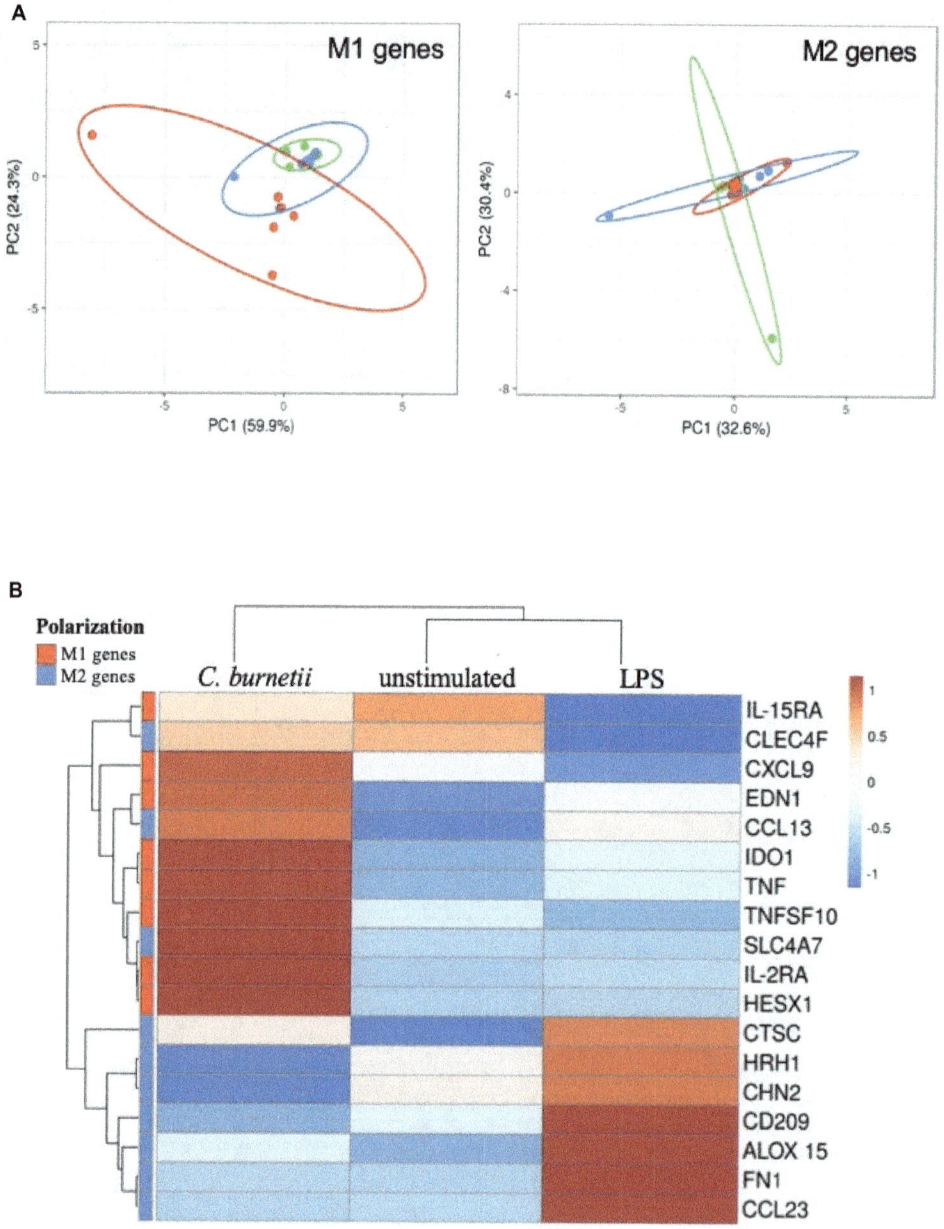

FIGURE 4 | Polarization profile of placental macrophages stimulated by *C. burnetii.* Placental macrophages (1×10^6 cells per assay) were incubated with *C. burnetii* (bacterium-to-cell ratio of 50:1) or 1 µg/ml LPS for 6 h, and their M1/M2 transcriptional response was analyzed by qRT-PCR. **(A)** A principal component analysis showed the repartition of unstimulated placental macrophages (in green, six placentas), *C. burnetii*-stimulated (in red, seven placentas), and LPS-stimulated macrophages (in blue, seven placentas) according to the expression of M1 genes (left panel) and M2 genes (right panel). **(B)** A heat-map analysis showed the modulation of the relative quantity expression of M1 genes (in red) and M2 genes (in blue) when placental macrophages were unstimulated or stimulated by *C. burnetii* or LPS.

DISCUSSION

In the present study, we first characterized CD14⁺ cells isolated from full-term placentas. We found that more than 97% of CD14⁺ placental cells expressed CD68, a marker associated with macrophage differentiation confirming that CD14⁺ placental cells were macrophages, not circulating monocytes (Pinhal-Enfield et al., 2012). Next, we quantified fetal and maternal cells in placental macrophages by genotyping. We found a mixed cell population with maternal and fetal origins, even if the proportion of fetal macrophages seemed to be higher than that of maternal cells. In previous studies, the origin of placental macrophages (Hofbauer cells *versus* decidual macrophages) was based on the location of these cells within the placenta tissue (Reyes and Golos, 2018). These findings highlight the phenotype and origin of placental macrophage populations.

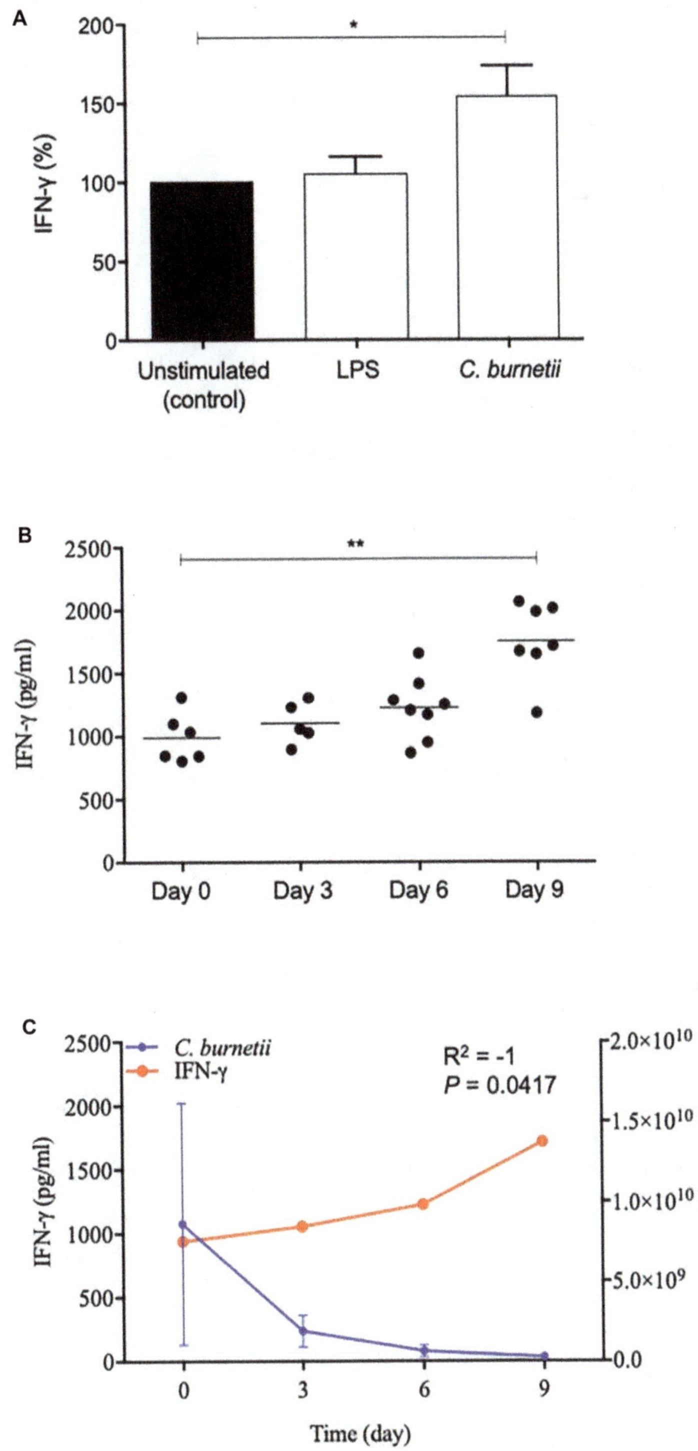

FIGURE 5 | IFN-γ release and *C. burnetii* infection. **(A** and **B)** Placental macrophages (1×10^6 cells per assay) were incubated or not with *C. burnetii* (bacterium-to-cell ratio of 50:1) or 1 μg/ml LPS for 4 h (day 0) and then washed to eliminate free bacteria. The release of IFN-γ was quantified at 0-, 3-, 6-, and 9-day post-infection or unstimulated cells as control when six placentas were used. **(C)** The release of IFN-γ by placental macrophages was correlated with *C. burnetii* survival ($R^2 = -1$, $p = 0.0417$) when four placentas were used. $^*p \leq 0.05$ and $^{**}p \leq 0.01$.

Here, we provided evidence that placental macrophages belong to the target cells for *C. burnetii,* as determined by the efficiency of bacterial uptake. This finding amplifies our previous observations that BeWo trophoblast cell line (Ben Amara et al., 2010) and decidual dendritic cells (Gorvel et al., 2014) are able to internalize *C. burnetii* whereas placental mast cells exhibit a powerful extracellular antimicrobial mechanism against the bacterium (Mezouar et al., 2019c,d). In contrast to BeWo trophoblast cell line, *C. burnetii* was eliminated by macrophages from full-term placentas. The use of macrophages from full-term placentas is consistent with the observation that the risk of fetal infection by *C. burnetii* is higher during the first and second trimesters than during the third trimester (Eldin et al., 2017).

C. burnetii did not prevent the spontaneous formation of MGCs, a peculiar property of placental macrophages (Ben Amara et al., 2013; Belhareth et al., 2018). This is distinct from infectious placental pathologies such as chorioamnionitis in which MGC formation is prevented (Ben Amara et al., 2013). Additionally, MGC formation and *C. burnetii* elimination were correlated, suggesting a microbicidal role of these cells derived from placental macrophages. This hypothesis is supported by the observation that MGCs from other origins can play an anti-microbial role (Enelow et al., 1992; Hernandez-Pando et al., 2000).

It is well known that the functional properties of macrophages including microbicidal activity are controlled by their microenvironment. We found that *C. burnetii* induced a transcriptional program consisting of M1-related genes. Surprisingly, LPS, a powerful M1 agonist of tissue macrophages, rather induced an M2 program, demonstrating that the placental microenvironment governs the inflammatory or the immunoregulatory activity of placental macrophages. This is distinct from our previous results with monocyte-derived macrophages that express an atypical M2 program in response to *C. burnetii* associated with bacterial persistence (Benoit et al., 2008a). We suggest that *C. burnetii* induces a M1 program in placental macrophages that, in turn, plays a role in the elimination of the bacteria.

Interestingly, we showed that two members of the TNF family, including TNF and TNFSF10, were up-modulated by *C. burnetii* infection compared to LPS stimulation. A large variety of anti-microbial responses have been attributed to genes of the TNF family such as direct killing of infected cells, inhibition of intracellular pathogen or induction of apoptosis (Rahman and McFadden, 2006). Here, we found an absence of cell apoptosis and a strong anti-microbial response. The anti-microbial role of TNF has been previously reported using mice model. Indeed, during *C. burnetii* infection TNF deficient mice presented a defect of infection control as for other pathogens such as *Listeria monocytogenes* or *Mycobacterium tuberculosis* (Rahman and McFadden, 2006; Andoh et al., 2007). Interestingly, during pregnancy an excess of TNF production by inflammatory immune cells leads to the abrogation of fetus tolerance and its rejection as observed in pregnant women with *C. burnetii* infection (Chabtini et al., 2013; Eldin et al., 2017). In contrast, other inflammatory cytokines such as IL-1β are not specifically modulated by *C. burnetii* (data not shown). All together these findings suggested that further investigations are needed to clarify the role of genes for TNF family in the placental response during *C. burnetii* infection.

We also found that *C. burnetii* stimulated the release of large amounts of IFN-γ by placental macrophages. IFN-γ is known to be produced by innate lymphoid cells, NK and Th1 cells but tissue macrophages are generally considered as poor producers of IFN-γ. The placental context plays likely an important role in the ability of placental cells to produce IFN-γ. Indeed, trophoblasts produce high levels of type III interferons (Aboagye-Mathiesen et al., 1994; Lee et al., 2001) that are likely to be involved in pregnancy. The role of the IFN-γ produced by placental macrophages remains elusive. Interestingly, the release of IFN-γ by placental macrophages and their microbicidal activity were significantly correlated, suggesting that an autocrine loop could lead to their microbicidal activity. Additionally, IFN-γ was found involved in the increased expression of IDO1 leading to the deprivation of tryptophan, as essential amino acid for bacteria (Nelp et al., 2018). Interestingly, we found an up modulation of IDO1 in *C. burnetii* infected placental macrophages. Indirectly it has been previously reported that this process lead the inhibition of bacterial growth (Pantoja et al., 2000). This result is reminiscent of the observations that the co-culture of decidual macrophages and NK cells increases the production of IFN-γ, which contributes to control the infection of macrophages with HIV (Quillay et al., 2016).

In conclusion, our results showed that macrophages from full-term placentas were resistant to *C. burnetii* infection; such resistance may be related to an autocrine effect of IFN-γ. This study provides new insight into the pathophysiology of Q fever disease at the placenta level and suggests the microbicidal role of MGCs.

AUTHOR CONTRIBUTIONS

SM and J-LM conceived and designed the experiments. SM, IB, AB, and AD performed experiments. CC, JB, and CB performed flow cytometry, genotype, and LDH assay experiments, respectively. SM, IB, AB, and AD analyzed the data. SM, PH, MK, and J-LM supervised the study. SM and J-LM wrote the paper.

ACKNOWLEDGMENTS

The authors thank Dr. Capo for his help and advice for the redaction of the manuscript.

REFERENCES

Aboagye-Mathiesen, G., Tóth, F. D., Zdravkovic, M., and Ebbesen, P. (1994). Production of interferons in human placental trophoblast subpopulations and their possible roles in pregnancy. *Clin. Diagn. Lab. Immunol.* 1, 650–659.

Andoh, M., Zhang, G., Russell-Lodrigue, K. E., Shive, H. R., Weeks, B. R., and Samuel, J. E. (2007). T cells are essential for bacterial clearance, and gamma interferon, tumor necrosis factor alpha, and B cells are crucial for disease development in *Coxiella burnetii* infection in mice. *Infect. Immun.* 75, 3245–3255. doi: 10.1128/IAI.01767-06

Belhareth, R., Mezouar, S., Ben Amara, A., Chartier, C., Azzouz, E. B., Chabrière, E., et al. (2018). Cigarette smoke extract interferes with placenta macrophage functions: a new mechanism to compromise placenta functions? *Reprod. Toxicol.* 78, 120–129. doi: 10.1016/j.reprotox.2018.04.009

Ben Amara, A., Ghigo, E., Le Priol, Y., Lépolard, C., Salcedo, S. P., Lemichez, E., et al. (2010). *Coxiella burnetii*, the agent of Q fever, replicates within trophoblasts and induces a unique transcriptional response. *PLoS One* 5:e15315. doi: 10.1371/journal.pone.0015315

Ben Amara, A., Gorvel, L., Baulan, K., Derain-Court, J., Buffat, C., Vérollet, C., et al. (2013). Placental macrophages are impaired in chorioamnionitis, an infectious pathology of the placenta. *J. Immunol.* 191, 5501–5514. doi: 10.4049/jimmunol.1300988

Benoit, M., Barbarat, B., Bernard, A., Olive, D., and Mege, J.-L. (2008a). *Coxiella burnetii*, the agent of Q fever, stimulates an atypical M2 activation program in human macrophages. *Eur. J. Immunol.* 38, 1065–1070. doi: 10.1002/eji.200738067

Benoit, M., Desnues, B., and Mege, J.-L. (2008b). Macrophage polarization in bacterial infections. *J. Immunol.* 181, 3733–3739. doi: 10.4049/jimmunol.181.6.3733

Brown, M. B., von Chamier, M., Allam, A. B., and Reyes, L. (2014). M1/M2 macrophage polarity in normal and complicated pregnancy. *Front. Immunol.* 5:606. doi: 10.3389/fimmu.2014.00606

Bulmer, J. N., Williams, P. J., and Lash, G. E. (2010). Immune cells in the placental bed. *Int. J. Dev. Biol.* 54, 281–294. doi: 10.1387/ijdb.082763jb

Carcopino, X., Raoult, D., Bretelle, F., Boubli, L., and Stein, A. (2007). Managing Q fever during pregnancy: the benefits of long-term cotrimoxazole therapy. *Clin. Infect. Dis.* 45, 548–555. doi: 10.1086/520661

Chabtini, L., Mfarrej, B., Mounayar, M., Zhu, B., Batal, I., Dakle, P. J., et al. (2013). TIM-3 regulates innate immune cells to induce fetomaternal tolerance. *J. Immunol.* 190, 88–96. doi: 10.4049/jimmunol.1202176

Eldin, C., Mélenotte, C., Mediannikov, O., Ghigo, E., Million, M., Edouard, S., et al. (2017). From Q fever to *Coxiella burnetii* infection: a paradigm change. *Clin. Microbiol. Rev.* 30, 115–190. doi: 10.1128/CMR.00045-16

Enelow, R. I., Sullivan, G. W., Carper, H. T., and Mandell, G. L. (1992). Cytokine-induced human multinucleated giant cells have enhanced candidacidal activity and oxidative capacity compared with macrophages. *J. Infect. Dis.* 166, 664–668.

Fong, G.-H. (2008). Mechanisms of adaptive angiogenesis to tissue hypoxia. *Angiogenesis* 11, 121–140. doi: 10.1007/s10456-008-9107-3

Gorvel, L., Ben Amara, A., Ka, M. B., Textoris, J., Gorvel, J.-P., and Mege, J.-L. (2014). Myeloid decidual dendritic cells and immunoregulation of pregnancy: defective responsiveness to *Coxiella burnetii* and *Brucella abortus*. *Front. Cell. Infect. Microbiol.* 4:179. doi: 10.3389/fcimb.2014.00179

Heikkinen, J., Möttönen, M., Alanen, A., and Lassila, O. (2004). Phenotypic characterization of regulatory T cells in the human decidua. *Clin. Exp. Immunol.* 136, 373–378. doi: 10.1111/j.1365-2249.2004.02441.x

Heikkinen, J., Möttönen, M., Komi, J., Alanen, A., and Lassila, O. (2003). Phenotypic characterization of human decidual macrophages. *Clin. Exp. Immunol.* 131, 498–505. doi: 10.1046/j.1365-2249.2003.02092.x

Hernandez-Pando, R., Bornstein, Q. L., Aguilar Leon, D., Orozco, E. H., Madrigal, V. K., and Martinez Cordero, E. (2000). Inflammatory cytokine production by immunological and foreign body multinucleated giant cells. *Immunology* 100, 352–358. doi: 10.1046/j.1365-2567.2000.00025.x

Houser, B. L. (2012). Decidual macrophages and their roles at the maternal-fetal interface. *Yale J. Biol. Med.* 85, 105–118.

Huang, C.-E., Ma, G.-C., Jou, H.-J., Lin, W.-H., Lee, D.-J., Lin, Y.-S., et al. (2017). Noninvasive prenatal diagnosis of fetal aneuploidy by circulating fetal nucleated red blood cells and extravillous trophoblasts using silicon-based nanostructured microfluidics. *Mol. Cytogenet.* 10:44. doi: 10.1186/s13039-017-0343-3

Joerink, M., Rindsjö, E., van Riel, B., Alm, J., and Papadogiannakis, N. (2011). Placental macrophage (Hofbauer cell) polarization is independent of maternal allergen-sensitization and presence of chorioamnionitis. *Placenta* 32, 380–385. doi: 10.1016/j.placenta.2011.02.003

Ka, M. B., Mezouar, S., Ben Amara, A., Raoult, D., Ghigo, E., Olive, D., et al. (2016). *Coxiella burnetii* induces inflammatory interferon-like signature in plasmacytoid dendritic cells: a new feature of immune response in Q fever. *Front. Cell. Infect. Microbiol.* 6:70. doi: 10.3389/fcimb.2016.00070

Lee, B. N., Hammill, H., Popek, E. J., Cron, S., Kozinetz, C., Paul, M., et al. (2001). Production of interferons and beta-chemokines by placental trophoblasts of HIV-1-infected women. *Infect. Dis. Obstet. Gynecol.* 9, 95–104. doi: 10.1155/S1064744901000175

Loegl, J., Hiden, U., Nussbaumer, E., Schliefsteiner, C., Cvitic, S., Lang, I., et al. (2016). Hofbauer cells of M2a, M2b and M2c polarization may regulate feto-placental angiogenesis. *Reproduction* 152, 447–455. doi: 10.1530/REP-16-0159

Mantovani, A., Biswas, S. K., Galdiero, M. R., Sica, A., and Locati, M. (2013). Macrophage plasticity and polarization in tissue repair and remodelling: macrophage plasticity and polarization in tissue repair and remodelling. *J. Pathol.* 229, 176–185. doi: 10.1002/path.4133

Mezouar, S., Ben Amara, A., Chartier, C., Gorvel, L., and Mege, J.-L. (2019a). A fast and reliable method to isolate human placental macrophages. *Curr. Protoc. Immunol.* 125:e77. doi: 10.1002/cpim.77

Mezouar, S., Ben Amara, A., Vitte, J., and Mege, J.-L. (2018). Isolation of human placental mast cells. *Curr. Protoc. Cell Biol.* 80:e52. doi: 10.1002/cpcb.52

Mezouar, S., and Mege, J.-L. (2018). "Gene expression profiling of placenta from normal to pathological pregnancies" in *Placenta*. ed. A. Gaber (IntechOpen).

Mezouar, S., Omar Osman, I., Melenotte, C., Slimani, C., Chartier, C., Raoult, D., et al. (2019b). High concentrations of serum soluble E-cadherin in patients with Q fever. *Front. Cell. Infect. Microbiol.* 9:219. doi: 10.3389/fcimb.2019.00219

Mezouar, S., Vitte, J., Gorvel, L., Ben Amara, A., Desnues, B., and Mege, J.-L. (2019c). Mast cell cytonemes as a defense mechanism against *Coxiella burnetii*. *MBio* 10. doi: 10.1128/mBio.02669-18

Mezouar, S., Vitte, J., and Mege, J.-L. (2019d). A role for placental mast cells in normal and complicated pregnancy. *Reprod. Immunol. Open Acc.* 3:37.

Nelp, M. T., Kates, P. A., Hunt, J. T., Newitt, J. A., Balog, A., Maley, D., et al. (2018). Immune-modulating enzyme indoleamine 2,3-dioxygenase is effectively inhibited by targeting its apo-form. *Proc. Natl. Acad. Sci.* 115, 3249–3254. doi: 10.1073/pnas.1719190115

Pantoja, L. G., Miller, R. D., Ramirez, J. A., Molestina, R. E., and Summersgill, J. T. (2000). Inhibition of *Chlamydia pneumoniae* replication in human aortic smooth muscle cells by gamma interferon-induced indoleamine 2,3-dioxygenase activity. *Infect. Immun.* 68, 6478–6481. doi: 10.1128/IAI.68.11.6478-6481.2000

Pinhal-Enfield, G., Leibovich, J., and Vas, N. (2012). "The role of macrophages in the placenta" in *Embryology – Updates and highlights on classic topics*. ed. L. V. Pereira (Intechopen).

Pongcharoen, S., Somran, J., Sritippayawan, S., Niumsup, P., Chanchan, P., Butkhamchot, P., et al. (2007). Interleukin-17 expression in the human placenta. *Placenta* 28, 59–63. doi: 10.1016/j.placenta.2006.01.016

Quillay, H., El Costa, H., Duriez, M., Marlin, R., Cannou, C., Madec, Y., et al. (2016). NK cells control HIV-1 infection of macrophages through soluble factors and cellular contacts in the human decidua. *Retrovirology* 13:39. doi: 10.1186/s12977-016-0271-z

Rahman, M. M., and McFadden, G. (2006). Modulation of tumor necrosis factor by microbial pathogens. *PLoS Pathog.* 2:e4. doi: 10.1371/journal.ppat.0020004

Raoult, D., Marrie, T., and Mege, J. (2005). Natural history and pathophysiology of Q fever. *Lancet Infect. Dis.* 5, 219–226. doi: 10.1016/S1473-3099(05)70052-9

Reyes, L., and Golos, T. G. (2018). Hofbauer cells: their role in healthy and complicated pregnancy. *Front. Immunol.* 9:2628. doi: 10.3389/fimmu.2018.02628

Roest, H.-J., van Gelderen, B., Dinkla, A., Frangoulidis, D., van Zijderveld, F., Rebel, J., et al. (2012). Q fever in pregnant goats: pathogenesis and excretion of *Coxiella burnetii*. *PLoS One* 7:e48949. doi: 10.1371/journal.pone.0048949

Shinar, S., Skornick-Rapaport, A., and Rimon, E. (2012). Placental abruption remote from term associated with Q fever infection. *Obstet. Gynecol.* 120, 503–505. doi: 10.1097/AOG.0b013e318260590f

Sobotta, K., Bonkowski, K., Liebler-Tenorio, E., Germon, P., Rainard, P., Hambruch, N., et al. (2017). Permissiveness of bovine epithelial cells from lung, intestine, placenta and udder for infection with *Coxiella burnetii*. *Vet. Res.* 48:23. doi: 10.1186/s13567-017-0430-9

Wang, X.-Q., Zhou, W.-J., Hou, X.-X., Fu, Q., and Li, D.-J. (2018). Trophoblast-derived CXCL16 induces M2 macrophage polarization that in turn inactivates NK cells at the maternal-fetal interface. *Cell. Mol. Immunol.* 15, 1038–1046. doi: 10.1038/s41423-018-0019-x

Zhang, Y.-H., He, M., Wang, Y., and Liao, A.-H. (2017). Modulators of the balance between M1 and M2 macrophages during pregnancy. *Front. Immunol.* 8:120. doi: 10.3389/fimmu.2017.00120

15

Human Placental Trophoblasts Infected by *Listeria monocytogenes* Undergo a Pro-Inflammatory Switch Associated with Poor Pregnancy Outcomes

Lauren J. Johnson[1,2], *Siavash Azari*[1,2], *Amy Webb*[3], *Xiaoli Zhang*[4], *Mikhail A. Gavrilin*[5], *Joanna M. Marshall*[1], *Kara Rood*[6] *and Stephanie Seveau*[1,2,7*]

Department of Microbial Infection and Immunity, The Ohio State University, Columbus, OH, United States, [2] *Department of Microbiology, The Ohio State University, Columbus, OH, United States,* [3] *Department of Biomedical Informatics, The Ohio State University, Columbus, OH, United States,* [4] *Department of Biomedical Informatics, Center for Biostatistics, The Ohio State University, Columbus, OH, United States,* [5] *Pulmonary, Critical Care and Sleep Medicine Division, Department of Internal Medicine, The Ohio State University, Columbus, OH, United States,* [6] *Department of Obstetrics and Gynecology, Division of Maternal Fetal Medicine, The Ohio State University, Columbus, OH, United States,* [7] *Infectious Diseases Institute, The Ohio State University, Columbus, OH, United States*

***Correspondence:**
Stephanie Seveau
seveau.1@osu.edu

The placenta controls the growth of the fetus and ensures its immune protection. Key to these functions, the syncytiotrophoblast (SYN) is a syncytium formed by fusion of underlying mononuclear trophoblasts. The SYN covers the placental surface and is bathed in maternal blood to mediate nutritional and waste exchanges between the mother and fetus. The bacterial pathogen *Listeria monocytogenes* breaches the trophoblast barrier and infects the placental/fetal unit resulting in poor pregnancy outcomes. In this work, we analyzed the *L. monocytogenes* intracellular lifecycle in primary human trophoblasts. In accordance with previous studies, we found that the SYN is 20-fold more resistant to infection compared to mononuclear trophoblasts, forming a protective barrier to infection at the maternal interface. We show for the first time that this is due to a significant reduction in *L. monocytogenes* uptake by the SYN rather than inhibition of the bacterial intracellular division or motility. We here report the first transcriptomic analysis of *L. monocytogenes*-infected trophoblasts (RNA sequencing). Pathway analysis showed that infection upregulated TLR2, NOD-like, and cytosolic DNA sensing pathways, as well as downstream pro-inflammatory circuitry (NF-κB, AP-1, IRF4, IRF7) leading to the production of mediators known to elicit the recruitment and activation of maternal leukocytes (IL8, IL6, TNFα, MIP-1). Signature genes associated with poor pregnancy outcomes were also upregulated upon infection. Measuring the release of 54 inflammatory mediators confirmed the transcriptomic data and revealed sustained production of tolerogenic factors (IL-27, IL-10, IL-1RA, TSLP) despite infection. Both the SYN and mononuclear trophoblasts produced cytokines, but surprisingly, some cytokines were predominantly produced by the SYN (IL-8, IL-6) or by non-fused trophoblasts (TNFα). Collectively, our data support that trophoblasts act as placental gatekeepers that limit and detect *L. monocytogenes* infection resulting in a pro-inflammatory response, which may contribute to the poor pregnancy outcomes if the pathogen persists.

Keywords: trophoblast, fusion, placenta, *Listeria monocytogenes*, infection, inflammation, RNAseq, pregnancy complications

INTRODUCTION

Listeria monocytogenes is a foodborne pathogen that primarily affects the elderly, pregnant women, and immuno-compromised individuals. During pregnancy, the mother generally experiences mild symptoms, but vertical transmission of *L. monocytogenes* occurs *via* breaching the placental barrier leading to fetal death, preterm birth, and severe infections of the newborn (1–7). Several studies support that *L. monocytogenes* enters the placenta *via* infection of epithelial cells that delineate the maternal/fetal interface: the syncytiotrophoblast (SYN) and extravillous trophoblasts (8–11). We studied the interplay between primary human trophoblasts, isolated from term pregnancies, and *L. monocytogenes* to gain understanding of their responses to infection and their potential role in poor pregnancy outcomes.

The placenta is an essential organ that nourishes, protects, and supports the growth of the fetus. Central to these functions, trophoblasts are epithelial cells derived from the outer layer of the blastocyst (trophectoderm) that play key roles in blastocyst implantation in the maternal uterine tissue, in the production of pregnancy hormones, and in placentation. Trophoblasts play essential roles in controlling fetal development and immunity (12). Various trophoblast subtypes specialize in distinct functions. The syncytiotrophoblast (SYN), formed by fusion of underlying mononuclear trophoblasts, is a syncytium that covers the ~12 m^2 surface of chorionic villi and is bathed in maternal blood to allow all nutritional and waste exchanges between mother and fetus (3, 13–16). The SYN also secretes pregnancy hormones and releases extracellular vesicles in maternal blood (17, 18). A second category of trophoblasts, the extravillous trophoblasts, are located at the tip of placental villi, forming columns of mononuclear cells that anchor villi into the maternal endometrium (12). A third type of trophoblasts, the endovascular trophoblasts, which differentiate from extravillous trophoblasts, remodel the maternal spiral arteries that provide the placenta with maternal blood (12). Due to their location at the interface with maternal cells, trophoblasts play critical roles in promoting immune tolerance of the semi-allogeneic fetal cells *via* controlling expression of immune modulatory surface receptors and releasing tolerogenic mediators (19–21).

The SYN has been shown to be less permissive to infection compared to mononuclear trophoblasts, but the underlying mechanisms are not fully elucidated (3, 22). Although the SYN, and other trophoblasts form an effective barrier to infection, some pathogens, such as *Toxoplasma gondii*, Zika virus, herpes simplex virus, cytomegalovirus, and *L. monocytogenes*, can breach this cell barrier with devastating consequences for the developing fetus (16, 22–30). The deleterious effects of infection are not solely due to the presence of the pathogen in the placental-fetal unit, but also derive from its consequential inflammation. Inflammation is a normal manifestation of the anti-infective host responses aimed at eliminating the pathogen, but placental inflammation can be particularly deleterious. Indeed, excessive placental inflammation (placentitis, placental villitis, and chorio-amnionitis) causes preterm birth by mimicking the rise of inflammatory mediators involved in labor and parturition (31–34). Also, misguided placental inflammation can disrupt the immunological tolerance of the semi-allogeneic fetus leading to fetal rejection and abortion (35). Therefore, establishing the trophoblast inflammatory responses to infectious agents and their potential contribution to placental immunity and inflammation is of paramount importance.

L. monocytogenes is a facultative intracellular pathogen that infects professional phagocytes and normally non-phagocytic cells, such as epithelial cells (8). In accordance with the notion that placental pathogens have an intracellular lifestyle, *L. monocytogenes* virulence factors involved in host cell invasion are also critical for placental infection, as demonstrated using small animal models (36–40). These virulence factors include the surface proteins InlA and InlB, which facilitate *L. monocytogenes* internalization into cells that express their receptors: the adherens junction protein E-cadherin and the HGF-receptor c-Met, respectively (8, 41, 42). The secreted pore-forming toxin listeriolysin O (LLO) and the surface protein ActA, are respectively critical for bacterial escape from the phagosome and cell-to-cell spreading. However, LLO and ActA are multifunctional as they both also promote bacterial internalization in some, but not all, host cells (43–45). Several placenta-specific virulence factors were identified including InlP, which is a secreted factor thought to play a role in *L. monocytogenes* crossing of the basement membrane of chorionic villi (46, 47). Placental infection by *L. monocytogenes* is accompanied by placental inflammation, as observed from clinical cases and animal studies (5, 7, 48–50). However, the cell types and mechanisms contributing to inflammation in the placenta have yet to be determined.

In the present work, we isolated primary human trophoblasts from healthy term placentas. These cells spontaneously fuse in cell culture, mimicking the SYN. We also used the human choriocarcinoma BeWo cell line that can fuse upon activation of adenylate cyclase by forskolin, as a surrogate trophoblast model (51, 52). We characterized the *L. monocytogenes* intracellular lifecycle in syncytia (fused) and non-fused trophoblasts to establish molecular mechanisms underlying

SYN resistance to infection. RNA sequencing (RNAseq) of *L. monocytogenes* infected trophoblasts in conjunction with monitoring cellular production of 54 inflammatory mediators established the trophoblast pro-inflammatory circuitry in response to *L. monocytogenes* infection.

MATERIALS AND METHODS

Human Cell Culture, Isolation, Purity, and Fusion Efficiency

Primary human trophoblasts (PHT) were isolated from healthy, singleton, term placentas collected by Caesarean section (OSU Wexner Medical Center, Columbus, Ohio) according to the Institutional Review Board protocol # 2017H0478. A total of 24 placentas were used in the presented studies. Tissue dissection, enzymatic digestion and cell separation were performed as previously described (53). Collected cells were plated at 10^6 cells/1.9 cm^2 (with glass coverslip for microscopy experiments) washed after 12 h to remove non-adherent cells, and cultured in Dulbecco's modified Eagle's medium containing F12 (DMEM/F12 Gibco), GlutaMAX, 10% heat-inactivated fetal bovine serum (HI-FBS, Atlanta Biologicals), 100 U/ml penicillin, and 100 µg/ml streptomycin (Invitrogen) at 37°C in 5% CO_2 humidified cell culture incubator. *Cell purity* was 95 ± 0.9% (n=8) (**Figure S1A**), as measured by fluorescence microscopy after 72 h of culture, which accounts for proliferation of contaminating fibroblasts at the time of all infection procedures carried out in this study. This method was preferred over flow cytometry that measures fluorescence intensities of detached, suspended cells. Indeed, microscopy allows measuring purity of attached cells, avoiding detaching strongly adherent cells and large syncytia, which would have caused major cell damage. For all fluorescence labeling, cells were fixed with 4% paraformaldehyde (PFA) in phosphate buffered saline (PBS) pH 7.4 for 20 min at room temperature (RT) and blocked for 1 h in PBS, 0.1 M glycine and 10% HI-FBS. For purity measurement, cells were co-labeled with primary mouse anti-cytokeratin 7 (Abcam, OV-TL 12/30, 1:100), rabbit anti-vimentin (Abcam, ab16700, 1:200), and secondary antibodies conjugated to Alexa Fluor dyes (Molecular Probes). Coverslips were mounted in Prolong Diamond Antifade (Molecular Probes) containing DAPI to label nuclei. Ten sets of phase-contrast and fluorescence images were randomly acquired, in duplicate, with a 40X objective, corresponding to at least 2200 cells (nuclei) per experiment. Purity was enumerated by counting the number of nuclei in cytokeratin 7 positive cells (trophoblasts, N_c) and in vimentin positive cells (macrophages and fibroblasts, N_v). Trophoblast purity was calculated as follows: $[N_c/(N_c + N_v)] \times 100$. Human chorionic gonadotropin (β-hCG) from cell culture supernatants was measured by ELISA (DRG international) as per manufacturers' instructions (**Figure S1B**). *Syncytia formation* (cell fusion) was also measured by fluorescence microscopy, by fluorescence labeling with mouse anti-E-cadherin (Abcam, HECD-1, 1:100), rabbit anti-cytokeratin 7 (Abcam, ab53123, 1:300), followed by labeling with Alexa Fluor-conjugated secondary antibodies, Alexa Fluor 488-Phalloidin, and DAPI (15, 54). A minimum of 2000 nuclei were counted per experiment and the percentage of cell fusion was calculated based on the number of nuclei in fused (N_f) and non-fused trophoblasts (N_{nf}) as follows: $[N_f/(N_f + N_{nf})] \times 100$. Only cells containing a minimum of three nuclei were considered to be fused. *The human choriocarcinoma cell line BeWo* (ATCC CCL-98) was a kind gift from Dr. John Mitchell Robinson (The Ohio State University, OH, USA). BeWo cells were mycoplasma-free and were authenticated by ATCC by short tandem repeat DNA profiling. BeWo cells were plated in DMEM/F12 supplemented with GlutaMAX plus 10% HI-FBS and penicillin/streptomycin at 5×10^4 cells/cm^2 for fused, and 2.5×10^4 cells/cm^2 for non-fused experimental conditions (55). Fusion was induced after 24 h of culture by daily addition of 20 µM forskolin (FSK, Sigma-Aldrich) for up to 72 h. Cell fusion was measured by β-hCG quantification (**Figure S1B**) by ELISA and by fluorescence microscopy (as described for PHT) at the following time points: 0 (after 24 h of culture), 24, 48, and 72 h after addition of FSK. *HeLa cells* (ATCC CCL-2) were mycoplasma-free and authenticated by ATCC, *via* short tandem repeat DNA profiling. They were plated in 24-well plates at 2×10^5 cells/well 24 h prior to infection in DMEM supplemented with 10% HI-FBS, 100 U/ml penicillin and 100 µg/ml streptomycin at 37°C in 5% CO_2 humidified cell culture incubator.

Listeria monocytogenes Strains and Culture

Wild-type (WT) *L. monocytogenes* (10403S) and isogenic Δ*inlA* (DP-L4405), Δ*inlB* (DP10403S), Δ*hly* (DP-L2161), Δ*actA* (DP-L3078) mutants were gifts from Dr. Daniel Portnoy (UC Berkeley, CA, USA). The isogenic p*actA*-RFP, which expresses the red fluorescent protein under the control of the *actA* promoter, was a gift from Dr. Anna I. Bakardjiev (UC San Francisco, CA, USA) (11). *L. monocytogenes* 10403S, a streptomycin-resistant derivative of strain 10403 (lineage II and serotype 1/2a), was originally isolated from a human skin lesion (56) (57, 58). For invasion assays, bacteria were grown overnight under agitation at 37°C in brain heart infusion broth (BHI; BD Biosciences) until OD_{600} of 0.7-0.9 was reached. Bacteria were washed three times at 37°C and suspended in cell culture medium without serum and antibiotics for infection experiments.

Fluorescence Microscopy Analysis of Trophoblast Invasion by *L. monocytogenes*

PHT and BeWo, cultured in 24-well plates, were infected in duplicate with 10^6 *listeria monocytogenes (Lm)*/well. Cell culture plates were centrifuged at RT for 2 min at 1500 x *g*, incubated 1 h at 37°C, then washed three times and incubated with DMEM/F12, 10% HI-FBS and 15 µg/ml gentamicin for 1 h at 37°C. For bacterial labeling, extracellular and total bacteria were labeled with rabbit anti-*Lm* (GeneTex, 1:100) and anti-rabbit Alexa Fluor-conjugated secondary antibodies as previously described (59). Briefly, extracellular bacteria were first labeled on nonpermeabilized cells with a first fluorochrome; whereas, total bacteria (extracellular plus intracellular) were labeled with a distinct fluorochrome following cell permeabilization with 0.3% Triton-X100. E-cadherin and F-actin (Alexa Fluor-phalloidin, Molecular Probes) labeling were performed in parallel to distinguish fused from non-fused cells. Ten sets of phase-contrast and fluorescence images were randomly acquired, in duplicate (20 image sets) for each experimental condition using a 100X objective. The numbers of total bacteria (N_t), extracellular bacteria (N_e), and DAPI-labeled nuclei (N_n) were enumerated in fused and non-fused cells. Bacterial association efficiency was calculated as N_t/N_n. The internalization efficiency was calculated as $100 \times (N_t - N_e)/N_t$. Typically, 1000 - 2500 host cell nuclei were counted for each experimental condition.

Live-Cell Fluorescence Microscopic Analysis of *L. monocytogenes* Intracellular Division Time and Motility

Trophoblasts were plated at $2x10^6$ cells per 35 mm diameter imaging dish (Ibidi) and cultured at 37°C in 5% CO_2 for 72 h. Cells were infected with *pactA-L. monocytogenes* at MOI of 1 for a total of 5 h (1 h infection, followed by 30 min treatment with 15 µg/ml gentamicin, and 3.5 h incubation in cell culture medium without antibiotics) then washed 3 times with PBS at 37°C. Cells were incubated at 37°C with 0.1X CellMask Deep Red (Invitrogen) plasma membrane dye and Hoechst 33342 (Thermo Scientific) at 0.1 µg/ml for 5 min in cell culture medium without phenol red and supplemented with L-glutamine and HEPES pH 7.4 (imaging medium). Cells were washed 3x with warm PBS and incubated in imaging medium on the microscope stage at 37°C. Fluorescent images were acquired as Z-stacks with the 100X objective every 5 sec for 5 min to measure bacterial motility. Bacteria were tracked through each plane of the Z-stack using the multi-line function of MetaMorph (Molecular Devices). Each plane is considered 5 sec and the total µm/min was calculated based on the total length of each bacterial track through the Z-stack.

To determine 2 h division time, infected areas were chosen with priority given to fused areas. Initial phase-contrast, DSRED (*L. monocytogenes*), CY5 (plasma membrane), and DAPI images were taken for at least four positions to make overlays. Z-stacks of each position in the DSRED color channel were taken at 5 h, 6 h and 7 h. The 2 hour division time was calculated based on the difference between the initial and final DSRED images using the following equations: growth rate (gr) = (ln [N(t)/N(0)])/t and doubling time = ln (2)/gr, where N(t) is the final number of bacteria, N(0) is the initial number of bacteria, and t is the time point in hours.

TLR2 Analyses

TLR2 labeling was performed on fixed and permeabilized cells using rabbit anti-TLR2 (Invitrogen, clone JM22-41, 1:100) primary antibodies. *TLR2 western blot*: 25 µg of protein from cell lysates of infected and non-infected PHT were loaded on a 10% tris-glycine polyacrylamide gel in reduced conditions and analyzed for TLR2 production by immunoblot using rabbit monoclonal antibody to TLR2 (Invitrogen, clone JM22-41, 1:1000) as detected by chemiluminescence for a 60 second exposure time.

L. monocytogenes Trophoblast Invasion Measured by Gentamicin Survival Assay

Cells were cultured in 6-well plates and infected with 8 x 10^6 WT *Lm*/well, centrifuged, and incubated 1 h at 37°C. Cells were then incubated for 30 min with gentamicin (15 µg/ml) and immediately washed and plated (1.5 h sample), or were pulsed with gentamicin for 30 min every 5 hours, for the time points 5, 10, 15, and 24 h. Cells were then washed three times in warm PBS and lysed by incubation with 0.2% Triton X-100 for 5 min at RT followed by plating of serial dilutions of the cell lysates on BHI agar plates for colony forming unit (CFU) determination. Apparent growth rate was calculated as ln $(CFUt/CFUt_0)/(t-t_0)$ and doubling time = ln(2)/gr.

Measurements of Bacterial Actin Tails and Clouds, and Bacterial Length

For measuring the formation of F-actin clouds and comet tails on cytosolic *L. monocytogenes*, PHT and HeLa cells, cultured in 24-well plates with glass coverslips, were infected with 10^6 bacteria/well *pactA*-RFP *L. monocytogenes* for 1 h, followed by 30 min treatment with gentamicin, and 3.5 h incubation in cell culture medium without antibiotic. E-cadherin (only performed on trophoblasts) and F-actin fluorescence labeling were performed on fixed and TX-100 permeabilized cells. *For measuring the length of intracellular L. monocytogenes*, PHT were infected in duplicate in 24 well plate, with 10^5 bacteria/well WT *L. monocytogenes* for 1 h, washed and incubated with gentamicin for 30 min. Cells were then continuously incubated with gentamicin for 24 h (no pulse), or cells were pulsed for 30 min with gentamicin every 5 hours. After 24 h, E-cadherin and bacteria were labeled as described above. Twenty sets of images were acquired per experimental condition. MetaMorph was used to measure the length in µm of RFP-fluorescent bacteria.

RNA Extraction and RNAseq Using the Illumina Platform NovaSeq SP Flowcell

PHT and BeWo cells were infected, or not, in 6 well-cell culture plates with 4 x 10^6 WT *Lm*/well for 1 h followed by 30 min gentamicin, and 3.5 h in gentamicin-free medium (5 h samples). Cells were pulsed with gentamicin for 30 min after 5 hours infection, and incubated in gentamicin free medium for another 5 hours (10 hours samples). Cells were lysed in TRIzol reagent (Invitrogen). PureLink RNA extraction kit with on-column DNase treatment (Invitrogen) was used to isolate RNA. Input RNA integrity number (RIN) were all > 7 and concentration was >100 ng/µl RNA, as determined with the Agilent 2100 Bioanalyzer (Agilent Technologies, Santa Clara, CA) and Qubit Fluorometer (Thermo Fisher). RNA-seq libraries were generated with NEBNext® Ultra™ II Directional RNA Library Prep Kit for Illumina (NEB #E7760L) and NEBNext® rRNA Depletion Kit with sample purification beads (NEB #E6350) with an input amount of 200 ng total RNA per sample. Libraries were pooled and sequenced on an Illumina NovaSeq SP flowcell in paired-end 150 bp format (Illumina, San Diego, CA) to a read yield between 70-80 million reads (equivalent to 35- 40 million clusters). Three independent experiments were performed to compare infected to non-infected, PHT and FSK-treated or not, BeWo cells.

RNAseq Data Analyses

Raw fastq was aligned to human reference genome GRCh38 with hisat2 v2.1.0 (60, 61). Alignment QC was assessed by RSeQC. Gene wise counts were generated with featureCounts from the subread package v1.5.1 for genes annotated by Ensembl GRCh38.92 (62). Counts normalization and differential expression were performed with edgeR using a negative binomial distribution with a generalized linear model with a paired design (63). Genes were tested if at least half of the samples had an expression of 2 counts per million (CPM). Significant genes were defined as those with a false discovery rate (FDR) < 0.05 and absolute value (log2FC) > 1. The fold change of a gene was considered positive when its CPM was higher in *L. monocytogenes*-infected cells than in non-infected cells. Heatmaps were generated in R using package ComplexHeatmap. GO term and KEGG enrichment were performed with DAVID 6.8 for genes that were differentially expressed (64, 65). Pathway analysis was performed in Ingenuity Pathway Analysis.

Quantitative Real-Time PCR

Cells were lysed in TRIzol and total RNA was isolated using PureLink RNA extraction kit with on-column DNase treatment (Invitrogen). Total RNA was quantified by spectrophotometry with a NanoDrop 2000 (Thermo Scientific) and 1-3 ug total RNA from each sample were reverse-transcribed into cDNA by ThermoScript RNase H^- reverse transcriptase (Invitrogen Life Sciences). Quantitative real-time PCR was performed using an equal amount of cDNA per sample on a Bio-Rad CFX Real-Time PCR Detection System, using primer sets specific to *IFNL1, IFNL2, IFNL3, TNF, IL1B, IL6, IL8*, and *IL10* with iQ SYBR Green Supermix. Primers were designed using an algorithm which we described earlier (66). Clustal Muscle 3.8 alignment for IFNL genes was used to verify specificity of primers. Primer's efficiency was calculated using the following equation: $E=10^{(-1/slope)}$. Gene expression was analyzed with the Bio-Rad CFX Maestro Software. Relative copy numbers (RCN) of selected genes of interest were normalized to the expression of two housekeeping genes (GAPDH and CAP-1) using the following equation: $RCN = E^{-\Delta Ct} \times 100$, where E is the efficiency of PCR and ΔCt is the $Ct_{(target)} - Ct_{(reference)}$ (reference=average of the two housekeeping genes) (66, 67).

Cytokine Array and Lambda Interferon ELISA

Cell culture supernatants were collected from infected and control non-infected PHT, and FSK-treated or not BeWo cells. Supernatants were immediately centrifuged and frozen at -80°C. Thawed samples were pooled from three independent experiments and cytokine production was measured using the V-PLEX Human Biomarker 54-Plex Kit (Meso Scale Discovery). IFNL1, IFNL2, and IFNL3 ELISAs were performed using the human IL-29 (DY7246), IL-28A (DY1587), and IL-28B (DY5259) DuoSet ELISA kits (R&D Systems) per the manufacturer's instructions.

Colocalization of Cytokines (IL-8, IL-6, TNFα) With Fused and Non-Fused Trophoblasts

Primary mouse anti-IL-6 (R&D Systems, clone #1936, 1:33) and anti-IL-8 (R&D Systems, clone #6217, 1:33) antibodies were used in combination with secondary fluorescent antibodies to label infected PHT following PFA fixation and permeabilization by 0.3% TX-100. To distinguish fused from non-fused PHT, cells were colabelled using primary rabbit and βhCG (Abcam) and secondary fluorescent antibodies. Primary rabbit anti-TNFα (a gift from Dr. Mark Wewers, The Ohio State University, 1:100) (68) and mouse anti-E-cadherin antibodies were used with secondary fluorescent antibodies to label infected PHT following PFA fixation and permeabilization by 0.3% TX-100. Cytosolic *L. monocytogenes* expressed RFP and the dye DAPI was added post-fixation to visualize the host cell nuclei. The specificity of cytokine labeled was ensured by performing labeling with isotype control antibodies in parallel experiments, which led to low level background fluorescence. At least 30 sets of fluorescence images (RFP-*Lm*, DAPI, GFP-E-cadherin or -βhCG, far-red-cytokine) were acquired in each experimental condition (each image includes ~ 300 host cell nuclei). Colocalization experiments between the cytokine and fusion marker (E-cadherin or βhCG), using the MetaMorph software, were performed on background corrected fluorescence images, and a threshold was applied to analyze the cytokine integrated fluorescence intensity relative to cell areas covered (colocalization), or not (segregation), by βhCG (highlights fused cells) or by E-cadherin (highlights non-fused cells). Data were expressed as average percentage colocalization ± SEM of one representative experiment (of 3 independent experiments with 3 placentas).

Microscope Equipment

Images were acquired on a motorized, atmosphere-controlled inverted wide-field fluorescence microscope (Axio Observer D1, TempModule S1, Heating Unit XL S; Zeiss) equipped with a PZ-2000 XYZ series automated nano stage (Applied Scientific Instruments), 20X Plan Neofluar (numerical aperture [NA] = 0.5), 40X Plan Neofluar (NA = 1.3), and 100x Plan Apo (NA = 1.4) objective lenses, a high-speed Xenon fluorescence emission device (Lambda DG-4, 300 W; Sutter Instrument Company), a Lambda 10-3 optical emission filter wheel for fluorescence imaging, a SmartShutter to control the illumination for phase-contrast imaging (Sutter Instrument Company), a back-illuminated, frame-transfer electron-multiplying charge-coupled device (EMCCD) camera (Cascade II:512; Photometrics), and an ORCA-FLASH 4.0 V2 digital complementary metal-oxide –semiconductor camera

(Hamamatsu). The filter sets for fluorescence were purchased from Chroma Technology Corporation and were as follows: DAPI (49000), Alexa Fluor 488 (49002), Alexa Fluor 568 (49005), and Cy5 (49006). Images were acquired and analyzed using MetaMorph imaging software (Molecular Devices).

Statistical Methods

All experimental work involved at least three independent experiments, each performed in duplicate. All statistical analyses were performed using GraphPad Prism 7 and 8. Secretion of hCG, bacterial association, bacterial internalization, and fusion percentages were presented as mean ± SEM. Statistical significance of association, internalization, and fusion was determined by linear mixed effects models and p-values were adjusted with Holm-Sidak's procedure, unless otherwise stated. For ELISA analysis, data were first normalized to internal controls or the loading standard to reduce variation before analysis. Statistical methods are indicated in figure legends, n indicates the number of independent experiments (each involving a different placenta).

RESULTS

InlA- and ActA-Mediated *L. monocytogenes* Uptake Are Ineffective in Syncytia

Two cell culture models were used to establish the mechanisms that confer syncytia enhanced resistance to *L. monocytogenes* infection in comparison to non-fused trophoblasts: (1) primary human mononuclear trophoblasts obtained from term placentas (PHT), which spontaneously form syncytia in culture, and (2) the BeWo cell line that forms syncytia upon forskolin (FSK) treatment (**Figure 1**) (52, 69). Syncytia formation was measured as the percentage of fused cells defined as cells with three or more nuclei, based on visualization of intercellular junctions (E-cadherin labeling) and number of nuclei per cell (DAPI labeling) (**Figures 1A, B**). PHT cultured for 72 h and BeWo cells treated with FSK for 48 h reached a similar percentage of fusion (~50%)(**Figure 1C**); therefore, these cell culture conditions were used in all experiments presented in this article. BeWo cells (FSK-treated or not) and PHT were infected for 1 h with isogenic wild-type (WT), Δ*inlA*, Δ*inlB*, Δ*hly*, and Δ*actA* *L. monocytogenes*. After chemical fixation and fluorescent labeling of bacteria and trophoblasts, the efficiencies of *L. monocytogenes* association and internalization into syncytia versus non-fused trophoblasts were measured by fluorescence microscopy (**Figure 2A**). Data showed that syncytia are significantly less susceptible (~20-fold) to *L. monocytogenes* infection than non-fused trophoblasts, as previously reported (**Figures 2B–E**) (70). As expected, this drastic decrease in syncytia invasion is primarily due to the significant decrease in InlA/E-cadherin-mediated *L. monocytogenes* invasion (8). We then dissected if the InlA/E-cadherin interaction mediates bacterial attachment and/or internalization. Not surprisingly, we found that bacterial association to non-fused PHT, which express high levels of E-cadherin, is InlA-dependent; whereas, WT and Δ*inlA* similarly display low association to syncytia, which express faint E-cadherin levels (**Figures 1B, 2B**). However, InlA/E-cadherin interaction did not play a role in bacterial internalization into PHT (**Figure 2C**). We show that *L. monocytogenes* internalization efficiency is significantly decreased in syncytia in comparison to non-fused cells (**Figures 2C, E**). We identified a significant role for ActA in bacterial internalization into non-fused PHT, but this role was no longer significant in syncytia (**Figure 2E**). Using the BeWo cell model, we observed that InlA controlled both *L. monocytogenes* association and internalization, whereas no role for ActA was observed in this cell line (**Figure S2**). Also, no role for LLO or InlB in *L. monocytogenes* association and internalization was observed in PHT or BeWo cells, as we and others previously reported with this bacterial strain (data not shown) (36, 71). In conclusion, our studies support that both InlA and ActA play a significant role in promoting *L. monocytogenes* uptake by mononuclear trophoblasts, but this role is lost in the SYN. The cell line BeWo does not constitute a model for the study of the role of ActA in trophoblast invasion, which highlights the importance of working with primary cells.

L. monocytogenes Cytosolic Doubling Time Is Similar in Syncytia and Non-Fused Trophoblasts

To evaluate the *L. monocytogenes* intracellular doubling time, a gentamicin survival assay was performed in PHT and BeWo cells infected for up to 24 h (**Table 1**). The bacterial load (CFUs) reached a plateau as early as 10 h post-infection, which reflects that cells were over-infected and/or became permeable to the antibiotic gentamicin used to kill extracellular bacteria. Comparison of CFUs between 1.5 h and 5 h infection led to the calculation of an apparent intracellular doubling time: 70.8 min ± 5.0 (SEM) in PHT, 69.0 min ± 5.5 (SEM) in FSK-treated BeWo, and 64.3 min ± 3.8 (SEM) in control non-fused BeWo cells. Because this method could not distinguish syncytia from non-fused cells in PHT, we also measured the bacterial doubling time by live-cell fluorescence microscopy. PHT were infected with p*actA*-RFP *L. monocytogenes*, which expresses the red fluorescent protein under the control of a promoter that is only active when bacteria have reached the cytosol (11). In these experiments, after 5 h of infection in the absence of gentamicin, cells were transferred to the atmosphere-controlled microscope, and the fluorescent dyes CellMask Deep Red and Hoechst 33342, were added to label the host cell plasma membrane and nuclei, respectively, thereby allowing us to distinguish fused from non-fused cells (**Figure S3**). We found, by counting the number of RFP-positive bacteria between 5 h and 7 h of infection, that the average doubling times of *L. monocytogenes* were similar in fused [190.0 min ± 39.4 (SEM)] and non-fused PHT [199.4 min ± 29.6 (SEM)](**Figure 3**). Surprisingly, we observed by fluorescence microscopy that a proportion of intracellular *L. monocytogenes* were elongated in both fused and non-fused PHT after 10 h of infection, which may be a manifestation of bacterial stress (72). This was not observed in extracellular bacteria or in BeWo cells, regardless of their fusion status and infection time, for up to 24 h (data not shown). To determine the potential contribution of

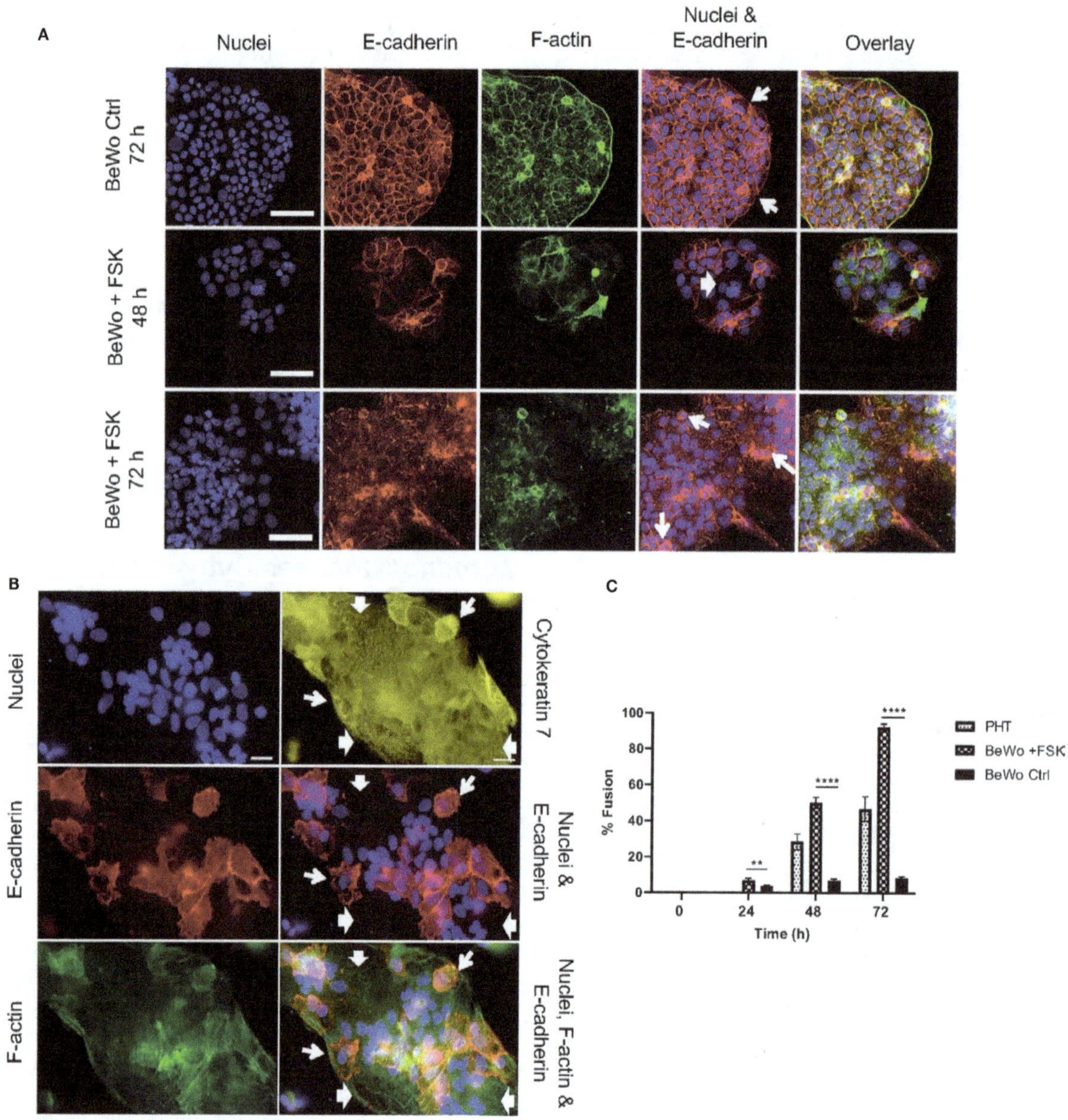

FIGURE 1 | Trophoblast culture models. **(A)** BeWo cells were cultured 24 h prior to daily treatment with 20 μM forskolin (BeWo +FSK), or with 0.1% control DMSO (BeWo Ctrl), for up to 72 h. Cells were fixed and fluorescently labeled to visualize nuclei (DAPI), F-actin (phalloidin-Alexa Fluor 568), and intercellular junctions (E-cadherin, Alexa Fluor 488-conjugated antibodies). Fluorescence images were acquired with a 20X objective (scale bar = 100 μm). **(B)** Primary human trophoblasts (PHT) were cultured for 72 h before fixation and fluorescence labeling to visualize nuclei (DAPI), intercellular junctions (E-cadherin, Alexa Fluor 568-conjugated antibodies), F-actin (phalloidin-AlexaFluor 488), and trophoblasts (cytokeratin 7, Alexa Fluor 647-conjugated antibodies). Fluorescence images were acquired with a 40X objective (scale bar = 50 μm). In **(A, B)**, wide arrows highlight examples of fused cells visualized by the absence of E-cadherin and the presence of multiple nuclei. Narrow arrows highlight some mononuclear non-fused cells delineated by continuous E-cadherin junctions. **(C)** PHT were analyzed after 48 h and 72 h of culture and BeWo cells were analyzed 0, 24, 48, and 72 h after FSK treatment. At least 2,000 – 3,000 nuclei were counted per experimental condition. Data are expressed as Percent Cell Fusion ± SEM. Statistical significance was determined using the Two-stage linear step-up procedure of Benjamini, Krieger and Yekutieli, with Q = 1%. Each row was analyzed individually, without assuming a consistent SD. **P = 0.0083, ****P < 0.000001 (n = 4 placentas for PHT, n = 3 for BeWo).

gentamicin, we measured the length of intracellular *L. monocytogenes* in PHT infected for 24 h, either continuously exposed to gentamicin or subjected to 30 min gentamicin pulses every 5 h (**Figure S4**). We found that the proportion of elongated bacteria was lower when cells were pulsed with gentamicin, reflecting that penetration of the antibiotic into the PHT could account for bacterial elongation, at least partially. In conclusion, *L. monocytogenes* intracellular doubling time is similar in the SYN

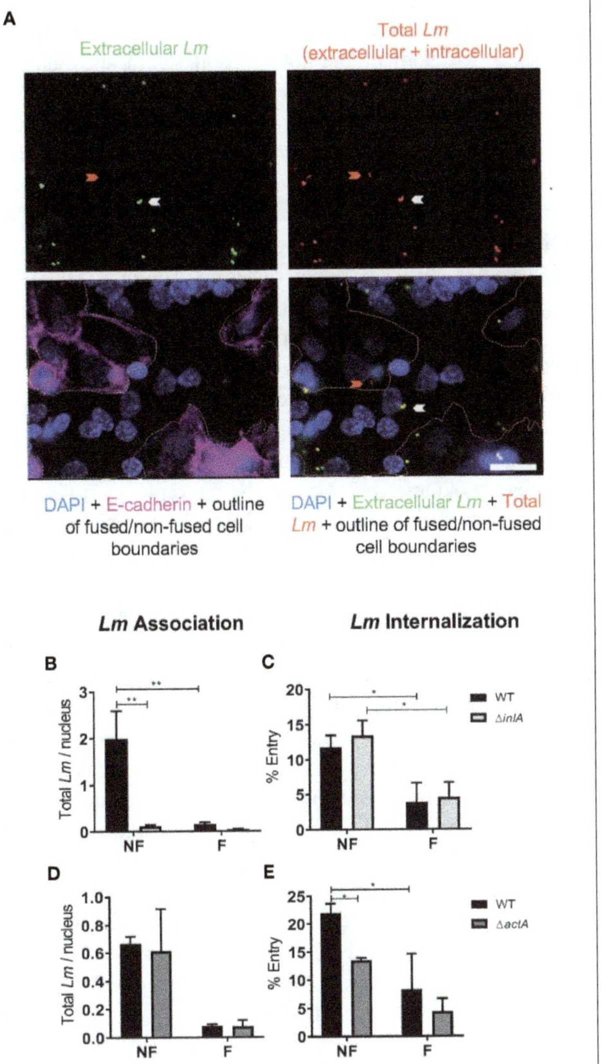

FIGURE 2 | *L. monocytogenes* association and internalization into primary human trophoblasts. PHT were infected with isogenic *L. monocytogenes* (*Lm*) WT, Δ*inlA*, or Δ*actA* at MOI 1 **(A–C)** or 0.5 **(D, E)** for 1 h at 37°C. Cells were washed, fixed and labeled to enumerate bacterial association and internalization into fused (F) and non-fused (NF) trophoblasts by fluorescence microscopy. Ten fields of phase-contrast and fluorescence images (DAPI, total *Lm*-Alexa Fluor 488, extracellular *Lm*-Alexa Fluor 568, and E-cadherin-Alexa Fluor 647) were randomly acquired from duplicate slides (20 image sets), for each experimental condition using a 100X objective. **(A)** Representative images. The red arrow points towards an intracellular *Lm* within a non-fused trophoblast. The white arrow points towards an extracellular *Lm* on a fused cell. A white outline was drawn on the overlay images to delineate the boundaries between non-fused and fused trophoblasts. Scale bar = 20 µm. **(B–E)** The numbers of total *Lm* (Nt), extracellular *Lm* (Ne), and DAPI-labeled host cell nuclei (Nn) were counted in fused and non-fused PHT. *Lm* Association **(B, D)** was calculated as Nt/Nn. *Lm* Internalization **(C, E)** was calculated as [(Nt – Ne)/Nt] x 100. Data are expressed as the average ± SEM (**B, C** n = 5) of 3 independent experiments (3 placentas) (**D, E** n = 3). Statistical significance was determined by 2-way ANOVA. P-values were adjusted using Holm-Sidak's multiple comparisons test, **P = 0.0024, *P = 0.0266 **(B, C)**; *P = 0.0304, 0.0486 **(E)**. All cell counts corresponding to data analysis of **Figure 2** are summarized in **Figure S9**.

and mononuclear trophoblasts (in PHT and BeWo) at least for the first 7 hours of infection. Interestingly, we observed that the division time significantly increases after 5 h of infection independently of the cell fusion status. In parallel, we observed bacterial elongation after 10 h of infection, but this phenotype was influenced, at least partially, by the presence of gentamicin in the cell culture medium.

The Proportion of Motile *L. monocytogenes* and the Average Bacterial Speeds Are Similar in Syncytia and Non-Fused Trophoblasts

ActA-mediated *L. monocytogenes* intracellular motility, *via* the assembly of the host actin cytoskeleton at one bacterial pole, promotes *L. monocytogenes* spreading from cell-to-cell (45). Because PHT syncytialization is paralleled with a decrease in actin stress fibers and an increase in the G-/F-actin ratio, we hypothesized that *L. monocytogenes* motility could be altered in syncytia (15, 69). We thus measured if *L. monocytogenes* could nucleate host actin as efficiently in syncytialized and non-fused PHT. As a control, we used HeLa cells in which *L. monocytogenes* motility has been extensively studied (73–75). PHT and HeLa cells were infected with p*actA*-RFP *L. monocytogenes*. In these assays, cells were treated with gentamicin for 30 min following infection and were then cultured in gentamicin-free medium for the remaining 3.5 h. After fixation and labeling, the percentage of cytosolic bacteria that could recruit actin clouds or comet tails was enumerated by fluorescence microscopy (**Figure 4A**). About 20% of RFP-expressing bacteria formed comet tails in PHT, similar to HeLa cells (**Figure 4B**). However, there was a significant difference in the percentages of bacteria decorated with actin clouds (about 44% in PHT and 65% in HeLa) and bacteria devoid of an actin coat (about 36% in PHT and 14% in HeLa). In syncytia, the percentage of actin tails was lower and the percentage of clouds higher in comparison to non-fused PHT, but these differences did not reach statistical significance (**Figure 4C**). As a more accurate method to assess bacterial motility, we measured cytosolic speed of RFP-expressing *L. monocytogenes* by live-cell fluorescence imaging 5 h post-infection. We found that the percentage of non-motile versus motile bacteria was 76.2% ± 2.9 vs 23.8% ± 2.9, respectively in non-fused and 74% ± 15.4 vs. 26% ± 15.4 in syncytia (n=4 placentas), confirming data obtained from fixed cells. The average speed of motile bacteria was also similar in syncytia and non-fused PHT (**Figure 4D**). Collectively, our data support that the barrier function of the SYN operates *via* blocking *L. monocytogenes* entry into the SYN, but not bacterial intracellular proliferation or motility, at least during the first 7 h of infection.

Transcriptome of Primary Trophoblasts Infected by *L. monocytogenes* Reveals a Pro-Inflammatory Switch With Upregulated Signature Genes Associated With Pregnancy Complications

We performed RNAseq analysis to determine how *L. monocytogenes* infection for 5 h affects the trophoblast transcriptome. Three

TABLE 1 | Gentamicin survival assay.

Time (h)	PHT	BeWo (+FSK)	BeWo (control)
1.5	4.3E6 ± 2.2E6	1.4E6 ± 7.2E5	2.7E6 ± 9.8E5
5	3.6E7 ± 1.6E7	1.1E7 ± 3.8E6	2.5E7 ± 4.7E6
10	2.5E7 ± 8.3E6	3.3E7 ± 3.9E6	2.8E7 ± 5.8E6
15	3.5E7 ± 1.6E7	2.5E7 ± 2.6E6	7.6E6 ± 7.1E6
24	1.1E7 ± 3.8E6	8.4E6 ± 2.9E6	1.4E6 ± 2.3E5

PHT and BeWo cells were infected with WT L. monocytogenes (MOI 1) for 1 h at 37°C followed by a 30 min incubation with gentamicin. Cells were washed and incubated for a total of 1.5, 5, 10, 15, and 24 h including 30 min gentamicin pulses performed every 5 h. Data are presented as the average CFUs/ml ± SEM (n = 3). Based on CFUs between 1.5 and 5 h, apparent doubling time from 1.5 to 5 h for PHT was 70.8 ± 5.0 min, for Fused BeWo 69.0 ± 5.5 min, and for Non-Fused (control) BeWo 64.3 ± 3.8 min.

independent experiments involving 3 different placentas were performed comparing infected to non-infected PHT. In parallel, we analyzed infected and non-infected FSK-treated and control BeWo cells (**Figures 5A, B**). We found that among the 12,275 detected PHT genes, corresponding to genes which expression was at least 2 counts per million (CPM) in half of the samples, a total of 385 genes were differentially expressed (DEG) upon infection (**Figures 5C, D**). These include 359 upregulated genes, whereas only 26 genes were downregulated. DEGs were defined as genes with $\log_2$ (FC) >1 or <-1, and FDR-adjusted $P < 0.05$ comparing non-infected and infected cells at time point 5 h. In contrast, FSK treatment, but not infection, significantly affected the BeWo cell transcriptome (**Figure 5B**). Importantly, RNAseq data were validated by real-time quantitative polymerase chain reaction (RT-qPCR) analysis of a collection of DE cytokine genes using 5 h infected versus non-infected trophoblasts (PHT isolated from 3 additional placentas and independent BeWo cell samples) (**Tables S1, S2**). As a first analysis of the transcriptomic changes, PHT DEG were grouped into functional categories (**Figures 5C, D**). The largest category of genes controls inflammation and immune functions (31% of total upregulated and 23% of total downregulated genes). The prevalence of immune genes was also illustrated by the top 50 DE protein-coding genes, defined as the highest absolute $\log_2$FC values, (**Table 2**), 76% of which have inflammatory and immune functions, with 60% of genes encoding cytokines, chemokines, their receptors and regulators. The second largest category includes genes controlling cell signaling (14% of upregulated and 27% of downregulated DEGs). The third category includes genes encoding transcription factors and co-activators, and enzymes controlling the epigenome (13% of upregulated and 19% of downregulated DEGs). We found that 41 upregulated DE genes encode transcriptional regulators (**Table S3**). Additional upregulated DEGs are involved in the regulation of apoptosis, metabolism, and the cytoskeleton. Of note, genes involved in cell signaling, transcription, and other categories cited above, include genes regulating immune responses, thereby leading to an underestimation of the overall proportion of genes involved in immune functions.

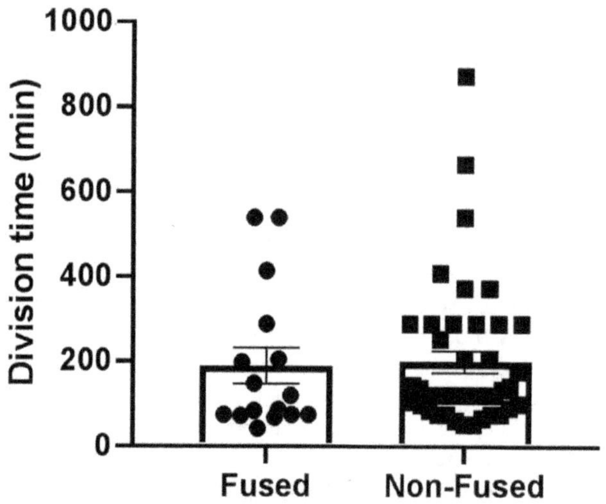

FIGURE 3 | *L. monocytogenes* cytosolic doubling time. PHT were plated in 35 mm diameter imaging dishes at $2x10^6$ cells/dish and cultured for 72 h. Cells were infected with pactA-RFP *L. monocytogenes* at MOI 1 for 5 h. Cells were transferred to the temperature-controlled microscope stage. The plasma membrane was labeled with CellMask Deep Red dye and the nuclei with Hoechst 33342 (**Figure S3**). At least four fields of view of infected fused and infected non-fused PHT were selected and memorized. Initial sets of phase-contrast and fluorescence (RFP, DAPI, Deep Red) images were acquired immediately and at 1 h time intervals at the four positions for 2 hours. Z-stacks of the fluorescent bacteria were acquired to facilitate bacterial counting in 3D. Division time was calculated based on the difference between the initial and final DSRED images using the following equations: growth rate (gr) = (ln [N(t)/N(0)])/t and doubling time = ln (2)/gr, where N(t) is the final number of bacteria, N(0) is the initial number of bacteria, and t is the time point in hours. (n = 3 placentas).

We then performed gene enrichment and functional annotation analysis to gain understanding of specific pathways affected in PHT upon *L. monocytogenes* infection. We used the DAVID Bioinformatics Resources (6.8, NIAID/NIH DAVID) to analyze the 330 upregulated protein-coding genes. The top biological processes (BP) were identified using P value and FDR<0.05, EASE value of 0.05 (**Table 3**). The BP were dominated by immune responses, inflammation, positive regulation of transcription, signal transduction, and negative regulation of apoptosis, which are in accordance with the gene functional categories reported in **Figure 5C**. The molecular functions also highlighted transcriptional regulation and cytokine-based signaling (**Table 3**). The Kyoto Encyclopedia of Genes and Genomes (KEGG) pathway analysis (P value and FDR<0.05, ease value 0.05) allowed us to identify the most significant immune signaling pathways (**Table 3**). Consistent with the detection of Gram-positive bacteria by pattern recognition receptors, these pathways include toll-like receptor and NOD-like signaling. The most significant pathways included bacterial detection *via* TLR2 leading to the transcriptional activation of genes such as CXCL8, CCL3, and CCL4 (among others) that encode potent neutrophil and monocyte chemokines, and genes encoding the pro-inflammatory cytokines TNFα, IL-6, and IL-1β (**Figure S5A**). This finding is in accordance with the expression of TLR2 by fused and non-fused PHT and on the SYN and trophoblasts of human placentas, as previously demonstrated by others (**Figures**

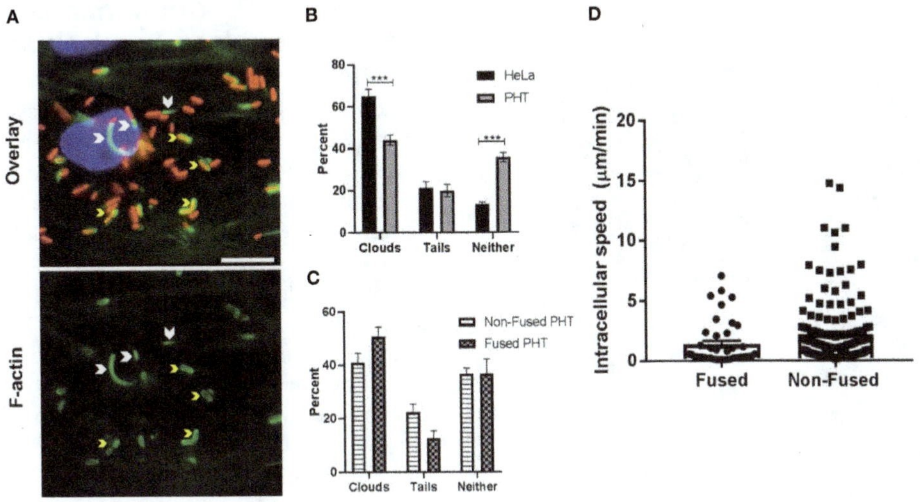

FIGURE 4 | Measure of F-actin clouds and comet tails. PHT and HeLa cells were infected with *pactA*-RFP *L. monocytogenes* for a total of 5 h (MOI 1). Cells were fixed and labeled with DAPI, phalloidin-Alexa Fluor 488, and anti-E-cadherin antibodies conjugated to Alexa Fluor 647 (PHT only). Fluorescence images were acquired with the 100X objective and analyzed for the presence of F-actin comet tails and clouds. **(A)** Representative images, arrowheads point out F-actin tails and yellow arrows depict F-actin clouds. Scale bar = 50 µm. **(B, C)** At least 190 bacteria were counted per experimental condition in each experiment. Data are presented as Average percentages ± SEM (n = 3 (3 placentas), each experiment performed in duplicate). Statistical significance was determined by two-way ANOVA, Holm-Sidak's procedure was used for multiple comparison adjustment. ***P = 0.0003, P = 0.0002 (left to right). **(D)** Intracellular L. monocytogenes speed was determined by acquiring Z-stacks with the 100x objective every 5 sec for 5 min to measure bacterial motility. Bacteria were tracked through each plane of the Z-stack using the multi-line function of Metamorph. Each plane is considered 5 sec and the total µm/min was calculated based on the total length of each bacterial track through the Z-stack.

S5B, C) (76). Autocrine stimulation by cytokines is expected to amplify the PHT inflammatory responses, with TNFα as a prevailing pathway (**Figure S6**). Also consistent with TLR2- and TNFα- pathways, MAPK, PI3K-Akt, JAK-STAT, and NF-κB genes were upregulated (**Table 3** and **Figures S5, S6**). Gene enrichment analysis *via* Genetic Association Database (GAD) revealed sets of signature genes associated with infectious diseases (syncytial virus, HIV), cancer (multiple myeloma, Hodgkin disease and ovarian cancer), and rheumatoid arthritis, which were predominantly pro-inflammatory genes. Most relevant to listeriosis in pregnancy, 32 inflammatory genes (including 13 genes present in the top 50 DEGs) were associated with chorioamnionitis, placental infection and premature birth (**Table 3** and **Table S4**). In conclusion, RNAseq analysis of *L. monocytogenes*-infected human trophoblasts indicated the bacterial sensing pathways and resulting pro-inflammatory transcriptional circuitry. Importantly, this analysis also identified in *L. monocytogenes* infected PHT signature genes associated with poor pregnancy outcomes.

The Secretome of *L. monocytogenes*-Infected Trophoblasts Confirms the Transcriptional Pro-Inflammatory Reprogramming and Revealed the Production of Tolerogenic Cytokines

In parallel to the preparation of PHT samples for RNAseq, cell culture supernatants were collected from infected and non-infected trophoblasts to measure the production of 54 inflammatory mediators. Cell culture supernatants were collected from 3 independent experiments and were pooled at the time of the assay. We used a V-PLEX Human Biomarker 54-Plex that includes 54 inflammatory mediators and growth factors that play key roles in inflammation and immunity. This assay was selected for its high dynamic range and sensitivity. Because primary trophoblasts have been shown to produce IFNλ and because *L. monocytogenes* was shown to induce the production of IFNλ by epithelial cell lines, we also used ELISA kits to measure IFNλ1, IFNλ2, and IFNλ3 (77, 78). *L. monocytogenes* infection for up to 10 h increased by at least 2-fold (average $\log_2$(FC)>1) the release of 12 mediators including chemokines (CXCL8, CCL3, CCL4, CCL20, CCL2, and CXCL10), pro-inflammatory cytokines (TNFα, IL-6, IL-1α, IL-1β), and anti-inflammatory cytokines (IL-10 and IL-1RA) (**Table 4**). Four immune mediators were produced in similar amounts by infected and non-infected PHTs (IL-27, VEGFR1, IFNλ3, and FGF2). Importantly, the fold-change of these mediators at the mRNA and protein levels were very similar 5 h post-infection, which supports that the increased production of cytokines and chemokines is most generally regulated at the transcriptional level (**Table 4**). Importantly, these findings also support the pro-inflammatory pathways identified by RNAseq, including the production of cytokines and chemokines. The transcripts encoding IFNλs were upregulated upon *L. monocytogenes* infection, as previously reported (78). IFNλ3 was constitutively produced by PHT, but its concentration remained unaffected by infection in our experimental conditions (**Table 4**). To rule out cell dysfunction or a failure to detect IFNλs, we infected PHTs

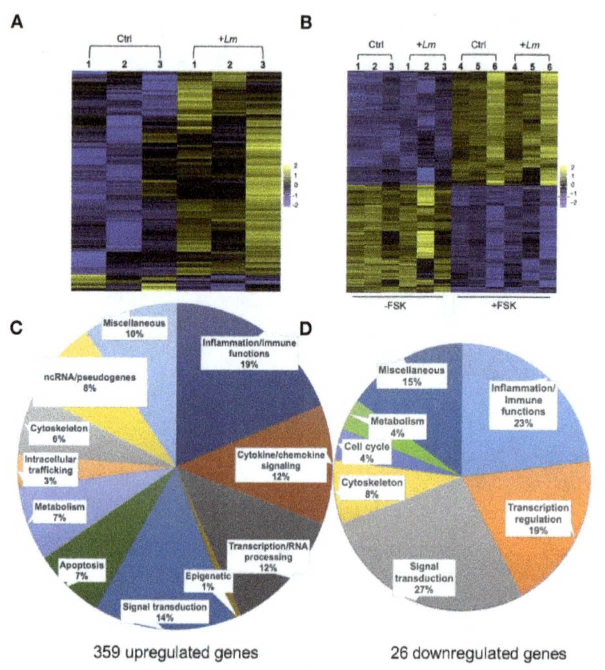

FIGURE 5 | RNAseq analysis of *L. monocytogenes* infected trophoblasts. Heatmaps of PHT **(A)**, and FSK-treated (+FSK) or DMSO-treated control (-FSK) BeWo cells **(B)**, infected for 5 h (*+Lm*) or control non-infected (Ctrl). RNA was extracted from infected and control cells for RNAseq analysis. RNA-seq counts were generated by featureCounts from subread-1.5.1 for genes annotated by GRCh38.92. Count normalization and differential expression was performed using edgeR. Heatmaps were generated by plotting genes with $log_2(FC) > 1$ and < -1 and p value < 0.05. Scale is based on $log_2(CPM)$ from -2 to +2 (n = 3 placentas, and 3 independent experiments involving BeWo cells). Genes were clustered based on similarity of expression profiles. **(C, D)** The upregulated and downregulated DEG were classified based on their known function.

with the Sendai virus from 5 h to 24 h, leading to the conclusion that viral infection significantly increased both transcripts and cytokine release (**Table S5**) (78). Overall, the PHT secretome is congruent with the transcriptomic data (with the exception of IFNλs) and supports the notion that trophoblasts play a role in the detection of *L. monocytogenes* and respond to this bacterium by producing pro-inflammatory mediators including cytokines and chemokines. Of importance, cytokines that play key roles in fetal tolerance, such as IL-27, IL-10, and IL-1RA, were also produced by infected trophoblasts, either at similar or increased levels compared to non-infected cells (**Table 4**) (79–81). The production of cytokines associated with pregnancy complications (premature birth and infections of the placental/fetal unit, **Table S4**) was also increased in *L. monocytogenes*-infected trophoblasts (CCL2, CCL3, IL-8, CSF2, IL-1α/β, IL-1RA, IL-10, GM-CSF, IL-6, and TNFα). This latter finding supports a potential role for trophoblasts in the generation of deleterious inflammation leading to poor pregnancy outcomes.

L. monocytogenes Induces Cytokine and Chemokine Production in Both Syncytia and Mononuclear Trophoblasts, but With Distinct Prevalence

We next established if the inflammatory mediators detected at the transcriptional and translational levels in infected PHT were expressed by both syncytia and non-fused trophoblasts, and if infected cells were exclusively responsible for expression of these mediators. Cells were infected with RFP-expressing *L. monocytogenes* for 5 h (same experimental conditions as in RNAseq). Cells were fixed, permeabilized, and fluorescently labeled for the cytokines (IL-6, IL-8, or TNFα), and βhCG or E-cadherin (**Figures 6, 7** and **S7**). E-cadherin and βhCG were selected as prototypical cell fusion markers since cell fusion is accompanied by loss of E-cadherin expression and gain of βhCG expression (15, 82). As a control, we performed E-cadherin and βhCG colabeling in PHT, confirming the segregation of these two fusion markers (**Figure S8**). We selected IL-6, IL-8, and TNFα as their production was markedly enhanced post-infection (**Table 4**). IL-8 was produced at basal level and its expression was enhanced upon infection, while the two others (IL-6, and TNFα) were mostly induced by *L. monocytogenes*. As expected, we found that *L. monocytogenes* predominantly infected non-fused PHT (E-cadherin-positive and βhCG-negative PHT) (**Figures 6, 7**). There was no correlation between cell infection and their cytokine expression level, as cytokines were detected in similar amount in both infected and non-infected cells (data not shown). We found that syncytia and non-fused trophoblasts both expressed the three cytokines. However, there was a correlation between the cell fusion status and the pattern of cytokine expression. Indeed, IL-8 strongly colocalized with βhCG-producing cells (~85%), which means that 85% of the total IL-8 fluorescence intensity was associated with fused PHT. IL-6 also colocalized with fused cells, but to a lesser extent than IL-8 (~70%). On the contrary, TNFα was expressed more evenly between fused and non-fused cells, with some enrichment (~66%) in non-fused PHT (E-cadherin expressing PHT). In conclusion, our data support that the transcriptional pathways analyzed by RNAseq are representative of both syncytia and non-fused trophoblasts and that PHT expressed pro-inflammatory cytokines independently of their fusion and infection status (at least for IL-6, IL-8, and TNFα). Interestingly, we show for the first time that syncytia and non-fused trophoblasts appear to be more portent at producing some cytokines than others in response to exposure to *L. monocytogenes*.

DISCUSSION

Trophoblasts are epithelial cells located at the maternal/fetal interface that play key immune roles by protecting the fetus from rejection by the maternal immune system and by forming an anti-infective barrier (12, 19, 83). We still have limited knowledge about the trophoblast antimicrobial and inflammatory roles during infection by *L. monocytogenes*. Our studies are in agreement with the notion that trophoblasts act as

TABLE 2 | Top 50 Induced Genes.

Ensembl Gene ID	gene_name	logTPM	logCPM	logFC	FDR	Ensembl Gene ID	gene_name	logTPM	logCPM	logFC	FDR
ENSG00000164400	CSF2	5.2	2.6	7.8	2.7E-47	ENSG00000125657	TNFSF9	3.4	1.9	4.4	1.6E-19
ENSG00000115009	CCL20	5.2	3.3	7.7	1.6E-67	ENSG00000124882	EREG	6.6	6.7	4.4	6.6E-35
ENSG00000275302	CCL4	6.0	4.7	7.4	8.6E-113	ENSG00000158050	DUSP2	5.2	4.0	4.3	1.3E-35
ENSG00000108342	CSF3	3.8	2.6	7.1	9.2E-35	ENSG00000143479	DYRK3	1.8	1.5	4.2	5.6E-16
ENSG00000117090	SLAMF1	2.6	2.2	7.1	4.2E-48	ENSG00000169429	CXCL8	10.2	9.1	4.2	3.8E-19
ENSG00000277632	CCL3	8.4	6.7	6.7	1.8E-72	ENSG00000134460	IL2RA	3.5	2.9	4.0	5.2E-30
ENSG00000050730	TNIP3	3.0	2.3	6.6	2.5E-36	ENSG00000090339	ICAM1	7.6	7.2	4.0	5.0E-42
ENSG00000125538	IL1B	8.3	7.6	6.5	3.0E-64	ENSG00000170209	ANKK1	4.7	3.7	4.0	1.4E-31
ENSG00000276085	CCL3L1	6.5	4.8	6.2	3.9E-54	ENSG00000023445	BIRC3	4.8	5.2	4.0	9.5E-56
ENSG00000123689	G0S2	6.6	4.1	6.2	4.3E-83	ENSG00000171174	RBKS	4.0	3.6	3.8	1.1E-37
ENSG00000110944	IL23A	6.1	4.0	6.0	9.9E-75	ENSG00000184371	CSF1	5.3	5.3	3.8	3.5E-38
ENSG00000276070	CCL4L2	5.2	3.4	5.9	1.4E-57	ENSG00000160326	SLC2A6	4.5	4.1	3.8	1.8E-42
ENSG00000126353	CCR7	6.4	5.4	5.9	4.5E-92	ENSG00000140379	BCL2A1	5.2	3.0	3.8	1.3E-26
ENSG00000197110	IFNL3	4.4	1.6	5.6	2.3E-17	ENSG00000172548	NIPAL4	3.2	3.2	3.7	8.2E-26
ENSG00000182393	IFNL1	3.9	1.3	5.5	2.3E-22	ENSG00000081041	CXCL2	7.5	5.9	3.7	1.8E-31
ENSG00000183709	IFNL2	4.8	1.8	5.5	5.2E-15	ENSG00000073756	PTGS2	6.2	6.3	3.5	1.7E-22
ENSG00000049249	TNFRSF9	3.3	3.5	5.3	1.5E-56	ENSG00000136244	IL6	6.1	5.0	3.5	5.8E-28
ENSG00000241794	SPRR2A	4.8	1.8	5.3	1.5E-23	ENSG00000137265	IRF4	1.3	1.5	3.4	1.8E-12
ENSG00000056558	TRAF1	5.4	5.8	5.1	9.9E-75	ENSG00000115008	IL1A	6.9	5.6	3.4	7.5E-15
ENSG00000123610	TNFAIP6	4.6	2.9	4.9	4.7E-43	ENSG00000109321	AREG	4.7	3.1	3.3	1.8E-23
ENSG00000232810	TNF	6.9	5.4	4.8	1.7E-45	ENSG00000026751	SLAMF7	4.7	4.6	3.2	1.3E-30
ENSG00000136634	IL10	3.1	1.8	4.7	3.8E-11	ENSG00000163735	CXCL5	2.3	1.2	3.1	1.1E-06
ENSG00000163734	CXCL3	7.1	5.9	4.6	9.3E-57	ENSG00000183484	GPR132	4.4	4.4	3.1	1.5E-35
ENSG00000172602	RND1	3.3	2.5	4.5	1.8E-30	ENSG00000135373	EHF	2.9	2.6	3.0	2.2E-11
ENSG00000163739	CXCL1	6.8	4.8	4.4	1.5E-49	ENSG00000136689	IL1RN	6.7	6.2	3.0	9.9E-22

The top 50 upregulated PHT DEG are represented based on log_2(FC) and FDR. Data are the average of three independent experiments. TPM, transcripts per million; CPM, counts per million; FDR, false discovery rate.

placental gatekeepers that limit *L. monocytogenes* infection, and act as immune sensors of infection. In response to infection by *L. monocytogenes*, trophoblasts produce pro-inflammatory cytokines (predominantly IL-6 and TNFα) as well as neutrophil, natural killer, and monocyte chemokines (predominantly IL8 and MIP-1α/β). In parallel, trophoblasts maintain or increase the production of cytokines such as IL-27, IL1-RA and IL-10, which are expected to balance the activation of the pro-inflammatory innate immune response with the suppression of the maternal anti-fetal adaptive immunity (79–81). However, a collection of upregulated cytokines and other inflammatory genes observed in our studies are associated with infection of the placental-fetal unit and pregnancy complications such as chorioamnionitis and preterm birth. These observations suggest that if *L. monocytogenes* is not cleared from the placenta, trophoblast responses are likely to become deleterious to pregnancy.

We found that syncytia of primary human trophoblasts and BeWo cells are about 20-fold more resistant to infection than non-fused trophoblasts. This is in accordance with previous reports showing that fusion of murine trophoblasts increased their resistance to *L. monocytogenes* by 25-fold and the SYN of human placental explants displayed low susceptibility to this pathogen (10, 70, 84). We propose for the first time that the SYN barrier function operates *via* blocking initial bacterial entry rather than limiting bacterial phagosomal escape or intracellular proliferation (**Figures 1–4** and **S2**). The loss of *L. monocytogenes* association to the SYN is explained by its faint level of E-cadherin expression, the receptor for the bacterial surface invasin InlA (**Figures 1A, B, 2** and **S2**) (8, 38).

Elucidating the roles of InlA and InlB in infection of the placental/fetal unit has been challenging due to the species-specificity of InlA and InlB. *In vivo* animal studies using E-cadherin-humanized mice and gerbils (permissive to InlA- and InlB-mediated invasion), *ex vivo* analysis of human placental explants, and epidemiological studies, support that InlA is important for placental infection (10, 39, 40, 85). Other studies using the guinea pig model (permissive to InlA, but not InlB), or an InlA-murinized *L. monocytogenes* strain in an oral murine infection model (permissive to InlB, but not InlA), concluded that InlA is dispensable for *L. monocytogenes* transmission to the placental/fetal unit (36, 38, 86). The discrepancies between these studies might be explained by differences in the species specificity of InlA and InlB, the infectious route, and by the bacterial strains used in these studies. Indeed, it was proposed that the role of InlA in crossing the placental barrier *in vivo* requires the conjugated action of InlA and InlB, which entry pathways are simultaneously functional in the murine humanized and gerbil models, but not in guinea pigs (87). However, the bacterial strain mostly used in these studies carries a mutation in the transcriptional regulator of virulence genes *prfA* leading to elevated expression of InlA/InlB (57). Also, mInlA, expressed by the InlA-murinized *L. monocytogenes* strain, was shown to bind to other receptors in addition to E-cadherin, which questions the relevance of this strain (37). It was proposed that InlA may contribute to low level of infection of the SYN (8) and/

TABLE 3 | Gene Enrichment and Annotation.

Biological Process	# of genes	P-value	FDR
Inflammatory response (GO: 0006954)	56	4.00E-34	8.40E-31
Immune response (GO: 0006955)	45	1.90E-21	2.00E-18
Positive regulation of transcription from RNAP II promoter (GO: 0045944)	49	2.20E-10	5.00E-08
Cell-cell signaling (GO: 0007267)	23	1.20E-09	2.00E-07
Signal transduction (GO: 0007165)	51	6.70E-09	1.00E-06
Positive regulation of gene expression (GO: 0010628)	21	6.00E-08	7.00E-06
Apoptotic process (GO: 0006915)	30	4.40E-07	4.10E-05
Innate immune response (GO: 0045087)	25	1.00E-06	7.80E-05
Negative regulation of apoptotic process (GO: 0043066)	25	2.70E-06	1.80E-04
Negative regulation of cell proliferation (GO: 0008285)	23	3.10E-06	2.00E-04
Molecular Function	**# of genes**	**P-value**	**FDR**
Cytokine activity (GO: 0005125)	24	9.10E-14	4.50E-11
Protein binding (GO: 0005515)	191	7.80E-05	9.50E-03
Transcription factor activity, sequence-specific DNA binding (GO: 0003700)	30	4.20E-03	1.60E-01
Identical protein binding (GO: 0042802)	23	1.60E-02	3.40E-02
KEGG Pathways Induced	**# of genes**	**P-value**	**FDR**
Cytokine-cytokine receptor interaction	41	1.00E-22	1.50E-20
TNF signaling pathway	27	2.90E-19	2.00E-17
NF-kappa B signaling pathway	20	2.20E-13	7.50E-12
Toll-like receptor signaling pathway	20	9.20E-12	2.10E-10
NOD-like receptor signaling pathway	15	5.10E-11	8.90E-10
Jak-STAT signaling pathway	18	9.70E-08	7.50E-07
Cytosolic DNA-sensing pathway	13	4.00E-08	3.30E-07
Chemokine signaling pathway	21	2.90E-08	2.70E-07
MAPK signaling pathway	19	5.50E-05	2.90E-04
Disease Ontology	**# of genes**	**P-value**	**FDR**
Chorioamnionitis|Fetal Membranes, Premature Rupture|Infection of amniotic sac and membranes	27	1.10E-14	2.60E-12
Inflammation|Premature Birth	21	1.70E-12	2.30E-10
Premature Birth	17	1.60E-10	1.30E-08

Analysis of the 330 upregulated DE protein-coding genes was performed with DAVID Bioinformatics Resources functional annotation. Significantly enriched activities from GO aspects for biological processes, molecular functions, KEGG pathways, and GAD for disease ontology. FDR are represented based on a -log_{10} scale (P value and FDR < 0.05 and EASE value of 0.05), the number of genes for each aspect is indicated as well as the corresponding FDR value, and the GO terms are between parentheses. DAVID, Database for annotation, visualization, andintegrated discovery; GO, gene ontology; KEGG, Kyoto Encyclopedia of Genes and Genomes; GAD, Genetic Association Disease Database; FDR, false discovery rate; EASE, expression analysis systematic explorer.

or to infection of other cell types that express higher levels of E-cadherin. These could be maternal cells that are infected before the bacterium reaches the placental/fetal unit, or placental endovascular trophoblasts and extravillous trophoblasts, which are present at the maternal/fetal interface (10). Also, it was proposed that *L. monocytogenes* could invade subsyncytial trophoblasts, expressing high E-cadherin levels, at locations where the SYN is damaged (10).

We did not identify a role for InlB in *L. monocytogenes* uptake by human trophoblasts using the *L. monocytogenes* strain 10403S [(71) and this work]. Similarly, other studies using the strain 10403S, made the same conclusion (10, 36). This is most likely due to the low level of InlB expressed by 10403S, as we and others have previously shown (57, 71, 88). Indeed, studies that used *L. monocytogenes* strains expressing higher InlB levels identified a role for InlB in invasion of cultured trophoblasts and in placental infection *in vivo* (39, 71, 89, 90).

The *L. monocytogenes* virulence factor ActA was previously shown to facilitate bacterial uptake by Caco-2, HeLa, MDCK, and Vero epithelial cells (44). Our study identified a previously unrecognized role for ActA in facilitating *L. monocytogenes* internalization into primary mononuclear trophoblasts, but not in syncytia (**Figure 2E**). The nature of the molecules involved in ActA-mediated *L. monocytogenes* internalization and how these molecules are altered in syncytia are unknown.

ActA most importantly promotes *L. monocytogenes* cytosolic motility for cell-to-cell spread and is required for placental-fetal infection of various small animals (91). Remodeling of the F-actin cytoskeleton in the SYN suggested that the *L. monocytogenes* intracellular motility could be altered (15). However, we found that the average percentage of motile *L. monocytogenes* and their average speed were similar in the SYN and non-fused trophoblasts (**Figure 4C**). A study using a murine SYN model, proposed that the high rigidity of the subcortical actin cytoskeleton in the SYN decreased *L. monocytogenes* cell-to-cell spreading to these cells (70). In accordance with these latter finding, we observed that fused cells in proximity to infectious foci of non-fused cells most often remained non-infected.

The bacterial cytosolic doubling time, measured between 1 and 5 h and between 5 and 7 h of infection, were similar in fused and non-fused trophoblasts (**Table 1** and **Figure 3**). Together with cell invasion experiments (**Figures 2** and **S2**), these data support that the anti-*L. monocytogenes* barrier function of the

TABLE 4 | PHT cytokine array.

	5 h			10 h			5 h RNAseq Log$_2$(FC)
Cytokine	**NI**	***+Lm***	**Log$_2$(FC)**	**NI**	***+Lm***	**Log$_2$(FC)**	
MIP-1α (*CCL3*)	<2.83*	832	≥8.20	<2.83*	1360	≥8.91	6.69
MIP-1β (*CCL4*)	3.17	516	7.35	0.34	444	10.34	7.42
IL-8 (*CXCL8*)	50	3860	6.27	135.60	12324	6.51	4.17
MIP-3α (*CCL20*)	1.36	44	5.01	3.30	76	4.52	7.72
MCP-1 (*CCL2*)	2.04	14.24	2.81	2.28	10.52	2.21	2.38
MCP-4 (*CCL13*)	7.56	23.92	1.66	<2.66*	30.16	≥3.50	–
IP-10 (*CXCL10*)	18.36	27.24	0.57	23.32	75.6	1.70	–
IL-1β	0.17	7.12	5.40	0.56	23.92	5.41	6.53
IL-1α	<0.16*	0.94	2.58	0.72	3.54	2.29	3.36
IL-1RA (*IL-1RN*)	50	268.80	2.43	77.6	456	2.55	2.99
TNFα	<0.06*	101.20	≥10.70	0.29	145.2	8.97	4.78
IL-10	0.27	57.60	7.71	0.66	44.4	6.08	4.70
GM-CSF (*CSF2*)	<0.065*	7.32	≥6.81	<0.065*	29.32	≥8.81	7.81
TSLP	<0.056*	0.97	≥4.10	0.056*	14.48	≥8.00	–
IL-6	9.28	116	3.64	11.76	367.2	4.96	3.47
IL-12/23p40 (*IL-12B*)	<0.06*	0.57	≥3.15	<0.06*	5.92	≥6.53	–
IL-13	<0.36*	7.00	≥4.92	0.36*	36.56	≥6.68	–
IL-27	1604	1648	0.039	2800	2180	-0.36	0.14
bFGF (*FGF2*)	11.52	10.08	-0.19	9.40	7.96	-0.24	–
Flt-1 (*VEGFR1*)	1464	1472	0.0079	3012	2752	-0.13	–
IL-28B (*IFNλ3*)	149.37	185.44	0.31	174.37	181.93	0.06	5.60

Cells were infected (+Lm), or not (NI), for a total of 5 and 10 h as in RNAseq experiments. The cell culture supernatants were collected, centrifuged and immediately and frozen. Cytokine production was measured using the V-PLEX Human Biomarker 54-Plex Kit (Meso Scale Discovery). Samples from 3 independent experiments were pooled and analyzed in duplicates, results are presented as the average cytokine concentration and fold change (FC) between infected and non-infected samples. IFNλ3 was measured by ELISA. (*): (Value < detection limit). (-): transcript below threshold of having an expression level of 2 counts per million in at least half of the samples in RNAseq.

SYN primarily consists in preventing bacterial entry and not the subsequent intracellular proliferation, at least during the first 7 h of infection.

Interestingly, we found that intracellular doubling time of *L. monocytogenes* increased in trophoblasts from ~ 70 min (1-5 h post-infection) to 200 min (5-7 h post-infection). The underlying mechanisms are currently unknown, do not involve the antibiotic gentamicin, and are not specific to trophoblasts. This appears to be a general feature, as *L. monocytogenes* doubling time was 180 min in MDCK infected for 6 to 22 h (92). We observed a population of *L. monocytogenes* in PHT (fused and non-fused) that were unable to nucleate the host cell actin, and the elongation of *L. monocytogenes* in PHT at late infection times (≥ 10 hours) (**Figure S4**). However, we found that bacterial elongation was influenced by the presence of gentamicin, which does not preclude that PHT may also limit bacterial growth at late infection times.

Previous studies analyzing primary human extravillous trophoblasts (first trimester pregnancy) showed that *L. monocytogenes* failed to escape the phagosome and to replicate in these cells (11). Therefore, extravillous trophoblasts, which express high E-cadherin levels, are more permissive to initial *L. monocytogenes* uptake, but then restrict intracellular bacterial proliferation, a property not shared with third trimester SYN and sub-syncytial trophoblasts (our study). In addition, decidual natural killer cells, which are in close proximity to extravillous trophoblasts at the chorionic villi anchoring sites, were recently shown to transfer granulysin into infected extravillous trophoblasts leading to the restriction of *L. monocytogenes* cytosolic growth (93).

We report the first RNAseq analysis of *L. monocytogenes*-infected trophoblasts. Trophoblast exposure to *L. monocytogenes* mainly resulted in the upregulation of 330 protein-coding genes. Gene enrichment analysis revealed that gene upregulation likely involves transcriptional activation *via* RNA polymerase II (**Figures 5C, D** and **Table 3**). The upregulated genes were predominantly related to immunity, inflammation, signaling, and transcription. Genes were enriched in pro-inflammatory pathways activated by pattern recognition receptors (PRRs) such as TLR2 and cytosolic receptors, and *via* autocrine stimulation by cytokines such as TNFα (**Table 3** and **Figures S5, S6**). Several studies showed that trophoblasts express various pattern recognition receptors to detect and respond to pathogens; thereby playing a role in placental immunity (19, 94). In particular, we found that the transcripts encoding TLR2, which recognizes bacterial lipoproteins, peptidoglycan, and lipoteichoic acid (95–98), RIG-I (DDX58) and MAD-5 (IFIH1), which are involved in the cytosolic detection of *L. monocytogenes* nucleotides (99, 100), were upregulated upon *L. monocytogenes* infection. Also, trophoblasts including the SYN are known to express TLR2 (**Figure S5**) (101). The immune signaling pathways involve the MAP kinases and JAK-STAT, among others, and converge toward NF-κB activation and other transcription factors (**Table S3**) leading to transcriptional activation of a collection of cytokines and chemokine genes (**Figures S5, S6**). Gene-disease mappings using the

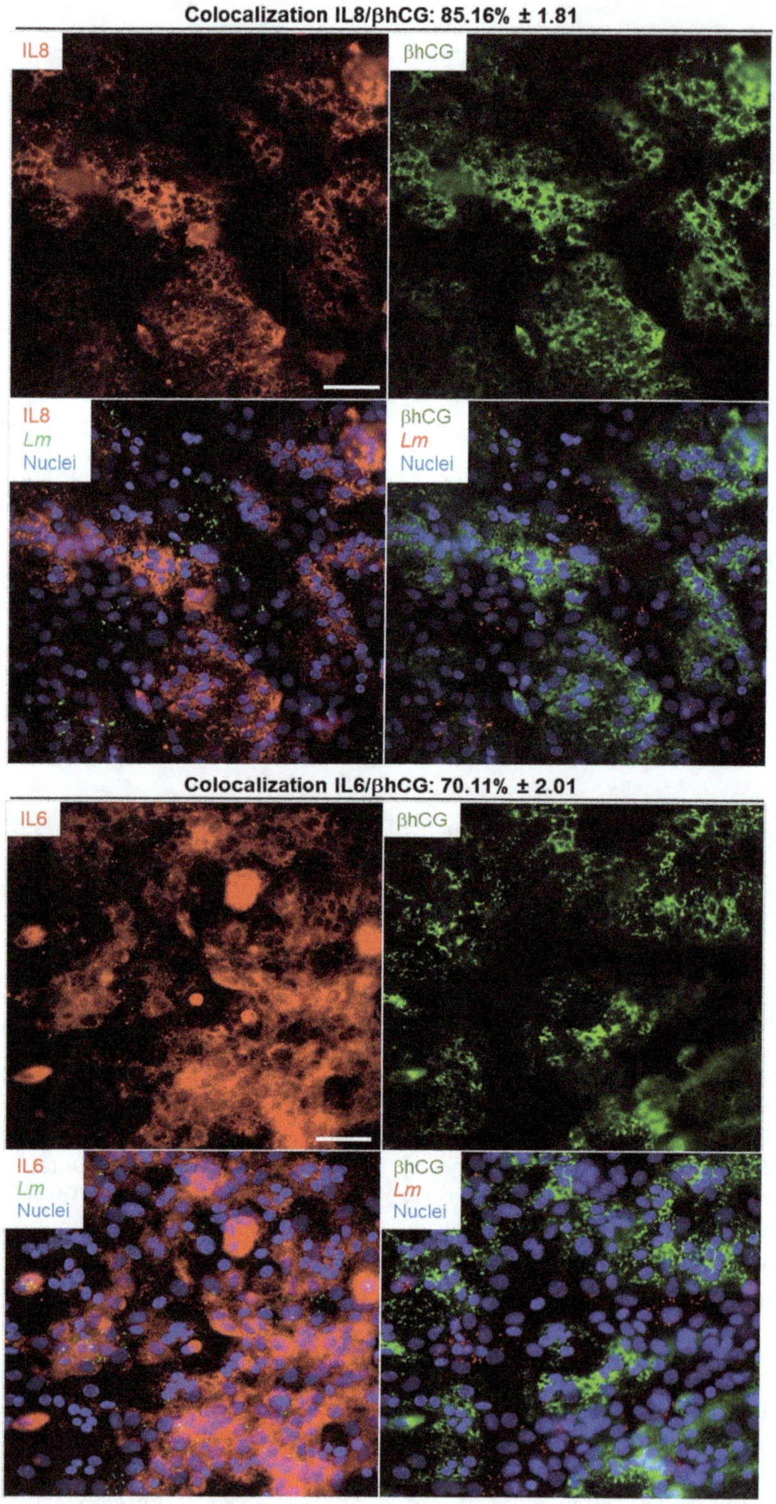

FIGURE 6 | IL-6 and IL-8 colabeling with βhCG in infected primary trophoblasts. PHT were infected with *pactA*-RFP *L. monocytogenes* (MOI 1) for 5 h using the same experimental procedure as the RNAseq infection experiments. Cells were fixed, permeabilized and labeled for IL-6 (mouse primary Ab and secondary Ab-Alexa Fluor 647), IL-8 (mouse primary Ab and secondary Ab-Alexa Fluor 647), βhCG (rabbit primary Ab and secondary Ab-Alexa Fluor 488), and nuclei were labeled with DAPI. At least thirty fluorescent images were randomly acquired with the 40X objective. Representative images are from one experiment. Scale bar = 50 μm. The Metamorph software was used to measure the percent colocalization between each cytokine and, βhCG the average colocalization ± SEM is indicated at the top of the images.

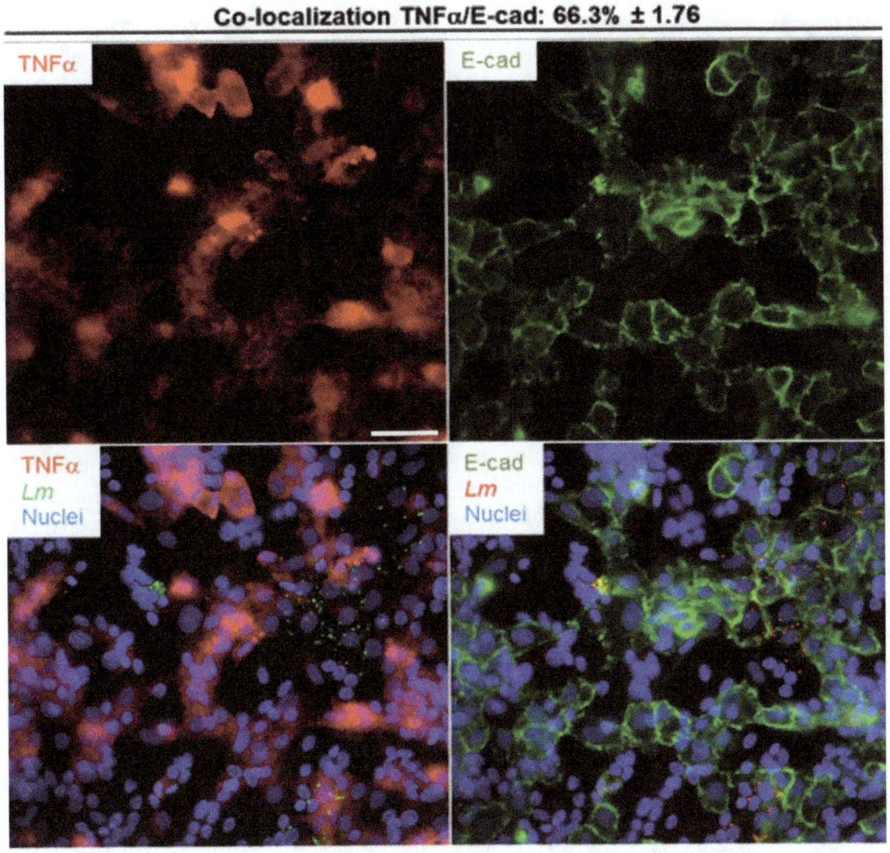

FIGURE 7 | TNFα colabeling with E-cadherin in infected primary trophoblasts. PHT were infected with *pactA*-RFP *L. monocytogenes* (MOI 1) for 5 h using the same experimental procedure as the RNAseq infection experiments. Cells were fixed, permeabilized and labeled for TNF-α (rabbit primary Ab and secondary Ab-Alexa Fluor 647) and for E-cadherin (mouse primary Ab and secondary Ab-Alexa Fluor 488). At least thirty fluorescent images were randomly acquired with the 40X objective. Representative images are from one experiment. Scale bar = 50 μm. The MetaMorph software was used to measure the percent colocalization between TNFα and E-cadherin, the average colocalization ± SEM is indicated at the top of the images.

"Genetic Association Database" highlighted common genes enriched in viral infections. At 5 h post-infection, infected or non-infected PHT, produced TNFα, IL-8 and IL-6 (**Figures 6, 7**). Together, these observations support that trophoblasts detected both extracellular and intracellular bacteria and mounted a pro-inflammatory response resulting in the release of inflammatory mediators (**Table 4**), which could stimulate neighboring cells. Importantly, there was congruence between the fold changes of transcripts and corresponding cytokines and chemokines detected in the trophoblast culture supernatants. For example, *L. monocytogenes* increased the production of MIP-1α/β (100- to 1000-fold), IL-8 (70-fold), TNFα (~1000-fold), IL-6 (30-fold), IL1-RA (6-fold), IL-1α/β (6- to 30-fold), GM-CSF (250-fold), IL-13 (100-fold), and IL-10 (200-fold). Trophoblasts isolated from term placentas have been previously shown to produce MIP-1α and MIP-1β along with IL-6, IL-8, IL-1β, TNFα, GM-CSF (*csf2*) (29, 102). Unlike primary cells, neither the BeWo transcriptome nor release of mediators were affected in a significant fashion upon *L. monocytogenes* infection, and therefore cannot be used as a trophoblast surrogate to study immune gene regulation downstream to *L. monocytogenes* infection.

Infection of small animal models by *L. monocytogenes* showed that neutrophils and other maternal leukocytes were massively recruited in the placenta (103). Our transcriptomic and cytokine data support that trophoblasts participate in the recruitment and activation of maternal leukocytes, neutrophils primarily, but also monocytes and T lymphocytes *via* the production of chemokines such as IL-8, MIP-1α and MIP-1β. The basal secretion of IL-8 (**Table 4**) and the predilection of the SYN for the production of this cytokine (**Figure 6**) are in accordance with elevated IL-8 levels in the SYN of healthy placentas (104, 105). TNFα plays an important role in *L. monocytogenes* immunity (106, 107). In mice infected with *L. monocytogenes*, TNFα was produced early in infection (108) and neutralization of TNFα exacerbated listeriosis (108). However, TNFα can induce trophoblast apoptosis (109). We did not observe any apoptotic cells based on nuclear structures observed by DAPI fluorescence for up to 24 h infection. RNAseq analysis showed the upregulation of 25 transcripts of anti-(BIRC2, BIRC3, FLIP, XIAP, SOCS3, PLAUR, etc.) and pro-(TRAILR2, BCL2, TNFRSF10A) apoptotic genes. However, pathway analysis revealed a negative regulation of apoptosis indicating that, together with the absence of apoptotic trophoblasts, anti-apoptotic signals prevailed. IL-6 is required for the control of *L. monocytogenes* in a non-pregnant murine model (110), therefore IL-6 production by trophoblasts may also have beneficial protective effects in placental immunity. As an important first line of defense, we found the transcripts for IL-1β, IL-18, GBP5, and caspase-1 to be significantly upregulated, supporting recent work showing that *L. monocytogenes* infection of placental villi activates the NLRP3 inflammasome, which provides placental anti-microbial protection (84). Accordingly, several studies initially reported NLRP3 stimulation by *L. monocytogenes* (111, 112) and barrier cells such as the intestinal epithelium and trophoblast cells produce the NLRP3 inflammasome (113, 114). However, activation of the NLRP3 inflammasome and IL-1 production can lead to embryo loss in *L. monocytogenes* infected mice (111). We found that trophoblasts produce IFNλ at basal level, as reported by others (78). Although the genes encoding IFNλs were all upregulated upon *L. monocytogenes* infection, we did not observe an increase in proteins for up to 24 h post-infection (**Table S5**). Of note, a study reported IFNλ production by epithelial cell lines infected by *L. monocytogenes*, but used a very high MOI of 50 to 100 for over 24 h (77). Therefore, increased IFNλ production may require high *L. monocytogenes* infection levels and prolonged infection times.

The placenta must tightly control inflammation to tolerate the semi-allogeneic fetus while maintaining host defense. Modulation of the immune response based on the microorganism is necessary to maintain growth of the fetus and limit pathogen invasion (115). In that respect, trophoblasts are unlike any other epithelial cells due to their tolerogenic functions (19). Interestingly, IL-27 is constitutively produced by trophoblasts and unaffected by *L. monocytogenes* infection (**Table 4**). IL-27 is known to promote T cell tolerance and modulate TLR expression (79, 116, 117). IL-10 is also an important anti-inflammatory cytokine that contributes to T cell tolerance, and its production was increased 200-fold 5 h post-infection upon *L. monocytogenes* infection (**Table 4**). Similarly, the IL-1 antagonist IL1-RA and the trophoblast-derived thymic stromal lymphopoietin (TSLP) production were increased upon *L. monocytogenes* infection (**Table 4**) (84). For infections such as listeriosis, for which sterilizing immunity requires T cell immunity, it is thought that the suppression of placental T cell responses for fetal tolerance is responsible for sustained infection of the placental-fetal unit despite the initial innate immune response. However, as the pathogen persists, placental inflammation may override suppression of maternal allo-reactive T cell responses. Indeed, bacterial and viral infections have been strongly associated with pregnancy disorders such as pre-eclampsia, intrauterine growth retardation, and spontaneous abortion (118). The fact that transcriptome of infected trophoblasts includes upregulation of signature genes involved in placental inflammation and preterm birth supports that the trophoblast pro-inflammatory responses may become deleterious. In conclusion, infected trophoblasts are balancing their pro-inflammatory activity by releasing tolerogenic factors in accordance with their known function of immune suppressor or of T cell activation. It is likely, that the initial inflammatory response of trophoblasts may have beneficial effects by recruiting and activating maternal neutrophils and monocytes, and by activation of NLRP3, but if infection is not cleared, prolonged and exacerbated production of pro-inflammatory mediators by trophoblasts may favor the known poor pregnancy outcomes of listeriosis.

AUTHOR CONTRIBUTIONS

LJ, SA, and JM carried out experiments. LJ performed numerical calculations and analyzed the data. AW processed RNAseq data. XZ consulted on statistical analysis. MG supervised RT-qPCR experiments. KR obtained placentae. LJ and SS wrote the manuscript with input from all other authors. SS supervised the project. All authors contributed to the article and approved the submitted version.

ACKNOWLEDGMENTS

The authors would like to thank Dr. John Mitchell Robinson (The Ohio State University) for his kind help and invaluable guidance throughout this work. Dr. Yoel Sadovsky (University of Pittsburgh) taught our lab the trophoblast isolation procedure and provided guidance for the development of this research project. The authors would like to thank Hannah Cackovic, RN, Sarah Buck-Davis, RN, Devra Mast, RN, and Jessica Russo, RDMS for their participation in consenting participants and collection of biological specimens.

REFERENCES

Goldenberg RL, Culhane JF, Johnson DC. Maternal Infection and Adverse Fetal and Neonatal Outcomes. *Clin Perinatol* (2005) 32(3):523–59. doi: 10.1016/j.clp.2005.04.006

Kell DB, Kenny LC. A Dormant Microbial Component in the Development of Preeclampsia. *Front Med (Lausanne)* (2016) 3:60. doi: 10.3389/ fmed.2016.00060

Robbins JR, Bakardjiev AI. Pathogens and the Placental Fortress. *Curr Opin Microbiol* (2012) 15(1):36–43. doi: 10.1016/j.mib.2011.11.006

Bakardjiev AI, Theriot JA, Portnoy DA. Listeria Monocytogenes Traffics From Maternal Organs to the Placenta and Back. *PloS Pathog* (2006) 2(6): e66. doi: 10.1371/journal.ppat.0020066

Charlier C, Disson O, Lecuit M. Maternal-Neonatal Listeriosis. *Virulence* (2020) 11(1):391–7. doi: 10.1080/21505594.2020.1759287

Madjunkov M, Chaudhry S, Ito S. Listeriosis During Pregnancy. *Arch Gynecol Obstet* (2017) 296(2):143–52. doi: 10.1007/s00404-017-4401-1

Lamont RF, Sobel J, Mazaki-Tovi S, Kusanovic JP, Vaisbuch E, Kim SK, et al. Listeriosis in Human Pregnancy: A Systematic Review. *J Perinat Med* (2011) 39(3):227–36. doi: 10.1515/jpm.2011.035

Lecuit M, Nelson DM, Smith SD, Khun H, Huerre M, Vacher-Lavenu M-C, et al. Targeting and Crossing of the Human Maternofetal Barrier by Listeria Monocytogenes: Role of Internalin Interaction With Trophoblast E-Cadherin. *PNAS* (2004) 101:6152–7. doi: 10.1073/pnas.0401434101

Lecuit M. Understanding How Listeria Monocytogenes Targets and Crosses Host Barriers. *Clin Microbiol Infect* (2005) 11(6):430–6. doi: 10.1111/j.1469-0691.2005.01146.x

Robbins JR, Skrzypczynska KM, Zeldovich VB, Kapidzic M, Bakardjiev AI. Placental Syncytiotrophoblast Constitutes a Major Barrier to Vertical

Transmission of Listeria Monocytogenes. *PloS Pathog* (2010) 6(1): e1000732. doi: 10.1371/journal.ppat.1000732

Zeldovich VB, Robbins JR, Kapidzic M, Lauer P, Bakardjiev AI. Invasive Extravillous Trophoblasts Restrict Intracellular Growth and Spread of Listeria Monocytogenes. *PloS Pathog* (2011) 11(3):e1002005. doi: 10.1371/journal.ppat.1002005

Knofler M, Haider S, Saleh L, Pollheimer J, Gamage T, James J. Human Placenta and Trophoblast Development: Key Molecular Mechanisms and Model Systems. *Cell Mol Life Sci* (2019) 76(18):3479–96. doi: 10.1007/ s00018-019-03104-6

Huppertz B. The Anatomy of the Normal Placenta. *J Clin Pathol* (2008) 61 (12):1296–302. doi: 10.1136/jcp.2008.055277

Gauster M, Maninger S, Siwetz M, Deutsch A, El-Heliebi A, Kolb-Lenz D, et al. Downregulation of P53 Drives Autophagy During Human Trophoblast Differentiation. *Cell Mol Life Sci* (2018) 75(10):1839–55. doi: 10.1007/ s00018-017-2695-6

Ishikawa A, Omata W, Ackerman ,W, Takeshita T, Vandre DD, Robinson JM. Cell Fusion Mediates Dramatic Alterations in the Actin Cytoskeleton, Focal Adhesions, and E-Cadherin in Trophoblastic Cells. *Cytoskeleton (Hoboken)* (2014) 71(4):241–56. doi: 10.1002/cm.21165

Ander SE, Rudzki EN, Arora N, Sadovsky Y, Coyne CB, Boyle JP. Human Placental Syncytiotrophoblasts Restrict Toxoplasma Gondii Attachment and Replication and Respond to Infection by Producing Immunomodulatory Chemokines. *MBio* (2018) 9(1):e01678–17. doi: 10.1128/mBio.01678-17

Sadovsky Y, Ouyang Y, Powell JS, Li H, Mouillet JF, Morelli AE, et al. Placental Small Extracellular Vesicles: Current Questions and Investigative Opportunities. *Placenta* (2020) 102:34–8. doi: 10.1016/j.placenta. 2020.03.002

Nwabuobi C, Arlier S, Schatz F, Guzeloglu-Kayisli O, Lockwood CJ, Kayisli UA. hCG: Biological Functions and Clinical Applications. *Int J Mol Sci* (2017) 18(10):2037. doi: 10.3390/ijms18102037

Liu J, Hao S, Chen X, Zhao H, Du L, Ren H, et al. Human Placental Trophoblast Cells Contribute to Maternal-Fetal Tolerance Through Expressing IL-35 and Mediating Itr35 Conversion. *Nat Commun* (2019) 10(1):4601. doi: 10.1038/ s41467-019-12484-z

Tersigni C, Meli F, Neri C, Iacoangeli A, Franco R, Lanzone A, et al. Role of Human Leukocyte Antigens at the Feto-Maternal Interface in Normal and Pathological Pregnancy: An Update. *Int J Mol Sci* (2020) 21(13):4756. doi: 10.3390/ ijms21134756

Wang XQ, Li DJ. The Mechanisms by Which Trophoblast-Derived Molecules Induce Maternal-Fetal Immune Tolerance. *Cell Mol Immunol* (2020) 17(11):1204–7. doi: 10.1038/s41423-020-0460-5

Arora N, Sadovsky Y, Dermody TS, Coyne CB. Microbial Vertical Transmission During Human Pregnancy. *Cell Host Microbe* (2017) 21 (5):561–7. doi: 10.1016/j. chom.2017.04.007

Maidji E, McDonagh S, Genbacev O, Tabata T, Pereira L. Maternal Antibodies Enhance or Prevent Cytomegalovirus Infection in the Placenta by Neonatal Fc Receptor-Mediated Transcytosis. *Am J Pathol* (2006) 168 (4):1210–26. doi: 10.2353/ajpath.2006.050482

Fisher S, Genbacev O, Maidji E, Pereira L. Human Cytomegalovirus Infection of Placental Cytotrophoblasts *In Vitro* and In Utero: Implications for Transmission and Pathogenesis. *J Virol* (2000) 74 (15):6808–20. doi: 10.1128/JVI.74.15.6808-6820.2000

Schwartz DA. The Origins and Emergence of Zika Virus, the Newest TORCH Infection: What's Old Is New Again. *Arch Pathol Lab Med* (2017) 141(1):18–25. doi: 10.5858/arpa.2016-0429-ED

Hemmings DG, Kilani R, Nykiforuk C, Preiksaitis J, Guilbert LJ. Permissive Cytomegalovirus Infection of Primary Villous Term and First Trimester Trophoblasts. *J Virol* (1998) 72(6):4970–9. doi: 10.1128/JVI.72.6.4970-4979.1998

Costa ML, de Moraes Nobrega G, Antolini-Tavares A. Key Infections in the Placenta. *Obstet Gynecol Clin North Am* (2020) 47(1):133–46. doi: 10.1016/ j.ogc.2019.10.003

Cao B, Mysorekar IU. Intracellular Bacteria in Placental Basal Plate Localizeto Extravillous Trophoblasts. *Placenta* (2014) 35(2):139–42. doi: 10.1016/ j.placenta.2013.12.007

Griesinger G, Saleh L, Bauer S, Husslein P, Knofler M. Production of Pro- and Anti-Inflammatory Cytokines of Human Placental Trophoblasts in Response to Pathogenic Bacteria. *J Soc Gynecol Investig* (2001) 8(6):334– 40. doi: 10.1016/ S1071-5576(01)00135-6

Koi H, Zhang J, Makrigiannakis A, Getsios S, MacCalman CD, Strauss JF, et al. Syncytiotrophoblast Is a Barrier to Maternal-Fetal Transmission of Herpes Simplex Virus. *Biol Reprod* (2002) 67(5):1572–9. doi: 10.1095/ biolreprod.102.004325

Cappelletti M, Presicce P, Kallapur SG. Immunobiology of Acute Chorioamnionitis. *Front Immunol* (2020) 11:649. doi: 10.3389/ fimmu.2020.00649

Tong M, Abrahams VM. Neutrophils in Preterm Birth: Friend or Foe?*Placenta* (2020) 102:17–20. doi: 10.1016/j.placenta.2019.12.010

Kim CJ, Romero R, Chaemsaithong P, Kim JS. Chronic Inflammation of the Placenta: Definition, Classification, Pathogenesis, and Clinical Significance. *Am J Obstet Gynecol* (2015) 213(4 Suppl):S53–69. doi: 10.1016/ j.ajog.2015.08.041

Heerema-McKenney A. Defense and Infection of the Human Placenta. *APMIS* (2018) 126(7):570–88. doi: 10.1111/apm.12847

Thellin O, Heinen E. Pregnancy and the Immune System: Between Tolerance and Rejection. *Toxicology* (2003) 185(3):179–84. doi: 10.1016/ S0300-483X(02)00607-8

Bakardjiev AI, Stacy BA, Fisher SJ, Portnoy DA. Listeriosis in the Pregnant Guinea Pig: A Model of Vertical Transmission. *Infect Immun* (2004) 72 (1):489–97. doi: 10.1128/IAI.72.1.489-497.2004

Tsai YH, Disson O, Bierne H, Lecuit M. Murinization of Internalin Extends Its Receptor Repertoire, Altering Listeria Monocytogenes Cell Tropism and Host Responses. *PloS Pathog* (2013) 9(5):e1003381. doi: 10.1371/ journal. ppat.1003381

Wollert T, Pasche B, Rochon M, Deppenmeier S, van den Heuvel J, Gruber AD, et al. Extending the Host Range of Listeria Monocytogenes by Rational Protein Design. *Cell* (2007) 129(5):891–902. doi: 10.1016/j.cell.2007.03.049

Disson O, Grayo S, Huillet E, Nikitas G, Langa-Vives F, Dussurget O, et al. Conjugated Action of Two Species-Specific Invasion Proteins for Fetoplacental Listeriosis. *Nature* (2008) 455(7216):1114–8. doi: 10.1038/ nature07303

Lecuit M, Vandormael-Pournin S, Lefort J, Huerre M, Gounon P, Dupuy C, et al. A Transgenic Model for Listeriosis: Role of Internalin in Crossing the Intestinal Barrier. *Science* (2001) 292(5522):1722–5. doi: 10.1126/ science.1059852

Mengaud J, Ohayon H, Gounon P, Mege RM, Cossart P. E-Cadherin is the Receptor for Internalin, a Surface Protein Required for Entry of L. Monocytogenes Into Epithelial Cells. *Cell* (1996) 84(6):923–32. doi: 10.1016/S0092-8674(00)81070-3

Shen Y, Naujokas M, Park M, Ireton K. InIB-Dependent Internalization of Listeria is Mediated by the Met Receptor Tyrosine Kinase. *Cell* (2000) 103 (3):501–10. doi: 10.1016/S0092-8674(00)00141-0

Vadia S, Arnett E, Haghighat AC, Wilson-Kubalek EM, Tweten RK, Seveau S. The Pore-Forming Toxin Listeriolysin O Mediates a Novel Entry Pathway of L. Monocytogenes Into Human Hepatocytes. *PloS Pathog* (2011) 7(11): e1002356. doi: 10.1371/journal.ppat.1002356

Suarez M, Gonzalez-Zorn B, Vega Y, Chico-Calero I, Vazquez-Boland JA. A Role for ActA in Epithelial Cell Invasion by Listeria Monocytogenes. *Cell Microbiol* (2001) 3(12):853–64. doi: 10.1046/j.1462-5822.2001.00160.x

Kocks C, Gouin E, Tabouret M, Berche P, Ohayon H, Cossart P. L. Monocytogenes-Induced Actin Assembly Requires the actA Gene Product, a Surface Protein. *Cell* (1992) 68(3):521–31. doi: 10.1016/0092-8674(92) 90188-I

Faralla C, Bastounis EE, Ortega FE, Light SH, Rizzuto G, Gao L, et al. Listeria Monocytogenes InlP Interacts With Afadin and Facilitates Basement Membrane Crossing. *PloS Pathog* (2018) 14(5):e1007094. doi: 10.1371/ journal.ppat.1007094

Faralla C, Rizzuto GA, Lowe DE, Kim B, Cooke C, Shiow LR, et al. InlP, a New Virulence Factor With Strong Placental Tropism. *Infect Immun* (2016) 84(12):3584–96. doi: 10.1128/IAI.00625-16

Lowe DE, Robbins JR, Bakardjiev AI. Animal and Human Tissue Models of Vertical Listeria Monocytogenes transmission and Implications for Other Pregnancy-Associated Infections. *Infect Immun* (2018) 86(6):e00801–17. doi: 10.1128/IAI.00801-17

Va⊠zquez-Boland JA, Krypotou E, Scortti M. Listeria Placental Infection. *MBio* (2017) 8(3):e00949–17. doi: 10.1128/mBio.00949-17

Benshushan A, Tsafrir A, Arbel R, Rahav G, Ariel I, Rojansky N. *Listeria Infection During Pregnancy: A 10 Year Experience. Isr Med Assoc J* (2002) 4 (10):776–80.

Drewlo S, Baczyk D, Dunk C, Kingdom J. Fusion Assays and Models for the Trophoblast. *Methods Mol Biol* (2008) 475:363–82. doi: 10.1007/978-1- 59745-250-2_21

Wice B, Menton D, Geuze H, Schwartz AL. Modulators of Cyclic AMP Metabolism Induce Syncytiotrophoblast Formation In Vitro. *Exp Cell Res* (1990) 186(2):306–16. doi: 10.1016/0014-4827(90)90310-7

Kliman HJ, Nestler JE, Sermasi E, Sanger JM, Strauss JF3rd. Purification, Characterization, and *In Vitro* Differentiation of Cytotrophoblasts From Human Term Placentae. *Endocrinology* (1986) 118(4):1567–82. doi: 10.1210/ endo-118-4-1567

Huppertz B, Gauster M. Trophoblast Fusion. *Adv Exp Med Biol* (2011) 713:81–95. doi: 10.1007/978-94-007-0763-4_6

Vandre DD, Ackerman ,W, Kniss DA, Tewari AK, Mori M, Takizawa T, et al. Dysferlin Is Expressed in Human Placenta But Does Not Associate With Caveolin. *Biol Reprod* (2007) 77(3):533–42. doi: 10.1095/biolreprod.107.062190

Edman DC, Pollock MB, Hall ER. Listeria Monocytogenes L Forms I. Induction, Maintenance, and Biological Characteristics1. *J Bacteriol* (1968) 96(2):352–7. doi: 10.1128/jb.96.2.352-357.1968

Be⊠cavin C, Bouchier C, Lechat P, Archambaud C, Creno S, Gouin E, et al. Comparison of Widely Used Listeria Monocytogenes Strains EGD, 10403S, and EGD-E Highlights Genomic Differences Underlying Variations in Pathogenicity. *mBio* (2014) 5:e00969–14. doi: 10.1128/mBio.00969-14

Bishop DK, Hinrichs DJ. Adoptive Transfer of Immunity to ListeriaMonocytogenes. The Influence of *In Vitro* Stimulation on Lymphocyte Subset Requirements. *J Immunol* (1987) 139(6):2005–9.

Haghighat AC, Seveau S. Quantification of Host-Microbe Interactions by Automated Fluorescence Microscopy. *J Immunol Methods* (2010) 352(1- 2):186–91. doi: 10.1016/j.jim.2009.11.013

Zheng-Bradley X, Streeter I, Fairley S, Richardson D, Clarke L, Flicek P. Alignment of 1000 Genomes Project Reads to Reference Assembly Grch38. *Gigascience* (2017) 6(7):1–8. doi: 10.1093/gigascience/gix038

Wong KHY, Ma W, Wei C-Y, Yeh E-C, Lin W-J, Wang EHF, et al. Towards a Reference Genome That Captures Global Genetic Diversity. *Nat Commun* (2020) 11(1):5482. doi: 10.1038/s41467-020-19311-w

Liao Y, Smyth GK, Shi W. Featurecounts: An Efficient General Purpose Program for Assigning Sequence Reads to Genomic Features. *Bioinformatics* (2013) 30(7):923–30. doi: 10.1093/bioinformatics/btt656

Lin Y, Golovnina K, Chen ZX, Lee HN, Negron YL, Sultana H, et al. Comparison of Normalization and Differential Expression Analyses Using RNA-Seq Data From 726 Individual Drosophila Melanogaster. *BMC Genomics* (2016) 17:28. doi: 10.1186/s12864-015-2353-z

Huang da W, Sherman BT, Lempicki RA. Systematic and Integrative Analysis of Large Gene Lists Using DAVID Bioinformatics Resources. *Nat Protoc* (2009) 4(1):44–57. doi: 10.1038/nprot.2008.211

Huang da W, Sherman BT, Lempicki RA. Bioinformatics Enrichment Tools: Paths Toward the Comprehensive Functional Analysis of Large Gene Lists. *Nucleic Acids Res* (2009) 37(1):1–13. doi: 10.1093/nar/gkn923

Gavrilin MA, Bouakl IJ, Knatz NL, Duncan MD, Hall MW, Gunn JS, et al. Internalization and Phagosome Escape Required for Francisella to Induce Human Monocyte IL-1Beta Processing and Release. *Proc Natl Acad Sci USA* (2006) 103(1):141–6. doi: 10.1073/pnas.0504271103

Fahy RJ, Exline MC, Gavrilin MA, Bhatt NY, Besecker BY, Sarkar A, et al. Inflammasome mRNA Expression in Human Monocytes During Early Septic Shock. *Am J Respir Crit Care Med* (2008) 177(9):983–8. doi: 10.1164/rccm.200703-418OC

Allen JN, Herzyk DJ, Allen ED, Wewers MD. Human Whole Blood Interleukin-1-Beta Production: Kinetics, Cell Source, and Comparison With TNF-Alpha. *J Lab Clin Med* (1992) 119(5):538–46.

Omata W, Ackerman WE, Vandre DD, Robinson JM. *Trophoblast Cell Fusion and Differentiation Are Mediated by Both the Protein Kinase C and A Pathways. PloS One* (2013) 8(11):e81003. doi: 10.1371/journal.pone.0081003

Zeldovich VB, Clausen CH, Bradford E, Fletcher DA, Maltepe E, Robbins JR, et al. Placental Syncytium Forms a Biophysical Barrier Against Pathogen Invasion. *PloS Pathog* (2013) 9(12):e1003821. doi: 10.1371/journal.ppat.1003821

Phelps CC, Vadia S, Arnett E, Tan Y, Zhang X, Pathak-Sharma S, et al. Relative Roles of Listeriolysin O, InlA, and InlB in Listeria Monocytogenes Uptake by Host Cells. *Infect Immun* (2018) 86(10):e00555-18. doi: 10.1128/ IAI.00555-18

Adler HI, Hardigree AA. Growth and Division of Filamentous Forms of Escherichia Coli. *J Bacteriol* (1965) 90(1):223–6. doi: 10.1128/jb.90.1.223- 226.1965

Wang J, King JE, Goldrick M, Lowe M, Gertler FB, Roberts IS. *Lamellipodin Is Important for Cell-To-Cell Spread and Actin-Based Motility in Listeria Monocytogenes. Infect Immun* (2015) p:3740–8. doi: 10.1128/IAI.00193-15

Czuczman MA, Fattouh R, van Rijn J, Canadien V, Osborne S, Muise AM, et al. Listeria Monocytogenes Exploits Efferocytosis to Promote Cell-to-Cell Spread. *Nature* (2014) 509(7499):230–4. doi: 10.1038/nature13168

Kortebi M, Milohanic E, Mitchell G, Pe⊠choux C, Prevost MC, Cossart P,et al. Listeria Monocytogenes Switches From Dissemination to Persistence by Adopting a Vacuolar Lifestyle in Epithelial Cells. *PloS Pathog* (2017) 13 (11):e1006734. doi: 10.1371/journal.ppat.1006734

Rindsjo E, Holmlund U, Sverremark-Ekstrom E, Papadogiannakis N, Scheynius A. Toll-Like Receptor-2 Expression in Normal and Pathologic Human Placenta. *Hum Pathol* (2007) 38(3):468–73. doi: 10.1016/j.humpath.2006.09.009

Bierne H, Travier L, Mahlakoiv T, Tailleux L, Subtil A, Lebreton A, et al. Activation of Type III Interferon Genes by Pathogenic Bacteria in Infected Epithelial Cells and Mouse Placenta. *PloS One* (2012) 7(6):e39080. doi: 10.1371/journal.pone.0039080

Bayer A, Lennemann NJ, Ouyang Y, Bramley JC, Morosky S, Marques ET, et al. Type III Interferons Produced by Human Placental Trophoblasts Confer Protection Against Zika Virus Infection. *Cell Host Microbe* (2016) 19 (5):705–12. doi: 10.1016/j.chom.2016.03.008

Coulomb-L'Hermine⊠ A, Larousserie F, Pflanz S, Bardel E, Kastelein RA, Devergne O. Expression of Interleukin-27 by Human Trophoblast Cells. *Placenta* (2007) 28(11-12):1133–40. doi: 10.1016/j.placenta.2007.06.004

Thaxton JE, Sharma S. Interleukin-10: A Multi-Faceted Agent of Pregnancy. *Am J Reprod Immunol* (2010) 63(6):482–91. doi: 10.1111/j.1600- 0897.2010.00810.x

Girard S, Tremblay L, Lepage M, Se⊠bire G. IL-1 Receptor Antagonist Protects Against Placental and Neurodevelopmental Defects Induced by Maternal Inflammation. *J Immunol* (2010) 184(7):3997–4005. doi: 10.4049/jimmunol.0903349

Orendi K, Gauster M, Moser G, Meiri H, Huppertz B. The Choriocarcinoma Cell Line BeWo: Syncytial Fusion and Expression of Syncytium-Specific Proteins. *Reproduction* (2010) 140(5):759–66. doi: 10.1530/REP-10-0221

Staud F, Karahoda R. Trophoblast: The Central Unit of Fetal Growth, Protection and Programming. *Int J Biochem Cell Biol* (2018) 105:35–40. doi: 10.1016/j.biocel.2018.09.016

Megli C, Morosky S, Rajasundaram D, Coyne CB. Inflammasome Signaling in Human Placental Trophoblasts Regulates Immune Defense Against Listeria Monocytogenes Infection. *J Exp Med* (2021) 218(1):e20200649. doi: 10.1084/jem.20200649

Jacquet C, Doumith M, Gordon JI, Martin PM, Cossart P, Lecuit M. A Molecular Marker for Evaluating the Pathogenic Potential of Foodborne Listeria Monocytogenes. *J Infect Dis* (2004) 189(11):2094–100. doi: 10.1086/ 420853

Holch A, Ingmer H, Licht TR, Gram L. Listeria Monocytogenes Strains Encoding Premature Stop Codons in inlA Invade Mice and Guinea Pig Fetuses in Orally Dosed Dams. *J Med Microbiol* (2013) 62(Pt 12):1799–806. doi: 10.1099/jmm.0.057505-0

Nikitas G, Deschamps C, Disson O, Niault T, Cossart P, Lecuit M. Transcytosis of Listeria Monocytogenes Across the Intestinal Barrier Upon Specific Targeting of Goblet Cell Accessible E-Cadherin. *J Exp Med* (2011) 208(11):2263–77. doi: 10.1084/jem.20110560

Ripio MT, Domınguez-Bernal G, Lara M, Sua⊠rez M, Vazquez-Boland JA. A Gly145Ser Substitution in the Transcriptional Activator PrfA Causes Constitutive Overexpression of Virulence Factors in Listeria Monocytogenes. *J Bacteriol* (1997) 179(5):1533–40. doi: 10.1128/jb.179.5.1533-1540.1997

Lamond NM, McMullen PD, Paramasvaran D, Visvahabrathy L, Eallonardo SJ, Maheswhari A, et al. Cardiotropic Isolates of Listeria Monocytogenes With Enhanced Vertical Transmission Dependent Upon the Bacterial Surface Protein InlB. *Infect Immun* (2021) 89(2):e00321–20. doi: 10.1128/ IAI.00321-20

Maruyama S, Shen H, Kanoh M, Matsumoto A, Asano Y. Differential Effect of Listeria Monocytogenes Infection on Cytokine Production and Cytotoxicity of CD8 T Cells. *Microbiol Immunol* (2007) 51(9):893–901. doi: 10.1111/j.1348-0421.2007.tb03972.x

Le Monnier A, Autret N, Join-Lambert OF, Jaubert F, Charbit A, Berche P, et al. ActA is Required for Crossing of the Fetoplacental Barrier by Listeria Monocytogenes. *Infect Immun* (2007) 75(2):950–7. doi: 10.1128/IAI.01570-06

Ortega FE, Koslover EF, Theriot JA. Listeria Monocytogenes Cell-to-Cell Spread in Epithelia is Heterogeneous and Dominated by Rare Pioneer Bacteria. *Elife* (2019) 8:e40032. doi: 10.7554/eLife.40032

Crespo AC, Mulik S, Dotiwala F, Ansara JA, Sen Santara S, Ingersoll K, et al. Decidual NK Cells Transfer Granulysin to Selectively Kill Bacteria in Trophoblasts. *Cell* (2020) 182(5):1125–1139 e18. doi: 10.1016/j.cell.2020.07.019

Olmos-Ortiz A, Flores-Espinosa P, Mancilla-Herrera I, Vega-Sanchez R, Diaz L, Zaga-Clavellina V. Innate Immune Cells and Toll-Like Receptor- Dependent Responses at the Maternal-Fetal Interface. *Int J Mol Sci* (2019) 20 (15):3654. doi: 10.3390/ijms20153654

Abrahams VM, Bole-Aldo P, Kim YM, Straszewski-Chavez SL, Chaiworapongsa T, Romero R, et al. Divergent Trophoblast Responses toBacterial Products Mediated by TLRs. *J Immunol* (2004) 173(7):4286–96. doi: 10.4049/jimmunol.173.7.4286

Holmlund U, Cebers G, Dahlfors AR, Sandstedt B, Bremme K, Ekstrom ES, et al. Expression and Regulation of the Pattern Recognition Receptors Toll-Like Receptor-2 and Toll-Like Receptor-4 in the Human Placenta. *Immunology* (2002) 107(1):145–51. doi: 10.1046/j.1365-2567.2002.01491.x

Yoshimura A, Lien E, Ingalls RR, Tuomanen E, Dziarski R, Golenbock D. Cutting Edge: Recognition of Gram-Positive Bacterial Cell Wall Components by the Innate Immune System Occurs *via* Toll-Like Receptor 2. *J Immunol* (1999) 163(1):1–5.

Schwandner R, Dziarski R, Wesche H, Rothe M, Kirschning CJ. Peptidoglycan- and Lipoteichoic Acid-Induced Cell Activation is Mediated by Toll-Like Receptor 2. *J Biol Chem* (1999) 274(25):17406–9. doi: 10.1074/jbc.274.25.17406

Hagmann CA, Herzner AM, Abdullah Z, Zillinger T, Jakobs C, Schuberth C, et al. RIG-I Detects Triphosphorylated RNA of Listeria Monocytogenes During Infection in Non-Immune Cells. *PloS One* (2013) 8(4):e62872. doi: 10.1371/journal.pone.0062872

Abdullah Z, Schlee M, Roth S, Mraheil MA, Barchet W, Bottcher J, et al. RIG- I Detects Infection With Live Listeria by Sensing Secreted Bacterial Nucleic Acids. *EMBO J* (2012) 31(21):4153–64. doi: 10.1038/emboj.2012.274

Mitsunari M, Yoshida S, Shoji T, Tsukihara S, Iwabe T, Harada T, et al. Macrophage-Activating Lipopeptide-2 Induces Cyclooxygenase-2 and Prostaglandin E(2) via Toll-Like Receptor 2 in Human Placental Trophoblast Cells. *J Reprod Immunol* (2006) 72(1-2):46–59. doi: 10.1016/ j.jri.2006.02.003

Moussa M, Roques P, Fievet N, Menu E, Maldonado-Estrada JG, Brunerie J, et al. Placental Cytokine and Chemokine Production in HIV-1-Infected Women: Trophoblast Cells Show a Different Pattern Compared to Cells From HIV-Negative Women. *Clin Exp Immunol* (2001) 125(3):455–64. doi: 10.1046/j.1365-2249.2001.01629.x

Guleria I, Pollard JW. The Trophoblast Is a Component of the Innate Immune System During Pregnancy. *Nat Med* (2000) 6(5):589–93. doi: 10.1038/75074

Germain SJ, Sacks GP, Sooranna SR, Sargent IL, Redman CW. Systemic Inflammatory Priming in Normal Pregnancy and Preeclampsia: The Role of Circulating Syncytiotrophoblast Microparticles. *J Immunol* (2007) 178 (9):5949–56. doi: 10.4049/jimmunol.178.9.5949

Messerli M, May K, Hansson SR, Schneider H, Holzgreve W, Hahn S, et al. Feto-Maternal Interactions in Pregnancies: Placental Microparticles Activate Peripheral Blood Monocytes. *Placenta* (2010) 31(2):106–12. doi: 10.1016/ j.placenta.2009.11.011

Havell EA. Production of Tumor Necrosis Factor During Murine Listeriosis. *J Immunol* (1987) 139(12):4225–31.

Nakane A, Minagawa T, Kato K. Endogenous Tumor Necrosis Factor (Cachectin) Is Essential to Host Resistance Against Listeria Monocytogenes Infection. *Infect Immun* (1988) 56(10):2563–9. doi: 10.1128/iai.56.10.2563-2569.1988

Havell EA. Evidence That Tumor Necrosis Factor has an Important Role in Antibacterial Resistance. *J Immunol* (1989) 143(9):2894–9.

Yui J, Garcia-Lloret M, Wegmann TG, Guilbert LJ. Cytotoxicity of Tumour Necrosis Factor-Alpha and Gamma-Interferon Against Primary Human Placental Trophoblasts. *Placenta* (1994) 15(8):819–35. doi: 10.1016/S0143-4004(05)80184-5

Lucke K, Yan I, Krohn S, Volmari A, Klinge S, Schmid J, et al. Control of Listeria Monocytogenes Infection Requires Classical IL-6 Signaling in Myeloid Cells. *PloS One* (2018) 13(8):e0203395. doi: 10.1371/ journal.pone.0203395

Li W, Chang Y, Liang S, Zhong Z, Li X, Wen J, et al. NLRP3 Inflammasome Activation Contributes to Listeria Monocytogenes-Induced Animal Pregnancy Failure. *BMC Vet Res* (2016) 12:36. doi: 10.1186/s12917-016-0655-2

Wu J, Fernandes-Alnemri T, Alnemri ES. Involvement of the AIM2, NLRC4, and NLRP3 Inflammasomes in Caspase-1 Activation by Listeria Monocytogenes. *J Clin Immunol* (2010) 30(5):693–702. doi: 10.1007/ s10875-010-9425-2

Winsor N, Krustev C, Bruce J, Philpott DJ, Girardin SE. Canonical and Noncanonical Inflammasomes in Intestinal Epithelial Cells. *Cell Microbiol* (2019) 21(11):e13079. doi: 10.1111/cmi.13079

Cheng SB, Nakashima A, Huber WJ, Davis S, Banerjee S, Huang Z, et al. Pyroptosis Is a Critical Inflammatory Pathway in the Placenta From Early Onset Preeclampsia and in Human Trophoblasts Exposed to Hypoxia and Endoplasmic Reticulum Stressors. *Cell Death Dis* (2019) 10(12):927. doi: 10.1038/s41419-019-2162-4

Mor G, Cardenas I. The Immune System in Pregnancy: A Unique Complexity. *Am J Reprod Immunol* (2010) 63(6):425–33. doi: 10.1111/ j.1600-0897.2010.00836.x

Hu X, Zhu Q, Wang Y, Wang L, Li Z, Mor G, et al. Newly Characterized Decidual Tim-3+ Treg Cells Are Abundant During Early Pregnancy and Driven by IL-27 Coordinately With Gal-9 From Trophoblasts. *Hum Reprod* (2020) 35(11):2454–66. doi: 10.1093/humrep/deaa223

Kourko O, Seaver K, Odoardi N, Basta S, Gee K. IL-27, IL-30, and IL-35: A Cytokine Triumvirate in Cancer. *Front Oncol* (2019) 9:969. doi: 10.3389/ fonc.2019.00969

Vrachnis N, Vitoratos N, Iliodromiti Z, Sifakis S, Deligeoroglou E, Creatsas G. Intrauterine Inflammation and Preterm Delivery. *Ann N Y Acad Sci 2010* (2010) 1205:118–22. doi: 10.1111/j.1749-6632.2010.05684.x

Edgar R, Domrachev M, Lash AE. Gene Expression Omnibus: NCBI Gene Expression and Hybridization Array Data Repository. *Nucleic Acids Res* (2002) 30(1):207–10. doi: 10.1093/nar/30.1.207

16

Trypanosoma cruzi Infection at the Maternal-Fetal Interface: Implications of Parasite Load in the Congenital Transmission and Challenges in the Diagnosis of Infected Newborns

*Patricia L. Bustos[1], Natalia Milduberger[1,2], Bibiana J. Volta[1], Alina E. Perrone[1], Susana A. Laucella[1] and Jacqueline Bua[1,2]**

[1]*Instituto Nacional de Parasitología "Dr. Mario Fatala Chaben" – ANLIS C. G. Malbrán, Buenos Aires, Argentina,*
[2]*Centro de Altos Estudios en Ciencias Humanas y de la Salud (CAECIHS), Universidad Abierta Interamericana, Buenos Aires, Argentina*

***Correspondence:**
Jacqueline Bua
jacbua@yahoo.com

Trypanosoma cruzi is the protozoan unicellular parasite that causes Chagas disease. It can be transmitted from infected mothers to their babies *via* the connatal route, thus being able to perpetuate even in the absence of Triatomine insect vectors. Chagas disease was originally endemic in Central and South America, but migration of infected women of childbearing age has spread the *T. cruzi* congenital infection to non-endemic areas like North America, Europe, Japan, and Australia. Currently, 7 million people are affected by this infection worldwide. This review focuses on the relevance of the *T. cruzi* parasite levels in different aspects of the congenital *T. cruzi* infection such as the mother-to-child transmission rate, the maternal and fetal immune response, and its impact on the diagnosis of infected newborns. Improvements in detection of this parasite, with tools that can be easily adapted to be used in remote rural areas, will make the early diagnosis of infected children possible, allowing a prompt trypanocidal treatment and avoiding the current loss of opportunities for the diagnosis of 100% of *T. cruzi* congenitally infected infants.

Keywords: *Trypanosoma cruzi*, mother-to-child transmission, parasitemia, infected pregnant women, congenitally infected infants, early diagnosis

EPIDEMIOLOGY OF THE CONNATAL CHAGAS DISEASE

The American trypanosomiasis, or Chagas disease, is caused by the protozoan parasite *Trypanosoma cruzi*, which affects about 6–7 million people worldwide, with most of the cases in Latin America (WHO | Chagas disease (American trypanosomiasis), 2019).

Given the great success in the control of *Triatoma infestans*, after which Brazil, Paraguay, Uruguay, and Chile were free of *T. cruzi* vectorial transmission, and appropriate control of blood supply that interrupted parasite infection through blood transfusion in most endemic countries, interruption of mother-to-child *T. cruzi* transmission became the new challenge in research and in public health policies. Around 9,000 babies are born to *T. cruzi*-infected mothers each year, and it is estimated that 1.1 million women of childbearing age are infected with *T. cruzi* in 21 countries from Mexico to Argentina, where this neglected tropical disease is endemic (WHO | Chagas disease (American trypanosomiasis), 2019).

Currently, *T. cruzi* infection is globally distributed and has been increasingly detected in countries where vector transmission is absent, mainly due to migration of infected individuals from Latin America. Among the non-endemic countries, the United States is home to the largest number of Chagas infection cases, estimated to be more than 300,000, of which a small number of cases were reported as autochthonous vector-borne transmission in the southern US (Bern et al., 2011; Manne-Goehler et al., 2016), whereas the number of *T. cruzi*-infected people has exceeded 100,000 in Europe (Strasen et al., 2013). It has had a smaller impact in Canada, Australia, and Japan (Buekens et al., 2008; Imai et al., 2014; Jackson et al., 2014). There is a substantial proportion of *T. cruzi*-infected women of childbearing age and congenitally infected infants among the Latin American migrants (Soriano-Arandes et al., 2016). Conversely, *T. cruzi* transmission through blood transfusion or organ transplants are of less epidemiological importance, since non-endemic countries with large immigrant populations have begun to intervene in blood-borne *T. cruzi* transmission (Gascon et al., 2010).

The outcome of congenital infection with *T. cruzi* is due to the result of complex interactions among the parasite, the placenta and the immune responses of the mother and the fetus, and studies about the mechanism of congenital infection are scarce. Understanding these relationships would help in successfully preventing congenital transmission of the parasite or facilitate better access to diagnosis and treatment of the newborns, which would eventually contribute to decreasing the number of cases of this disease around the world.

T. cruzi MOTHER-TO-CHILD TRANSMISSION

It has been reported that *T. cruzi* maternal-fetal transmission occurs in about 1–12% of the pregnancies, taking into account reports with the largest number of infected pregnant women studied in endemic areas (Russomando et al., 1998; Torrico et al., 2005; De Rissio et al., 2010; Salas Clavijo et al., 2012; Bua et al., 2013). The rate of parasite transmission is variable in different countries: 6% in Argentina, 4.1% in Bolivia, and 4.3% in Paraguay (Carlier and Truyens, 2015), 1.7% in Brazil (Martins-Melo et al., 2014), and between 0.8 and 4.08 in Mexico (Cardoso et al., 2012; Montes-Rincón et al., 2016), with an average rate of around 5% (Howard et al., 2014). The wide variation in the reported rates is probably due to studies performed in different areas with and without vector transmission, with heterogeneous populations, experimental conditions and different diagnostic methods.

MATERNAL PARASITEMIA AND VECTOR EXPOSURE

The vertical transmission rate of *T. cruzi* is different in areas with or without the presence of insect vectors, as geographic regions where the disease is endemic are twice as likely to have congenital transmission, compared to the countries free of transmission vectors, 5.0 vs. 2.7% respectively, according to studies performed mainly in Spain (Howard et al., 2014). It was intuitive that parasite load would be enhanced under continuous vector exposure in endemic areas, increasing the risk of parasite congenital transmission (Dias et al., 2002; Torrico et al., 2006). However, it was also demonstrated that infected women living in houses under active vector control had significantly higher parasite loads compared to those women who lived in infested houses (Sánchez Negrette et al., 2005; Rendell et al., 2015). This is probably due to repeated parasite inoculations, which induce an enhanced immune response that helps to control the parasite levels (Rendell et al., 2015).

MATERNAL PARASITEMIA AND RISK OF CONNATAL PARASITE TRANSMISSION

A correlation between high parasitemia in pregnant women and the risk of maternal-fetal *T. cruzi* transmission was observed when the blood from mothers of infected children showed a higher frequency of positive parasite hemocultures (Hermann et al., 2004). A higher parasitemia was also observed in the blood buffy coats of women that transmitted the parasite to their offspring compared to those who did not (Salas et al., 2007; Brutus et al., 2010). A higher frequency of vertical parasite transmission was observed in *T. cruzi* acute infection, which is usually associated with an increased parasitemia (Moretti et al., 2005). Among the studies that quantified parasite load in seropositive pregnant women, mothers of infected babies had significantly higher parasitemia, compared to the mothers of non-infected babies (Virreira et al., 2007; Bern et al., 2009; Bua et al., 2012; Kaplinski et al., 2015; Rendell et al., 2015). When the parasitic load, quantified by quantitative polymerase chain reaction (qPCR), was correlated with the parasite transmission rate in 128 *T. cruzi*-infected pregnant women from Bolivia, researchers found that 31.3% of women with a high parasite load (35 Pe/mL or more) delivered infected children, compared to 15.4% in women with a moderate parasite load (between 1 and 34 Pe/mL), and 0% in women with a parasite load of less than 1 Pe/mL (Rendell et al., 2015). Similar results were obtained in another study in Spain, with migrants from Bolivia and Paraguay, where 31% of pregnant women with detectable *T. cruzi* DNA by conventional PCR delivered infected children, whereas a 0% parasite transmission rate was observed in babies born to chronic infected mothers with negative PCR findings (Murcia et al., 2013).

A high *T. cruzi* parasite load was also detected in patients co-infected with HIV (Rosemberg et al., 1992), and a 100% parasite transmission rate was observed in children born to mothers with reactivated Chagas disease, due to immunosuppression in four different studies (Freilij and Altcheh, 1995; Nisida et al., 1999; Scapellato et al., 2009; Agosti et al., 2012).

Congenital *T. cruzi* infection cannot be prevented during pregnancy as there are no studies on the possible teratogenic effects in pregnant women treated with trypanocidal drugs, benznidazole or nifurtimox. However, six different retrospective studies showed that no congenital infection was detected in infants delivered from a total of 243 infected women that had been treated with benznidazole or nifurtimox prior to pregnancy, in childhood or even in early adulthood (Sosa-estani et al., 2009; Murcia et al., 2013, 2017; Fabbro et al., 2014; Moscatelli et al., 2015; Álvarez et al., 2017).

Altogether, research in this field has strongly supported that parasitemia during pregnancy is a key factor for *T. cruzi* connatal transmission, considering that 100% of the infants were born infected with *T. cruzi* when their mothers displayed high parasitemia during pregnancy. On the other hand, 100% of the children born to drug-treated women or women with naturally very low or no parasitemia were uninfected (Murcia et al., 2013; Rendell et al., 2015). These studies reinforce the notion that decreasing the parasite load might be beneficial in avoiding congenital infection, and supports the idea that either a specific trypanocidal treatment or a possible preconceptional therapeutic vaccine with *T. cruzi* recombinant proteins in near future (Dumonteil et al., 2019) should be offered to women of childbearing age who could potentially transmit the infection to their babies.

PARASITEMIA AND MATERNAL IMMUNE RESPONSE

Interferon-gamma (IFN-γ) and tumor necrosis factor (TNF) are key mediators that control *T. cruzi* infection. IFN-γ activates monocytes/macrophages and stimulates, in synergy with TNF-α, the generation of nitric oxide which kills the parasite (Carlier and Truyens, 2015).

Regarding the maternal immune response during pregnancy, it has been observed that mothers that gave birth to infected children have decreased plasma levels of TNF-α (Cardoni et al., 2004; García et al., 2008) and moderately decreased circulating levels of soluble TNF receptor 1 (sTNF-R1), compared to mothers of uninfected children. Soluble TNF receptors downregulate the biological activity of TNF-α by competing with its membrane receptors (García et al., 2008).

A decrease in production of IFN-γ, in response to parasite antigens, was found in the blood cells derived from the mothers of infected children before and after delivery. However, similar levels of intracellular IFN-γ, within $CD3^+$ cells derived from both groups of infected mothers, were found after polyclonal activation, indicating that they have a comparable ability to produce IFN-γ. Mothers that gave birth to infected children also showed decreased percentages of activated T lymphocytes and monocytes, compared to those who did not transmit the infection to their offspring (Hermann et al., 2004).

Another study that compared cytokine production in *T. cruzi*-infected women that gave birth to uninfected children showed that the mothers with detectable parasitemia presented increased levels of IFN-γ and TNF-α in peripheral, placental and cord blood (Cuna et al., 2009), compared to infected mothers with undetectable parasitemia. These results indicate that, when a higher parasite load is associated with a more robust but pro-inflammatory response, there is no congenital transmission.

Altogether, these findings indicate that the ability to control the infection through an appropriate innate and adaptive immune response against *T. cruzi* to maintain a low parasite load in mothers is associated with lower rates of vertical transmission. Alterations in the control of the inflammatory response may have direct consequences on the congenital transmission and on the children's immune response. Taking into account the challenges related to congenital Chagas diagnosis, the identification of immunological mediators could be very useful for the development of new biomarkers of vertical transmission risk.

PARASITEMIA AND FETAL IMMUNE RESPONSE

T. cruzi infection in pregnant women can induce the activation of T lymphocytes in the fetus *in utero*, as supported by the production of proinflammatory cytokines like interleukin (IL) 1β, IL-6 and TNF-α, in response to *T. cruzi* antigens in uninfected infants born to *T. cruzi*-infected mothers (Vekemans et al., 2000; Hermann et al., 2002; García et al., 2008).

The study of serum cytokines showed a distinct immune profile in congenitally infected infants, with a vigorous innate immune response skewed towards a Th17 profile. Decreased levels of IFN-γ, but increased levels of IL-17A, monokine induced by gamma interferon (MIG) and monocyte chemoattractant protein-1 (MCP-1), were revealed as early predictors of *T. cruzi* infection in the presence of either high or low parasitemia, while *T. cruzi*-infected infants also displayed increased levels of IL-6 and IL-17F, but only in the presence of low parasitemia (Volta et al., 2016).

These demonstrations of a distinct and polarized profile of cytokines and chemokines in the circulation of infants born to *T. cruzi*-infected mothers, and its correlation with the newborn parasite load, reinforce the role of the immune system in restricting the severity of this parasitic infection, preventing the morbidity and mortality of a possible congenital Chagas disease.

PARASITE DIVERSITY AND THE PLACENTAL BARRIER

T. cruzi parasites display genetic differences that have been defined by molecular markers and can be differentiated into six discrete typing units or DTUs (TcI to TcVI), with a localized geographical distribution (Zingales et al., 2012). Although efforts have been made to correlate the different *T. cruzi* DTUs with parasite virulence or clinical manifestations in humans, there has not been any clear association so far (Del Puerto et al., 2010).

T. cruzi parasites from almost all DTUs, except TcIV, have been found in babies born to infected mothers. TcV is the predominant DTU reported in the congenital cases in the Southern cone countries of Latin America (Burgos et al., 2007; Virreira et al., 2007; Corrales et al., 2009). In our laboratory, 38 parasite isolates were obtained from 382 *T. cruzi*-infected pregnant women, which represents 10% positive hemocultures in this group. All of the isolated parasites were identified as

TcV, among which only six belonged to mothers who have gave birth to infected children (Bua et al., 2012); thus, we were not able to associate any parasite DTU with connatal transmission. Nevertheless, it would be interesting to study the genetic differences between parasites isolated from mothers who did not transmit the infection in two or even three different pregnancies and those parasites isolated from infected children (Bua et al., 2013), looking at other biomarkers that would probably help in discriminating the divergences in virulence and pathogenicity under the DTU classification.

Many studies have tried to mimic the human maternal-fetal *T. cruzi* transmission in experimental models with rare offspring infections (Carlier and Truyens, 2015), but some studies with TcI, TcII and TcVI strains revealed that infected pups were obtained only from acutely infected mice with Y and Tulahuen strains which were TcII and TcVI, respectively (Cencig et al., 2013). This suggests that the connatal transmission in experimental models were related more to mice parasitemia than DTU differences. It was possible to obtain a congenital transmission rate of 3.7% in chronically infected mice with the *T. cruzi* strain RA (TcVI), although maternal parasitemia in those mice was significantly higher than the mice infected with K98 clone/TcI, from which no congenitally infected offspring were obtained (Solana et al., 2002).

Another interesting study on the genetic response of the placenta in chronic experimental infections in mice compared the virulence of *T. cruzi* K98 clone with an isolated parasite from a congenitally infected child (VD/TcVI), and demonstrated that the murine placental infection with the VD isolated parasite was associated with upregulation of genes related to components of the innate immune system and IFN-γ. Even so, no congenital transmission was observed in pups born to infected mice with VD nor K98 parasites (Juiz et al., 2017). The VD/TcVI parasite proved to be more infective in the human trophoblast-derived cell line BeWo compared to the *T. cruzi* Y strain/TcII (Medina et al., 2018), probably due to a higher virulence and placental tropism, as it was isolated from a human case of congenital infection (Risso et al., 2004). Nevertheless, no significantly different infection levels could be observed on placental explants with a *T. cruzi* isolated from a congenitally-infected newborn (Lucky, TcII/VI) compared to the Tulahuen strain (TcVI), although the isolated parasite Lucky showed a greater survival rate in a deleterious placental milieu (Triquell et al., 2009). It was demonstrated that a high inoculum of these two parasites resulted in increased infection of placental explants, producing structural and physiological changes through nitric oxide synthase and oxidative-nitrosative stress of the placental barrier (Triquell et al., 2018).

The human placenta forms an anatomical barrier between the maternal blood and fetal tissue, and when infected by *T. cruzi,* a reorganization of the extracellular matrix occurs (Duaso et al., 2012), and a differential expression of pro-inflammatory and immune-modulating cytokines has been observed in infected human placental explants (Castillo et al., 2018), confirming the important role of this organ in avoiding parasite infectivity (Liempi et al., 2014; Díaz-Luján et al., 2016; Juiz et al., 2017).

PARASITEMIA AND DIAGNOSIS IN CONGENITALLY INFECTED INFANTS

Since most *T. cruzi*-infected pregnant women and children are asymptomatic, this parasite infection can go undetected. Additionally, there is a current under-diagnosis of this infection due to losses of opportunities in the prenatal care and proper child follow-up by the health system surveillance programs (Carlier et al., 2015).

The diagnosis of *T. cruzi* congenitally infected children under 8–10 months of age relies primarily on the detection of the parasite, usually live parasites in blood by microscopic methods, as specific antibodies are usually transferred by their seropositive mothers. Only when parasitological assays fail to detect the infection are infants required to be monitored over time for the detection of parasite-specific antibodies, which confirm additional cases of *T. cruzi* infection when maternal antibodies disappear (De Rissio et al., 2010).

In most of the Latin American countries, an early diagnosis of infants born to *T. cruzi*-infected pregnant women relies on the direct examination of the buffy coat from fresh blood samples collected in microhematocrit heparinized tubes or microtubes. This micromethod has limited analytical sensitivity (40–50 parasites/mL) and strongly depends on trained operators (Freilij and Altcheh, 1995; De Rissio et al., 2010), due to the fact that this method needs a minimal 30 min of microscopic observation per sample. Since the micromethod only detects 40–60% of congenitally infected newborns, it is necessary to perform additional serological tests at 8–10 months of age, a period in which around 40–60% of the children do not complete the follow-up for the final diagnosis of this infection (De Rissio et al., 2010; Bua et al., 2013).

MOLECULAR APPROACHES FOR THE PARASITOLOGICAL DIAGNOSIS OF THE CONNATAL *T. cruzi* INFECTION

T. cruzi nucleic acid amplification by PCR has been utilized since 1998 (Russomando et al., 1998) for the detection of *T. cruzi* in congenitally infected babies, offering a higher sensitivity and specificity than parasitological methods involving direct microscopic examination of blood buffy coat samples (Schijman et al., 2003; Virreira et al., 2003; Mora et al., 2005). Later, qPCR technology was developed (Piron et al., 2007; Virreira et al., 2007; Duffy et al., 2009, 2013; Ramírez et al., 2015) and was able to detect 0.85 or 0.43 parasite equivalents per mL (Pe/mL) of satellite DNA and kinetoplastid DNA, respectively, providing more sensitivity than the conventional PCR technique (Cura et al., 2017). qPCR emerged as a potential tool for an accurate and early diagnosis of congenital *T. cruzi* infection (Virreira et al., 2007; Bua et al., 2013). However, a positive amplification of parasitic DNA in newborns could be ambiguously interpreted as a result of maternal parasite DNA debris not related to the passage of live parasites (Virreira et al., 2007), and thus for a positive DNA amplification in babies close to birth it would not be confirmative of parasite infection (Carlier et al., 2015).

This represents a disadvantage over microscopic detection methods, which rely on the observation of viable and motile parasites (Freilij et al., 1983). To avoid misinterpretations, PCR diagnosis would be more reliable at 1 month after delivery (Bua et al., 2013) or for the confirmation of diagnosis with a subsequent blood sample (Murcia et al., 2017).

It is important to highlight that qPCR requires highly equipped laboratories and robust quality controls, frequently found in urban areas or reference health centers but rarely available in maternities or primary point of care units in endemic areas (Porrás et al., 2015; Messenger and Bern, 2018; Picado et al., 2018). In fact, PCR is not included as a tool for diagnosis of congenital *T. cruzi* infection in the Latin American guidelines, with the exception of Chile, although its use is sometimes recommended (Picado et al., 2018). In Argentina, this molecular technique is in the process of being transferred to different laboratories of the national public health network (Cura et al., 2017).

Other molecular methods that could be implemented for the *T. cruzi* diagnosis are the techniques based on isothermal amplification of DNA. These methods overcome the needs for specialized PCR equipment and have been proven to amplify the *T. cruzi* DNA successfully. Loop-mediated isothermal amplification (LAMP) can be performed at a constant temperature of 60–65°C with a simple heat-block (Besuschio et al., 2017; Rivero et al., 2017), and the recombinase polymerase amplification (RPA) can be run at 37–42°C (Castellanos-Gonzalez et al., 2018) with a sensitivity similar to that of the quantitative PCR amplification (Besuschio et al., 2017; Jimenez-Coello et al., 2018). These new molecular approaches await the necessary standardization and validation, but, as with all molecular techniques, the main issue is that parasite DNA amplification cannot be performed without purification of DNA from patient blood samples, which cannot be performed easily in health centers in rural areas, as it requires experienced operators, infrastructure and the necessary quality controls recommended by good practice guidelines.

PARASITEMIA IN *T. cruzi* INFECTED-CHILDREN AT A 1-YEAR FOLLOW-UP STUDY

Parasitemia levels in infants congenitally infected with *T. cruzi* are significantly higher at birth than in their infected mothers, who are usually in the chronic phase of this infection (Schijman et al., 2003; Virreira et al., 2007; Bern et al., 2009; Bua et al., 2012), and no correlation has been observed between the parasitemia of pregnant women and their babies (Bua et al., 2012).

Parasite load was quantified by qPCR in 51 infected babies born to *T. cruzi*-infected mothers in a retrospective study. These babies were grouped according to the time and method in which congenital infection was diagnosed during 1-year follow-up after delivery. A group of 19 newborns diagnosed by micromethod at 1 month showed the highest median parasitemia, around 1,700 Pe/mL. The infected infants that came back for a second parasitological diagnosis at 6 months of age showed a median parasitemia of around 20 Pe/mL in the sample obtained at 1 month of age, which was under the threshold of the micromethod sensitivity. This group of 10 infants could be diagnosed by microscopy at 6 months of age because parasitemia increased up to 500 Pe/mL. In the infants (22/51) negative for the first and second parasitological control, who required serological diagnosis at around 1 year of age, the median parasite load was 5,800 and 20 Pe/mL in the blood samples obtained at 1, 6, and 12 months after delivery, respectively. This study helped to understand the differences among diverse groups of *T. cruzi* congenitally infected children during 1 year follow-up in centers where molecular techniques are not available (Bua et al., 2013). An infected child that is not diagnosed at 8–10 months after delivery and not treated will experience a drastic decrease of parasitemia, indicating the transition from the acute phase to the chronic phase of the *T. cruzi* infection, and most importantly, will be excluded from the possibility of being treated with trypanocidal drugs.

Although DNA amplification has shown great sensitivity for the detection of cases of *T. cruzi* mother-to-child transmission, qPCR does not detect 100% of congenital cases, and in case of negative PCR findings, it is necessary to detect the congenital infection by serology at 8–10 months of age. Quantitative PCR was able to detect *T. cruzi* infection in 50/51 babies in the first control visit, and we did not observe any false positive PCR in the babies diagnosed by micromethod at 1 month after delivery (Bua et al., 2013). The only *T. cruzi*-infected infant that could not be diagnosed by qPCR at 20 days nor at 6 months of age was infected by a TcI *T. cruzi* parasite that was isolated by hemoculture at 7 months of age, a period in which the specific anti-*T. cruzi* serology was also positive (Volta et al., 2018).

SEARCH OF BIOMARKERS FOR THE EARLY SEROLOGICAL DIAGNOSIS OF THE CONNATAL *T. cruzi* INFECTION

As mentioned, the detection of anti-*T. cruzi* specific antibodies in infants born to seropositive mothers can be performed when they are 8–10 months of age, when maternal passively transferred antibodies are no longer detectable (Moya et al., 1989). A positive serological result at this time is a conclusive diagnosis for the *T. cruzi* congenital infection in infants where previous parasitological methods failed to detect the parasite. Unfortunately, only 40–60% of congenitally infected children complete the required 1-year follow-up (Sosa-Estani, 2005; De Rissio et al., 2010). Efforts are being made to find specific serological markers to diagnose this infection at an earlier stage and overcome the loss of opportunities to detect 100% of the *T. cruzi* infected children as soon as they are born.

The *T. cruzi* Shed Acute Phase Antigen (SAPA) (Affranchino et al., 1989) proved to be a reliable and highly sensitive marker for the early parasite detection of congenital *T. cruzi* infection (Reyes et al., 1990). An ELISA test available in Paraguay detects anti-SAPA IgG antibodies in children born to infected mothers at 3 months of age (Russomando et al., 2010). The anti-SAPA IgG levels in binomial blood samples from seropositive mothers and their babies also allowed for diagnosis in 90.5% of the *T. cruzi*-infected children at around 1 month of age (Volta et al., 2015) by subtracting the anti-SAPA OD value of the mother from the one in the child (Mallimaci et al., 2010). We observed a positive correlation between parasitemia levels in mothers and infants, evaluated by qPCR, and the anti-SAPA IgG antibody titers detected by ELISA, which more likely accounts for the secretion of SAPA antigen by the trypomastigotes in the bloodstream (Volta et al., 2015).

Trypomastigote secreted/excreted (TESA) protein bands of 120–200 kDa were blotted on membranes (Umezawa et al., 1996) and recognized by anti-SAPA IgM antibodies in acute and congenital *T. cruzi*-infected children, but with lower sensitivity than qPCR (Messenger et al., 2017). Western blotting with TESA antigen helped discriminate the chronic maternal infection by detecting IgG bound to TESA (a single 150–160 kDa band) from the blood of newborns with acute infection, highlighting the presence of four to six SAPA-specific protein bands between 120 and 200 kDa on the IgM TESA-blot (Noazin et al., 2018). Although the sensitivity of the anti-SAPA IgM on TESA blots reached 80% in *T. cruzi*- infected newborns (Noazin et al., 2018), the immunodetection of membrane strips has several issues of reproducibility and standardization in care units outside urban areas (Messenger and Bern, 2018).

The SAPA antigen has been considered as a promising biomarker for the diagnosis of *T. cruzi* infection, and some new approaches for the development of diagnostic assays which include detection of SAPA along with other antigenic determinants in single multiplex assays, to confirm the *T. cruzi* infection in humans, are being developed (Granjon et al., 2016). SAPA has also been included in the design of chimeric molecules, named as CP1 and CP3, which were sensitive enough to circumvent inconclusive diagnosis in subjects with serodiscordant findings (Peverengo et al., 2018). These multi-epitope constructs are currently being tested for an improved detection of congenital infected newborns (Dr. Ivan Marcipar, personal communication).

Another recent development was to span *T. cruzi* linear B-cell epitopes and design antigenic short peptides to achieve an accurate diagnosis of this infection in chronic human samples by ELISA (Mucci et al., 2017). The next step is to extend this approach with the aim of an early accurate diagnosis for congenital infection (Dr. Fernán Agüero, personal communication).

In summary, the current search for highly sensitive serological diagnostic tests based on multiple antigenic determinants in multiplex assays could offer the possibility to detect *T. cruzi*-infected children born to seropositive women. A prompt diagnosis may prevent dropout during the 1-year serological follow-up after delivery required for the accurate diagnosis of *T. cruzi* infection. Ideally, serological diagnosis for early parasite detection in newborns could be available as a lateral flow immunochromatographic test, with an affordable cost for public health systems, easily performed by operators with minimal training, without the need of any specialized and costly equipment, no reagent preparations, with immediate results and easy adaptability for use in primary health care facilities, public hospitals or maternities in endemic area. As established by WHO, *T. cruzi* infection is curable if treatment is initiated soon after infection (Carlier et al., 2011; WHO | Chagas disease (American trypanosomiasis), 2019). Many reports have shown that benznidazole and nifurtimox treatments are well tolerated in children and resulted in undetectable parasite load (Russomando et al., 1998; Blanco et al., 2000; Schijman et al., 2003; Altcheh et al., 2005; Luquetti et al., 2005).

Infants who fail to complete the required follow-up period for parasite diagnosis will be deprived of access to immediate drug treatment and parasite clearance and will become *T. cruzi*-infected adults. It is crucial to develop improved, rapid and simple diagnostic methods for a timely detection of *T. cruzi* congenital infection, soon after birth and before the newborn leaves the care unit, especially in rural areas where access to the health system can be limited.

CONCLUSION

Mother-to-child transmission of *T. cruzi* infection represents a challenge in controlling parasite dissemination in endemic and non-endemic regions. Parasitemia in infected women plays a key role in congenital Chagas outcome, as it directly affects transmission rate and maternal and fetal protective immune response against the parasite. In fact, decreasing parasite load by trypanocidal treatment administered to women of childbearing age proved to be highly efficient in avoiding congenital infection. Parasite levels in congenitally infected newborns have a direct impact on their diagnosis, so it is crucial to develop improved diagnostic methods to facilitate access to treatment.

AUTHOR CONTRIBUTIONS

PB, NM, BV, AP, SL, and JB wrote the manuscript and approved its final version.

REFERENCES

Affranchino, J. L., Ibañez, C. F., Luquetti, A. O., Rassi, A., Reyes, M. B., Macina, R. A., et al. (1989). Identification of a *Trypanosoma cruzi* antigen that is shed during the acute phase of Chagas' disease. *Mol. Biochem. Parasitol.* 34, 221–228. doi: 10.1016/0166-6851(89)90050-9

Agosti, M. R., Ercoli, P., Dolcini, G., Andreani, G., Martínez Peralta, L., and González Ayala, S. (2012). Two cases of mother-to-child transmission of HIV and *Trypanosoma cruzi* in Argentina. *Braz. J. Infect. Dis.* 16, 398–399. doi: 10.1016/j.bjid.2012.06.008

Altcheh, J., Biancardi, M., Lapeña, A., Ballering, G., and Freilij, H. (2005). Congenital Chagas disease: experience in the Hospital de Niños, Ricardo Gutiérrez, Buenos Aires, Argentina. *Rev. Soc. Bras. Med. Trop.* 38(Suppl. 2), 41–45. Available at: http://www.ncbi.nlm.nih.gov/pubmed/16482812

Álvarez, M. G., Vigliano, C., Lococo, B., Bertocchi, G., and Viotti, R. (2017). Prevention of congenital Chagas disease by benznidazole treatment in reproductive-age women. An observational study. *Acta Trop.* 174, 149–152. doi: 10.1016/j.actatropica.2017.07.004

Bern, C., Kjos, S., Yabsley, M. J., and Montgomery, S. P. (2011). *Trypanosoma cruzi* and Chagas' disease in the United States. *Clin. Microbiol. Rev.* 24, 655–681. doi: 10.1128/CMR.00005-11 Review.

Bern, C., Verastegui, M., Gilman, R. H., LaFuente, C., Galdos-Cardenas, G., Calderon, M., et al. (2009). Congenital *Trypanosoma cruzi* transmission in Santa Cruz, Bolivia. *Clin. Infect. Dis.* 49, 1667–1674. doi: 10.1086/648070

Besuschio, S. A., Llano Murcia, M., Benatar, A. F., Monnerat, S., Cruz Mata, I., Picado de Puig, A., et al. (2017). Analytical sensitivity and specificity of a loop-mediated isothermal amplification (LAMP) kit prototype for detection of *Trypanosoma cruzi* DNA in human blood samples. *PLoS Negl. Trop. Dis.* 11, 1–18. doi: 10.1371/journal.pntd.0005779

Blanco, S. B., Segura, E. L., Cura, E. N., Chuit, R., Tulián, L., Flores, I., et al. (2000). Congenital transmission of *Trypanosoma cruzi*: an operational outline for detecting and treating infected infants in northwestern Argentina. *Trop. Med. Int. Health* 5, 293–301. doi: 10.1046/j.1365-3156.2000.00548.x

Brutus, L., Castillo, H., Bernal, C., Salas, N. A., Schneider, D., Santalla, J. A., et al. (2010). Short report: detectable *Trypanosoma cruzi* parasitemia during pregnancy and delivery as a risk factor for congenital Chagas disease. *Am. J. Trop. Med. Hyg.* 83, 1044–1047. doi: 10.4269/ajtmh.2010.10-0326

Bua, J., Volta, B. J., Perrone, A. E., Scollo, K., Velázquez, E. B., Ruiz, A. M., et al. (2013). How to improve the farly diagnosis of *Trypanosoma cruzi* infection: relationship between validated conventional diagnosis and quantitative DNA amplification in congenitally infected children. *PLoS Negl. Trop. Dis.* 7, 12–14. doi: 10.1371/journal.pntd.0002476

Bua, J., Volta, B. J., Velazquez, E. B., Ruiz, A. M., De Rissio, A. M., and Cardoni, R. L. (2012). Vertical transmission of *Trypanosoma cruzi* infection: quantification of parasite burden in mothers and their children by parasite DNA amplification. *Trans. R. Soc. Trop. Med. Hyg.* 106, 623–628. doi: 10.1016/j.trstmh.2012.03.015

Buekens, P., Almendares, O., Carlier, Y., Dumonteil, E., Eberhard, M., Gamboa-Leon, R., et al. (2008). Mother-to-child transmission of Chagas' disease in North America: why don't we do more? *Matern. Child Health J.* 12, 283–286. doi: 10.1007/s10995-007-0246-8

Burgos, J. M., Altcheh, J., Bisio, M., Duffy, T., Valadares, H. M. S., Seidenstein, M. E., et al. (2007). Direct molecular profiling of minicircle signatures and lineages of *Trypanosoma cruzi* bloodstream populations causing congenital Chagas disease. *Int. J. Parasitol.* 37, 1319–1327. doi: 10.1016/j.ijpara.2007.04.015

Cardoni, R. L., García, M. M., and De Rissio, A. M. (2004). Proinflammatory and anti-inflammatory cytokines in pregnant women chronically infected with *Trypanosoma cruzi*. *Acta Trop.* 90, 65–72. doi: 10.1016/j.actatropica.2003.09.020

Cardoso, E. J., Valdéz, G. C., Campos, A. C., Sanchez, R. d. l. L., Mendoza, C. R., Hernández, A. P., et al. (2012). Maternal fetal transmission of *Trypanosoma cruzi*: a problem of public health little studied in Mexico. *Exp. Parasitol.* 131, 425–432. doi: 10.1016/j.exppara.2012.05.013

Carlier, Y., Sosa-Estani, S., Luquetti, A. O., and Buekens, P. (2015). Congenital Chagas disease: an update. *Mem. Inst. Oswaldo Cruz* 110, 363–368. doi: 10.1590/0074-02760140405

Carlier, Y., Torrico, F., Sosa-Estani, S., Russomando, G., Luquetti, A., Freilij, H., et al. (2011). Congenital Chagas disease: recommendations for diagnosis, treatment and control of newborns, siblings and pregnant women. *PLoS Negl. Trop. Dis.* 5, 4–6. doi: 10.1371/journal.pntd.0001250

Carlier, Y., and Truyens, C. (2015). Congenital Chagas disease as an ecological model of interactions between *Trypanosoma cruzi* parasites, pregnant women, placenta and fetuses. *Acta Trop.* 151, 103–115. doi: 10.1016/j.actatropica.2015.07.016

Castellanos-Gonzalez, A., White, A. C., Melby, P., and Travi, B. (2018). Molecular diagnosis of protozoan parasites by recombinase polymerase amplification. *Acta Trop.* 182, 4–11. doi: 10.1016/j.actatropica.2018.02.002

Castillo, C., Carrillo, I., Libisch, G., Juiz, N., Schijman, A., Robello, C., et al. (2018). Host-parasite interaction: changes in human placental gene expression induced by *Trypanosoma cruzi*. *Parasit. Vectors* 11, 1–13. doi: 10.1186/s13071-018-2988-0

Cencig, S., Coltel, N., Truyens, C., and Carlier, Y. (2013). Fertility, gestation outcome and parasite congenital transmissibility in mice infected with TcI, TcII and TcVI genotypes of *Trypanosoma cruzi*. *PLoS Negl. Trop. Dis.* 7:e2271. doi: 10.1371/journal.pntd.0002271

Corrales, R. M., Mora, M. C., Negrette, O. S., Diosque, P., Lacunza, D., Virreira, M., et al. (2009). Congenital Chagas disease involves *Trypanosoma cruzi* sub-lineage IId in the northwestern province of Salta, Argentina. *Infect. Genet. Evol.* 9, 278–282. doi: 10.1016/j.meegid.2008.12.008

Cuna, W. R., Herrera Choque, A. G., Passera, R., and Rodriguez, C. (2009). Pro-inflammatory cytokine production in chagasic mothers and their uninfected newborns. *J. Parasitol.* 95, 891–894. doi: 10.1645/GE-1927.1

Cura, C. I., Ramírez, J. C., Rodríguez, M., Lopez-Albízu, C., Irazu, L., Scollo, K., et al. (2017). Comparative study and analytical verification of PCR methods for the diagnosis of congenital Chagas disease. *J. Mol. Diagn.* 19, 673–681. doi: 10.1016/j.jmoldx.2017.05.010

De Rissio, A. M., Riarte, A. R., García, M. M., Esteva, M. I., Ruiz, A. M., and Quaglino, M. (2010). Congenital *Trypanosoma cruzi* infection. Efficacy of its monitoring in an urban reference health center in a non-endemic area of Argentina. *Am. J. Trop. Med. Hyg.* 82, 838–845. doi: 10.4269/ajtmh.2010.08-0383

Del Puerto, R., Nishizawa, J. E., Kikuchi, M., Iihoshi, N., Roca, Y., Avilas, C., et al. (2010). Lineage analysis of circulating *Trypanosoma cruzi* parasites and their association with clinical forms of Chagas disease in Bolivia. *PLoS Negl. Trop. Dis.* 4, 1–6. doi: 10.1371/journal.pntd.0000687

Dias, J., Silveira, A., and Schofield, C. (2002). The impact of Chagas disease control in Latin America - A review. *Mem. Inst. Oswaldo Cruz* 97, 603–612. doi: 10.1590/S0074-02762002000500002

Díaz-Luján, C., Triquell, M. F., Castillo, C., Hardisson, D., Kemmerling, U., and Fretes, R. E. (2016). Role of placental barrier integrity in infection by *Trypanosoma cruzi*. *Acta Trop.* 164, 360–368. doi: 10.1016/j.actatropica.2016.09.021

Duaso, J., Yanez, E., Castillo, C., Galanti, N., Cabrera, G., Corral, G., et al. (2012). Reorganization of extracellular matrix in placentas from women with asymptomatic Chagas disease: mechanism of parasite invasion or local placental defense? *J. Trop. Med.* 2012:758357. doi: 10.1155/2012/758357

Duffy, T., Bisio, M., Altcheh, J., Burgos, J. M., Diez, M., Levin, M. J., et al. (2009). Accurate real-time PCR strategy for monitoring bloodstream parasitic loads in Chagas disease patients. *PLoS Negl. Trop. Dis.* 3:e419. doi: 10.1371/journal.pntd.0000419

Duffy, T., Cura, C. I., Ramirez, J. C., Abate, T., Cayo, N. M., Parrado, R., et al. (2013). Analytical performance of a multiplex real-time PCR assay using TaqMan probes for quantification of *Trypanosoma cruzi* satellite DNA in blood samples. *PLoS Negl. Trop. Dis.* 7:e2000. doi: 10.1371/journal.pntd.0002000

Dumonteil, E., Herrera, C., and Buekens, P. (2019). A therapeutic preconceptional vaccine against Chagas disease: a novel indication that could reduce congenital transmission and accelerate vaccine development. *Trop. Dis.* 13:e0006985. doi: 10.1371/journal.pntd.0006985

Fabbro, D. L., Danesi, E., Olivera, V., Codebó, M. O., Denner, S., Heredia, C., et al. (2014). Trypanocide treatment of women infected with *Trypanosoma cruzi* and its effect on preventing congenital Chagas. *PLoS Negl. Trop. Dis.* 8:e3312. doi: 10.1371/journal.pntd.0003312

Freilij, H., and Altcheh, J. (1995). Congenital Chagas' disease: diagnostic and clinical aspects. *Clin. Infect. Dis.* 21, 551–555. doi: 10.1093/clinids/21.3.551

Freilij, H., Muller, L., and Gonzalez Cappa, S. M. (1983). Direct micromethod for diagnosis of acute and congenital Chagas' disease. *J. Clin. Microbiol.* 18, 327–330. Available at: https://www.ncbi.nlm.nih.gov/pubmed/6413530

García, M. M., De Rissio, A. M., Villalonga, X., Mengoni, E., and Cardoni, R. L. (2008). Soluble tumor necrosis factor (TNF) receptors (sTNF-R1 and -R2) in pregnant women chronically infected with *Trypanosoma cruzi* and their children. *Am. J. Trop. Med. Hyg.* 78, 499–503. doi: 10.4269/ajtmh.2008.78.499

Gascon, J., Bern, C., and Pinazo, M. J. (2010). Chagas disease in Spain, the United States and other non-endemic countries. *Acta Trop.* 115, 22–27. doi: 10.1016/j.actatropica.2009.07.019

Granjon, E., Dichtel-Danjoy, M. L., Saba, E., Sabino, E., Campos de Oliveira, L., and Zrein, M. (2016). Development of a novel multiplex immunoassay multi-cruzi for the serological confirmation of Chagas disease. *PLoS Negl. Trop. Dis.* 10:e0004596. doi: 10.1371/journal.pntd.0004596

Hermann, E., Truyens, C., Alonso-Vega, C., Even, J., Rodriguez, P., Berthe, A., et al. (2002). Human fetuses are able to mount an adultlike CD8 T-cell response. *Blood* 100, 2153–2158. Available at: http://bloodjournal.hematologylibrary.org/misc/rights.dtl#repub_requests

Hermann, E., Truyens, C., Alonso-Vega, C., Rodriguez, P., Berthe, A., Torrico, F., et al. (2004). Congenital transmission of *Trypanosoma cruzi* is associated with maternal enhanced parasitemia and decreased production of interferon-γ in response to parasite antigens. *J. Infect. Dis.* 189, 1274–1281. doi: 10.1086/382511

Howard, E. J., Xiong, X., Carlier, Y., Sosa-Estani, S., and Buekens, P. (2014). Frequency of the congenital transmission of *Trypanosoma cruzi*: a systematic review and meta-analysis. *BJOG* 121, 22–33. doi: 10.1111/1471-0528.12396

Imai, K., Maeda, T., Sayama, Y., Mikita, K., Fujikura, Y., Misawa, K., et al.

(2014). Mother-to-child transmission of congenital Chagas disease, Japan. *Emerg. Infect. Dis.* 20, 146–148. doi: 10.3201/eid2001.131071

Jackson, Y., Pinto, A., and Pett, S. (2014). Chagas disease in Australia and New Zealand: risks and needs for public health interventions. *Trop. Med. Int. Health* 19, 212–218. doi: 10.1111/tmi.12235

Jimenez-Coello, M., Shelite, T., Castellanos-Gonzalez, A., Saldarriaga, O., Rivero, R., Ortega-Pacheco, A., et al. (2018). Efficacy of recombinase polymerase amplification to diagnose *Trypanosoma cruzi* infection in dogs with cardiac alterations from an endemic area of Mexico. *Vector-Borne Zoonotic Dis.* 18, 417–423. doi: 10.1089/vbz.2017.2258

Juiz, N. A., Solana, M. E., Acevedo, G. R., Benatar, A. F., Ramirez, J. C., da Costa, P. A., et al. (2017). Different genotypes of *Trypanosoma cruzi* produce distinctive placental environment genetic response in chronic experimental infection. *PLoS Negl. Trop. Dis.* 11, 1–19. doi: 10.1371/journal.pntd.0005436

Kaplinski, M., Jois, M., Galdos-Cardenas, G., Rendell, V. R., Shah, V., Do, R. Q., et al. (2015). Sustained domestic vector exposure is associated with increased Chagas cardiomyopathy risk but decreased parasitemia and congenital transmission risk among young women in Bolivia. *Clin. Infect. Dis.* 61, 918–926. doi: 10.1093/cid/civ446

Liempi, A., Castillo, C., Duaso, J., Droguett, D., Sandoval, A., Barahona, K., et al. (2014). *Trypanosoma cruzi* induces trophoblast differentiation: a potential local antiparasitic mechanism of the human placenta? *Placenta* 35, 1035–1042. doi: 10.1016/j.placenta.2014.09.017

Luquetti, A. O., Dias, J. C. P., and Prata, A. (2005). Diagnosis and treatment of congenital infection caused by *Trypanosoma cruzi* in Brazil. *Rev. Soc. Bras. Med. Trop.* 38(Suppl. 2), 27–28. Available at: http://www.ncbi.nlm.nih.gov/pubmed/16482809

Mallimaci, M. C., Sosa-Estani, S., Russomando, G., Sanchez, Z., Sijvarger, C., Alvarez, I. M., et al. (2010). Short report: early diagnosis of congenital *Trypanosoma cruzi* infection, using shed acute phase antigen, in Ushuaia, Tierra del Fuego. Argentina. *Am. J. Trop. Med. Hyg.* 82, 55–59. doi: 10.4269/ajtmh.2010.09-0219

Manne-Goehler, J., Umeh, C. A., Montgomery, S. P., and Wirtz, V. J. (2016). Estimating the burden of Chagas disease in the United States. *PLoS Negl. Trop. Dis.* 10, 1–7. doi: 10.1371/journal.pntd.0005033

Martins-Melo, F. R., da Silveira Lima, M., Ramos, A. N., Alencar, C. H., and Heukelbach, J. (2014). Systematic review: prevalence of Chagas disease in pregnant women and congenital transmission of *Trypanosoma cruzi* in Brazil: a systematic review and meta-analysis. *Trop. Med. Int. Health* 19, 943–957. doi: 10.1111/tmi.12328

Medina, L., Castillo, C., Liempi, A., Herbach, M., Cabrera, G., Valenzuela, L., et al. (2018). Differential infectivity of two *Trypanosoma cruzi* strains in placental cells and tissue. *Acta Trop.* 186, 35–40. doi: 10.1016/j.actatropica.2018.07.001

Messenger, L. A., and Bern, C. (2018). Congenital Chagas disease: current diagnostics, limitations and future perspectives. *Curr. Opin. Infect. Dis.* 31, 415–421. doi: 10.1097/QCO.0000000000000478

Messenger, L. A., Gilman, R. H., Verastegui, M., Galdos-Cardenas, G., Sanchez, G., Valencia, E., et al. (2017). Toward improving early diagnosis of congenital Chagas disease in an endemic setting. *Clin. Infect. Dis.* 65, 268–275. doi: 10.1093/cid/cix277

Montes-Rincón, L. M., Galaviz-Silva, L., González-Bravo, F. E., and Molina-Garza, Z. J. (2016). *Trypanosoma cruzi* seroprevalence in pregnant women and screening by PCR and microhaematocrit in newborns from Guanajuato, Mexico. *Acta Trop.* 164, 100–106. doi: 10.1016/j.actatropica.2016.08.029

Mora, M. C., Negrette, O. S., Marco, D., Barrio, A., Ciaccio, M., Segura, M. A., et al. (2005). Early diagnosis of congenital *Trypanosoma cruzi* infection using PCR, hemoculture, and capillary concentration, as compared with delayed serology. *J. Parasitol.* 91, 1468–1473. doi: 10.1645/GE-549R.1

Moretti, E., Basso, B., Castro, I., Paez, M. C., Chaul, M., Barbieri, G., et al. (2005). Chagas' disease: study of congenital transmission in cases of acute maternal infection. *Rev. Soc. Bras. Med. Trop.* 38, 53–55. doi: 10.1590/S0037-86822005000100010

Moscatelli, G., Moroni, S., García-Bournissen, F., Ballering, G., Bisio, M., Freilij, H., et al. (2015). Prevention of congenital Chagas through treatment of girls and women of childbearing age. *Mem. Inst. Oswaldo Cruz* 110, 507–509. doi: 10.1590/0074-02760140347

Moya, P., Moretti, E., Paolasso, R., Basso, B., Blanco, S., Sanmartino, C., et al. (1989). Neonatal Chagas disease: laboratory diagnosis during the first year of life. *Medicina* 49, 595–599. Available at: http://www.ncbi.nlm.nih.gov/pubmed/2518645

Mucci, J., Carmona, S. J., Volcovich, R., Altcheh, J., Bracamonte, E., Marco, J. D., et al. (2017). Next-generation ELISA diagnostic assay for Chagas disease based on the combination of short peptidic epitopes. *PLoS Negl. Trop. Dis.* 11, 1–19. doi: 10.1371/journal.pntd.0005972

Murcia, L., Carrilero, B., Munoz-Davila, M. J., Thomas, C. M., López, M. C., and Segovia, M. (2013). Risk factors and primary prevention of congenital Chagas disease in a nonendemic country. *Clin. Infect. Dis.* 56, 496–502. doi: 10.1093/cid/cis910

Murcia, L., Simón, M., Carrilero, B., Roig, M., and Segovia, M. (2017). Treatment of infected women of childbearing age prevents congenital *Trypanosoma cruzi* infection by eliminating the parasitemia detected by PCR. *J. Infect. Dis.* 215, 1452–1458. doi: 10.1093/infdis/jix087

Nisida, I. V. V., Neto, V. A., Braz, L. M. A., Duarte, M. I. S., and Umezawa, E. S. (1999). A survey of congenital Chagas' disease, carried out at three health institutions in São Paulo city, Brazil. *Rev. Inst. Med. Trop. Sao Paulo* 41, 305–311. doi: 10.1590/S0036-46651999000500007

Noazin, S., Lee, J. A., Malaga, E. S., Ayala, E. V., Condori, B. J., Roca, C., et al. (2018). Trypomastigote excretory secretory antigen (TESA) blot is associated in neonates with parasite load and detects congenital *T. cruzi* infection using anti-SAPA IgM. *J. Infect. Dis.* 219, 609–618 doi: 10.1093/infdis/jiy562

Peverengo, L. M., Garcia, V., Rodeles, L. M., Mendicino, D., Vicco, M., Lagier, C., et al. (2018). Development and assessment of an improved recombinant multiepitope antigen-based immunoassay to diagnose chronic Chagas disease. *Parasitology* 145, 1594–1599. doi: 10.1017/S0031182018000458

Picado, A., Cruz, I., Redard-Jacot, M., Schijman, A. G., Torrico, F., Sosa-Estani, S., et al. (2018). The burden of congenital Chagas disease and implementation of molecular diagnostic tools in Latin America. *BMJ Glob. Heal.* 3:e001069. doi: 10.1136/bmjgh-2018-001069

Piron, M., Fisa, R., Casamitjana, N., López-Chejade, P., Puig, L., Vergés, M., et al. (2007). Development of a real-time PCR assay for *Trypanosoma cruzi* detection in blood samples. *Acta Trop.* 103, 195–200. doi: 10.1016/j.actatropica.2007.05.019

Porrás, A. I., Yadon, Z. E., Altcheh, J., and Britto, C. (2015). Target product profile (TPP) for Chagas disease point-of-care diagnosis and assessment of response to treatment. *PLoS Negl. Trop. Dis.* 9:e0003697. doi: 10.1371/journal.pntd.0003697

Ramírez, J. C., Cura, C. I., da Cruz Moreira, O., Lages-Silv, E., Juiz, N., Velázquez, E., et al. (2015). Analytical validation of quantitative real-time PCR methods for quantification of *Trypanosoma cruzi* DNA in blood samples from Chagas disease patients. *J. Mol. Diagn.* 17, 605–615. doi: 10.1016/j.jmoldx.2015.04.010

Rendell, V. R., Gilman, R. H., Valencia, E., Galdos-Cardenas, G., Verastegui, M., Sanchez, L., et al. (2015). *Trypanosoma cruzi*-infected pregnant women without vector exposure have higher parasitemia levels: implications for congenital transmission risk. *PLoS One* 10, 1–9. doi: 10.1371/journal.pone.0119527

Reyes, M. B., Lorca, M., Muñoz, P., and Frasch, A. C. (1990). Fetal IgG specificities against *Trypanosoma cruzi* antigens in infected newborns. *Proc. Natl. Acad. Sci. U. S. A.* 87, 2846–2850. doi: 10.1073/pnas.87.7.2846

Risso, M. G., Garbarino, G. B., Mocetti, E., Campetella, O., González Cappa, S. M., Buscaglia, C. A., et al. (2004). Differential expression of a virulence factor, the trans- sialidase, by the main *Trypanosoma cruzi* phylogenetic lineages. *J. Infect. Dis.* 189, 2250–2259. doi: 10.1086/420831

Rivero, R., Bisio, M., Velazquez, E., Esteva, M. I., Scollo, K., Gonzalez, N., et al. (2017). Rapid detection of *Trypanosoma cruzi* by colorimetric loop-mediated isothermal amplification (LAMP): A potential novel tool for the detection of congenital Chagas infection. *Diagn. Microbiol. Infect. Dis.* 89, 26–28. doi: 10.1016/j.diagmicrobio.2017.06.012

Rosemberg, S., Chaves, C. J., Higuchi, M. L., Lopes, M. B., Castro, L. H., and Machado, L. R. (1992). Fatal meningoencephalitis caused by reactivation of *Trypanosoma cruzi* infection in a patient with AIDS. *Neurology* 42, 640–642. doi: 10.1212/WNL.42.3.640

Russomando, G., De Tomassone, M. M. C., De Guillen, I., Acosta, N., Vera, N., Almiron, M., et al. (1998). Treatment of congenital Chagas' disease diagnosed and followed up by the polymerase chain reaction. *Am. J. Trop. Med. Hyg.* 59, 487–491. doi: 10.4269/ajtmh.1998.59.487

Russomando, G., Snchez, Z., Meza, G., and De Guillen, Y. (2010). Shed acute-phase antigen protein in an ELISA system for unequivocal diagnosis of congenital Chagas disease. *Expert. Rev. Mol. Diagn.* 10, 705–707. doi: 10.1586/erm.10.70

Salas Clavijo, N. A., Postigo, J. R., Schneider, D., Santalla, J. A., Brutus, L., and Chippaux, J. P. (2012). Prevalence of Chagas disease in pregnant women and incidence of congenital transmission in Santa Cruz de la Sierra, Bolivia. *Acta Trop.* 124, 87–91. doi: 10.1016/j.actatropica.2012.06.012

Salas, N. A., Cot, M., Schneider, D., Mendoza, B., Santalla, J. A., Postigo, J., et al. (2007). Risk factors and consequences of congenital Chagas disease in Yacuiba, south Bolivia. *Trop. Med. Int. Health* 12, 1498–1505. doi: 10.1111/j.1365-3156.2007.01958.x

Sánchez Negrette, O., Mora, M. C., and Basombrío, M. Á. (2005). High prevalence of congenital Trypanosoma cruzi infection and family clustering in Salta, Argentina. *Pediatrics* 115, e668–e672. doi: 10.1542/peds.2004-1732

Scapellato, P. G., Bottaro, E. G., and Rodríguez-Brieschke, M. T. (2009). Mother-child transmission of Chagas disease: could coinfection with human immunodeficiency virus increase the risk? *Rev. Soc. Bras. Med. Trop.* 42, 107–109. doi: 10.1590/S0037-86822009000200002

Schijman, A. G., Altcheh, J., Burgos, J. M., Biancardi, M., Bisio, M., Levin, M. J., et al. (2003). Aetiological treatment of congenital Chagas' disease diagnosed and monitored by the polymerase chain reaction. *J. Antimicrob. Chemother.* 52, 441–449. doi: 10.1093/jac/dkg338

Solana, M. E., Celentano, A. M., Tekiel, V., Jones, M., and González Cappa, S. M. (2002). *Trypanosoma cruzi*: effect of parasite subpopulation on murine pregnancy outcome. *J. Parasitol.* 88, 102–106. doi: 10.1645/0022-3395(2002)088[0102:TCEOPS]2.0.CO;2

Soriano-Arandes, A., Angheben, A., Serre-Delcor, N., Treviño-Maruri, B., Gómez i Prat, J., and Jackson, Y. (2016). Control and management of congenital Chagas disease in Europe and other non-endemic countries: current policies and practices. *Trop. Med. Int. Health* 21, 590–596. doi: 10.1111/tmi.12687

Sosa-Estani, S. (2005). Congenital transmission of *Trypanosoma cruzi* infection in Argentina. *Rev. Soc. Bras. Med. Trop.* 38(Suppl. 2), 29–32. Available at: http://www.ncbi.nlm.nih.gov/pubmed/16482810

Sosa-estani, S., Cura, E., and Velazquez, E. (2009). Etiological treatment of young women infected with *Trypanosoma cruzi*, and prevention of congenital transmission. *Rev. Soc. Bras. Med. Trop.* 42, 484–487. doi: 10.1590/S0037-86822009000500002

Strasen, J., Williams, T., Ertl, G., Zoller, T., Stich, A., and Ritter, O. (2013). Epidemiology of Chagas disease in Europe: many calculations, little knowledge. *Clin. Res. Cardiol.* 103, 1–10. doi: 10.1007/s00392-013-0613-y

Torrico, F., Alonso-Vega, C., Suarez, E., Rodríguez, P., Torrico, M.-C., Dramaix, M., et al. (2005). Endemic level of congenital *Trypanosoma cruzi* infection in the areas of maternal residence and the development of congenital Chagas disease in Bolivia. *Rev. Soc. Bras. Med. Trop.* 38(Suppl. 2), 17–20. Available at: http://www.ncbi.nlm.nih.gov/pubmed/16482806 (Accessed February 11, 2019).

Torrico, F., Vega, C. A., Suarez, E., Tellez, T., Brutus, L., Rodriguez, P., et al. (2006). Are maternal re-infections with *Trypanosoma cruzi* associated with higher morbidity and mortality of congenital Chagas disease? *Trop. Med. Int. Health* 11, 628–635. doi: 10.1111/j.1365-3156.2006.01623.x

Triquell, M. F., Díaz-Luján, C., Freilij, H., Paglini, P., and Fretes, R. E. (2009). Placental infection by two subpopulations of *Trypanosoma cruzi* is conditioned by differential survival of the parasite in a deleterious placental medium and not by tissue reproduction. *Trans. R. Soc. Trop. Med. Hyg.* 103, 1011–1018. doi: 10.1016/j.trstmh.2009.03.004

Triquell, M. F., Díaz-Luján, C., Romanini, M. C., Ramirez, J. C., Paglini-Oliva, P., Schijman, A. G., et al. (2018). Nitric oxide synthase and oxidative-nitrosative stress play a key role in placental infection by *Trypanosoma cruzi*. *Am. J. Reprod. Immunol.* 80:e12852. doi: 10.1111/aji.12852

Umezawa, E. S., Nascimento, M. S., Kesper, N., Coura, J. R., Borges-Pereira, J., Junqueira, A. C., et al. (1996). Immunoblot assay using excreted-secreted antigens of *Trypanosoma cruzi* in serodiagnosis of congenital, acute, and chronic Chagas' disease. *J. Clin. Microbiol.* 34, 2143–2147. Available at: https://www.ncbi.nlm.nih.gov/pubmed/8862574

Vekemans, J., Truyens, C., Torrico, F., Solano, M., Torrico, M., Rodriguez, P., et al. (2000). Maternal *Trypanosoma cruzi* infection upregulates capacity of uninfected neonate cells to produce pro- and anti-inflammatory cytokines. *Infect. Immun.* 68, 5430–5434. doi: 10.1128/IAI.68.9.5430-5434.2000

Virreira, M., Torrico, F., Truyens, C., Alonso-vega, C., Solano, M., Carlier, Y., et al. (2003). Comparison of polymerase chain reaction methods for reliable and easy detection of congenital *Trypanosoma cruzi* infection. *Am. J. Trop. Med. Hyg.* 68, 574–582. doi: 10.4269/ajtmh.2003.68.574

Virreira, M., Truyens, C., Alonso-Vega, C., Brutus, L., Jijena, J., Torrico, F., et al. (2007). Comparison of *Trypanosoma cruzi* lineages and levels of parasitic DNA in infected mothers and their newborns. *Am. J. Trop. Med. Hyg.* 77, 102–106. doi: 10.4269/ajtmh.2007.77.102

Volta, B. J., Bustos, P. L., Cardoni, R. L., De Rissio, A. M., Laucella, S. A., and Bua, J. (2016). Serum cytokines as biomarkers of early *Trypanosoma cruzi* infection by congenital exposure. *J. Immunol.* 196, 4596–4602. doi: 10.4049/jimmunol.1502504

Volta, B. J., Perrone, A. E., Rivero, R., Scollo, K., Bustos, P. L., and Bua, J. (2018). Some limitations for early diagnosis of congenital chagas infection by PCR. *Pediatrics* 141(Suppl. 5), S451–S455. doi: 10.1542/peds.2016-3719

Volta, B. J., Russomando, G., Bustos, P. L., Scollo, K., De Rissio, A. M., Sánchez, Z., et al. (2015). Diagnosis of congenital *Trypanosoma cruzi* infection: a serologic test using Shed Acute Phase Antigen (SAPA) in mother-child binomial samples. *Acta Trop.* 147, 31–37. doi: 10.1016/j.actatropica.2015.03.026

WHO | Chagas disease (American trypanosomiasis) (2019). WHO. Available at: https://www.who.int/chagas/en/ (Accessed February 12, 2019).

Zingales, B., Miles, M. A., Campbell, D. A., Tibayrenc, M., Macedo, A. M., Teixeira, M. M. G., et al. (2012). The revised *Trypanosoma cruzi* subspecific nomenclature: rationale, epidemiological relevance and research applications. *Infect. Genet. Evol.* 12, 240–253. doi: 10.1016/j.meegid.2011.12.009

17

Malaria in Pregnancy: From Placental Infection to its Abnormal Development and Damage

Caroline Lin Lin Chua[1], Sebastian Kah Ming Khoo[2], Jun Long Ernest Ong[2], Gaurav Kumar Ramireddi[3], Tsin Wen Yeo[2,4,5] and Andrew Teo[2,6]**

[1] School of Biosciences, Taylor's University, Subang Jaya, Malaysia, [2] Lee Kong Chian School of Medicine, Nanyang Technological University, Singapore, Singapore, [3] Department of Medicine, Monash University, Victoria, VIC, Australia, [4] National Center for Infectious Diseases, Singapore, Singapore, [5] Department of Infectious Diseases, Tan Tock Seng Hospital, Singapore, Singapore, [6] Department of Medicine at Royal Melbourne Hospital, Peter Doherty Institute, University of Melbourne, Melbourne, VIC, Australia

****Correspondence:***
Caroline Lin Lin Chua
linlin.chua@taylors.edu.my
Andrew Teo
andrewcc.teo@ntu.edu.sg

Malaria remains a global health burden with *Plasmodium falciparum* accounting for the highest mortality and morbidity. Malaria in pregnancy can lead to the development of placental malaria, where *P. falciparum*-infected erythrocytes adhere to placental receptors, triggering placental inflammation and subsequent damage, causing harm to both mother and her infant. Histopathological studies of *P. falciparum*-infected placentas revealed various placental abnormalities such as excessive perivillous fibrinoid deposits, breakdown of syncytiotrophoblast integrity, trophoblast basal lamina thickening, increased syncytial knotting, and accumulation of mononuclear immune cells within intervillous spaces. These events in turn, are likely to impair placental development and function, ultimately causing placental insufficiency, intrauterine growth restriction, preterm delivery and low birth weight. Hence, a better understanding of the mechanisms behind placental alterations and damage during placental malaria is needed for the design of effective interventions. In this review, using evidence from human studies and murine models, an integrated view on the potential mechanisms underlying placental pathologies in malaria in pregnancy is provided. The molecular, immunological and metabolic changes in infected placentas that reflect their responses to the parasitic infection and injury are discussed. Finally, potential models that can be used by researchers to improve our understanding on the pathogenesis of malaria in pregnancy and placental pathologies are presented.

Keywords: low birth weight, preterm birth, malaria, pregnancy, *Plasmodium falciparum*, syncytiotrophoblast, placental insufficiency, fetal growth restriction

INTRODUCTION

Malaria is a blood-borne disease caused by *Plasmodium* spp., with *Plasmodium falciparum* (*P. falciparum*) being the most deadly species (World Health Organization [WHO], 2020). Pregnant women, especially first-time mothers, are at high risk of severe malaria due to *P. falciparum*, hence *P. falciparum*-related malaria in pregnancy (MiP) will be the focus of this review. Long-term childhood exposure to the parasites can result in the development of protective antibodies; however, first-time pregnant mothers become susceptible again (Teo et al., 2016). Their susceptibility can be attributed to the *P. falciparum* erythrocyte membrane protein-1 (PfEMP1), a major variant surface antigen displayed on the surface of *P. falciparum*-infected erythrocytes (IEs) that serves as an adhesin (Lennartz et al., 2019; Wang et al., 2021). Each parasite has up to 60 *var* genes that encode the PfEMP1 molecules, and only a single variant is expressed at any one time (Smith et al., 2001). Switching of this *var* gene expression enables *P. falciparum* to evade host immunity. Consequently, IEs can sequester in organs and avoid splenic clearance, which then promotes inflammation and/or microvasculature obstruction (Biggs et al., 1991; Dondorp et al., 2008; Chua et al., 2021b). VAR2CSA is a PfEMP1 molecule that is expressed during MiP, and it mediates the binding of IEs to placental receptors such as chondroitin sulfate A found on placental syncytiotrophoblast (SCT) (Salanti et al., 2003; Tuikue Ndam et al., 2005). As a result, IEs accumulate within the placenta, triggering an inflammation in the placental intervillous spaces; the infected and inflamed placenta is commonly termed as placental malaria (PM). PM is particularly common amongst first-time pregnant women, due to their lack of immunity against placental-binding IEs, and this is likely to adversely impact the placenta, leading to poor outcomes in MiP (Fried et al., 1998; Staalsoe et al., 2001; Tran et al., 2020). However, our understanding on the physical and physiological changes to the infected placentas during PM is still rather limited, mainly due to the invasive nature of studying placental tissues during pregnancy and the limitations associated with existing animal models of MiP.

In this review, we will first provide a general overview of a successful pregnancy, followed by a detailed discussion on MiP and its deleterious impact on the placenta. The different immunological, molecular and metabolic changes in the infected placentas following parasitic infection, which are subsequently linked to placental injury and its dysregulated physiology, will be reviewed. We will include findings from several established rodent models of MiP which have enhanced our understanding on the topic, albeit there are differences between humans and rodents, as described in **Table 1**. Lastly, we discuss potential models that can be used by researchers to better understand the pathogenesis of MiP and the mechanisms underlying placental damage and injury in this disease.

A SUCCESSFUL PREGNANCY

A successful pregnancy requires proper development of the placenta and its sustenance throughout pregnancy. In the first trimester, T_h1 pro-inflammatory responses promote proper tissue remodeling and angiogenesis; dysregulated immune responses have been associated with increased risk of early pregnancy failures (Wang et al., 2020). Subsequent shift toward a T_h2 environment during the second trimester, characterized by increased anti-inflammatory cytokine levels and expansion of regulatory T cells, allows for rapid fetal growth and prevents fetal rejection (Aluvihare et al., 2004; Wang et al., 2020). At the end of pregnancy, there is a shift back to the pro-inflammatory environment with increased IL-1β, IL-6, and IL-8 expression, which are essential for parturition (Christiaens et al., 2008; Rinaldi et al., 2017). However, elevated T_h1-type responses in the third trimester can increase the risk of pre-term birth (Romero et al., 2014; Fried et al., 2017).

Various immune tolerance mechanisms in the placenta play crucial roles to prevent fetal rejection. For example, placental trophoblasts do not express the classical major histocompatibility complex (MHC) molecules, which can otherwise trigger a pro-inflammatory immune cascade. Instead, they widely express the non-classical human leukocyte antigen (HLA)-G and HLA-E molecules that protect the placenta from $CD8^+$ T cell and decidual natural killer cell cytotoxicity (Tersigni et al., 2020; Xu et al., 2020). The placenta can also secrete exosomes with immuno-regulatory functions, such as inducing the differentiation of macrophages to display characteristics of decidual cells that play important roles at the maternal-fetal interface (Bai et al., 2021). In addition, Hofbauer cells, which are fetal-derived placental macrophages in the chorionic villi, display M2 phenotype and express IL-10 (Yang et al., 2017). IL-10 is an anti-inflammatory cytokine expressed throughout pregnancy, with higher expression levels detected during first and second trimesters, and the lack of this cytokine was associated with poor pregnancy outcomes such as growth restriction and preterm birth (Cheng and Sharma, 2015). However, clinical studies and rodent models, increased IL-10 levels at delivery have been associated with poor birth outcomes, suggesting possible impairment in parasite clearance that may contribute to poor outcomes (Megnekou et al., 2013, 2015a). Overall, the dysregulation of either T_h1 or T_h2 responses during pregnancy may contribute to adverse outcomes and maintaining a balance between pro- and anti-inflammatory immune responses is crucial for a healthy pregnancy.

THE DEVELOPMENT OF THE HUMAN PLACENTA

The placenta is a highly specialized organ that regulates the exchange of metabolites between fetal blood in the chorionic villi and maternal blood within the intervillous spaces. Defective placental development can lead to placental insufficiency, contributing to fetal growth restriction (FGR), miscarriage and stillbirth (Brosens et al., 2011). Critically, placental development is a complex and yet delicate process. In the first trimester, the trophoblast, a specialized group of cells, differentiates to form blastocyst, and the outer layer termed trophectoderm fuses to the uterine endometrium to form the primary syncytium. The primary syncytium then further divides and differentiates into the cytotrophoblasts (inner core) and SCT (outer layer). Around 6–8 weeks after implantation, the SCT rapidly expands, forming branching villous trees that invade maternal intervillous spaces and endometrial glands, subsequently allowing the perfusion of intervillous spaces with maternal blood. Toward the second trimester, the cytotrophoblasts continue to expand, giving rise to extravillous trophoblasts that will further invade the decidua and maternal uterine spiral arteries (**Figure 1**). The

TABLE 1 | Comparison between humans and rodent models of malaria in pregnancy.

	Human	Rodent	References
Parasitemia	• Infection is through the bite of an infective mosquito, transmitting sporozoites during a blood meal. This triggers a complex pathway of inflammation; however, case of extreme parasitemia is rarely observed in pregnant women. This is presumably due to the use of effective antimalarials and the acquisition of protective antibodies during subsequent pregnancies.	• Infection is often through blood-stage inoculation; this may trigger different pathways of inflammation. Blood-stage infection results in high parasitemia that is often lethal. Because of the shorter duration of pregnancy, immunity during pregnancy is harder to investigate.	Humans protective antibodies—(Fried et al., 1998; Ndam et al., 2015). Mouse models—(Poovassery and Moore, 2006; Neres et al., 2008) Mouse models of immunity—(Marinho et al., 2009; Megnekou et al., 2009)
Placental anatomy	• Placenta is comprised of tree branch-like villi. • Placental invasion is mediated by extravillous trophoblast cells that are highly invasive. • Placenta is hemomonochorial, where maternal blood is in direct contact with fetal villi, separated only by the syncytiotrophoblast layer.	• Placenta is comprised of labyrinth villous structure. • Placental invasion is mediated by trophoblast giant cells that are modestly invasive. • Placenta is hemotrichorial, where maternal blood is separated from fetal blood via three thin layers of trophoblastic cells (cytotrophoblasts and two layers of syncytiotrophoblasts).	Differences in placental anatomy—(Takata et al., 1997; Georgiades et al., 2002; Cline et al., 2014; Schmidt et al., 2015; Soncin et al., 2015)
Parasite antigens	Parasites that infect pregnant women express *var* genes coding for VAR2CSA proteins, which are expressed on IEs and are responsible for binding to placental receptors such as chondroitin sulfate A.	Rodent parasites express antigens transcribed by the multigenic *Plasmodium* interspersed repeats (*pir*) superfamily. Their function in MiP and PM is unknown.	VAR2CSA—(Salanti et al., 2003; Tuikue Ndam et al., 2005; Duffy et al., 2006) *pir* multigene—(Janssen et al., 2004; Hall et al., 2005)
IE sequestration	• IEs can sequester in placental intervillous spaces, mediated by their binding to the syncytiotrophoblast, and this is the hallmark of placental malaria. • Infection may be "hidden" in the placenta, as higher parasite density has been found in the placenta compared to maternal peripheral circulation.	• Evidence of IE binding to the placenta is less prominent, likely due to the lack of VAR2CSA homologs. However, IEs are often observed to accumulate in the placenta. • High parasite density observed in the placenta may be due to overall high parasitemia in maternal peripheral blood, resulting in the circulation of parasites into the placenta.	Human studies on placental sequestration—(Fried and Duffy, 1996; Ordi et al., 1998) Mouse models of placental parasite accumulation—(Neres et al., 2008; Sharma et al., 2016; Morffy Smith et al., 2019)
Placental inflammation and pathology	• Excessive immune cell accumulation in placental intervillous spaces, termed intervillositis, has been observed in chronic cases, and is associated with poor placenta development and birth outcomes. • Human pregnancy has a longer gestation period. Thus, inflammation at different trimesters which disrupt the cytokines/chemokines balance may disrupt placental development or/and function, depending on the stage of pregnancy.	• Mice challenged with *P. chabaudi* sporozoites displayed little evidence of immune cell accumulation; however, when challenged with blood-stage *P. chabaudi* or *P. berghei*, massive accumulation of immune cells has been observed. • Experimental infection of mice often takes place later in pregnancy when the placenta is fully developed, as infection early in pregnancy results in mortality and loss of pregnancy.	Intervillositis in human—(Ordi et al., 1998; Rogerson et al., 2003b; Muehlenbachs et al., 2010) Mononuclear cells infiltration in mice—(Neres et al., 2008; Poovassery et al., 2009; Sarr et al., 2015; Rahmah et al., 2019) Lack of monocytes and macrophages accumulation in placentas of mice—(Poovassery and Moore, 2006; Sharma et al., 2016)

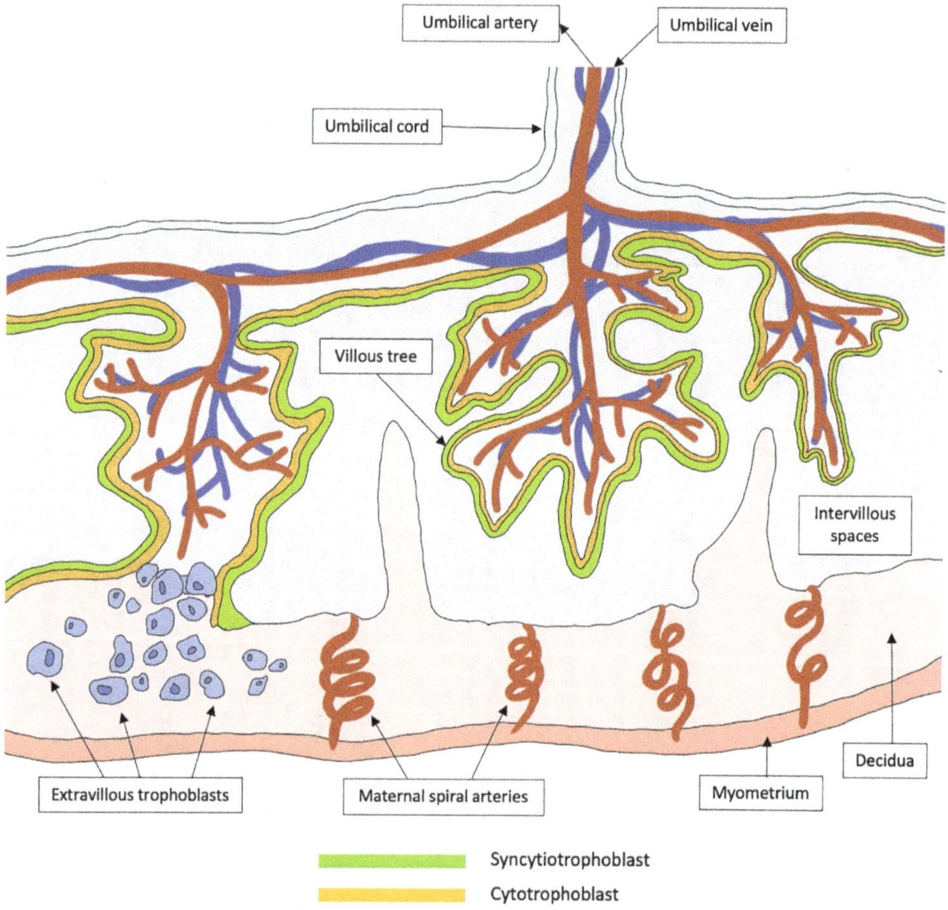

FIGURE 1 | Schematic representation of a healthy functional unit of the human placenta. The placenta is a specialized organ that is primarily involved in the exchange of metabolites between the mother and her fetus. In the early trimester, the trophoblast differentiates to form primary syncytium that further divides into the cytotrophoblast and syncytiotrophoblast. The syncytiotrophoblast will then expand to form a continuous layer of tree-like villous that are in contact with maternal blood in the intervillous spaces. These villous trees greatly increase the surface areas available for the exchange of metabolites. Cytotrophoblasts can further differentiate into extravillous trophoblasts that invade the decidua, which is the maternal uterine tissue, to promote immune tolerance between the mother and her fetus. The extravillous trophoblasts also migrate up the maternal spiral arteries and promote spiral artery remodeling, to form large vessels of low resistance that is required to sustain a healthy pregnancy.

uterine spiral arteries then undergo extracellular remodeling through degradation and rebuilding, a process which is critical for ensuring adequate blood supply to the placenta during pregnancy. This complex process involves various immunological cells such as decidual macrophages, regulatory T cells and uterine natural killer cells (Staff et al., 2020), as well as angiogenic, vascular, and placental growth factors (Hanna et al., 2006; Lash et al., 2006).

PLACENTAL PATHOLOGIES DURING MALARIA IN PREGNANCY

Dysregulated Placental Vascularization and Angiogenesis

Bilateral uterine artery notching and concomitant vascular resistance are signs of disruption to the utero-placental hemodynamics and these have been observed in *P. falciparum*-infected placentas (Dorman et al., 2002). Placental vascularization begins as early as eight gestational weeks (GW) (Leijnse et al., 2018), hence infection during and after this period may affect the development of placental vasculature and its blood flow. In placentas from Tanzanian women, MiP before 15 GW was associated with decreased volume of transport villi and increased diffusion distance in diffusion vessels, suggesting impairment of placental vascular development (Moeller et al., 2019). Furthermore, Doppler ultrasound studies showed that infection before 20 GW in primigravids was associated with increased umbilical artery resistance, an indirect measurement of resistance flow within the placenta (Griffin et al., 2012; Ome-Kaius et al., 2017). A study on a cohort of Malawian pregnant women revealed that MiP infection between 13 and 23 GW was associated with dysregulation of various angiogenic factors and metabolic hormones, which play vital roles in placental vascularization (Elphinstone et al., 2019). Impaired trophoblast differentiation, represented by shallow trophoblast invasion and narrow spiral arteries formation, may contribute to increased umbilical artery resistance and poor placental perfusion, leading to preeclampsia (Roland et al., 2016; Obiri et al., 2020). MiP before 18 GW was associated with reduced trophoblast invasion and migration *in vitro*, suggesting possible reduction in placental blood circulation that might contribute to later pregnancy complications (Abrahams et al., 2005; Umbers et al., 2013). Interestingly, MiP infection in later pregnancy, 32–35 GW, was also associated with increased uterine artery resistance (Dorman et al., 2002). Given that the invasion of trophoblasts is usually complete around 19–20 GW, this pathology is more likely to be due to damaged trophoblasts and/or their impaired function in producing angiogenic factors to sustain exponential fetal growth in the third trimester (Pollheimer et al., 2018). Additionally, in one study, women with PM were reported to be four times more likely to have low placental weight, which is a risk factor for FGR (Singoei et al., 2021). This may be related to the dysregulation of angiopoietins, where women with higher levels of Angiopoietin-2 (Ang-2) were at higher risk of having low placental weight, and in PM, increased levels of Ang-2 in both peripheral and placental blood at delivery have been reported (Silver et al., 2010; McDonald et al., 2016; Singh et al., 2020).

Irreversible Damage and Abnormal Placental Structure

Irreversible placental damage and abnormal placental structure have been reported in MiP, regardless of the timing of infection. Placentas from women who were infected in their first trimester showed signs of damage at delivery, including reduced transport villi, increased syncytial knotting and increased placental lesions (Crocker et al., 2004; Elphinstone et al., 2019; Moeller et al., 2019). Active infection at delivery was associated with reduced villous area and vascularity, increased basal membrane thickening, syncytial damage, increased syncytial knotting, and fibrinoid necrosis (Crocker et al., 2004; Chaikitgosiyakul et al., 2014). Collectively, the accumulation of fibrin in the intervillous spaces coupled with dysregulation of angiogenesis in placenta can result in inadequate perfusion to the placenta, causing necrosis (Burton and Jauniaux, 2018). Necrotic cell death has been observed in infected placentas, with extensive syncytial breaks in some cases of active PM leading to denudation of the villi, vacuolation, and complete destruction of villous integrity (Crocker et al., 2004). Chronic placental infection at delivery is characterized by increased accumulation of phagocytes in the intervillous spaces and sparse villi numbers, which are likely to reduce nutrient and protein transport across the placenta (**Figure 2**; Lybbert et al., 2016; Chua et al., 2021a).

Hemozoin, the insoluble product of *Plasmodium* parasites, is commonly observed in the intervillous spaces, either trapped in fibrin or within maternal macrophages (McGready et al., 2002). The presence of hemozoin in infected placentas can further cause placental damage through its immunomodulatory properties. For instance, hemozoin may fuel placental inflammation by reducing parasite clearance, as phagocytes that have ingested hemozoin were shown to have reduced phagocytic capacity and increased cytokine secretion (Tyberghein et al., 2014). Furthermore, an *in vitro* study reported that hemozoin can activate SCT to produce cytokines and chemokines such as Tumor necrosis factor (TNF)-α, IL-8, CCL3, and CCL4; consequently, this may sustain an inflammatory response that contributes to increased inflammatory cell infiltration and fibrinoid deposits in the placenta (Lucchi et al., 2008).

Apoptosis in the Placenta

Apoptosis is a physiological response that is involved in normal placental growth and development. The apoptosis of placental villi is observed throughout pregnancy, with increasing percentage of apoptosis being reported as the pregnancy progresses to third trimester (Smith et al., 1997b). High rates of apoptosis in the placenta have been associated with several pathological conditions including spontaneous abortion, intrauterine growth restriction, and preeclampsia (Smith et al., 1997a; He et al., 2013). Interestingly, active parasitemia at delivery was not associated with increased placental apoptosis despite being associated with significantly lower birth weights compared to healthy placentas (Crocker et al., 2004). Instead, the study reported reduced apoptosis in placentas with past infections. In contrast, another study showed that apoptotic gene expressions were increased in women with past infections and increased oxidative insults may trigger apoptosis in the placenta (Kawahara et al., 2019). The discrepancies could be because the latter study was based on a larger sample size and the authors performed molecular studies instead of histological analysis to detect apoptosis. In a mouse model of PM, increased oxidative stress, determined by increased levels of malondialdehyde (MDA) and reduced levels of antioxidant enzyme catalase, were associated with enhanced apoptosis in the placentas of mice with active infection (Sharma et al., 2012). Similarly, apoptosis markers were observed in maternal blood and junctional zone trophoblasts in *P. chabaudi*-infected pregnant mice (Sarr et al., 2015). Of note, the junctional zone trophoblasts are cells that are only found in mice placentas; it is unknown if specific types of human trophoblasts similarly undergo apoptosis during infection. In women with PM, similar findings of increased MDA and reduced antioxidant enzyme levels were also reported in placental tissues, suggesting that oxidative stress may contribute to pathophysiology of the placenta; however, whether or not this was mediated through placental apoptosis is unclear (Megnekou et al., 2015b). Further investigations are required to understand the mechanisms of apoptosis and its impact on placental function and outcomes at delivery in MiP.

MECHANISMS UNDERLYING PLACENTAL PATHOLOGIES IN MALARIA IN PREGNANCY

Disruption to Placental Blood Vessels Formation

Decreased villous area and vascularity were observed in active *P. falciparum* infected-placentas compared to both healthy and

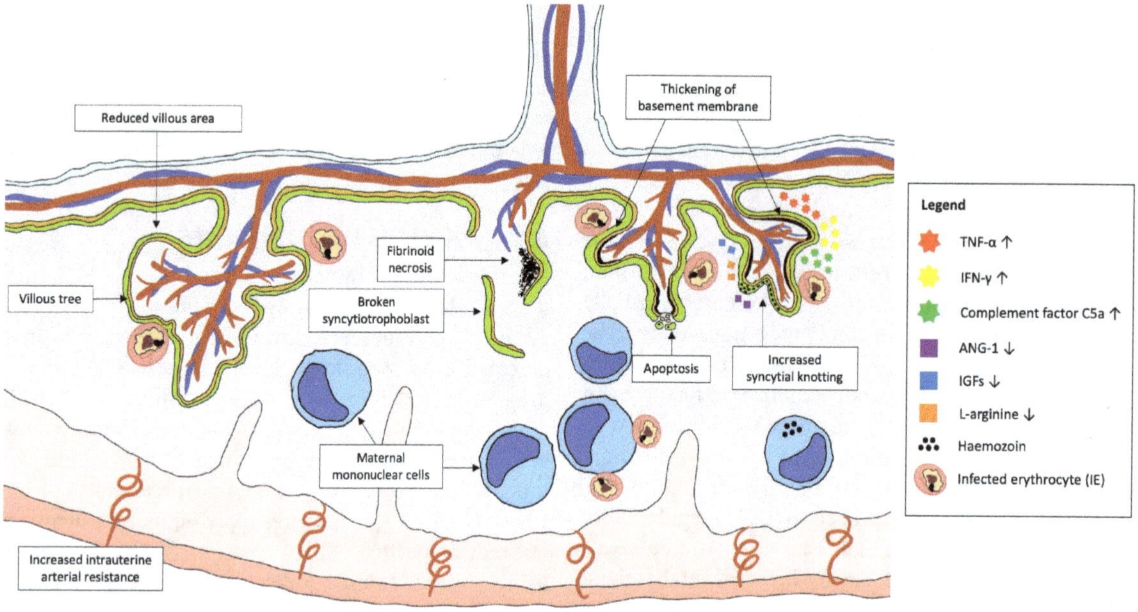

FIGURE 2 | *Plasmodium* parasite infection in the placenta that cause abnormal placental development and damage. Placental malaria is an infection in the placenta by *Plasmodium* spp., commonly *P. falciparum*. Emerging evidence suggests that pregnant women are at the highest risk of PM in the first trimester, which coincides with the period of placental growth and development. Abnormalities in the placenta during PM include permanent damage to placental structures such as broken syncytiotrophoblast, thickening of basement membrane, increased syncytial knotting, increased areas of fibrinoid necrosis and dysregulated apoptosis of trophoblasts. This can result in placental insufficiency that contributes to the increased risk of fetal growth restriction, low birth weight and pre-eclampsia. The pathology is mainly associated with the activation of a local inflammatory response, characterized by the accumulation of activated maternal mononuclear cells within the intervillous spaces. The subsequent pathways leading to placental pathologies include the increased production of pro-inflammatory cytokines, chemokines, and complement proteins, as well as reduced levels of important angiogenic and placental growth factors. Together, these factors may disrupt the development of placenta if infection takes place early in pregnancy, leading to shallow spiral artery development and increased intrauterine arterial resistance.

previously treated malaria cases (Chaikitgosiyakul et al., 2014). While the underlying mechanism has yet to be fully understood, it is hypothesized that activated maternal complement system during infection may play a role. C5a levels assayed from placental blood correlated negatively to Ang-1 levels, and positively to Ang-2, vascular endothelial growth factor (VEGF) (required for early vessel formation) and sFLt-1 (inhibits angiogenesis by binding to VEGF), suggesting that alterations in angiogenic factor expression may contribute to poor birth outcomes (Conroy et al., 2013; Singh et al., 2020). Increase in the Ang-2:Ang-1 ratio in women with a positive episode of parasitemia during pregnancy has been reported and sustained Ang-2 levels during pregnancy may result in the formation of new blood vessels instead of vessel maturation; this may explain the excessive fetal vessels observed in infected placentas (Leke et al., 2004; Silver et al., 2010). Importantly, in healthy pregnancies, a gradual increase and decrease in Ang-1 and Ang-2 levels, respectively, across pregnancy, enables the initial branching and subsequent maturation of blood vessels to promote normal placental vascular development (Geva et al., 2002). Altered L-arginine level was also proposed as a contributor to dysregulated placental angiogenesis. L-arginine is a precursor of nitric oxide (NO), which plays a central role in promoting endothelial growth, regulating the expression of placental growth factors and angiopoietins (Krause et al., 2011). In Malawi, MiP before 28 GW was associated with lower L-arginine levels and increased levels of NO inhibitors; these in turn, were associated with small for gestational age babies (McDonald et al., 2018). In a mouse model of MiP, supplementation of L-arginine reduced C5 protein and Ang-2 expression, while Ang-1 level was upregulated (McDonald et al., 2018). Furthermore, L-arginine supplementations led to an increase in total number of placental vessel segments and small-diameter vessels ($<50\ \mu m$) compared to infected controls without supplementation, and this correlated with improved birth weight (McDonald et al., 2018). Of note, these small-diameter vessels are important in vascular remodeling during pregnancy (Geva et al., 2002). Overall, these findings suggest a potential intervention in improving vascularization in the placenta, but whether L-arginine supplementation is useful in pregnant women remains to be investigated.

DISRUPTION TO PLACENTAL DEVELOPMENT AND UTERO-PLACENTAL HEMODYNAMICS

The Role of Cytokines

The production of pro-inflammatory cytokines during pregnancy is a double-edged sword. While timely production of these inflammatory mediators assists placental remodeling and growth, dysregulated production may cause irreversible damage to its structure and function. For example, although IFN-γ plays an important role in the remodeling of uterine spiral artery, excessive levels of the cytokine may be detrimental for fetal growth (Ashkar et al., 2000; Suguitan et al., 2003a). In a mouse model of PM, increased IFN-γ levels, and IFN-γ receptor 1 signaling were linked to reduced numbers of vascular branches in the labyrinth of the placentas compared to IFN-γ receptor 1 knocked-out (KO) mice (Niikura et al., 2017). In normal pregnancy, TNF-α expression in the placenta was detectable across all trimesters but was highest in the second trimester (Basu et al., 2016). In MiP, the levels of TNF-α were further elevated and often associated with poor birth outcomes (Rogerson et al., 2003a). Previous *in vitro* studies reported that TNF-α can exert various effects on the placenta such as inhibiting extravillous trophoblast invasion through promoting apoptosis and downregulating human chorionic gonadotropin (hCG) expression by cytotrophoblasts to cause suppressed trophoblast growth and increased apoptosis (Leisser et al., 2006; Otun et al., 2011). These mechanisms could ultimately result in the inhibition of extravillous trophoblast invasion; however, they have yet to be proven in MiP models. Additionally, in a mouse model of PM, increased expression of TNF-α in the placenta was found to induce the expression of tissue factor, which correlated to hemorrhage, fibrin and thrombi formation in the placenta; interestingly, placental architecture can be preserved in mice treated with anti-TNF antibodies (Poovassery et al., 2009).

In *P. falciparum*-infected placentas, increased inflammasome activation was also associated with increase in necrotic areas, fibrioid necrosis and syncytial aggregates (Reis et al., 2020). In the same study, using murine PM model, it was revealed that inflammasome activation led to downstream increase in IL-1β signaling, which contributed to decreased expression of nutrient transporters including SNAT1, SNAT2, and GLUT1 gene expression in *P. berghei*-infected placentas (Reis et al., 2020). In PM, decreased activities of amino acid and glucose transporters have been reported, but it is unclear whether these are similarly mediated through inflammasome activation (Boeuf et al., 2013; Chandrasiri et al., 2014). Furthermore, in mice treated with an IL-1 receptor antagonist or in IL-1β KO mice, nutrient transporter expression was comparable to uninfected controls, suggesting that targeting the IL-1 pathway could be a possible therapeutic approach in MiP (Reis et al., 2020).

The Role of Placental Hormones and Chemokines

A complex network of placental hormones ensures a functional placenta. Insulin-like growth factor (IGFs) are produced by placental cells and play pivotal roles in placental survival and promoting fetal development (Han et al., 1996). Lack of IGFs was associated with decreased proliferation and poor survival of placental fibroblasts, which can predispose to FGR (Miller et al., 2005; Forbes et al., 2008). In PM, pregnant women were reported to have reduced levels IGF-1, IGF-2, and IL-8, and increased levels of invasion-inhibitory factors including hCG and IL-10 in peripheral blood samples; these factors can inhibit trophoblast invasion and migration (Jovanović et al., 2010; Umbers et al., 2013). In addition, the levels of fetal insulin-like growth factor-binding protein-1 (IGFBP-1) were elevated in PM; this molecule negatively regulates IGFs expression and is associated with placental insufficiency (Shibuya et al., 2011; Umbers et al., 2011; Nawathe et al., 2016). Hypothetically, the dysregulated levels of these growth factors during early trimesters MiP may reduce trophoblast invasion and migration, subsequently affecting the transformation of maternal spiral arteries leading to FGR (Lyall et al., 2013). Healthy placental development also requires chemokines that will recruit immune cells into the decidua during early stage of pregnancy; different chemokines may be needed at different stages of placental development (Ramhorst et al., 2016). However, PM is known to cause elevated levels of chemokines within the intervillous spaces. CCL2 (MCP-1), CCL3 (MIP- 1α), CCL4, CXCL8, CXCL9, CXCL13, and CXCL16 have been observed in the placentas of women with PM, and CXCL9, CXCL13, and CCL4 were associated with adverse pregnancy outcomes such as low birth weight (Ioannidis et al., 2014; Fried et al., 2017). In addition, increased levels of chemokines produced by maternal cells during infection is likely to result in the accumulation of phagocytic cells within the placenta (Suguitan et al., 2003b; Megnekou et al., 2015a). Together, the recruitment of immune cells to the placenta due to infection rather than for the purpose of promoting placental growth, is likely to overdrive inflammation, thus adversely impact on the development of the organ.

The Role of Complement Proteins

The placenta's ability to synthesize both complement proteins and their relevant inhibitors suggest that a tightly regulated complement system is essential for a successful pregnancy (Bulla et al., 2009; Lokki et al., 2014). For example, in murine pregnancy model, C1q is synthesized by migrating extravillous trophoblasts to promote trophoblast migration and adhesion, whereas C1q deficiency was associated with impaired labyrinth development (Agostinis et al., 2010). Dysregulated C5a levels may have pathological consequence, as increased C5a expression has been observed in the trophoblasts of pre-eclamptic placentas and C5a-stimulated trophoblasts demonstrated an anti-angiogenic phenotype *in vitro* (Ma et al., 2018). In PM, increased peripheral and placental levels of C5a have been associated with poor birth outcomes in women from all gravidities (Conroy et al., 2009, 2013). In a mouse model of PM, increased C5a and C5a receptor (C5aR) expressions were observed. Interaction between C5a and C5aR was found to impair vascular remodeling necessary to compensate for the placental insult and C5aR blockade improved vasculature development, further highlighting the impact of complement on placental vascularization (Conroy et al., 2013). Of note, these studies were conducted at delivery; hence future studies investigating infection at earlier trimesters are required to further improve understanding on the impact of complement system activation in placental development.

The Role of Activated Coagulation Cascade

Several studies have shown that MiP induces a pro-coagulative state in the placenta, characterized by perivillous fibrin deposits, elevated biomarkers of coagulation such as tissue factor and D-Dimer, as well as reduced levels of fibrinolysis biomarkers including protein-C, antithrombin-III, and tissue factor pathway inhibitor (Avery et al., 2012; Mostafa et al., 2015). Tissue factor is primarily expressed by macrophages that are found in abundance in *P. falciparum*-infected placentas, particularly those with chronic PM, and may be the reason for increased fibrin deposition in these placentas (Hohensinner et al., 2021). High levels of plasminogen activator inhibitor-1 (PAI-1) can suppress fibrinolysis, leading to increased fibrin deposition and pathological effects on tissues. Interestingly, pregnant women with submicroscopic infections, presumably due to having lower parasite density, had increased levels of PAI-1 but not fibrin deposition; PAI-1 levels were comparable to that of PM detected by microscopy (Avery et al., 2012). The authors also found low levels of inflammation in the submicroscopic cases, suggesting that fibrin deposition/coagulation is likely to be triggered only in chronic infection. Indeed, increase in fibrin deposits was more common in placentas from primigravids, who are usually unable to effectively clear infection due to lack of immunity (Rogerson et al., 2003b). Given that coagulation may play a role in placental pathology, therapeutics that target the inflammatory-coagulation pathways may be useful in preventing placental injury. *In vivo*, the treatment of *P. chabaudi*-infected pregnant mice with low molecular heparin (an anticoagulant), showed absence of placental hemorrhage, tissue necrosis and large fibrin deposit in placentas (Avery et al., 2012). More studies are required to determine if similar effects can be achieved in humans.

DYSREGULATED AUTOPHAGY AND HEAT SHOCK PROTEINS IN RESCUE MECHANISMS

Autophagy is an important mechanism in normal pregnancy as it plays an important role in embryogenesis, implantation and placentation (Nakashima et al., 2019). Autophagy is activated in extravillous trophoblasts during the invasion and vascular remodeling process early in pregnancy. In addition, it appears to be a protective mechanism against cellular senescence in trophoblasts (Burton et al., 2017). However, increased autophagic activities in the villous trophoblasts have been associated with FGR and preterm labor (Nakashima et al., 2019). In placental biopsies, PM with intervillositis increased autophagosome (an upstream pathway of autophagy) formation but not autophagy, and the density of autophagosome formation correlated negatively with amino acid uptake, suggesting that impaired autophagy may reduce transplacental amino acid transport (Dimasuay et al., 2017b). In another study, mRNA expression of autophagic genes were reduced in women with PM and was associated with low birth weight delivery (Lima et al., 2019). The triggers of autophagic responses in MiP remains unclear, although hypoxia or inflammation are likely candidates (Oh and Roh, 2017). The effect of MiP on autophagy in earlier stages of pregnancy is also unknown, as current studies employed the use of term placentas.

Heat shock proteins (HSPs) are produced by cells to promote recovery from an injury or stress. HSPs 27, 60, 70, and 90 are also found to be in abundance in the endometrial and uterine cells especially in the first trimester, suggesting that they may be involved in placental development (Jee et al., 2021). Their roles in pregnancy may include maintaining the integrity of decidual cells, promote syncytialization and provide protection from preterm deliveries (Jee et al., 2021). On the other hand, elevated levels of certain HSPs have been associated with adverse pregnancy outcomes including FGR and preterm deliveries, suggesting that abnormally high levels of HSPs may indicate excessive tissue damage (Tan et al., 2007). In *P. berghei* PM model, levels of HSP 90, 70, 60, and 25 were increased in the placenta during infection, and levels of HSPs 70, 60, 25 but not HSP 90 decreased gradually with increasing disease severity (Sharma et al., 2014). The decrease in HSPs 70, 60, and 25 was proposed to be responsible for placental necrosis, while increased HSP 90 appears to be a compensatory mechanism to repair damaged placental cells (Sharma et al., 2012, 2014). The mechanisms leading to altered HSP levels and how the repair mechanisms of these proteins are affected in MiP require further attention.

In vitro and *in vivo* Models to Delineate Pathways in the Placenta During Malaria in Pregnancy

Models that can recapitulate features of MiP are required for studying mechanisms underlying placental pathologies, as well as for testing potential therapies. Monolayer cell lines including primary human trophoblast, Swan 71 and BeWo cells have been used in MiP research, and some findings from these 2D models were successfully translated to *in vivo* findings (Boeuf et al., 2013; Umbers et al., 2013; Dimasuay et al., 2017a). However, there are still major limitations associated with these models; continuous cell lines have chromosomal abnormalities and single-cell model lacks the immunological stimuli that are usually present in the placentas during PM. Pehrson et al. (2016) reported that a novel *ex vivo* placental perfusion model can be used to investigate receptor-ligand interactions and they demonstrated the accumulation of parasites in the placenta. This may be a useful model to study real-time pathological changes in the placental tissues at later stage in pregnancy, albeit with some limitations such as requiring highly skilled personnel and specialized equipment. *In vivo* rodent models have been used to study PM, but their transferability to humans remains an issue. Mouse models were able to replicate certain consequences of PM including dysregulated immunological factors, imbalanced angiogenesis and vasculogenesis factors, and poor outcomes in offsprings (Megnekou et al., 2013; Doritchamou et al., 2017; McDonald et al., 2018). Additionally, structural similarities and presence of analogous placental cell types between rodents and humans make them an attractive model for MiP (Georgiades et al., 2002). However, there are differences in their placental structures, and certain features of placental inflammation such as monocytes/macrophages accumulation were not seen (Poovassery and Moore, 2006; Sharma et al., 2016). In addition, the lack of hemozoin accumulation in mouse placentas suggests that the model may be suitable for studying acute rather than past and/or chronic infection (Boareto et al., 2019). There are other limitations associated with rodent models including the absence of pre-existing immunity in mice which is not reflective of the conditions of pregnant women living in malarious regions, as well as difference in the degree of parasite sequestration and mode of infection between rodents and humans (**Table 1**). On the other hand, while non-human primate models are more similar to humans in terms of physiology, high cost and sustainability issues arises. The suitability of animal models in MiP has been extensively discussed in many recent reviews, thus will not be further discussed here (Doritchamou et al., 2017; Barateiro et al., 2019).

MiP in the first trimester can cause suboptimal development and irreversible damage to the placenta, hence it is crucial to study the effects of MiP during early pregnancy (Chaikitgosiyakul et al., 2014; Moeller et al., 2019; Obiri et al., 2020). However, this proves to be a huge challenge, as existing models fail to replicate infection during early trimester. In recent years, newer models such as placental organoids have been used to study the placenta. Organoids are miniaturized *in vitro* tissue construct that are isolated from stem cells and the *in vitro* culture is usually representative of the organ *in vivo*. Placental organoids can be isolated from first-trimester trophoblasts and with appropriate growth factors and conditions, they can differentiate into SCT and extravillous trophoblasts that closely resemble first trimester placentas (Haider et al., 2018; Okae et al., 2018; Turco et al., 2018). This would provide vast experimental opportunities on two major trophoblast layers that are involved in early placental development. For example, a recent study was able to establish innate immune signaling pathways during Zika infection using maternal-derived organoids and key roles of antiviral immunity at the maternal-fetal interface can be elucidated (Yang et al., 2021). The use of trophoblast organoids to study early impact of MiP would allow real-time precise identification of placental responses during infection. Experimental design that includes a co-culture system of the organoids with immune cells can provide a better representation of the placental response, and specific cell populations that are responsible for placental damage or impaired placental development can be identified. This model can also be considered for the study of cytotoxicity and efficacy of potential therapeutics for early trimester MiP.

CONCLUSION

MiP remains a huge threat to the well-being of pregnant women and their developing fetus in malaria-endemic regions. Pregnant women are at the highest risk of MiP in the first trimester, which often results in poor placental development and irreversible placental structure damages that contribute to poor birth outcomes. Dysregulated levels of various soluble mediators have been associated with placental pathologies, including cytokines, chemokines, complement proteins, and growth factors. However, our current understanding of the pathogenetic mechanisms in the placenta relies either on a single time point during pregnancy, usually at delivery, or on animal models, which have their own limitations. Hence, there is a need to develop better models of the placenta to obtain a more comprehensive understanding of the pathogenesis of MiP during early pregnancy and follow through the disease progression. These efforts will ultimately enable the design of targeted strategies to aid placenta recovery and minimize the impact of MiP.

AUTHOR CONTRIBUTIONS

All authors listed have made a substantial, direct and intellectual contribution to the work, and approved it for publication.

REFERENCES

Abrahams, V. M., Visintin, I., Aldo, P. B., Guller, S., Romero, R., and Mor, G. (2005). A role for TLRs in the regulation of immune cell migration by first trimester trophoblast cells. *J. Immunol.* 175, 8096–8104. doi: 10.4049/jimmunol.175.12.8096

Agostinis, C., Bulla, R., Tripodo, C., Gismondi, A., Stabile, H., Bossi, F., et al. (2010). An alternative role of C1q in cell migration and tissue remodeling: contribution to trophoblast invasion and placental development. *J. Immunol.* 185, 4420–4429. doi: 10.4049/jimmunol.0903215

Aluvihare, V. R., Kallikourdis, M., and Betz, A. G. (2004). Regulatory T cells mediate maternal tolerance to the fetus. *Nat. Immunol.* 5, 266–271. doi: 10.1038/ni1037

Ashkar, A. A., Di Santo, J. P., and Croy, B. A. (2000). Interferon gamma contributes to initiation of uterine vascular modification, decidual integrity, and uterine natural killer cell maturation during normal murine pregnancy. *J. Exp. Med.* 192, 259–270. doi: 10.1084/jem.192.2.259

Avery, J. W., Smith, G. M., Owino, S. O., Sarr, D., Nagy, T., Mwalimu, S., et al. (2012). Maternal malaria induces a procoagulant and antifibrinolytic state that is embryotoxic but responsive to anticoagulant therapy. *PLoS One* 7:e31090. doi: 10.1371/journal.pone.0031090

Bai, K., Li, X., Zhong, J., Ng, E. H. Y., Yeung, W. S. B., Lee, C. L., et al. (2021). Placenta-derived exosomes as a modulator in maternal immune tolerance during pregnancy. *Front. Immunol.* 12:671093. doi: 10.3389/fimmu.2021.671093

Barateiro, A., Pereira, M. L. M., Epiphanio, S., and Marinho, C. R. F. (2019). Contribution of murine models to the study of malaria during pregnancy. *Front. Microbiol.* 10:1369.

Basu, J., Agamasu, E., Bendek, B., Salafia, C. M., Mishra, A., Benfield, N., et al. (2016). Placental tumor necrosis factor-α protein expression during normal human gestation. *J. Matern. Fetal Neonatal Med.* 29, 3934–3938. doi: 10.3109/14767058.2016.1156668

Biggs, B. A., Goozé, L., Wycherley, K., Wollish, W., Southwell, B., Leech, J. H., et al. (1991). Antigenic variation in *Plasmodium falciparum*. *Proc. Natl. Acad. Sci. U. S. A.* 88, 9171–9174. doi: 10.1073/pnas.88.20.9171

Boareto, A. C., Gomes, C., Centeno Müller, J., da Silva, J. G., Vergara, F., Salum, N., et al. (2019). Maternal and fetal outcome of pregnancy in Swiss mice infected with *Plasmodium berghei* ANKA(GFP). *Reprod. Toxicol.* 89, 107–114. doi: 10.3389/fmicb.2019.01369

Boeuf, P., Aitken, E. H., Chandrasiri, U., Chua, C. L., McInerney, B., McQuade, L., et al. (2013). *Plasmodium falciparum* malaria elicits inflammatory responses that dysregulate placental amino acid transport. *PLoS Pathog.* 9:e1003153. doi: 10.1371/journal.ppat.1003153

Brosens, I., Pijnenborg, R., Vercruysse, L., and Romero, R. (2011). The "Great Obstetrical Syndromes" are associated with disorders of deep placentation. *Am. J. Obstet. Gynecol.* 204, 193–201. doi: 10.1016/j.ajog.2010.08.009

Bulla, R., Bossi, F., Agostinis, C., Radillo, O., Colombo, F., De Seta, F., et al. (2009). Complement production by trophoblast cells at the feto-maternal interface. *J. Reprod. Immunol.* 82, 119–125. doi: 10.1016/j.jri.2009.06.124

Burton, G. J., and Jauniaux, E. (2018). Pathophysiology of placental-derived fetal growth restriction. *Am. J. Obstet. Gynecol.* 218, S745–S761. doi: 10.1016/j.ajog.2017.11.577

Burton, G. J., Yung, H. W., and Murray, A. J. (2017). Mitochondrial - Endoplasmic reticulum interactions in the trophoblast: stress and senescence. *Placenta* 52, 146–155. doi: 10.1016/j.placenta.2016.04.001

Chaikitgosiyakul, S., Rijken, M. J., Muehlenbachs, A., Lee, S. J., Chaisri, U., Viriyavejakul, P., et al. (2014). A morphometric and histological study of placental malaria shows significant changes to villous architecture in both *Plasmodium falciparum* and *Plasmodium vivax* infection. *Malar J.* 13:4. doi: 10.1186/1475-2875-13-4

Chandrasiri, U. P., Chua, C. L., Umbers, A. J., Chaluluka, E., Glazier, J. D., Rogerson, S. J., et al. (2014). Insight into the pathogenesis of fetal growth restriction in placental malaria: decreased placental glucose transporter isoform 1 expression. *J. Infect. Dis.* 209, 1663–1667. doi: 10.1093/infdis/jit803

Cheng, S. B., and Sharma, S. (2015). Interleukin-10: a pleiotropic regulator in pregnancy. *Am. J. Reprod. Immunol.* 73, 487–500. doi: 10.1111/aji.12329

Christiaens, I., Zaragoza, D. B., Guilbert, L., Robertson, S. A., Mitchell, B. F., and Olson, D. M. (2008). Inflammatory processes in preterm and term parturition. *J. Reprod. Immunol.* 79, 50–57. doi: 10.1016/j.jri.2008.04.002

Chua, C. L. L., Ng, I. M. J., Yap, B. J. M., and Teo, A. (2021b). Factors influencing phagocytosis of malaria parasites: the story so far. *Malar J.* 20:319. doi: 10.1186/s12936-021-03849-1

Chua, C. L. L., Hasang, W., Rogerson, S. J., and Teo, A. (2021a). Poor birth outcomes in malaria in pregnancy: recent insights into mechanisms and prevention approaches. *Front. Immunol.* 12:621382. doi: 10.3389/fimmu.2021.621382

Cline, J. M., Dixon, D., Ernerudh, J., Faas, M. M., Göhner, C., Häger, J. D., et al. (2014). The placenta in toxicology. Part III: pathologic assessment of the placenta. *Toxicol. Pathol.* 42, 339–344. doi: 10.1177/0192623313482207

Conroy, A., Serghides, L., Finney, C., Owino, S. O., Kumar, S., Gowda, D. C., et al. (2009). C5a enhances dysregulated inflammatory and angiogenic responses to malaria *in vitro*: potential implications for placental malaria. *PLoS One* 4:e4953. doi: 10.1371/journal.pone.0004953

Conroy, A. L., Silver, K. L., Zhong, K., Rennie, M., Ward, P., Sarma, J. V., et al. (2013). Complement activation and the resulting placental vascular insufficiency drives fetal growth restriction associated with placental malaria. *Cell Host Microbe* 13, 215–226. doi: 10.1016/j.chom.2013.01.010

Crocker, I. P., Tanner, O. M., Myers, J. E., Bulmer, J. N., Walraven, G., and Baker, P. N. (2004). Syncytiotrophoblast degradation and the pathophysiology of the malaria-infected placenta. *Placenta* 25, 273–282. doi: 10.1016/j.placenta.2003.09.010

Dimasuay, K. G., Gong, L., Rosario, F., McBryde, E., Spelman, T., Glazier, J., et al. (2017b). Impaired placental autophagy in placental malaria. *PLoS One* 12:e0187291. doi: 10.1371/journal.pone.0187291

Dimasuay, K. G., Aitken, E. H., Rosario, F., Njie, M., Glazier, J., Rogerson, S. J., et al. (2017a). Inhibition of placental mTOR signaling provides a link between placental malaria and reduced birthweight. *BMC Med.* 15:1. doi: 10.1186/s12916-016-0759-3

Dondorp, A. M., Ince, C., Charunwatthana, P., Hanson, J., van Kuijen, A., Faiz, M. A., et al. (2008). Direct *in vivo* assessment of microcirculatory dysfunction in severe falciparum malaria. *J. Infect. Dis.* 197, 79–84. doi: 10.1086/523762

Doritchamou, J., Teo, A., Fried, M., and Duffy, P. E. (2017). Malaria in pregnancy: the relevance of animal models for vaccine development. *Lab. Anim. (NY)* 46, 388–398. doi: 10.1038/laban.1349

Dorman, E. K., Shulman, C. E., Kingdom, J., Bulmer, J. N., Mwendwa, J., Peshu, N., et al. (2002). Impaired uteroplacental blood flow in pregnancies complicated by falciparum malaria. *Ultrasound Obstet. Gynecol.* 19, 165–170. doi: 10.1046/j.0960-7692.2001.00545.x

Duffy, M. F., Maier, A. G., Byrne, T. J., Marty, A. J., Elliott, S. R., O'Neill, M. T., et al. (2006). VAR2CSA is the principal ligand for chondroitin sulfate A in two allogeneic isolates of *Plasmodium falciparum*. *Mol. Biochem. Parasitol.* 148, 117–124. doi: 10.1016/j.molbiopara.2006.03.006

Elphinstone, R. E., Weckman, A. M., McDonald, C. R., Tran, V., Zhong, K., Madanitsa, M., et al. (2019). Early malaria infection, dysregulation of angiogenesis, metabolism and inflammation across pregnancy, and risk of preterm birth in Malawi: a cohort study. *PLoS Med.* 16:e1002914. doi: 10.1371/journal.pmed.1002914

Forbes, K., Westwood, M., Baker, P. N., and Aplin, J. D. (2008). Insulin-like growth factor I and II regulate the life cycle of trophoblast in the developing human placenta. *Am. J. Physiol. Cell Physiol.* 294, C1313–C1322. doi: 10.1152/ajpcell.00035.2008

Fried, M., and Duffy, P. E. (1996). Adherence of *Plasmodium falciparum* to chondroitin sulfate A in the human placenta. *Science* 272, 1502–1504. doi: 10.1126/science.272.5267.1502

Fried, M., Kurtis, J. D., Swihart, B., Pond-Tor, S., Barry, A., Sidibe, Y., et al. (2017). Systemic inflammatory response to malaria during pregnancy is associated with pregnancy loss and preterm delivery. *Clin. Infect. Dis.* 65, 1729–1735. doi: 10.1093/cid/cix623

Fried, M., Nosten, F., Brockman, A., Brabin, B. J., and Duffy, P. E. (1998). Maternal antibodies block malaria. *Nature* 395, 851–852. doi: 10.1038/27570

Georgiades, P., Ferguson-Smith, A. C., and Burton, G. J. (2002). Comparative developmental anatomy of the murine and human definitive placentae. *Placenta* 23, 3–19. doi: 10.1053/plac.2001.0738

Geva, E., Ginzinger, D. G., Zaloudek, C. J., Moore, D. H., Byrne, A., and Jaffe, R. B. (2002). Human placental vascular development: vasculogenic and angiogenic (branching and nonbranching) transformation is regulated by vascular endothelial growth factor-A, angiopoietin-1, and angiopoietin-2. *J. Clin. Endocrinol. Metab.* 87, 4213–4224. doi: 10.1210/jc.2002-020195

Griffin, J. B., Lokomba, V., Landis, S. H., Thorp, J. M. Jr., Herring, A. H., Tshefu, A. K., et al. (2012). *Plasmodium falciparum* parasitaemia in the first half of pregnancy, uterine and umbilical artery blood flow, and foetal growth: a longitudinal Doppler ultrasound study. *Malar J.* 11:319. doi: 10.1186/1475-2875-11-319

Haider, S., Meinhardt, G., Saleh, L., Kunihs, V., Gamperl, M., Kaindl, U., et al. (2018). Self-renewing trophoblast organoids recapitulate the developmental program of the early human placenta. *Stem Cell Rep.* 11, 537–551. doi: 10.1016/j.stemcr.2018.07.004

Hall, N., Karras, M., Raine, J. D., Carlton, J. M., Kooij, T. W., Berriman, M., et al. (2005). A comprehensive survey of the *Plasmodium* life cycle by genomic, transcriptomic, and proteomic analyses. *Science* 307, 82–86. doi: 10.1126/science.1103717

Han, V. K., Bassett, N., Walton, J., and Challis, J. R. (1996). The expression of insulin-like growth factor (IGF) and IGF-binding protein (IGFBP) genes in the human placenta and membranes: evidence for IGF-IGFBP interactions at the feto-maternal interface. *J. Clin. Endocrinol. Metab.* 81, 2680–2693. doi: 10.1210/jcem.81.7.8675597

Hanna, J., Goldman-Wohl, D., Hamani, Y., Avraham, I., Greenfield, C., Natanson-Yaron, S., et al. (2006). Decidual NK cells regulate key developmental processes at the human fetal-maternal interface. *Nat. Med.* 12, 1065–1074. doi: 10.1038/nm1452

He, G., Xu, W., Chen, Y., Liu, X., and Xi, M. (2013). Abnormal apoptosis of trophoblastic cells is related to the up-regulation of CYP11A gene in placenta of preeclampsia patients. *PLoS One* 8:e59609. doi: 10.1371/journal.pone.0059609

Hohensinner, P. J., Mayer, J., Kichbacher, J., Kral-Pointner, J., Thaler, B., Kaun, C., et al. (2021). Alternative activation of human macrophages enhances tissue factor expression and production of extracellular vesicles. *Haematologica* 106, 454–463. doi: 10.3324/haematol.2019.220210

Ioannidis, L. J., Nie, C. Q., and Hansen, D. S. (2014). The role of chemokines in severe malaria: more than meets the eye. *Parasitology* 141, 602–613. doi: 10.1017/S0031182013001984

Janssen, C. S., Phillips, R. S., Turner, C. M., and Barrett, M. P. (2004). *Plasmodium* interspersed repeats: the major multigene superfamily of malaria parasites. *Nucleic Acids Res.* 32, 5712–5720. doi: 10.1093/nar/gkh907

Jee, B., Dhar, R., Singh, S., and Karmakar, S. (2021). Heat shock proteins and their role in pregnancy: redefining the function of "Old Rum in a New Bottle". *Front. Cell Dev. Biol.* 9:648463. doi: 10.3389/fcell.2021.648463

Jovanović, M., Stefanoska, I., Radojcić, L., and Vićovac, L. (2010). Interleukin-8 (CXCL8) stimulates trophoblast cell migration and invasion by increasing levels of matrix metalloproteinase (MMP)2 and MMP9 and integrins alpha5 and beta1. *Reproduction* 139, 789–798. doi: 10.1530/REP-09-0341

Kawahara, R., Rosa-Fernandes, L., Dos Santos, A. F., Bandeira, C. L., Dombrowski, J. G., Souza, R. M., et al. (2019). Integrated proteomics reveals apoptosis-related mechanisms associated with placental malaria. *Mol. Cell Proteomics* 18, 182–199. doi: 10.1074/mcp.RA118.000907

Krause, B. J., Hanson, M. A., and Casanello, P. (2011). Role of nitric oxide in placental vascular development and function. *Placenta* 32, 797–805. doi: 10.1016/j.placenta.2011.06.025

Lash, G. E., Schiessl, B., Kirkley, M., Innes, B. A., Cooper, A., Searle, R. F., et al. (2006). Expression of angiogenic growth factors by uterine natural killer cells during early pregnancy. *J. Leukoc Biol.* 80, 572–580. doi: 10.1189/jlb.0406250

Leijnse, J. E. W., de Heus, R., de Jager, W., Rodenburg, W., Peeters, L. L. H., Franx, A., et al. (2018). First trimester placental vascularization and angiogenetic factors are associated with adverse pregnancy outcome. *Pregnancy Hypertens.* 13, 87–94. doi: 10.1016/j.preghy.2018.04.008

Leisser, C., Saleh, L., Haider, S., Husslein, H., Sonderegger, S., and Knöfler, M. (2006). Tumour necrosis factor-alpha impairs chorionic gonadotrophin beta-subunit expression and cell fusion of human villous cytotrophoblast. *Mol. Hum. Reprod.* 12, 601–609. doi: 10.1093/molehr/gal066

Leke, R. F. G., Cadigan, T. J., Mbu, R., Leke, R. I. J., Fogako, J., Megnkou, R., et al. (2004). *Plasmodium falciparum* infection in pregnant Cameroonian women: an assessment of changes in the placenta of low birth weight infants. *J. Cameroon Acad. Sci.* 2, 203–212.

Lennartz, F., Smith, C., Craig, A. G., and Higgins, M. K. (2019). Structural insights into diverse modes of ICAM-1 binding by *Plasmodium falciparum*-infected erythrocytes. *Proc. Natl. Acad. Sci. U. S. A.* 116, 20124–20134. doi: 10.1073/pnas.1911900116

Lima, F. A., Barateiro, A., Dombrowski, J. G., de Souza, R. M., Costa, D. S., Murillo, O., et al. (2019). *Plasmodium falciparum* infection dysregulates placental autophagy. *PLoS One* 14:e0226117. doi: 10.1371/journal.pone.0226117

Lokki, A. I., Heikkinen-Eloranta, J., Jarva, H., Saisto, T., Lokki, M. L., Laivuori, H., et al. (2014). Complement activation and regulation in preeclamptic placenta. *Front. Immunol.* 5:312. doi: 10.3389/fimmu.2014.00312

Lucchi, N. W., Peterson, D. S., and Moore, J. M. (2008). Immunologic activation of human syncytiotrophoblast by *Plasmodium falciparum*. *Malar J.* 7:42. doi: 10.1186/1475-2875-7-42

Lyall, F., Robson, S. C., and Bulmer, J. N. (2013). Spiral artery remodeling and trophoblast invasion in preeclampsia and fetal growth restriction: relationship to clinical outcome. *Hypertension* 62, 1046–1054. doi: 10.1161/HYPERTENSIONAHA.113.01892

Lybbert, J., Gullingsrud, J., Chesnokov, O., Turyakira, E., Dhorda, M., Guerin, P. J., et al. (2016). Abundance of megalin and Dab2 is reduced in syncytiotrophoblast during placental malaria, which may contribute to low birth weight. *Sci. Rep.* 6:24508. doi: 10.1038/srep24508

Ma, Y., Kong, L. R., Ge, Q., Lu, Y. Y., Hong, M. N., Zhang, Y., et al. (2018). Complement 5a-mediated trophoblasts dysfunction is involved in the development of pre-eclampsia. *J. Cell Mol. Med.* 22, 1034–1046. doi: 10.1111/jcmm.13466

Marinho, C. R., Neres, R., Epiphanio, S., Gonçalves, L. A., Catarino, M. B., and Penha-Gonçalves, C. (2009). Recrudescent *Plasmodium berghei* from pregnant mice displays enhanced binding to the placenta and induces protection in multigravida. *PLoS One* 4:e5630. doi: 10.1371/journal.pone.0005630

McDonald, C. R., Cahill, L. S., Gamble, J. L., Elphinstone, R., Gazdzinski, L. M., Zhong, K. J. Y., et al. (2018). Malaria in pregnancy alters l-arginine bioavailability and placental vascular development. *Sci. Transl. Med.* 10:eaan6007. doi: 10.1126/scitranslmed.aan6007

McDonald, C. R., Darling, A. M., Liu, E., Tran, V., Cabrera, A., Aboud, S., et al. (2016). Angiogenic proteins, placental weight and perinatal outcomes among pregnant women in Tanzania. *PLoS One* 11:e0167716. doi: 10.1371/journal.pone.0167716

McGready, R., Brockman, A., Cho, T., Levesque, M. A., Tkachuk, A. N., Meshnick, S. R., et al. (2002). Haemozoin as a marker of placental parasitization. *Trans. R. Soc. Trop. Med. Hyg.* 96, 644–646. doi: 10.1016/s0035-9203(02)90339-1

Megnekou, R., Djontu, J. C., Bigoga, J. D., Lissom, A., and Magagoum, S. H. (2015a). Role of some biomarkers in placental malaria in women living in Yaoundé, Cameroon. *Acta Trop.* 141, 97–102. doi: 10.1016/j.actatropica.2014.10.007

Megnekou, R., Djontu, J. C., Bigoga, J. D., Medou, F. M., Tenou, S., and Lissom, A. (2015b). Impact of placental *Plasmodium falciparum* malaria on the profile of some oxidative stress biomarkers in women living in Yaoundé, Cameroon. *PLoS One* 10:e0134633. doi: 10.1371/journal.pone.0134633

Megnekou, R., Hviid, L., and Staalsoe, T. (2009). Variant-specific immunity to *Plasmodium berghei* in pregnant mice. *Infect. Immun.* 77, 1827–1834. doi: 10.1128/IAI.01321-08

Megnekou, R., Staalsoe, T., and Hviid, L. (2013). Cytokine response to pregnancy-associated recrudescence of *Plasmodium berghei* infection in mice with pre-existing immunity to malaria. *Malar J* 12:387. doi: 10.1186/1475-2875-12-387

Miller, A. G., Aplin, J. D., and Westwood, M. (2005). Adenovirally mediated expression of insulin-like growth factors enhances the function of first trimester placental fibroblasts. *J. Clin. Endocrinol. Metab.* 90, 379–385. doi: 10.1210/jc.2004-1052

Moeller, S. L., Nyengaard, J. R., Larsen, L. G., Nielsen, K., Bygbjerg, I. C., Msemo, O. A., et al. (2019). Malaria in early pregnancy and the development of the placental vasculature. *J. Infect. Dis.* 220, 1425–1434. doi: 10.1093/infdis/jiy735

Morffy Smith, C. D., Russ, B. N., Andrew, A. K., Cooper, C. A., and Moore, J. M. (2019). A novel murine model for assessing fetal and birth outcomes following transgestational maternal malaria infection. *Sci. Rep.* 9:19566.

Mostafa, A. G., Bilal, N. E., Abass, A. E., Elhassan, E. M., Mohmmed, A. A., and Adam, I. (2015). Coagulation and fibrinolysis indicators and placental palaria infection in an area characterized by unstable malaria transmission in Central Sudan. *Malar Res. Treat.* 2015:369237. doi: 10.1155/2015/369237

Muehlenbachs, A., Fried, M., McGready, R., Harrington, W. E., Mutabingwa, T. K., Nosten, F., et al. (2010). A novel histological grading scheme for placental malaria applied in areas of high and low malaria transmission. *J. Infect. Dis.* 202, 1608–1616. doi: 10.1086/656723

Nakashima, A., Tsuda, S., Kusabiraki, T., Aoki, A., Ushijima, A., Shima, T., et al. (2019). Current understanding of autophagy in pregnancy. *Int. J. Mol. Sci.* 20:2342. doi: 10.3390/ijms20092342

Nawathe, A. R., Christian, M., Kim, S. H., Johnson, M., Savvidou, M. D., and Terzidou, V. (2016). Insulin-like growth factor axis in pregnancies affected by fetal growth disorders. *Clin. Epigenetics* 8:11. doi: 10.1186/s13148-016-0178-5

Ndam, N. T., Denoeud-Ndam, L., Doritchamou, J., Viwami, F., Salanti, A., Nielsen, M. A., et al. (2015). Protective antibodies against placental palaria and poor outcomes during pregnancy, Benin. *Emerg. Infect. Dis.* 21, 813–823. doi: 10.3201/eid2105

Neres, R., Marinho, C. R., Goncalves, L. A., Catarino, M. B., and Penha-Goncalves, C. (2008). Pregnancy outcome and placenta pathology in *Plasmodium berghei* ANKA infected mice reproduce the pathogenesis of severe malaria in pregnant women. *PLoS One* 3:e1608. doi: 10.1371/journal.pone.0001608

Niikura, M., Inoue, S. I., Mineo, S., Asahi, H., and Kobayashi, F. (2017). IFNGR1 signaling is associated with adverse pregnancy outcomes during infection with malaria parasites. *PLoS One* 12:e0185392. doi: 10.1371/journal.pone.0185392

Obiri, D., Erskine, I. J., Oduro, D., Kusi, K. A., Amponsah, J., Gyan, B. A., et al. (2020). Histopathological lesions and exposure to *Plasmodium falciparum* infections in the placenta increases the risk of preeclampsia among pregnant women. *Sci. Rep.* 10:8280. doi: 10.1038/s41598-020-64736-4

Oh, S. Y., and Roh, C. R. (2017). Autophagy in the placenta. *Obstet. Gynecol. Sci.* 60, 241–259. doi: 10.5468/ogs.2017.60.3.241

Okae, H., Toh, H., Sato, T., Hiura, H., Takahashi, S., Shirane, K., et al. (2018). Derivation of human trophoblast stem cells. *Cell Stem Cell* 22, 50–63.e6.

Ome-Kaius, M., Karl, S., Wangnapi, R. A., Bolnga, J. W., Mola, G., Walker, J., et al. (2017). Effects of *Plasmodium falciparum* infection on umbilical artery resistance and intrafetal blood flow distribution: a Doppler ultrasound study from Papua New Guinea. *Malar J.* 16:35. doi: 10.1186/s12936-017-1689-z

Ordi, J., Ismail, M. R., Ventura, P. J., Kahigwa, E., Hirt, R., Cardesa, A., et al. (1998). Massive chronic intervillositis of the placenta associated with malaria infection. *Am. J. Surg. Pathol.* 22, 1006–1011. doi: 10.1097/00000478-199808000-00011

Otun, H. A., Lash, G. E., Innes, B. A., Bulmer, J. N., Naruse, K., Hannon, T., et al. (2011). Effect of tumour necrosis factor-α in combination with interferon-γ on first trimester extravillous trophoblast invasion. *J. Reprod. Immunol.* 88, 1–11. doi: 10.1016/j.jri.2010.10.003

Pehrson, C., Mathiesen, L., Heno, K. K., Salanti, A., Resende, M., Dzikowski, R., et al. (2016). Adhesion of *Plasmodium falciparum* infected erythrocytes in ex vivo perfused placental tissue: a novel model of placental malaria. *Malar J.* 15:292. doi: 10.1186/s12936-016-1342-2

Pollheimer, J., Vondra, S., Baltayeva, J., Beristain, A. G., and Knöfler, M. (2018). Regulation of placental extravillous trophoblasts by the maternal uterine environment. *Front. Immunol.* 9:2597. doi: 10.3389/fimmu.2018.02597

Poovassery, J., and Moore, J. M. (2006). Murine malaria infection induces fetal loss associated with accumulation of *Plasmodium chabaudi* AS-infected erythrocytes in the placenta. *Infect. Immun.* 74, 2839–2848. doi: 10.1128/IAI.74.5.2839-2848.2006

Poovassery, J. S., Sarr, D., Smith, G., Nagy, T., and Moore, J. M. (2009). Malaria-induced murine pregnancy failure: distinct roles for IFN-gamma and TNF. *J. Immunol.* 183, 5342–5349. doi: 10.4049/jimmunol.0901669

Rahmah, Z., Wahju-Sardjono, T., Enggar-Fitri, L., Ulfiati, A., Ungu, B., Zulhaidah-Arthamin, M., et al. (2019). Accumulation of CD4 and CD8 T Cells in Placenta of Malaria Infected Mice Induces the Expression of Hypoxia Inducible Factor-1α (HIF-1α) and Low Birth Weight (LBW) of the Fetus. *Iran J. Parasitol.* 14, 604–613.

Ramhorst, R., Grasso, E., Paparini, D., Hauk, V., Gallino, L., Calo, G., et al. (2016). Decoding the chemokine network that links leukocytes with decidual cells and the trophoblast during early implantation. *Cell Adh. Migr.* 10, 197–207. doi: 10.1080/19336918.2015.1135285

Reis, A. S., Barboza, R., Murillo, O., Barateiro, A., Peixoto, E. P. M., Lima, F. A., et al. (2020). Inflammasome activation and IL-1 signaling during placental malaria induce poor pregnancy outcomes. *Sci. Adv.* 6:eaax6346. doi: 10.1126/sciadv.aax6346

Rinaldi, S. F., Makieva, S., Saunders, P. T., Rossi, A. G., and Norman, J. E. (2017). Immune cell and transcriptomic analysis of the human decidua in term and preterm parturition. *Mol. Hum. Reprod.* 23, 708–724. doi: 10.1093/molehr/gax038

Rogerson, S. J., Brown, H. C., Pollina, E., Abrams, E. T., Tadesse, E., Lema, V. M., et al. (2003a). Placental tumor necrosis factor alpha but not gamma interferon is associated with placental malaria and low birth weight in Malawian women. *Infect. Immun.* 71, 267–270. doi: 10.1128/IAI.71.1.267-270.2003

Rogerson, S. J., Pollina, E., Getachew, A., Tadesse, E., Lema, V. M., and Molyneux, M. E. (2003b). Placental monocyte infiltrates in response to *Plasmodium falciparum* malaria infection and their association with adverse pregnancy outcomes. *Am. J. Trop. Med. Hyg.* 68, 115–119. doi: 10.4269/ajtmh.2003.68.1.0680115

Roland, C. S., Hu, J., Ren, C. E., Chen, H., Li, J., Varvoutis, M. S., et al. (2016). Morphological changes of placental syncytium and their implications for the pathogenesis of preeclampsia. *Cell Mol. Life Sci.* 73, 365–376. doi: 10.1007/s00018-015-2069-x

Romero, R., Dey, S. K., and Fisher, S. J. (2014). Preterm labor: one syndrome, many causes. *Science* 345, 760–765. doi: 10.1126/science.1251816

Salanti, A., Staalsoe, T., Lavstsen, T., Jensen, A. T. R., Sowa, M. P. K., Arnot, D. E., et al. (2003). Selective upregulation of a single distinctly structured var gene in chondroitin sulphate A-adhering *Plasmodium falciparum* involved in pregnancy-associated malaria. *Mol. Microbiol.* 49, 179–191. doi: 10.1046/j.1365-2958.2003.03570.x

Sarr, D., Bracken, T. C., Owino, S. O., Cooper, C. A., Smith, G. M., Nagy, T., et al. (2015). Differential roles of inflammation and apoptosis in initiation of mid-gestational abortion in malaria-infected C57BL/6 and A/J mice. *Placenta* 36, 738–749. doi: 10.1016/j.placenta.2015.04.007

Schmidt, A., Morales-Prieto, D. M., Pastuschek, J., Fröhlich, K., and Markert, U. R. (2015). Only humans have human placentas: molecular differences between mice and humans. *J. Reprod. Immunol.* 108, 65–71. doi: 10.1016/j.jri.2015.03.001

Sharma, A., Conteh, S., Langhorne, J., and Duffy, P. E. (2016). Heterologous infection of pregnant mice induces low birth weight and modifies offspring susceptibility to malaria. *PLoS One* 11:e0160120. doi: 10.1371/journal.pone.0160120

Sharma, L., Kaur, J., and Shukla, G. (2012). Role of oxidative stress and apoptosis in the placental pathology of *Plasmodium berghei* infected mice. *PLoS One* 7:e32694. doi: 10.1371/journal.pone.0032694

Sharma, L., Kaur, J., and Shukla, G. (2014). Expression of heat shock protein 90, 70, 60 and 25 in the placenta of *Plasmodium berghei* infected BALB/c mice. *Asian Pac. J. Trop. Dis.* 4, S442–S444. doi: 10.1016/S2222-1808(14)60487-4

Shibuya, H., Sakai, K., Kabir-Salmani, M., Wachi, Y., and Iwashita, M. (2011). Polymerization of insulin-like growth factor-binding protein-1 (IGFBP-1) potentiates IGF-I actions in placenta. *J. Cell Physiol.* 226, 434–439. doi: 10.1002/jcp.22349

Silver, K. L., Zhong, K., Leke, R. G. F., Taylor, D. W., and Kain, K. C. (2010). Dysregulation of angiopoietins is associated with placental malaria and low birth weight. *PLoS One* 5:e9481. doi: 10.1371/journal.pone.0009481

Singh, P. P., Bhandari, S., Sharma, R. K., Singh, N., and Bharti, P. K. (2020). Association of angiopoietin dysregulation in placental malaria with adverse birth outcomes. *Dis. Markers* 2020:6163487. doi: 10.1155/2020/6163487

Singoei, M., Obimbo, M. M., Odula, P. O., Gitaka, J., and Ongidi, I. H. (2021). Changes in the structure of chorioamniotic membrane in patients with malaria in pregnancy. *Placenta* 114, 42–49. doi: 10.1016/j.placenta.2021.08.054

Smith, J. D., Gamain, B., Baruch, D. I., and Kyes, S. (2001). Decoding the language of var genes and *Plasmodium falciparum* sequestration. *Trends Parasitol.* 17, 538–545. doi: 10.1016/s1471-4922(01)02079-7

Smith, S. C., Baker, P. N., and Symonds, E. M. (1997b). Placental apoptosis in normal human pregnancy. *Am. J. Obstet. Gynecol.* 177, 57–65. doi: 10.1016/s0002-9378(97)70438-1

Smith, S. C., Baker, P. N., and Symonds, E. M. (1997a). Increased placental apoptosis in intrauterine growth restriction. *Am. J. Obstet. Gynecol.* 177, 1395–1401. doi: 10.1016/s0002-9378(97)70081-4

Soncin, F., Natale, D., and Parast, M. M. (2015). Signaling pathways in mouse and human trophoblast differentiation: a comparative review. *Cell Mol. Life Sci.* 72, 1291–1302. doi: 10.1007/s00018-014-1794-x

Staalsoe, T., Megnekou, R., Fievét, N., Ricke, C. H., Zornig, H. D., Leke, R., et al. (2001). Acquisition and decay of antibodies to pregnancy-associated variant antigens on the surface of *Plasmodium falciparum*-infected erythrocytes that protect against placental parasitemia. *J. Infect. Dis.* 184, 618–626. doi: 10.1086/322809

Staff, A. C., Fjeldstad, H. E., Fosheim, I. K., Moe, K., Turowski, G., Johnsen, G. M., et al. (2020). Failure of physiological transformation and spiral artery atherosis: their roles in preeclampsia. *Am. J. Obstet. Gynecol.* 21, 31116–31119. doi: 10.1016/j.ajog.2020.09.026

Suguitan, A. L. Jr., Cadigan, T. J., Nguyen, T. A., Zhou, A., Leke, R. J., Metenou, S., et al. (2003a). Malaria-associated cytokine changes in the placenta of women with pre-term deliveries in Yaounde, Cameroon. *Am. J. Trop. Med. Hyg.* 69, 574–581. doi: 10.4269/ajtmh.2003.69.574

Suguitan, A. L. Jr., Leke, R. G. F., Fouda, G., Zhou, A., Thuita, L., Metenou, S., et al. (2003b). Changes in the levels of chemokines and cytokines in the placentas of women with *Plasmodium falciparum* malaria. *J. Infect. Dis.* 188, 1074–1082. doi: 10.1086/378500

Takata, K. G. U., Fujikura, K., and Shin, B. C. (1997). Ultrastructure of the rodent placental labyrinth: a site of barrier and transport. *J. Reprod. Dev.* 43, 13–24. doi: 10.1262/jrd.43.13

Tan, H., Xu, Y., Xu, J., Wang, F., Nie, S., Yang, M., et al. (2007). Association of increased heat shock protein 70 levels in the lymphocyte with high risk of adverse pregnancy outcomes in early pregnancy: a nested case-control study. *Cell Stress Chaperones* 12, 230–236. doi: 10.1379/csc-266.1

Teo, A., Feng, G., Brown, G. V., Beeson, J. G., and Rogerson, S. J. (2016). Functional antibodies and protection against blood-stage malaria. *Trends Parasitol.* 32, 887–898. doi: 10.1016/j.pt.2016.07.003

Tersigni, C., Meli, F., Neri, C., Iacoangeli, A., Franco, R., Lanzone, A., et al. (2020). Role of human leukocyte antigens at the feto-maternal interface in normal and pathological pregnancy: an update. *Int. J. Mol. Sci.* 21:4756. doi: 10.3390/ijms21134756

Tran, E. E., Cheeks, M. L., Kakuru, A., Muhindo, M. K., Natureeba, P., Nakalembe, M., et al. (2020). The impact of gravidity, symptomatology and timing of infection on placental malaria. *Malar J.* 19:227. doi: 10.1186/s12936-020-03297-3

Tuikue Ndam, N. G., Salanti, A., Bertin, G., Dahlbäck, M., Fievet, N., Turner, L., et al. (2005). High level of var2csa transcription by *Plasmodium falciparum* isolated from the placenta. *J. Infect. Dis.* 192, 331–335. doi: 10.1086/430933

Turco, M. Y., Gardner, L., Kay, R. G., Hamilton, R. S., Prater, M., Hollinshead, M. S., et al. (2018). Trophoblast organoids as a model for maternal-fetal interactions during human placentation. *Nature* 564, 263–267. doi: 10.1038/s41586-018-0753-3

Tyberghein, A., Deroost, K., Schwarzer, E., Arese, P., and Van den Steen, P. E. (2014). Immunopathological effects of malaria pigment or hemozoin and other crystals. *Biofactors* 40, 59–78. doi: 10.1002/biof.1119

Umbers, A. J., Boeuf, P., Clapham, C., Stanisic, D. I., Baiwog, F., Mueller, I., et al. (2011). Placental malaria-associated inflammation disturbs the insulin-like growth factor axis of fetal growth regulation. *J. Infect. Dis.* 203, 561–569. doi: 10.1093/infdis/jiq080

Umbers, A. J., Stanisic, D. I., Ome, M., Wangnapi, R., Hanieh, S., Unger, H. W., et al. (2013). Does malaria affect placental development? Evidence from in vitro models. *PLoS One* 8:e55269. doi: 10.1371/journal.pone.0055269

Wang, K., Dagil, R., Lavstsen, T., Misra, S. K., Spliid, C. B., Wang, Y., et al. (2021). Cryo-EM reveals the architecture of placental malaria VAR2CSA and provides molecular insight into chondroitin sulfate binding. *Nat. Commun.* 12:2956. doi: 10.1038/s41467-021-23254-1

Wang, W., Sung, N., Gilman-Sachs, A., and Kwak-Kim, J. (2020). T Helper (Th) Cell Profiles in Pregnancy and Recurrent Pregnancy Losses: Th1/Th2/Th9/Th17/Th22/Tfh Cells. *Front. Immunol.* 11:2025. doi: 10.3389/fimmu.2020.02025

World Health Organization [WHO] (2020). *World Malaria Report 2020.* Geneva: World Health Organization.

Xu, X., Zhou, Y., and Wei, H. (2020). Roles of HLA-G in the maternal-fetal immune microenvironment. *Front. Immunol.* 11:592010. doi: 10.3389/fimmu.2020.592010

Yang, L., Megli, C., and Coyne, C. B. (2021). Innate immune signaling in trophoblast and decidua organoids defines differential antiviral defenses at the maternal-fetal interface. *bioRxiv* [Preprint]. doi: 10.1101/2021.03.29.437467

Yang, S. W., Cho, E. H., Choi, S. Y., Lee, Y. K., Park, J. H., Kim, M. K., et al. (2017). DC-SIGN expression in Hofbauer cells may play an important role in immune tolerance in fetal chorionic villi during the development of preeclampsia. *J. Reprod. Immunol.* 124, 30–37. doi: 10.1016/j.jri.2017.09.012

Permissions

All chapters in this book were first published by Frontiers; hereby published with permission under the Creative Commons Attribution License or equivalent. Every chapter published in this book has been scrutinized by our experts. Their significance has been extensively debated. The topics covered herein carry significant findings which will fuel the growth of the discipline. They may even be implemented as practical applications or may be referred to as a beginning point for another development.

The contributors of this book come from diverse backgrounds, making this book a truly international effort. This book will bring forth new frontiers with its revolutionizing research information and detailed analysis of the nascent developments around the world.

We would like to thank all the contributing authors for lending their expertise to make the book truly unique. They have played a crucial role in the development of this book. Without their invaluable contributions this book wouldn't have been possible. They have made vital efforts to compile up to date information on the varied aspects of this subject to make this book a valuable addition to the collection of many professionals and students.

This book was conceptualized with the vision of imparting up-to-date information and advanced data in this field. To ensure the same, a matchless editorial board was set up. Every individual on the board went through rigorous rounds of assessment to prove their worth. After which they invested a large part of their time researching and compiling the most relevant data for our readers.

The editorial board has been involved in producing this book since its inception. They have spent rigorous hours researching and exploring the diverse topics which have resulted in the successful publishing of this book. They have passed on their knowledge of decades through this book. To expedite this challenging task, the publisher supported the team at every step. A small team of assistant editors was also appointed to further simplify the editing procedure and attain best results for the readers.

Apart from the editorial board, the designing team has also invested a significant amount of their time in understanding the subject and creating the most relevant covers. They scrutinized every image to scout for the most suitable representation of the subject and create an appropriate cover for the book.

The publishing team has been an ardent support to the editorial, designing and production team. Their endless efforts to recruit the best for this project, has resulted in the accomplishment of this book. They are a veteran in the field of academics and their pool of knowledge is as vast as their experience in printing. Their expertise and guidance has proved useful at every step. Their uncompromising quality standards have made this book an exceptional effort. Their encouragement from time to time has been an inspiration for everyone.

The publisher and the editorial board hope that this book will prove to be a valuable piece of knowledge for researchers, students, practitioners and scholars across the globe.

List of Contributors

André Barateiro and Claudio R. F. Marinho
Department of Parasitology, Institute of Biomedical Sciences, University of São Paulo, São Paulo, Brazil

Marcelo L. M. Pereira
Department of Parasitology, Institute of Biomedical Sciences, University of São Paulo, São Paulo, Brazil
Institute of Bio systems and Integrative Sciences, Faculty of Sciences, University of Lisbon, Lisbon, Portugal

Xiao-Ai Zhang, Jin-Jin Chen, Yang Yuan, Zi-Wei Zhou, Yu-Na Wang, Hai-Yang Zhang, Pan-He Zhang and Li-Qun Fang
State Key Laboratory of Pathogen and Biosecurity, Beijing Institute of Microbiology and Epidemiology, Beijing, China

Rui-Qiu Zhao, Xiang Tang, Luo Ren, En-Mei Liu and Hong-Mei Xu
Children's Hospital of Chongqing Medical University, Chongqing, China

Qin-Bin Lu
Department of Laboratorial Science and Technology, School of Public Health, Peking University, Beijing, China

Hai-Sheng Zhou
Key Laboratory of Dermatology, Anhui Medical University, Hefei, China
Department of Biochemistry and Molecular Biology, Anhui Medical University, Hefei, China

Wei Liu
State Key Laboratory of Pathogen and Biosecurity, Beijing Institute of Microbiology and Epidemiology, Beijing, China
Beijing Key Laboratory of Vector Borne and Natural Focus Infectious Diseases, Beijing, China

Bryce Wolfe
Department of Pathology and Laboratory Medicine, University of Wisconsin - Madison, Madison, WI, United States
Wisconsin National Primate Research Center, University of Wisconsin - Madison, Madison, WI, United States

Andres Mejia and Heather A. Simmons
Wisconsin National Primate Research Center, University of Wisconsin - Madison, Madison, WI, United States

Andrea R. Kerr
Department of Comparative Biosciences, School of Veterinary Medicine, University of Wisconsin - Madison, Madison, WI, United States

Charles J. Czuprynski
Department of Pathobiological Sciences, School of Veterinary Medicine, University of Wisconsin -Madison, Madison, WI, United States

Thaddeus G. Golos
Wisconsin National Primate Research Center, University of Wisconsin - Madison, Madison, WI, United States
Department of Comparative Biosciences, School of Veterinary Medicine, University of Wisconsin - Madison, Madison, WI, United States
Department of Obstetrics and Gynecology, University of Wisconsin - Madison, Madison, WI, United States

Yash Pandya and Carlos Penha-Gonçalves
Instituto Gulbenkian de Ciência, Oeiras, Portugal

Mila W. Reginatto, Klaus Novaes Fontes, Victoria R. S. Monteiro, Natalia L. Silva, Cherley Borba Vieira Andrade, Hanailly Ribeiro Gomes, Flavia Fonseca Bloise and Tania M. Ortiga-Carvalho
Laboratory of Translational Endocrinology, Institute of Biophysics Carlos Chagas Filho, Universidade Federal do Rio de Janeiro, Rio de Janeiro, Brazil

Guinever E. Imperio
Laboratory of Translational Endocrinology, Institute of Biophysics Carlos Chagas Filho, Universidade Federal do Rio de Janeiro, Rio de Janeiro, Brazil
Department of Physiology, Faculty of Medicine, University of Toronto, Toronto, ON, Canada
Lunenfeld-Tanenbaum Research Institute of Medical, Sinai Health System, Toronto, ON, Canada

George Eduardo Gabriel Kluck and Georgia Correa Atella
Laboratory of Lipids and Lipoproteins Biochemistry, Institute of Medical Biochemistry Leopoldo de Meis, Universidade Federal do Rio de Janeiro, Rio de Janeiro, Brazil

Stephen G. Matthews
Department of Physiology, Faculty of Medicine, University of Toronto, Toronto, ON, Canada
Lunenfeld-Tanenbaum Research Institute of Medical, Sinai Health System, Toronto, ON, Canada
Department of Obstetrics and Gynecology, Faculty of Medicine, University of Toronto, Toronto, ON, Canada
Department of Medicine, Faculty of Medicine, University of Toronto, Toronto, ON, Canada

Enrrico Bloise
Department of Morphology, Universidade Federal de Minas Gerais, Belo Horizonte, Brazil

Fernanda C. da Silva, Fernanda M. Magaldi and Estela Bevilacqua
Department of Cell and Developmental Biology, Institute of Biomedical Sciences, University of São Paulo, São Paulo, Brazil

Helena K. Sato
Secretaria do Estado de São Paulo, Epidemiological Surveillance Center, Department of Health, São Paulo, Brazil

Rina Ikeda, Nanako Ushio and Yoshifumi Nishikawa
National Research Center for Protozoan Diseases, Obihiro University of Agriculture and Veterinary Medicine, Obihiro, Japan

Ahmed M. Abdou
National Research Center for Protozoan Diseases, Obihiro University of Agriculture and Veterinary Medicine, Obihiro, Japan
Department of Forensic Medicine and Toxicology, Faculty of Veterinary Medicine, South Valley University, Qena, Egypt

Hidefumi Furuoka
Division of Pathobiological Science, Department of Basic Veterinary Medicine, Obihiro University of Agriculture and Veterinary Medicine, Obihiro, Japan

Renato Barboza
Departamento de Ciências Biológicas, Universidade Federal de São Paulo, Diadema, Brazil

Lutero Hasenkamp, Oscar Murillo, Erika Paula Machado Peixoto, Flávia Afonso Lima, Aramys Silva Reis and Lígia Antunes Gonçalves
Departamen to de Parasitologia, Instituto de Ciências Biomédicas, Universidade de São Paulo, São Paulo, Brazil

Sabrina Epiphanio
Departamento de Análises Clínicas e Toxicológicas, Faculdade de Ciências Farmacêuticas, Universidade de São Paulo, São Paulo, Brazil
Department of Clinical Analysis and Toxicology, Faculty of Pharmaceutical Sciences, University of São Paulo, São Paulo, Brazil

Ulrike Kemmerling
Programa de Anatomía y Biología del Desarrollo, Instituto de Ciencias Biomédicas, Facultad de Medicina, Universidad de Chile, Santiago, Chile
Instituto de Ciencias Biomédicas, Facultad de Medicina, Universidad de Chile, Santiago, Chile

Antonio Osuna
Grupo de Bioquímica y Parasitología Molecular, Departamento de Parasitología, Instituto de Biotecnología, Universidad de Granada, Granada, Spain

Alejandro Gabriel Schijman
Molecular Biology of Chagas Disease Laboratory, Genetic Engineering and Molecular Biology Research Institute Dr. Héctor Torres (INGEBI-CONICET), Buenos Aires, Argentina

Carine Truyens
Laboratory of Parasitology, Faculty of Medicine, Université Libre de Bruxelles, Brussels, Belgium

Maura Rojas-Pirela
Instituto de Ciencias Biomédicas, Facultad de Medicina, Universidad de Chile, Santiago, Chile
Instituto de Biología, Pontificia Universidad Católica de Valparaíso, Valparaíso, Chile
Facultad de Farmacia y Bioanálisis, Universidad de Los Andes, Mérida, Venezuela

Lisvaneth Medina, Ana Isabel Liempi and Jesús Guerrero-Muñoz
Instituto de Ciencias Biomédicas, Facultad de Medicina, Universidad de Chile, Santiago, Chile

Maria Verónica Rojas
Instituto de Biología, Pontificia Universidad Católica de Valparaíso, Valparaíso, Chile

Elizabeth Pérez-Pérez
Facultad de Farmacia y Bioanálisis, Universidad de Los Andes, Mérida, Venezuela

Christian Castillo
Instituto de Ciencias Biomédicas, Facultad de Medicina, Universidad de Chile, Santiago, Chile
Núcleo de Investigación Aplicada en Ciencias Veterinarias y Agronómicas, Facultad de Medicina Veterinaria y Agronomía, Universidad de Las Américas, Santiago, Chile

Sebastian Araneda
Instituto de Ciencias Biomédicas, Facultad de Medicina, Universidad de Chile, Santiago, Chile
Facultad de Salud y Odontología, Universidad Diego Portales, Santiago, Chile

Andrea M. Weckman and Julie Wright
Department of Laboratory Medicine and Pathobiology, University of Toronto, Toronto, ON, Canada

Michelle Ngai and Chloe R. McDonald
SAR Laboratories, Sandra Rotman Centre for Global Health, University Health Network-Toronto General Hospital, Toronto, ON, Canada

Kevin C. Kain
Department of Laboratory Medicine and Pathobiology, University of Toronto, Toronto, ON, Canada
SAR Laboratories, Sandra Rotman Centre for Global Health, University Health Network-Toronto General Hospital, Toronto, ON, Canada
Tropical Disease Unit, Division of Infectious Diseases, Department of Medicine, University of Toronto, Toronto, ON, Canada

Wanbo Tai, Denis Voronin, Jiawei Chen, Weili Bao, Debra A. Kessler, Beth Shaz, Karina Yazdanbakhsh and Lanying Du
Lindsley F. Kimball Research Institute, New York Blood Center, New York, NY, United States

Shibo Jiang
Lindsley F. Kimball Research Institute, New York Blood Center, New York, NY, United States
Key Laboratory of Medical Molecular Virology of MOE/MOH, Fudan University, Shanghai, China

Georgia Fakonti, Paschalia Pantazi, Vladimir Bokun and Beth Holder
Institute of Reproductive and Developmental Biology, Department of Metabolism, Digestion and Reproduction, Imperial College London, London, United Kingdom

Soraya Mezouar, Imene Benammar, Asma Boumaza, Aïssatou Bailo Diallo and Céline Chartier
Aix-Marseille Université, MEPHI, IRD, APHM, Marseille, France
IHU-Méditerranée Infection, Marseille, France

Christophe Buffat
APHM, Biochemistry and Molecular Biology, Hôpital de la Conception, Marseille, France

John Boudjarane
INSERM U1251, Centre de Génétique Médicale MMG, APHM, Hôpital de la Timone, Aix-Marseille Université, Marseille, France

Philippe Halfon
Laboratoire Alphabio, Hôpital Européen, Marseille, France

Maria Katsogiannou
Department of Obstetrics and Gynecology, Hôpital Saint Joseph, Marseille, France

Jean-Louis Mege
Aix-Marseille Université, MEPHI, IRD, APHM, Marseille, France
IHU-Méditerranée Infection, Marseille, France
APHM, UF Immunologie, Marseille, France

Joanna M. Marshall
Department of Microbial Infection and Immunity, The Ohio State University, Columbus, OH, United States

Lauren J. Johnson and Siavash Azari
Department of Microbial Infection and Immunity, The Ohio State University, Columbus, OH, United States
Department of Microbiology, The Ohio State University, Columbus, OH, United States

Amy Webb
Department of Biomedical Informatics, The Ohio State University, Columbus, OH, United States

Xiaoli Zhang
Department of Biomedical Informatics, Center for Biostatistics, The Ohio State University, Columbus, OH, United States

Mikhail A. Gavrilin
Pulmonary, Critical Care and Sleep Medicine Division, Department of Internal Medicine, The Ohio State University, Columbus, OH, United States

Kara Rood
Department of Obstetrics and Gynecology, Division of Maternal Fetal Medicine, The Ohio State University, Columbus, OH, United States

Stephanie Seveau
Department of Microbial Infection and Immunity, The Ohio State University, Columbus, OH, United States
Department of Microbiology, The Ohio State University, Columbus, OH, United State
Infectious Diseases Institute, The Ohio State University, Columbus, OH, United States

Patricia L. Bustos, Bibiana J. Volta, Alina E. Perrone and Susana A. Laucella
Instituto Nacional de Parasitología "Dr. Mario Fatala Chaben" - ANLIS C. G. Malbrán, Buenos Aires, Argentina

Natalia Milduberger and Jacqueline Bua
Instituto Nacional de Parasitología "Dr. Mario Fatala Chaben" - ANLIS C. G. Malbrán, Buenos Aires, Argentina
Centro de Altos Estudios en Ciencias Humanas y de la Salud (CAECIHS), Universidad Abierta Interamericana, Buenos Aires, Argentina

Caroline Lin Lin Chua
School of Biosciences, Taylor's University, Subang Jaya, Malaysia

Sebastian Kah Ming Khoo and Jun Long Ernest Ong
Lee Kong Chian School of Medicine, Nanyang Technological University, Singapore, Singapore

Gaurav Kumar Ramireddi
Department of Medicine, Monash University, Victoria, VIC, Australia

Tsin Wen Yeo
Lee Kong Chian School of Medicine, Nanyang Technological University, Singapore, Singapore
National Center for Infectious Diseases, Singapore, Singapore
Department of Infectious Diseases, Tan Tock Seng Hospital, Singapore, Singapore

Andrew Teo
Lee Kong Chian School of Medicine, Nanyang Technological University, Singapore, Singapore
Department of Medicine at Royal Melbourne Hospital, Peter Doherty Institute, University of Melbourne, Melbourne, VIC, Australia

Index

www.ingramcontent.com/pod-product-compliance
Lightning Source LLC
LaVergne TN
LVHW061513220926
848485LV00018B/1025